Contemporary Pediatric Nursing

A Conceptual Approach

Contemporary Pediatric Nursing
A Conceptual Approach

JUDITH M. McFARLANE, R.N., M.N.
Doctoral Candidate, School of Public Health,
The University of Texas Health Science Center at Houston
Formerly Assistant Professor and Clinical Specialist in Pediatric Hematology
Medical College of Georgia, Augusta, Georgia

BETTY JO WHITSON, R.N., M.N.
Clinical Specialist—Pediatric Nursing
Associate Professor of Pediatric Nursing
Department of Nursing
University of South Carolina at Aiken

LUCY M. HARTLEY, R.N., M.N.
Assistant Professor
University of South Carolina, College of Nursing, Columbia, S.C.

A WILEY MEDICAL PUBLICATION
JOHN WILEY & SONS
New York · Chichester · Brisbane · Toronto

Library of Congress Cataloging in Publication Data:

McFarlane, Judith.
Contemporary pediatric nursing.

Includes index.
1. Pediatric nursing. I. Whitson, Betty Jo, joint author. II. Hartley, Lucy M., joint author. III. Title. [DNLM: 1. Pediatric nursing. WY159 M145c]

RJ245.M25 610.73'62 79-18463
ISBN 0-471-03908-X

Printed in the United States of America

10 9 8 7 6 5 4 3 2 1

To my husband Robert, for listening, nurturing, and enduring.

—J.M.McF.

To my parents, Jack and Josephine Phillips, who taught me to love children, and to my own, Kelly and Brian.

—B.J.W.

To Lewie, Skipper, and Jason, for tolerating.

—L.M.H.

Preface

The sum of knowledge and skills that constitutes pediatric nursing is constantly growing, influenced by a vast quantity of new information from the natural and applied sciences. The primary objective of this book is to integrate this ever-changing body of knowledge, and to present it to the beginning student of pediatric nursing in a concise, specific, and easily understood manner.

Part I is an introduction to contemporary pediatric nursing and the factors that have influenced its current scope. The parent-child unit is introduced as the recipient of nursing care, and the family is mentioned throughout the text in connection with various sources of physical and emotional stress arising from deviations in the child's health.

The focus of Part II is the physiological, emotional, and cognitive development of the well child. This information is incorporated into discussions of the hospitalized child, and of the types of accidents common to each developmental stage and the corresponding preventive measures.

The child's health needs provide the conceptual framework of Part III. The first chapter in each section discusses the normal adaptive process that meets the identified need; subsequent chapters describe the symptoms, diagnostic procedures and treatments, and nursing care specific to various deviations from health.

Each chapter begins with a set of behavioral objectives and a list of key terms and concepts that will provide the reader with explicit learning goals. Specific disorders are presented in tables at the ends of chapters wherever the subject matter lends itself to a brief summary for easy reference. Over 200 illustrations, most of them prepared especially for this book, will further add to the student's understanding. Detailed instructions regarding specific procedures will be found in *The Pediatric Nursing Skills Manual.* John Wiley & Sons, 1980, referred to in this book as "the Skills Manual," a companion volume that will be useful to practicing pediatric nurses as well as students.

Throughout the text, the nurse is referred to as *she,* and in most cases, the child is referred to as *he.* This has been done for the sake of clarity; no discrimination against male nursing students and nurses or female patients is intended.

Students of pediatric nursing need a clear and concise text that will enable them to synthesize pertinent knowledge and apply it to the clinical setting. We believe that *Contemporary Pediatric Nursing* fulfills that need.

J.M.McF.
B.J.W.
L.M.H.

Acknowledgments

Completing this book required the assistance and support of many people. We are indebted to each of them. We extend special thanks to the Wiley staff, especially Cathy Somer for initiating, sustaining, and bringing the project to fruition, Don Schott for his meticulous editing and creative probing of the manuscript, which contributed to the clarity and relevance of the text, and Eileen Tommaso for providing the energy and keen attention to details, crucial for the production of the text.

We wish to thank the following persons for reviewing portions of the manuscript: Carol L. Baecher, Assist. Prof. of Medical-Surgical Nursing, University of South Carolina at Aiken; Beverly Belk, M.D., Assoc. Prof. of Pediatrics, Medical College of Georgia, Augusta, Georgia, and Coordinator of Pediatric Education, University Hospital, Augusta, Georgia; Van Inglett, R.N., B.S.N., Director of Pediatric Nursing, University Hospital, Augusta, Georgia; Carl Jelenko, III, Professor, Community Medicine, Director, Emergency Medicine Group, and Professor of Surgery, Wright State University School of Medicine, Dayton, Ohio; Judith B. Matthews, R.N., B.S.N., B.S.Ed., Coordinator, Paramedic Education, Greene Memorial Hospital, Xenia, Ohio; Paul B. Pritchard, III, M.D., Assistant Professor of Neurology, Medical University of South Carolina, Charleston, South Carolina; Lawrence Weiner, M.D., Dept. of Immunology and Allergy, School of Medicine, University of South Carolina, Columbia, South Carolina; our colleagues, for their support and encouragement—Betty M. Johnson, R.N., PhD.: Juanita Bowsher, R.N., M.S.N.; Larry L. Hedgepath, M.D.: Rita Jacques, R.N., Pauline H. Barton, R.N., Ed.D., Graduate Coordinator, College of Nursing, University of Florida, Gainesville, Florida; F.N.P.; Pat Christensen, R.N., M.S.N.; Esther E. Starkey, R.N., M.N.Ed.; Karen Sullivan, R.N., B.S.N.; Josephine A. Phillips, R.N.; Peggy Ryals; Anne Donnelly; The Division of Health Communications, Medical College of Georgia, Augusta, Georgia, especially staff members Karen Waldo, David Peace, David Mascaro, Jean Stewart, Ken Andruck, Virginia Schoonover, and Russ Baltzgar; The Department of Bio-Medical Communications, The University of Texas Health Science Center at Houston, especially staff member Cindy Lopez; photographers Tom Chumley and Henry Greene, University Hospital, Augusta, Georgia; also, Lewie Hartley, Robert McFarlane, Stan Whitson, Warren Whitson, Dobie and Leo Zimmerman; typists Aileen Craig, Sarah Grayson, Karen Harley, JoAnn Johnson, Elizabeth Odum, and Glenda Webb; our students, for their enthusiasm and inquisitiveness; our family and friends, for their support, love, and humor that contributed to our mental health during the preparation of this book; and very special thanks to our teachers—all the children and their families it has been our privilege to know.

J.M.McF.
B.J.W.
L.M.H.

Contents

Section 3: Growth

Section 4: Oxygenation

Section 5: Mobility

Section 6: Fluid and Electrolyte Balance

PART I

Pediatric Nursing Today

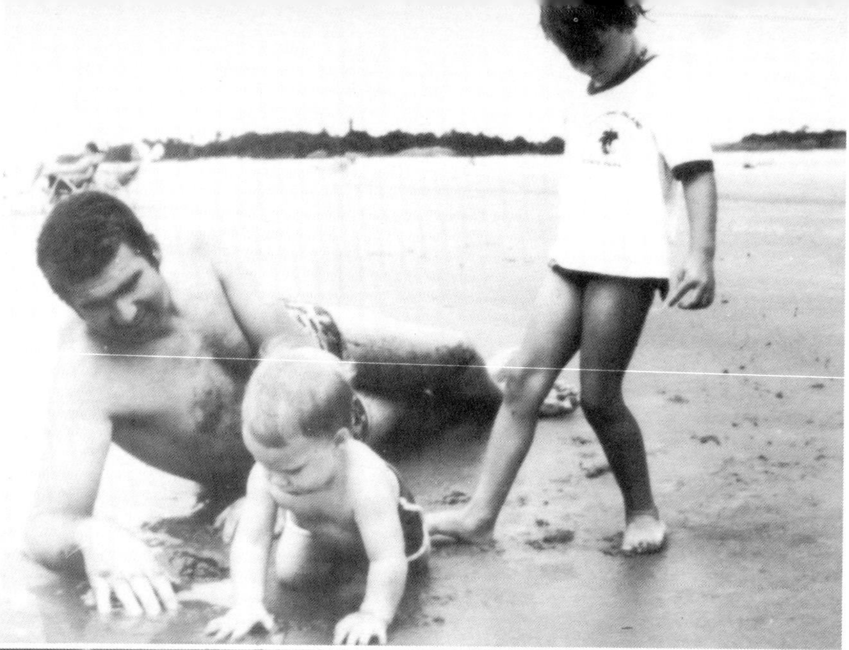

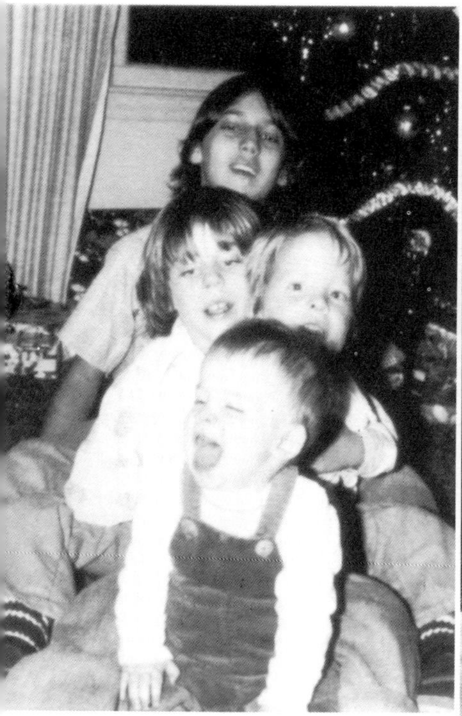

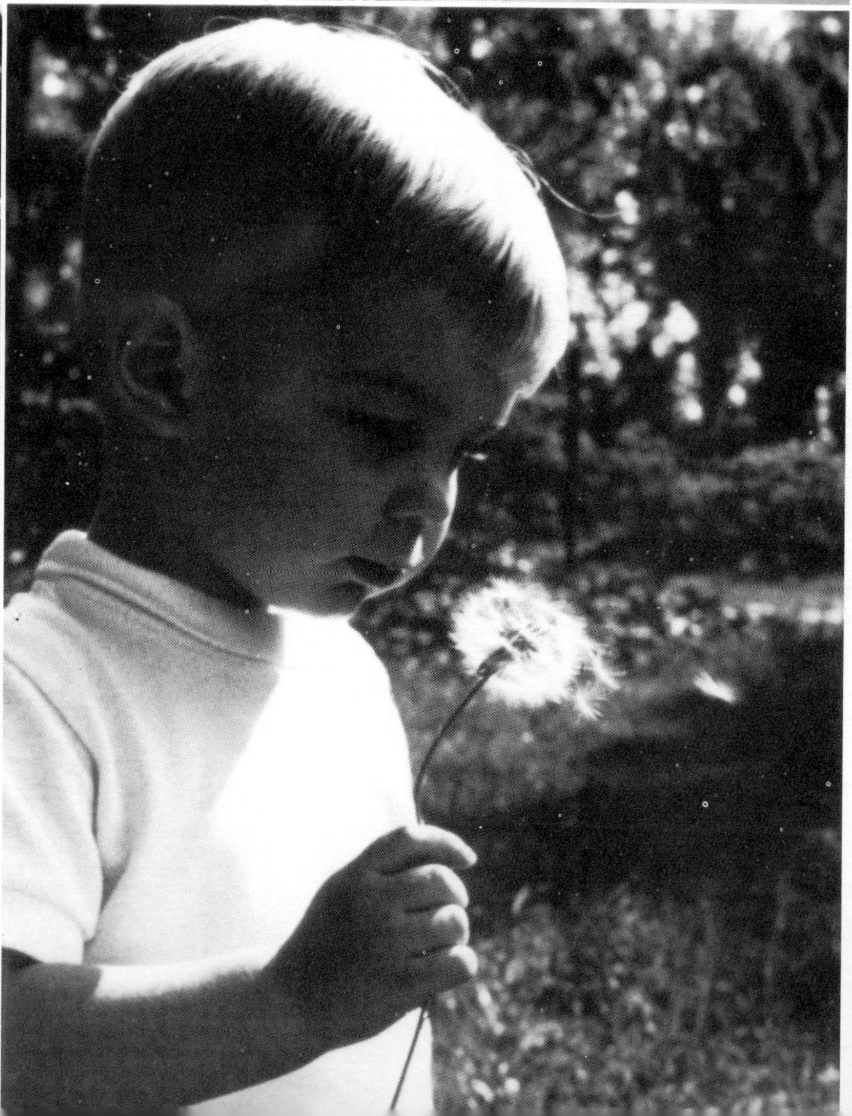

CHAPTER **1**

Pediatric Nursing Today

A cluster of young people listen as reproduction and contraception are discussed. Questions about abortion, the use of a diaphragm, and gonorrhea are answered by the adolescent nurse-specialist who organized and conducts the daily sex-education sessions at a walk-in clinic for teenagers.

The children are rolled in the grass, tickled, and hugged. Then each child is taken to a nearby tree where each small finger is slowly moved over the rough bark. Fragrant blooming honeysuckle is waved under each child's nose; the group is then settled on the grass to be fed lunch.

The stimulation program for retarded children was begun six months ago and is coordinated by a nurse who carefully notes daily changes in the behavior and ability of each child. The observations are shared with the children's parents, who reinforce the day's experiences in a home stimulation program, also begun and taught by the nurse.

The 7 P.M. phone call was not a surprise. Mrs. Brown had called the hospital in the afternoon to speak to Jim, the Browns' primary care nurse, when Keven, aged four, registered an elevated temperature and vomited his noon meal. Kevin's temperature did not respond to aspirin, and after he began to complain of severe abdominal pain and refused all liquids, his mother brought him to the hospital. Arriving at the hospital, Mrs. Brown listed Jim as Kevin's primary care nurse, Jim was notified and as he drove to the hospital, he reflected on his two years of working with the Brown family, and the special problems of Kevin, who has cancer. At the hospital, Jim completed the admission assessment, outlined an immediate care plan (which he discussed with family and staff), and received a report on his five other primary care inpatients before returning home.

The focus of contemporary pediatric nursing is on responding to the health needs of children in a variety of settings. Because the needs of children and their families are changing, pediatric nursing has seen the evolution of new and expanded roles, including that of the pediatric nurse practitioner and pediatric clinical nurse specialist.

The pediatric nurse practitioner (PNP) is a registered nurse who has completed a nurse practitioner program or a master's program in pediatric nursing. The PNP provides primary care in several settings, including private practice with a pediatrician or general family practitioner, public health departments, outpatient clinics, and hospitals. Her functions include monitoring well-child care, conducting physical examinations, ordering laboratory tests, treating minor illnesses, and referring children with serious conditions to a doctor (Figure 1–1). The PNP also teaches parents about growth and development and advises the whole family on preventive health care.

In contrast, the pediatric clinical nurse specialist is a registered nurse who has a master's degree in pediatric nursing and extensive clinical experience in a subspecialty of pediatrics. For example, a pediatric clinical nurse specialist in oncology

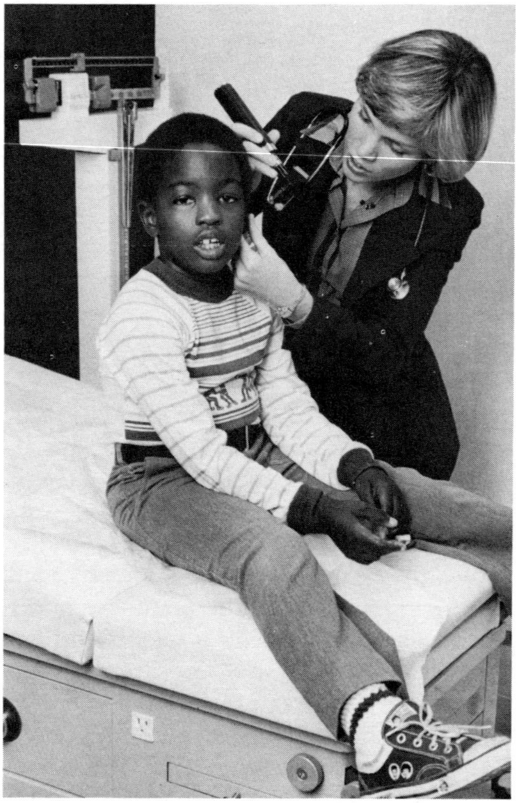

Figure 1-1. *Physical assessment is one of the special skills of the pediatric nurse practitioner.*

coordinates and supervises the care of children with cancer. She also performs a variety of specialized technical tasks and is active in research and the development and implementation of standards of nursing care for children with cancer. The clinical nurse specialist works in the same variety of settings as the nurse practitioner.

The environment in which the developing child is nurtured has been altered: in 1940, less than one of every ten mothers of children under age eighteen worked, whereas in 1972, four out of ten mothers worked; and it is projected that by 1985, 6.6 million mothers with children under age five will be gainfully employed outside the home. That a mother works is not harmful, but the environment and persons to which the child is exposed during the mother's working hours are crucial. More children are being exposed to more persons and situations at an earlier age. Once sequestered in an extended family that provided sex-role and task education and that met social and economic needs, the child now grows in the environment of the small nuclear family, consisting of one or two parents and children, living in a highly mobile, mechanized society in which a variety of persons and services—from day care to television—sustain the family. What are the needs of children today? What challenges confront pediatric nursing?

Until the 1940's, health programs were concerned primarily with the control of communicable diseases and the accompanying epidemics of typhoid fever, diphtheria, whooping cough, and poliomyelitis. With antibiotics, immunizations, and improved sanitation, most of the dreaded diseases of the past are no longer a threat. Yet we continue to hear and read about the high U.S. mortality rate, the large number of children lacking basic medical care, and the poor nutritional state of school-age children and adolescents. What is the relationship between these medical issues of morbidity and mortality and the biological, economic, and social environment of the growing child?

First we need to take a close look at what mortality figures mean. The *infant mortality rate* is expressed in terms of the number of deaths before the first birthday per 1,000 live births in a given calendar year. Aside from the face value of the statistic itself, the infant mortality rate is a valuable indicator of the quality of health services available to families, as well as of the existence of various socioeconomic factors. It has been recognized for some time that maternal age and health affect infant birth weight and health, but social and economic forces such as income, education, and occupation also influence the health of the newborn and growing child. A discussion of the increasing number of births to teenage mothers will serve to illustrate the relationship between biological, social, and economic factors and child health.

A mother between the ages of fifteen and nineteen has a 13 percent greater risk of dying as a direct result of pregnancy or childbirth than does the woman in her early twenties, and for the mother aged fourteen or younger, the maternal death rate is 60 percent higher than for the woman in her twenties. Infant offspring of teenagers are three times more likely to die in their first year than are infants of older women. The incidence of prematurity and low birth weight is considerably higher among teenage pregnancies, as is the risk of the child having a chronic condition such as mental retardation or epilepsy. Since about 20 percent of all births in a year are to teenage mothers, one of every five infants enters life with a drastically reduced chance of surviving the first year. However, health risks for the infant of a young mother do not stop at birth. Since the majority of teenage mothers have no work experience and 80 percent never complete high school, they are disadvantaged in competition for jobs and in income potential. Teenage mothers are more likely to be unemployed and to be receiving welfare than women who postpone their childbearing until their twenties. Among teenagers who marry after becoming pregnant, about one third of the marriages dissolve within two years. The child of the teenage mother begins and continues life in a less-than-optimal environment.

Poverty is an additional influence on a child's existing and potential health. Studies have shown that in low-income neighborhoods, more than 50 percent of the children are not completely immunized. Although this has caused widely publicized epidemics of such contagious diseases as measles, the important fact is that inadequate immunization is often only one of the problems arising from a deficit in overall health care. The indicators are clear that many children, especially those of low-income or young mothers, are *not* receiving continual health supervision. Health care for these children and their families is sporadic and usually crisis-oriented. An unanticipated hospitalization or emergency-room visit may be the child's first contact with health care.

Naturally, our high infant mortality rate cannot be simply explained as the result of poverty and teenage pregnancies—the issue is far more complex. For example, the sudden infant death syndrome (see Ch. 3), a poorly understood condition that claims over 10,000 infants a year, is still seemingly unpredictable and unpreventable as of this writing.

Social factors, such as family income and education, also influence the morbidity and mortality rates of children beyond infancy. For example, the well-known phenomenon of lead poisoning arising from the ingestion of lead-based paint in tenements is a major cause of disease and death among children of inner-city families. Accidents such as falls from staircases without railings or burns sustained in fires caused by faulty wiring are also clearly income-related to the extent that the poorly maintained apartments and houses of the poor make a higher incidence of such occurrences virtually inevitable. If the number of accidents is to be reduced, considerable amounts of energy and money must be spent on parent education, product safety, and adequate child supervision. We have not yet enacted the preventive measures needed to reduce childhood mortality caused by accidents.

Morbidity rates as well as mortality rates are significantly higher among children of low-income families. Historically, the programs for increasing child health and welfare have been targeted at economically deprived families. The child health programs (noted in the historical review on page 7) have reduced the infant mortality rate. For example, in Birmingham, Alabama, the infant death rate dropped from 25.4 per 1,000 live births in 1964 to 14.3 in 1969; and in Denver, Colorado, the reduction during the same period was from 34.2 to 21.5 in areas served by maternal and infant care programs. Community-based programs, however, cannot serve the estimated 300,000 children of migrant families that lack legal residence and community ties. How can consistent health care be offered to migrant children, who are frequently anemic and malnourished and have severe dental, respiratory, and gastrointestinal problems? This is one of the many health delivery problems facing pediatric care.

The middle-class child is also frequently deprived of consistent health supervision. An increasing number of families have moved from urban to suburban centers during the twentieth century. Geographic and social transitions have placed new social, economic, and environmental stresses on the family. Gender roles and tasks are no longer clearly defined. A father may stay home with young children while a mother works, or both parents may work, and the child is placed in a day care facility.

After the 1960's, when many policies and programs aimed at promoting the health and integrity of the nuclear family were implemented, the 1970's witnessed many legislative actions and lawsuits designed to clarify and secure the rights of minors. For example, the diagnosis and treatment of venereal disease in minors was customarily offered only if parental consent had been given. However, by the late 1970's all 50 states offered care for venereal disease without requiring parental consent. Some states have enacted statutes that obviate the acquisition of parental consent in such other matters as seeking treatment for drug abuse. The battle to secure the rights of minors in obtaining contraceptives, abortions, and general health services is on an upswing and will undoubtedly continue as lobbyists, legislators, and plaintiffs continue in the struggle to define and guarantee the rights of minors.

Informed consent for minors presupposes that the minor understands the nature of the health problem and the contemplated solution. Assessing the youth's level of understanding is difficult, and since children at each developmental age have different capacities and decision-making abilities (*and* children of the same developmental age may vary considerably in their mental abilities), clear rules on informed consent for minors will not be formulated quickly or easily.

The goal of contemporary pediatric nursing is to assist each child in obtaining his or her optimal physical and mental potential. Nursing is holistic in that it is concerned equally with the biological, psychological, social, and spiritual fulfillment of each child. How can health care be delivered so that infant mortality is reduced, immunization rates increased, accidents prevented, and the family in stress identified and assisted? If neighborhood-based health programs are emphasized, then health facilities will be socioeconomically segregated more often than not. Do we strive for equal or better services for low-income, high-risk families, or should we concentrate on establishing integrated, high-quality programs? And how can health education, disease prevention, and health care delivery be directed at the child as a person, not just at a problem such as a handicapping condition, teenage pregnancy, or delinquent behavior? Can we implement health care programs that are not devoted to specialized services and problems?

Demographic information on the child's circumstances is crucial to the delivery of health care to children, whether the child lives in a large city or a small community. We need to know the social, environmental, and biological forces affecting the child. Equally important, what are the health needs of young people as perceived by them?

When health programs are enacted in response to public demand, the design of the program is frequently based on aggregate data that do not reflect differences among the different racial and socioeconomic groups in the community. Before high quality community care can be offered, needs must be assessed and aggregate data unraveled to reveal the true health needs of youth in the community to be served. The accurate assessment, planning, implementation, and evaluation of health care for children are the challenges confronting pediatric nursing today.

As you learn about child health and practice pediatric nursing, identify the social, economic, and environmental factors affecting each child's health. Question what the child's nurturing environment is like. Assess what stresses are placed on the child and his family. Ascertain how the family unit is coping, what supports are helping to maintain the family unit, and what you can do to improve family integrity. Pediatric nursing continues to change to meet the different and expanding needs of each child and his family. You are part of the exciting evolution of pediatric care.

Historical Review of Policy Relating to the Health and Welfare of Children and Adolescents, 1855–1978.

1855 Children's Hospital of Philadelphia founded. First hospital in the U.S. devoted to the care of children.

1860 First children's clinic established in New York City.

1899 Initiation of juvenile courts as distinguished from adult courts.

1909 White House Conference convened by President T. Roosevelt. During this conference and subsequent ones held every 10 years, representatives from voluntary organizations, citizens' groups, and local, state, national, and federal agencies met to study and make recommendations for the creation and continuation of programs directed toward the needs and care of children.

1912 Children's Bureau established. The Bureau sponsors conferences and influences the direction of policy on child health and nutrition.

1917 First Federal Child Labor Law passed.

1933 Birthrate in the U.S. is 16 per 1,000 population compared to 20 in 1928, and 25 in 1919. Infant mortality rises to 58 per 1,000 live births.

1935 Social Security Act, amended many times in the future, provides for aid to dependent children, maternal and child health programs, child welfare services, and crippled children's services.

1946 The United Nations International Children's Emergency Fund (UNICEF) created by the United Nations. Postwar "baby boom" begins. Birthrate rises from 19 live births per 1,000 population in 1940 to 24 per 1,000 in 1964.
Social Security Act amended to provide larger grants for child and maternal health and child welfare programs. National School Lunch Act provides for money to states to establish and maintain school lunch programs.

1948 The World Health Organization (WHO) founded by the United Nations.
The Children's Bureau becomes a clearing house for research concerned with children and begins publishing *Research Relating To Children*.

1950 National Association For Retarded Children established. Mid-Century White House Conference on Children And Youth focuses on how to provide children with opportunities to achieve a healthy personality.

1953 Department of Health, Education, and Welfare (HEW) established. Six of the operating agencies are components of the Public Health Service. Three other large agencies are the Health Care Financing Administration, The Social Security Administration, and the Educational Division. All HEW agencies have health-related programs.

1956 Social Security Act amended to provide benefits to disabled children and adults over age eighteen (whose disability began before age eighteen).

1959 Assembly of United Nations adopts Declaration of the Rights of the Child.

1960 As a result of the "baby boom" children under age fifteen make up 31 percent of the total U.S. population. Children's Bureau and Women's Bureau have national conference on daycare. Following the conference the National Committee for Day Care is established to initiate standards of care.

1962 Congress approves Vaccination Assistance Act to help states and communities develop immunization programs. Stricter control of the release of new drugs following surge of birth defects in Europe caused by Thalidomide.

1962 Proposals for legislation that would
1965 require physicians to notify law officers of suspected child abuse cases.

1963 Measles vaccine deemed effective and licensed for manufacture in U.S.
Maternal and Child Health and Mental Retardation Planning Amendments to the Social Security Act are passed by Congress. Projects are established to deal with infant mortality, retardation, premature births, and other problems of mothers and infants.

1964 Economic Opportunity Act provides educational and occupational training programs for out-of-school and unemployed youth, aged sixteen to twenty-one.

1965 Median age of U.S. population is 28; 36 percent of U.S. population is under age 20.
Social Security Act revised to add Medicare and Medicaid benefits that have provisions for comprehensive health care for children in low-income families.

1966 U.S. infant mortality rate drops for first time in 10 years to 23.7 per 1,000 live births, a 4 percent decrease from the previous year.
Comprehensive Health Planning and Public Health Services Amendments. Grants of 75 percent matching federal funds for children and youth programs at state and community levels. Child Nutrition Act provides for continuation of school lunch program and addition of school breakfast program. Child Protection Act bans certain toys deemed hazardous.

1967 Child Health Act adds infant care, family planning, and dental care to the Social Security Act.
Number of families receiving Aid To Financially Dependent Children (AFDC) increases 73 percent since 1960. One of every ten white children and four of every ten nonwhite children live in poverty.

1969 Office of Child Development established to coordinate and administer Headstart and the Children's Bureau functions.

1970 White House Conference on Children and Youth organized into two conference groups, one for persons interested in the care of children and one for youth to speak out and make recommendations for actions.

1971 Congress passes Comprehensive Child Care Act intended to make day care available to all children.
Nurse-midwives endorsed by American College of Obstetricians and Gynecologists.

1972 Target year for implementation of 1967 Title XIX Social Security Act amendment that required early and periodic screening, diagnosis, and treatment (EPSDT). Women's, Infant's, and Children's (WIC) Program to provide nutritional supplement to pregnant women and to infants and young children who are at risk because of inadequate nutrition and income.
Birthrate decreases to 14.9 live births per 1,000 population; infant mortality rate decreases to 17.7 deaths per 1,000 live births.

1973 1,200 nurse midwives practicing in hospital delivery rooms, three times as many as 1963.

1974 Child Abuse Prevention and Treatment Act, National Health Planning and Resources Development Act, and Sudden Infant Death Syndrome Act passed.
Office of Handicapped founded.

1975 Title XX of Social Security Act includes funds for family planning services, child care services, protective services, and foster care services.

1976 Main-Stream Act, entitling each child to an education for his needs, regardless of handicaps, passed.
Toxic Substances Control Act passed to assess and control the development, production, and marketing of

synthetic chemicals, many of which are used in the production of children's toys, clothes, and foods.

1977 Following a plateau in the mid-1950's to mid-1960's infant mortality rate declined steadily for past ten years for both white and nonwhite infants; however, among children and youth aged one to nineteen who die, accidents account for more deaths than any single disease.
Birthrate rises from 14.8 in 1976 to 15.3.

1978 The sale of lead paint for most consumer uses, and its use in any toys, furniture, and other household products is prohibited to help prevent lead poisoning among children.

Bibliography

Births, Marriages, Divorces, and Deaths for 1977. Monthly Vital Statistics Report: Statistics from the National Center for Health Statistics. 26: March, 1978.

Bremner, R. (ed). *Children and Youth in America: A Documentary History,* vol. 3, 1933–1973. Cambridge, Harvard University Press., 1974

Children in Pursuit of Justice. A Rockefeller Foundation Conference. New York, N.Y., 1977.

Green, C.P., Potterger, K. Teenage Pregnancy: A Major Problem for Minors, *Zero Population Growth.* Washington, D.C., August, 1977.

Hull, W. and Denis, G. *Quality Assurance in Social Services in Health Programs for Mothers and Children.* Health Education and Welfare and University of Pittsburgh Graduate School of Public Health and Public Health Social Work, 1977.

Health in the United States 1976–77. U.S. Dept. of Health, Education and Welfare. National Center for Health Statistics. Publ. No. 77–1232. Hyattsville, Md., 1977.

Reported Morbidity and Mortality in the U.S.: Annual Summary: 1977. Center for Disease Control, 26:September, 1978.

Schmidt, W.M. The Development of Health Services for Mothers and Children in the U.S. *American Journal of Public Health* 63:419, 1973.

Senn, M.J. *Speaking Out for America's Children.* New Haven, Conn., Yale University Press, 1977.

Studies On Delivery Systems. U.S. Dept. of Health Education and Welfare. Publ. No. 77–5703 Rockville, Md., 1977.

Wilner, D., Walkley, R., O'Neill, E. *Introduction to Public Health,* ed. 7. New York, MacMillan Co., 1978.

CHAPTER 2

The Nursing Process Applied to Children

BEHAVIORAL OBJECTIVES

After studying this chapter you will be able to:

- Discuss the concept of parent-child nursing.
- Identify and explain the anatomical, physiological, and behavioral differences between the child and the adult.
- Discuss how you will involve the child's parents in his care.
- Describe the child-centered pediatric unit.
- Describe the procedure for admitting a child to the pediatric unit.
- Complete a pediatric assessment, using an assessment tool.
- Actively prepare a child for a diagnostic, therapeutic, or surgical procedure.
- Plan and implement a play session for a hospitalized child.
- Assess a child's reaction to pain.
- Explain the proper approach for administering both oral and intramuscular medications to a child.
- Plan a child's discharge from the hospital with the child's parents.

TERMS AND CONCEPTS

Parent-child unit
Play
Pain
Pediatric assessment

INTRODUCTION

Contemporary pediatric nursing involves not only the child, but the *parent-child unit*. The promotion and maintenance of health, as well as acute care nursing and follow-up, are not adequate unless focus is placed on the entire unit. The six-month-old infant cannot be expected to take his own medications, nor can the five-year-old prepare his special diet. Parental involvement is necessary, as well as highly desirable.

In 1973, the American Nurses' Association established standards for the practice of maternal and child nursing that relate to health promotion, maintenance, and acute care nursing, as well as continuity of care. The ANA considers knowledge of human growth and development to be essential to the practice of pediatric nursing. Familiarity with the norm will enable you to recognize deviations from the norm and to intervene as necessary.

The essential components of the nursing process—assessment, planning, implementation, evaluation, and re-planning—are constant whether an adult or a child is the client. However, because the child is not considered a "little adult," the nursing process must be adapted to fit his special needs and those of his parents.

This chapter discusses the nursing process as it applies to the child. The uniqueness of the child and how he differs from the adult are presented. A pediatric assessment tool is provided, along with guidelines for its use and suggestions for a successful interview. The admission and discharge of the child from the hospital are discussed, as well as vital nursing interventions during hospitalization, such as preparation for procedures, *play* as a diversion, play therapy, and administering medications. The assessment of *pain* is also discussed. The importance of including the parents in all aspects of the child's care is stressed throughout.

DIFFERENCES BETWEEN THE CHILD AND THE ADULT

Anatomical Differences

The most obvious difference between the child and the adult is physical size. The most important nursing implication arising from this difference is that there is less margin for error with the child than with the adult, especially in relation to medications and intravenous infusions. Although a loss of fluids and electrolytes is more devastating to the child, he can be overloaded too quickly with fluids, causing cardiac failure.

The smaller size of the child's body necessitates the use of smaller equipment. Many types of treatment and surgery are more difficult because of the child's smaller size, but this difference is an advantage in that the child is easier to observe and move. Techniques commonly used in adult nursing must be adapted for use with the child. For example, a mummy restraint is not necessary when tube-feeding an adult, but it is generally required with the infant.

Another important anatomical difference is in the eustachian tube; in the infant, it is shorter, wider, and straighter than in the adult. This leads to more ear infections following nasopharyngitis in the young child because the bacteria or virus travels more easily and quickly to the child's ear. Also, because the infant's cardiac sphincter is more lax, he may tend to regurgitate his feedings.

Physiological Differences

Because of the child's physiological immaturity, he responds differently to disease processes and medications than does the adult. The younger the child, the more different his reaction from the adult's. The newborn, especially, is vulnerable to drug reactions. He is far more susceptible to allergies and lacks immunity to a number of disease processes.

The child's temperature control is less effective than the adult's; the child tends to show greater fluctuations in temperature. The infant under three months of age may be seriously ill and not run a temperature, while the young child tends to convulse with high fevers, while the adult reaction may be chills with high fevers.

As a rule, the child reacts quickly to disease, becoming sicker faster and recovering more rapidly than the adult. The child must be observed carefully because dangerous complications occur more rapidly, too. His faster metabolic rate requires more fluid, calories and oxygen and affects his vital signs more dramatically. What would be considered bradycardia in the adult may be seen in a normal child, especially the adolescent athlete. Sinus arrhythmias (irregularities of heartbeat) may occur when the heart rate increases with inspiration and decreases with exhalation; this is also nonpathologic in the child.

Behavioral Differences

Behavioral differences between the child and the adult contribute to the challenge of parent-child nursing. The child may not be capable of expressing his needs, wants, and hurts verbally; therefore, the nurse must be alert to nonverbal communications. For example, the infant cannot say, "I have an earache," but he may rub his head on the bed and cry. Similarly, although the child has not learned to hid his feelings, he may not have the verbal skills to express himself; therefore, the nurse must be alert to such overt behavioral manifestations of discomfort as crying, aggression, hostility, and withdrawal, and must permit the child to play out his feelings in a nonthreatening environment.

Because the child may unknowingly place himself in danger, the nurse must anticipate his actions and take steps to ensure his safety. For example, side rails are a must for the young child's bed, and restraints are often necessary to prevent his pulling out an intravenous infusion.

Because the child is constantly growing and progressing through developmental stages, what constitutes adequate treatment and nursing intervention for a child of a given age may not be appropriate for a child of a different age. A consideration of the child's stage of development is a very necessary part of parent-child nursing; it will affect his emotional and physical response to illness or injury, and also influences how well he can communicate with you, the nurse.

You will learn in later chapters that the child reacts with greater anxiety to illness and confinement. Fantasy and magical thinking (ch. 6) contribute to his fear and misinterpretation of the hospital environment and procedures. Be aware of these factors and correct misinterpretations as necessary.

PARENT-CHILD PEDIATRIC NURSING

The beliefs that the child needs his parents (especially during such stressful times as hospitalization) and that the parents need support are central to contemporary pediatric nursing. Fostering the continuity of the parent-child relationship is a desirable and necessary goal on any pediatric unit.

There are tragic and far-reaching effects of depriving the young child of his parent (usually the mother). The child under five years of age is most vulnerable and at the greatest psychological risk. The primary source of anxiety in a child of this age is separation from his parents; his immature ego cannot sustain him. Separation often interrupts emotional development and may result in loss of trust and self-esteem. This loss, coupled with the feeling that hospitalization is a punishment for a real or imagined wrongdoing, can permanently impair the child's ability to form a close relationship with others. His mother's presence enables him to tolerate intrusive and painful procedures, to continue to develop, and to avoid emotional trauma. The mother is the liaison between child and staff. Her presence during painful procedures assures the child that he has not been abandoned. She is better able to interpret and explain what is happening to him, and to comfort and reassure him.

It is a misconception that the unhappy, maladjusted child will fare better in the hospital, away from his parents. In fact, he is less able to deal with separation than is the happy, secure child, because he does not have the inner strength and reassurances of his parents' love to sustain him. Rather, he may equate hospitalization with abandonment, which may have been a threat before the hospitalization.

Despite the more-than-adequate documentation of the above facts, many hospitals still do not permit parental participation in the child's care. However, there have been advances, ranging from more liberal visiting hours to 24-hour rooming-in. Unfortunately, even in the most liberal institutions, parents are often not encouraged to participate actively as team members in the child's care; family-centered care is thus thwarted.

In the truly family-centered unit, the parents are expected to become team members. At admission, or earlier if possible, parents are encouraged to stay with the child. The nurse will explain that it is their right to stay and that their presence is highly desirable. Some hospitals offer a discount in daily rates if one parent will stay with the child. The parents are made to feel welcome and are provided with space (lockers or closets) for their belongings, and a place to shower and sleep. Their strengths and coping patterns, as well as the child's, are assessed. The nurse asks what aspects of care they would like to be involved in and then explains what is expected of them. Rather than merely sitting with the child and being otherwise excluded from his daily care, the parents may bathe him, take his vital signs, monitor his intake and output, and so on. As their confidence grows, they may wish to take increasing responsibility for their child's care. However, the parents are never made to feel as though they are responsible for all of the child's physical care.

Becausc the parents are available as team members around the clock, there is more time for them to talk with the other members of the health care team, they are more knowledgable about their child's condition, and more confident in their ability to care for him (see Figure 2–1). This greatly enhances teaching them about post-hospitalization care. Under these circumstances, both the child and his parents tend to fare better after discharge. Liberal sibling visitation is also desirable; it decreases both the sibling's anxiety over the child's condition and the parents' anticipation of family disharmony when the sick child returns home.

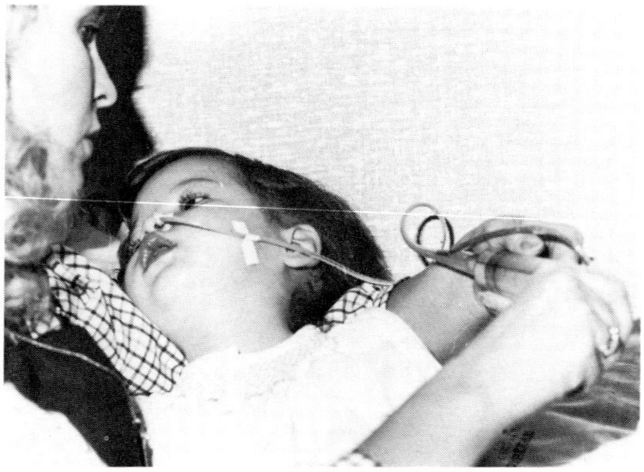

Figure 2–1. *This mother is gaining confidence in her ability to care for her hospitalized child.*

It may seem that parental participation makes the nurse unnecessary; not true! In fact, parental participation requires *more* nursing hours; parents need support, encouragement, education, and preparation before they can participate in the nursing care of their child. Parental anxiety is highly contagious: if the parent is anxious, the child is anxious. Nurses must be alert to signs of parental anxiety (see ch. 3) and take immediate steps to reduce it. An anxious parent is more prone to misunderstand directions, and is therefore more likely to endanger the child.

Parents who help to care for their child are usually less anxious and more self-confident of their ability to help. Many a parent-child unit suffers because the mother is afraid to touch her child, let alone pick him up and cuddle him. This is especially true if the child is in an oxygen tent or is getting an intravenous infusion. Explain to the mother that she *can* hold her baby, then help her to get comfortable, hand her the child, and stay with her until she feels comfortable holding him. Hand her the call bell so that she can call you when she is ready to return the child to bed. The rationale for encouraging the mother's involvement is the belief that the child in an oxygen tent or on bed rest is frequently better off resting quietly in his mother's arms if he is upset. However, if the child must be on absolute bed rest or must remain in the oxygen tent at all times, reassure the mother that it is all right to caress the child and talk or sing to him. Then, as soon as the child is physically able, get him up and into his mother's arms.

Turning a child's care over to unprepared, unsupervised, and unsupported parents can be disastrous. Parents must be taught such procedures as measuring intake and output and checking for adequate circulation. They may have to be shown how to read a thermometer. Careful and continuing assessment of parental participation in the care of the child is a necessary part of nursing care (see Figure 2–2).

Under some circumstances, it may be best for parents *not* to participate; if they are abusive, for example, or overanxious, they may be unable to contribute to the child's care. However, once it is established that the parent is to participate, the nurse must resist the temptation to perform procedures rather than to teach the parent to do them, even though the former course may be the easier. Of course, some procedures will be too complex for the parent and must be done by the nurse.

In some instances it may not be possible for the parents to stay. The family may live 200 miles away and may have no one else to look after other children at home; the hospitalization might arise from an accident that necessitates the hospitalization of the parents themselves. If, for whatever reason, it is not feasible for the parent(s) to stay, do not make them feel guilty for having to leave the child alone. Nursing care will have to be altered to the extent that it will be necessary to arrange for one primary caretaker to be with the child, acting as a surrogate mother. When parent and child must be separated, be sure to alert the parents to changes in the child's behavior that can be expected after discharge. The child's senses of trust and autonomy will have to be restored; he may withdraw, rejecting his parents and resisting their efforts to care for him; he may cling to them, whine, and demand their attention; or he may exhibit both types of behavior. It is important that the parents understand that this is normal behavior, and that with loving care, attention to the child's needs, and patience, his behavior will gradually return to normal.

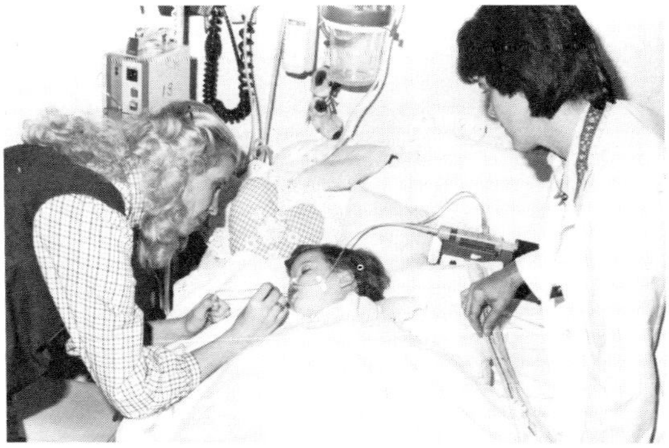

Figure 2–2. *A mother suctions her child's oropharynx under the careful supervision of the nurse.*

THE PEDIATRIC UNIT

The child-centered pediatric unit, ward, or hospital is as homelike as possible. Each child is allowed to decorate his room or space with his personal belongings and mementos. Some units reserve space for the child to paint or color on the lower walls in the playroom. After the walls are covered, they are repainted or washed, and the process begins again. If your institution does not or will not permit this graffiti, provide paper and finger paints or crayons so that the child can express himself; hang the finished works on the child's door or in his room (see the later section of this chapter on play).

The child is permitted to wear his own clothing or pajamas when possible; this helps him to maintain his sense of identity. Parents are encouraged to use the unit kitchen to prepare food for themselves and for their child if they so desire. This policy is especially helpful if the parents live a great distance from the hospital, and it also ensures adequate food and fluid intake for the child.

Telephones are provided, and the child is encouraged to call family and friends to help maintain home and community ties. The parents are asked to leave a family picture with the child as well as his favorite toy or blanket. If the parents cannot stay, provide them with a cassette tape recorder and a blank tape so that they can record a favorite story or song, or just talk to the child. The recorder is left with the child so that he can play the tape of the familiar voice whenever he wishes. This serves to strengthen his memory of his family and his attachment to them. The young child may cry when he hears the tape; if so, console him with love, attention, and physical contact, such as holding him close and rocking him. His memory is short and he may not be able to remember that his mother will come for him; the tape helps to remind him of his mother, even though he may cry when he hears it.

If the parents cannot stay, they should be encouraged to tell the child they are leaving and not to slip away "so he won't cry." If they leave without saying good-bye the child will wonder where they have gone and may fear they have abandoned him. Telling the child they are leaving before they do so may make him cry, but this honest approach is psychologically much better. Ask them when they will return and relate this to the child in terms he can understand. "Mommy will be back after your nap," is easier for the child to understand than the abstract "Mommy will be back about 4 o'clock." Encourage the parents to telephone if they cannot visit.

Staff members on the unit wear colored uniforms or colorful smocks over their white uniforms. If street clothes are worn, a lab coat or jacket worn over the clothes will help parents distinguish very quickly who the nurses are—often a concern of parents when street clothes are worn, particularly if their child is very young or very sick.

The adolescent client is housed in a separate unit of the hospital in an effort to place him with people his own age. Whenever possible, his roommate will also be someone of the same sex and with a similar diagnosis. The adolescent client is kept informed of his health status and is expected to participate in the planning and implementation of his care.

ADMISSION

The hospital is a strange and foreboding place to the average person. It is a place of hurtful and mutilating procedures and often, a place of death. How the child reacts to hospitalization depends on a number of factors. One of these is the child's previous experience with hospitals, which may range from a total lack of exposure, to a previous traumatic hospitalization, to hearing that a loved one died in the hospital. Or, the child may have a friend who boasted of the ice cream served after a tonsillectomy.

The child's age and stage of development also affect how he reacts to hospitalization, as does how often he's been left in the care of a person other than his parents. The child who has never left his mother's side or been exposed to an environment other than his own home will often have a more difficult time adjusting to the hospital, with or without the support of his mother. The strange environment is traumatic enough for the young child; therefore, he should never be separated from his mother during the hospitalization if this is possible.

The child's level of preparedness also influences his reaction to the hospital. If he has been told about his hospitalization and given a simple explanation of the need for it, it will be easier for him to adjust than it would be for the child who is not forewarned. The better prepared the child, the more positive his reaction. Unfortunately, a child will occasionally be admitted having being told by his parents that he is going "to visit Grandma." Not only is this deception cruel, but it undermines the child's faith in his own parents and sets the tone for a traumatic hospital experience.

When you admit a child to the unit, squat down to speak to him at eye level. Spend a few minutes talking with him and his parent to let him get used to you. Meet him empty-handed so that he can see that you mean him no harm and have nothing that can be used to hurt him (such as a syringe or thermometer). Take the child and his parent on a tour of the unit. Point out the play area, the parents' lounge, the unit kitchen, the child's room, and above all, the nurse's station; knowing where a nurse will be is important to the child's sense of security. Explain when he can visit the playroom and that his mother can use the kitchen to prepare food and drinks for him (if this is true in your institution).

Acquaint the child with the call bell in his room, and let him use it in your presence to call another nurse so that he can be assured that it does work and that he won't be left alone if he needs or wants someone (Figure 2–3). Show him how his bed works and let him play with it for a few minutes. Explain that the side rails will be used (especially at night) to keep him from falling out of bed. He may say that he's not a baby and doesn't need them; if so, acknowledge that he *is* a big boy, and that you're sure he wouldn't fall out of his bed at home, but that this is a strange bed and it's higher off the floor, and the side rails will protect him. Be sure the child understands the television controls and can reach the telephone and call bell from his bed. Show him and his parents where the bathroom is. Tell them what time meals will be served and that if the child is able, he may dine in the playroom with other children.

Checking vital signs is always a part of the admission routine and is particularly traumatic when the child is separated from his mother. Remember that not only are the people strange to the child, but the place is strange also. To add intrusive procedures,

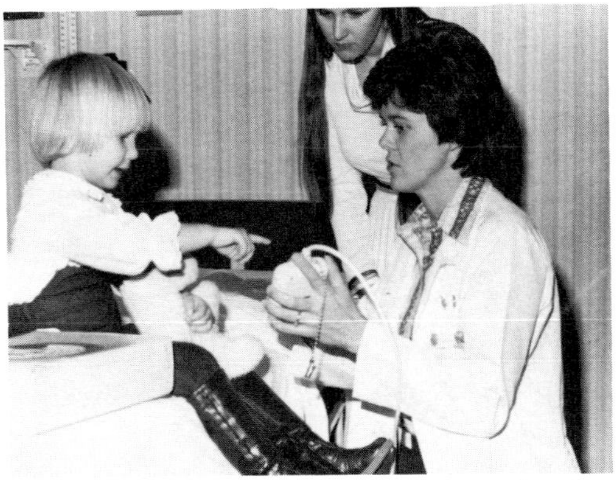

Figure 2–3. *The nurse acquaints a newly admitted child and her mother with the call bell.*

performed by a stranger, to the trauma of adjusting to a new place with new people is often unnecessarily cruel. The trauma can be reduced by letting the mother change the child's clothes and take his temperature.

If the child's admission is not an emergency and there are no contraindications to his playing in the playroom, you may begin your nursing assessment by interviewing the parents while the child plays.

PEDIATRIC ASSESSMENT

Assessment tools used in adult nursing are not adequate for a nursing assessment of the child. For this reason, many institutions have a separate form to use when admitting or assessing a child. Although the details of the tool vary with the institution, the information that should be obtained is uniform. A pediatric assessment tool is shown in Figure 2–4. A separate set of guidelines for its use is shown in Figure 2–5. The guidelines will aid the beginning interviewer to obtain the desired information and can serve as a checklist until the interviewer becomes comfortable with using the assessment tool alone.

The nursing assessment is made upon admission, unless the seriousness of the child's condition dictates otherwise. The nursing assessment makes caring for the parent-child unit an easier and more rewarding task. Knowing the child's usual daily routines enables the nurse to abide by them as much as possible, thus making the hospitalization more homelike and, hopefully, less traumatic for the child.

Interview the parents in a comfortable setting. If the admission is scheduled, the playroom may be ideal because the child

Figure 2–4. **Pediatric Assessment Tool**

Child's appearance (initial impression)

Present illness (parents' own words)

Previous hospitalizations
- Parents' perceptions
- Child's perception

Present hospitalization
- Parents' expectations
- Child's expectations
  - What does he know?
  - How has he been prepared?

Habits
- Eating
- Sleeping
- Elimination
- Mobility

Personal-social history
- Play
- Communication
- Temperament
- Behavior
- Level of independence
- Discipline
- Sociocultural

Physical assessment
- Vital signs/statistics
- Perceptual problems
- Skin integrity
- Past medical history
- Immunizations
- Allergies
- Medications

Figure 2–5. Pediatric Assessment Tool: Guidelines for Use

Child's Appearance/Initial Impression

Present Illness (let the parents tell their story)

Previous Hospitalizations

Reason Dates Outcome

Parents' Perceptions
"How do/did you feel about the hospitalization?"
"Why?"

Child's Perception
"How did Billy feel about the hospitalization?"
"How did he react?" [or ask child directly]

Present Hospitalization

Reason:
Parents' expectations:
Child's expectations:
What does he know? ("Billy, why are you in the hospital?")
How was child prepared? *or*
How did you find out that you were coming to the hospital?

Habits

Eating

Breast _____ Bottle _____ Baby foods _____ Finger foods _____ Table foods _____ Feeds self _____ Needs help _____ Does family eat together (dine) _____ Says grace _____ How many meals does he eat per day _____ Eats at table _____ Infant seat _____ High chair _____ Snacks _____ Good eater _____ Poor eater _____ Messy _____ Tidy _____ Uses spoon _____ Fork _____ Pica (paint, sand, soap) _____ Food allergies (include type of reaction):

Food preferences (include snacks):

Dislikes:

Sleeping

Morning nap _____ length _____ Afternoon nap _____ Length _____ Bedtime prayers _____ Sleeps alone _____ With others _____ Type of bed (crib, twin, full, mattress on floor, side rails) _____ Sleeps with others in room _____ Others in bed _____ Takes toy to bed _____ What _____ Gets up to bathroom during night _____ Used to being "tucked in" and kissed goodnight _____ Bedtime _____ Sleeps how long _____ Talks in sleep _____ Walks in sleep _____ Dreams _____ Nightmares _____ Wets bed _____

Child's reaction to nightmares/bed wetting?
How do parents handle situation?

focuses on the problem at hand and frequently helps put them at ease as they tell you in their own words what has happened to their child. In this part of the interview you will ascertain how well they understand the illness and the events leading up to it.

As has been said, previous hospitalizations affect how the child will react to the present one. Ask about the parents' perceptions as well as the child's.

The perceptions of parents and child regarding the present hospitalization are equally important. What do they expect to happen? Was the child prepared for this hospitalization? If so, how? Ask the child why he is in the hospital and what he thinks will happen to him. Typically, the child views illness as punishment, although he is not going to tell you that he is here because he "hit his little sister," for example. That the child sees the hospitalization as punishment is more easily understood in the case of the child who was burned because he played with matches against his parents' orders, or the child who was told to be careful when riding his skateboard, but decided to try a jumping turn and fell, breaking his leg.

Daily habits are assessed next. If you learn that the child goes to sleep with his teddy bear after being rocked and read to, provide these things at bedtime. If he shares a bare mattress and blanket on the floor with four siblings, don't expect him to sleep well while alone in a high bed with crisp linen and side rails.

If you know that the child gets out of bed and goes to the bathroom at night, you may be able to prevent bedwetting if you lower his bed as much as possible and leave a light on in the bathroom, or simply place the call bell so that he can reach it and ask the latter, make sure someone comes immediately, or he may climb over the side rails or wet the bed. Such an accident is not only ego-deflating for the child (especially the young child who has just learned to control his bladder and bowel), but it also increases the workload of the nurse who must change the wet linen. Never diaper a potty-trained child to prevent "accidents"; this is a severe blow to his ego and his independence, and serves only to make the nurses's workload lighter (i.e., she doesn't have to change wet sheets). Instead of diapering the child, provide a potty-chair in his room and be sure that his pants have an elastic waistband so that he can get them down in a hurry. This approach fosters the child's independence during hospitalization, and lessens his anxiety by permitting him to regain a measure of control over his situation.

Knowing the words the child uses to convey his wants and needs is also important, especially his words for urine and feces.

Jenny, two and half years old, was hospitalized with diarrhea. Her favorite toy, a stuffed "Winnie the Pooh," was clutched in her hand constantly. Jenny had recently been potty-trained, which was discovered during the nursing assessment by Ms. Taylor, Jenny's primary nurse. Jenny's mother had to return home briefly to check on her other children and left Jenny in the care of Ms. Taylor. Ms. Taylor elected to let Jenny keep her jeans and sweat shirt on, knowing that the change to a gown would be less traumatic if Jenny's mother changed her when she returned. Jenny began to cry "poo-poo, poo-poo" after her mother left. Ms. Taylor assumed Jenny was referring to her Pooh-bear and began to rock her and talk to her about the bear. Jenny then had a loose bowel movement that soaked through her pants and Ms. Taylor's uniform.

The child moves around to help reduce his anxiety and gain some control over his environment. The hospital may thwart this tendency if the child's condition requires immobilization. Ask if he crawls, creeps, or walks, if he walks on his toes, seems hyperactive, or has bizarre body movements.

Personal-social development is assessed next. Knowing how the child handles himself and interacts with others will give the nurse an idea of how well he can cope with his current situation.

Knowing with whom the child plays and what types of activities he enjoys will give you an idea of the type of diversion you may wish to use while he is hospitalized. What is his favorite toy and does he have it with him? If not, ask if someone can bring it to the hospital. How well does the child communicate with others? Does he speak well? How does he make his wants known (i.e., does he cry, point, grunt)?

Regarding the child's temperament, ask if he is easy-going and good-natured, or irritable and demanding. Is his behavior within normal limits according to his age and stage of development? Does he exhibit unusual behaviors such as repetitive movements, rocking, or head-banging? If he intentionally hurts other children, your goal will be to watch him carefully to prevent him from doing so.

How independent is the child? Ask if he can do most things for himself and what activities he needs help with. How does he react when he is separated from his parent? How does the parent respond?

A social history provides insight into the child's interpersonal relationships and an avenue of communication, especially with the school-aged child. He is interested in his peer group and activities outside the home. Knowing that he is a boy scout, for example, will permit you to discuss scouting with him.

Physical assessment includes vital statistics, perceptual problems, skin integrity, allergies, and the like. If the child is deaf, hard of hearing, or has visual problems, for example, this part of the nursing assessment will make note of the problem. Skin integrity refers to obvious bruises, cuts, abrasions, rashes, etc. Ask about his past illnesses, including dental problems. Has he had all of his immunizations to date, and what are his allergies, if any? Also ascertain if he is currently taking any medications.

PLAY

Play is the language and work of childhood. It is discussed in later chapters as it relates to specific stages of growth and development. In addition to fostering such aspects of physical development as eye-hand coordination and control of fine and gross motor movements, play also contributes to the development of the child's personality as he acts out various roles. In play, he imitates adults and rehearses the activities of daily living; he distinguishes the real from the unreal and learns spatial relationships. Play is also an important coping mechanism for the child.

The hospitalized child has the same emotional and social needs as the well child; he also has additional needs resulting from his illness and hospitalization, immobility and/or confinement, and separation from home. The young child is not able to express his emotions verbally, especially if they involve abstract concepts. Through play, he is able to express his emotions, to give vent to forbidden impulses, and to act out fantasies. Play provides a means for the child to reveal his fears, wants, and grievances with the adult world. It serves as an outlet for pent-up tensions and permits him to release aggression safely.

Every hospitalized child needs ample opportunity to play. Many hospitals have playrooms fully equipped with a variety of toys, building materials, and props. Water, sand, modeling clay, nonallergenic pets, and medical clothing and equipment are part of the well-stocked play area. His condition permitting, the child may be in the playroom at any time unless he is undergoing tests or treatment. The bed or crib can be rolled to the play area if the child is not ambulatory. The child is encouraged to spend some time each day in play; if he cannot go to the play area, play is permitted in his room.

The hospital may have a "play lady" who supervises and coordinates play activity. She is different from a *play therapist,* one who has training in providing and interpreting therapeutic play. The play therapist is likely to have a toy hospital completely equipped with dolls and props. The child is permitted to play with the hospital and equipment as he sees fit, the only limits being that he cannot hurt anyone or destroy the toys (Figure 2–6). Many times the child will perform acts of aggression against the nurse and doctor dolls. He may jab them with needles, saying exactly what he has heard—"Now be still, this won't hurt. Don't you cry." He may undress the dolls to perform tests. However, a child may be so anxious that he is not able to engage in a specific type of play, such as needle play.

Lisa, a five year old admitted for open-heart surgery, had five play sessions before she could pick up a syringe. Her father had repeatedly told her that she was *not* scared and that shw *would not* cry. Yet, her therapeutic play sessions showed her extreme anxiety.

Your hospital does not have to have the latest equipment and a full-time play

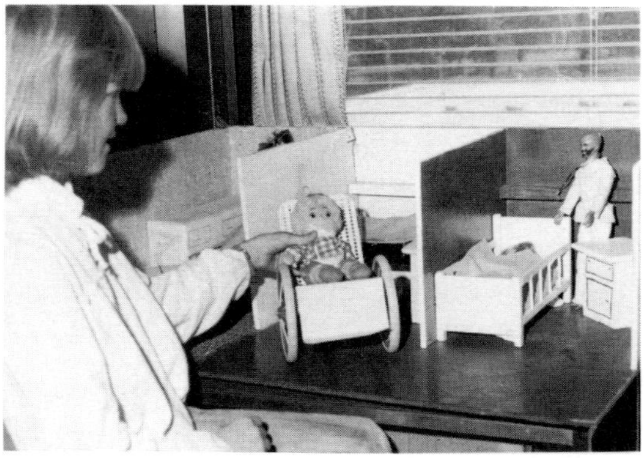

Figure 2–6. *A play session with a toy hospital.*

therapist for the children in your care to benefit from play. If the child has an IV, use a vial of sterile water and a small feeding tube to make an IV for his teddy bear (Figure 2–7). If the child's IV must be restarted in another extremity, let him first "change" his teddy bear's IV. These simple techniques and others you will think of (such as letting the child change bandages on his teddy bear as his own bandage is changed) will enable the child to "play out" some of his fears and feelings about his treatment.

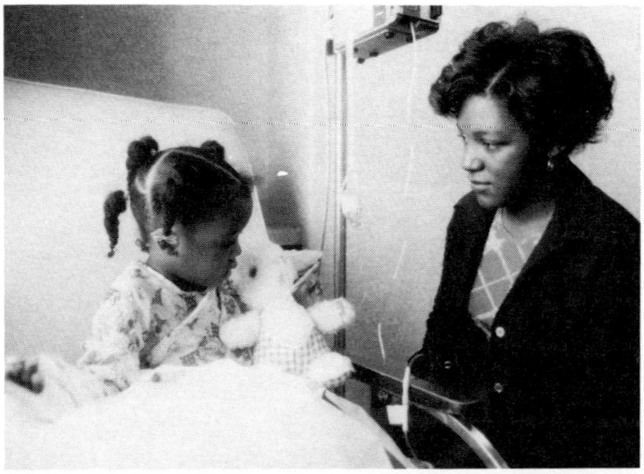

Figure 2–7. *Tolerating her IV will likely be less traumatic for this child, whose stuffed animal has been fitted with a toy IV made from a vial of water.*

They do not require a therapist, take very little time, and often work wonders. Needle play is permitted in many institutions as long as adequate supervision is provided. Even chubby three- and four-year-old hands become quite adept at handling syringes, withdrawing sterile water from a vial, and giving "injections" to dolls and teddy bears. Remember, though, to take the needle with you when you leave.

Kelly, five years old, was busily engaged in needle play with her doll. The nurse was silently watching as Kelly repeatedly filled the syringe and jabbed the needle forcefully into the doll baby. Kelly began humming the tune of "Merrily We Roll Along," and finally the words to her song were audible as she sang, "The nurse had a great big needle, a great big needle, a great big needle, and I grabbed it and jabbed it in her."

A punching bag (or a large, heavy balloon) tied to the traction frame is handy for the child in traction. He can punch the bag at will and thus release some of his aggression. Pounding and shaping modeling clay, pounding a peg board, and playing bean bag tic-tac-toe are also good for helping to release pent-up aggression.

All kinds of makeshift toys can be made if toys are not readily available. Colored medicine cards and gauze can be used to make a mobile for an infant; an empty disposable diaper box, with cups for wheels and gauze for a string, makes a fine pull-toy for a toddler; a tongue-blade airplane will keep a preschooler busy; and for the school-age child, you can make checkers from medicine cups, a puzzle cut up from a magazine picture, or a medical kit stocked with clean odds and ends found on the unit (syringe, tape, gauze, disposable tourniquet, etc.). You may be able to enlist the help of the adolescent patient in entertaining the younger child, or in constructing airplanes or trains. Use bath time to provide water play, but be prepared to get wet (cover your uniform with a scrub dress). If no tub toys are available, make the child a boat and give him at least two cups for pouring water back and forth. Remember to make sure that the child's diversion and stimulation are safe and age-appropriate (refer to the section on hospitalization in chs. 4–8).

PAIN

The child's response to pain differs from the adult's. Typically, the young child expresses pain through four modes of behavior: aggression, dependency, verbalization, and physiological response.

Aggression is seen when the child's usual mode of coping with stress is thwarted. Pain interrupts his play, which is the major way in which the young child (particularly the preschooler) copes with stress. His stress is therefore twofold: he must cope not only with the pain but also with the lack of his usual coping mechanism, play. When his coping behavior is interrupted, he becomes angry and reacts with aggressive behavior. Active aggression may be verbal (yelling or screaming) or nonverbal (jumping on the bed, hitting the nurse, or throwing things). Passive aggression, such as refusal to eat or take medicine, may also be seen.

The young child may associate physical pain with the pain of separation anxiety. Naturally, these two types of pain often occur at the same time when the child is hospitalized. Anxiety and uncertainty arising from separation cause dependent behavior in the young child.

Dependency may include forms of regression. Reverting to earlier behaviors is common. For example, the child may want to be held or rocked rather than play. Dependent behavior brings a nurturing adult close to the child out of necessity; the child needs emotional support, and his behavior assures that he will get it. It is important for the nurse to recognize the child's need for close, loving attention and to take steps to provide it.

The young child, in particular, will not be able to express his pain verbally since he lacks the language skills needed to do so. Therefore, you must be alert to nonverbal expressions of pain. The infant, for example, may pull on his ear or rub his head against the bed if his ear hurts. Of course, he also characteristically responds to pain by crying. With experience, the pediatric nurse learns to distinguish the cry of pain from the cry of hunger or a wet diaper. Crying is naturally easier for the parents to interpret since they know their child better; this is one of the many advantages of having the parents stay with the child. Even if the child's language skills do permit him to tell you he hurts, he may be unable to describe the exact location and nature of the pain. On the other hand, the child may deny feeling pain in an attempt to avoid an intramuscular injection, only to clench his teeth, grimace, and refuse to cough, breathe deeply, or change position. These are all signs of discomfort, as are whimpering, whining and irritability.

Physiological responses to pain include flushing of the skin, increased pulse and respirations, restlessness, dilated pupils, vomiting, and sighing.

Predetermined factors contribute in large part to the child's responses to pain. These factors, assessed upon admission, include the child's level of development and his past experience with illness, injury, doctors, nurses, and hospitals. Physical pain is closely interwoven with such emotions as fear, anxiety, anger, and loneliness, and what appear to be reactions to pain may be elicited by these emotions as much as by any physical discomfort.

Be sure to ask the parents how the child typically responds to pain when he is in a familiar environment (i.e., at home with his parents). Also important is what the child *perceives* to be happening. (For example, the child whose leg is being sutured under local anesthesia after an accident may cry out in pain every time he feels pressure from the suture needle. He does not actually feel pain, yet he responds as if he does. In such a case, respond to his behavior.) Help the child acknowledge and verbalize his pain by eliciting a description of its location and severity. Ask what you can do to make him more comfortable. If he refuses pain medication, accept his decision but explain that the medication will enable him to move and breathe easier and thus hasten his recovery and return home. Allow him a few minutes to think it over, then offer the medication again. He will probably take it when it is offered a second time. You have permitted him to "save face" by choosing to take his medication on his own terms.

MEDICATING THE CHILD

Administering medication to the hospitalized child is not the most pleasurable part of a pediatric nurse's day, but it is a necessary and most important job. Before you attempt to medicate the child, you must know not only the proper techniques, but also the proper approach to use. A few helpful hints are offered here.

First, never approach the child for the first time with something (syringe, thermometer, stethoscope) in your hand. Spend some time with him first, just getting acquainted. The admonition "look but don't touch" applies here. If the child is suspicious or scared of you, simply hold your hands up and say, "Look, I don't have anything in my hands. I'm not going to hurt you. I'm just going to talk." This will usually calm the child down.

When it is time for the child's medication, approach him in a matter-of-fact manner and say, "It is time for your medicine." If the medicine is an injection, you may say, "It is time for your injection," or "It is time for the medicine that you get with a needle."

This approach is preferable, although nurses sometimes make the mistake of approaching the child with a question (e.g., "Are you ready for your medicine now?"); this implies that you will honor the child's answer, and you must do so. If the child replies that he is not ready, you must retreat, return a few minutes later, and say "It is time for your medicine now."

An important part of good nursing is to allow the child as many choices as are appropriate, giving him some control over his care. For example, offer the child a choice of beverages after his injection, or, if appropriate, ask him which site he would like the injection in.

Aside from getting the child to cooperate when he is receiving medication, you will have to determine how well he can cope. Approach him with a positive attitude, and let him know you believe he can cope even though the experience may be unpleasant. Knowing that his nurse believes in him when the medicine tastes bad or the injection hurts is often support enough. You may say, "Jerry, it is time for your injection. You will need to hold still while I give it to you, but you may whistle, say 'ouch', or cry. If you need some help, we can help you hold still." Never threaten the child by saying, "If you don't hold still I'll have to stick you again." Also, do not tell him, "Big boys don't cry." This statement adds an additional stress to the primary one of a painful injection. If the child is in pain (or is scared) he may have a real need to cry and express his displeasure verbally. However, avoid encouraging him to the point that he begins to revel in self-pity. The happy medium is to provide an atmosphere of trust that permits the child to express whatever he is feeling.

There is a *big* difference between "helping you to hold still" and "holding you down." The former approach conveys respect to the child and allows him to maintain some control over his situation. Restraining him without permitting him to participate in the decision is a negative solution and is often more upsetting than the actual injection.

Always ask another nurse to go with you if you have to administer an injection. The parent may be perfectly capable of helping, but it is best to let her soothe and talk to her child while another nurse helps him to hold still. In the case of the infant or toddler, a brief explanation, followed by swift action, is often the best technique. The child will probably scream and struggle as soon as he realizes it is time for his injection; trying to reason with him may only prolong an upsetting situation. (See the Skills Manual.)

Administering oral medication to the child is usually less of a challenge than are intramuscular injections. However, a child may spit the medicine out, knock it out of your hand, or hold his lips tightly closed in refusal. Approaching the child in a pleasant manner and offering a choice of beverages after the medicine is correct procedure and usually elicits cooperation. The child or his parent may hold the cup for him to drink liquids, or if the child is an infant, you may wish to give the medicine via a nipple or needleless syringe (see the Skills Manual). If you want to offer the toddler or preschooler his medicine in a syringe, be sure to show him first that it has no needle. Occasionally, tablets will have to be crushed and mixed with syrup or honey. Offer the mixture on a spoon for the child to lick like a lollipop. Avoid mixing medications with nutritious substances such as apple sauce or orange juice; the unpleasant taste of the medicine will be associated with the food, and the child may later refuse to eat that food as part of a balanced diet.

After administering oral or parenteral medications, offer the child a drink of his choice (unless contraindicated by his condition). He is usually thirsty anyway, and this is a good time to promote adequate fluid intake. Never walk out leaving an upset child. Remember to return at other times during the day with nothing in your hands so that the child does not always associate your presence with the frustration and pain of medications.

PREPARATION FOR PROCEDURES

The traumatic aspect of hospitalization has already been mentioned (Figure 2–8). The child fantasizes about the unknown, frequently imagining far worse happenings than actually lie in store for him. He may think the x-ray machine will slowly lower to crush him, or that the purpose of surgery is to cut off his genitals. Proper preparation for all procedures—diagnostic, surgical, and therapeutic—will greatly reduce the

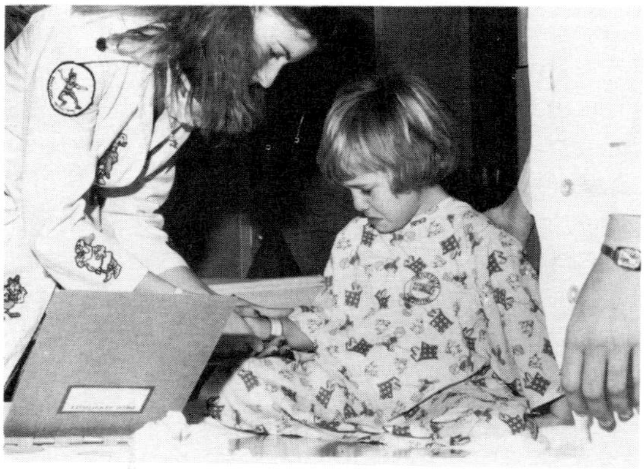

Figure 2–8. *The traumatic aspect of hospitalization is evident in this child's face.*

child's anxiety and permit him to master his fears. Later chapters on the hospitalization of children of various age groups will discuss preparation in more detail; an overview is offered here.

Before presenting the parent-child unit with the necessary information about the procedure to follow, you must determine what they already know. Your initial nursing assessment will provide clues about what they understand about the child's illness and hospitalization. Their perceptions may be wholly or partly accurate or totally inaccurate. Also, the parents may not wish you to tell the child about his illness or treatment, fearing that he will become upset. This reaction stems from the parents' anxiety, which they tend to project onto the child. In this situation, you will need to spend extra time with the parents, explaining the procedure and emphasizing that, in the physician's opinion, the hospitalization and treatment regimen are necessary.

Before the preparation session, be sure you know specific facts about the procedure: How long is it likely to take? How long will the child be in the recovery room? Where are the parents allowed to wait?

How far can they go with him when he leaves the room? Depending on the institution, the parents may have to say good-bye in the child's room; they may be able to ride on the elevator to the operating suite; or they may be able to carry the child in their arms or push his stretcher and stay until he is anesthetized, or until after the x-ray procedure. Usually, the child under ten will be anesthetized with a mask; an IV is used for those over ten. Check the policy in your own institution to avoid giving erroneous information.

The child is permitted to take his favorite toy with him for the procedure. After he is anesthetized, the toy may be taken away, but be sure that it is with him when he awakens. Some hospitals require that the child wear no underpants during surgery; this may be especially traumatic and is not necessary unless the garment interferes with the surgical site.

Belinda, eight years old, was scheduled for a secondary cleft palate repair and was extremely anxious and uncooperative. Her nurse observed that Belinda was obviously upset; Belinda agreed. Further questioning by the nurse revealed that Belinda was terrified because "they" would not let her wear her underpants to the operating room. She was sure "they" had lied about her surgery and were going to "cut up my privates."

Frequently, the staff may not wish the child to be prepared for his surgery, thinking that "it will only upset him." They assume that the concern with mutilation, death, and abandonment, frequently expressed by the child during pre-procedural teaching sessions, is produced by the teaching session itself. It should be kept in mind that the sessions do not produce these thoughts; they merely uncover them and promote their expression.

Willie, six years old, was scheduled for his fourteenth operation on his legs. The staff was upset when they discovered that the student nurse had given Willie a puppet show to prepare him for surgery. They said, "Surgery will have to be canceled. Willie always spikes a temp when he knows he's going to surgery. The doctor will be furious that you told him. We have to surprise Willie, we just go get him when it's time for him to go and he doesn't have tisme to spike a temp." Needless to say, Willie's trip to surgery was not canceled; for the first time, he did not "spike a temp." He also developed a trusting relationship for the first time since his hospitalization months earlier (with the student nurse who was honest with him).

Lack of proper equipment in an institution is no excuse for letting any child suffer through a procedure unprepared (except, of course, when emergency situations do not permit ample time). Hospital auxiliary workers are often looking for a way to help; recruit them to make puppets, or, if need be, you and the child can create your own with tongue blades, crayons, and construction paper. Sock puppets are easy to make, and other toys and props can be fashioned from tinker toys, feeding tubes, clean syringes, etc. Gradually, your unit can build a supply: a disposable oxygen mask, an inexpensive stethoscope, an IV made with a vial of sterile water. All of these props can be stored in a brightly colored beach bag and taken to the child's bedside as needed (Figure 2–9). The important thing is to prepare the child and his parents; how you do it will depend on the child's age and stage of development.

It is not necessary to be very detailed in your description, rather, concentrate on what the child will see, hear, and feel before, during, and after the procedure. Mention such things as the preoperative injection (it will hurt), the oxygen mask (it will smell like nail polish), the green masks and

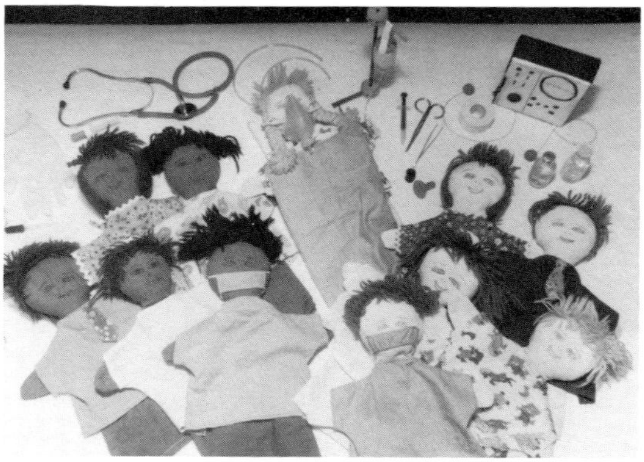

Figure 2–9. *These puppets and props are used to prepare the child for procedures and can be brought to the bedside as needed.*

gowns the personnel will wear, and any postoperative bandages and pain. Assure him that he can have medicine to relieve the pain. Remember, though, that the child will learn more if he can actually participate, so do not merely tell him what will happen; let him breathe through the oxygen mask, give a doll an "injection," and put a puppet on his hand and take part in the show. He may want to "put Mommy (or Daddy) to sleep." Emphasize that the sleep is a special sleep and that he will not wake up during surgery, but he *will* wake up when the doctor is all through. It is important that you not use the phrase "put to sleep" because of the possible association with an animal being "put to sleep," or mercifully killed.

After the teaching session, let the child practice with the equipment, cough, turn, and use blow bottles (or breathe deeply). Use this time to reinforce your teaching and to clarify any misconceptions the child or his parents may have. Chart the preparation so that others will know what you have done. If your hospital does not have a pediatric preoperative psychological checklist to accompany the standard preoperative checklist, you may wish to help design one. Be sure to include all of the necessary components of pre-procedural teaching, for example: tell child about preoperative medication; explain oxygen mask/IV for anesthesia; explain bandages, tubing, or monitors; explain the special wake-up room, and the like. Allow space on your checklist for additional comments and to record the child's selection of a toy to accompany him.

SURGERY

Preoperative Care

The child should be well hydrated, and any electrolyte imbalance corrected, before surgery. Intravenous infusions or total parenteral nutrition will be started to supply fluids and calories to maintain the child or to correct a deficit if one exists. Blood transfusions may be necessary to correct anemia. (See Chapter 29 for nursing care of the child who is receiving fluid therapy.)

If the child is not hydrated and in good condition for surgery several days may be needed to restore his fluid and electrolyte balance, administer antibiotics, and raise his hemoglobin preoperatively. Weight is measured daily to help determine the child's response to therapy. Urine output is measured, specific gravity checked, and stools counted, described, and recorded to assess the state of dehydration.

The restriction "NPO" (Latin *null per os,* meaning "nothing by mouth") is explained to both parents and child. Often, the parents do not realize the importance of going to surgery with an empty stomach and will give the child a drink of water. Tell them that vomiting can cause pneumonia. Also, fluid is sometimes silently regurgitated into the respiratory tract during surgery, also causing pneumonia. An infant's stomach normally empties in four hours, thus oral intake is withheld at least four hours before surgery; intake for the older child is withheld for eight hours.

Colon preparation, including cleansing enemas, is necessary before some procedures, such as a colostomy. Tap water is not used as an enema solution because of the danger of water intoxication (see ch. 29). Because enemas are psychologically traumatic to the child, the physician may order an oral cathartic and a stimulating suppository (Dulcolax). (See the Skills Manual.)

The newborn's body temperature fluctuates in response to environmental temperature. If the environmental temperature falls, the newborn's peripheral vessels constrict, he exhibits muscular hyperactivity, and has an increased oxygen need. His respiratory rate increases in order to take in more oxygen. He loses fluid through the expired air and the skin and is soon exhausted. Severe metabolic acidosis follows hypothermia in the newborn. Incubator temperature is kept at 27.8°C–29.4°C (82°F–84.9°F) for maximum energy conservation in the full-term infant. Record the incubator temperature once each shift. A persistently low body temperature, in the presence of an increase in incubator temperature, usually indicates sepsis.

The older child should be placed away from drafts and should be covered adequately with pajamas and bed linens. If his temperature is below normal when he returns from surgery, cover him with blankets and monitor his temperature until it returns to normal, then remove all but one of the blankets. All fluids, such as enemas, intravenous infusions, blood transfusions, and the like, should be warmed before administering them to the child.

If the child's temperature is elevated, remove his bed linens and excessive clothing, reduce the incubator temperature, administer antipyretics and/or sponge the child in lukewarm water to reduce fever (see the Skills Manual). Antibiotics are ordered if an infection is suspected of causing the elevated temperature.

Care must be taken to prevent infection in the child; he may be weakened by his condition and is therefore more susceptible to infection. The best defense is a clean environment and personnel who adhere to hospital routines that prevent the spread of infection, such as careful handwashing and isolation techniques.

Infants are usually kept in an isolette prior to surgery. The controlled temperature helps maintain body heat and the high humidity liquifies bronchial secretions. A neonatal intensive care center (NICC) is used as an alternative to the isolette (Figure 2–10). It is an open bed with overhead radiant heat, light, and life support systems all in one unit. It provides a safe heat source that is easily controlled and an accessible environment for infant care. Nasopharyngeal suctioning may be necessary to keep the child's airway clear, and oxygen is necessary for some infants.

Before surgery, the child (including the neonate) is introduced to restraints if these will be necessary in the postoperative period. Fit him correctly with the proper restraints and let him wear them for a few hours at a time before surgery. If special feeding techniques are to be used postoperatively, feed the child with them prior

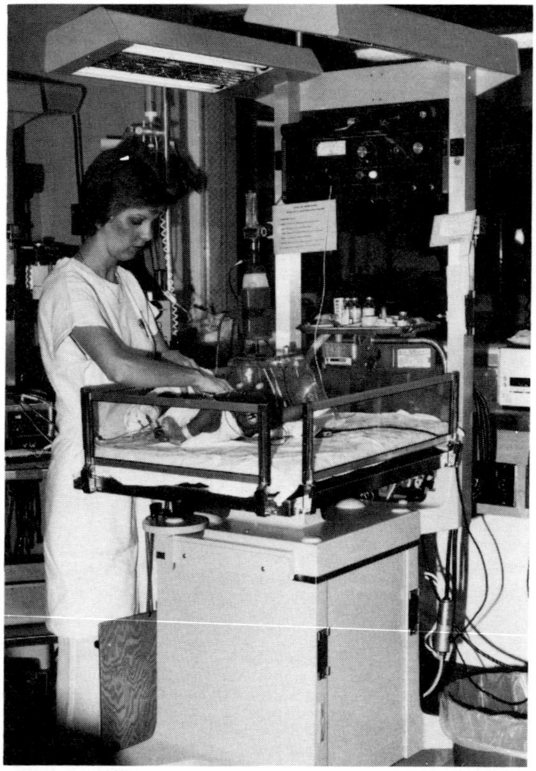

Figure 2–10. *A neonatal intensive care center.*

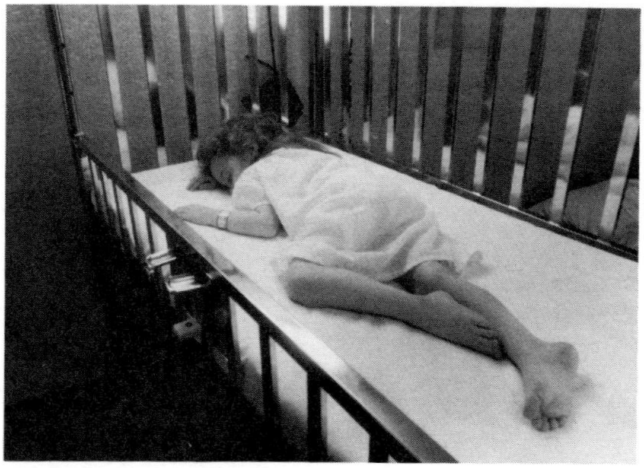

Figure 2–11. *Proper positioning of the child immediately after surgery.*

to surgery to accustom him to his new routine; this makes adaptation easier after surgery.

Postoperative Care

When the child returns from surgery, he is positioned on his side or abdomen with his head resting on his arm to allow secretions to drain and to prevent the tongue from obstructing the pharynx (Figure 2–11). Until the child is wide awake and talking, you must be certain that his airway is patent. Use oropharyngeal suction as needed to keep the airway clear. Respirations, pulse, blood pressure, and skin color are monitored every 15 minutes until the child is awake and his vital signs are stable. Note any change in vital signs, since this may be an indication of airway obstruction.

After simple surgery, such as a hernia repair, the child may awaken rapidly, look for his mother, and ask for a drink. He may want to play as soon as a few hours after surgery. On the other hand, he may be frightened upon awakening and may need comforting. A nurse should be present until the child awakens completely. Although pain relief and sedation usually are not necessary after less extensive surgery, the child will rest better if he has a mild analgesic. Morphine is the drug of choice for pain relief, but it is not given until the child is fully awake and his vital signs stable. If there is any evidence of pulmonary complication, narcotics are used sparingly because of their tendency to depress the cough reflex.

Respiratory complications are frequent postoperatively, especially within the first 48 hours after surgery. Tracheal irritation is due to the endotracheal tube used to ventilate the child during surgery. It lasts for a few days and is relieved by the inhalation of humidified air. Atelectasis and pneumonia occur when the child hypoventilates and does not adequately remove bronchial secretions. These complications are more severe in the child who has a respiratory problem before surgery (e.g., asthma or cystic fibrosis). The obese or debilitated child will have a less effective cough as will the child who has a thoracic or upper abdominal incision. This incision may be so painful that it restricts normal breathing.

Anticipate respiratory problems before they occur. Begin with preoperative teaching so that the child knows how to cough and breathe deeply and can understand the necessity for doing it after surgery.

Observe the child closely to detect early signs of respiratory complications such as increased respiratory rate, weak cry, an anxious expression, and restlessness. Late signs of respiratory distress include extreme restlessness and apprehension, labored respirations and retractions, nasal flaring, tachypnea, and cyanosis. Look for cyanosis in the mucous membranes and nail beds, especially in darkly pigmented children.

Encourage the child to cough, turn, and deep-breathe every two hours after surgery. Crying helps the infant to breathe deeply. Nasopharyngeal suctioning is used if the child's cough is ineffective. A bulb syringe, adequate for suctioning a normal newborn, is not effective for the child in respiratory distress; a catheter and suction machine is used to suction the mouth and pharynx of the child, and the procedure is repeated as necessary. Permit the child to rest and breathe oxygen between aspirations. Pain, or the fear of it, is a deterrent to effective coughing and deep breathing; offer the child his pain medication 20 to 30 minutes before asking him to cough and breathe deeply.

Oxygen and humidity provide comfort and help prevent respiratory problems in the child who has undergone surgery. The infant is kept in an isolette or an open bed with radiant heat as he was preoperatively. The older child may have a mist tent, a hood, or a face tent. (See chapter 23 for care of the child with respiratory problems.)

Antibiotics are not routinely administered after surgery. However, if there is any danger of pulmonary or wound infection, or if there was spillage of intestinal contents during surgery, then antibiotics are administered.

Intravenous fluids are usually maintained until the child is able to take oral feedings without vomiting or causing stress to suture lines. One or two ounces of clear fluids are offered initially; if this is tolerated, rapid progression is made to a more nutritious diet. Extra caution is taken if gastrointestinal surgery has been performed; the abdomen must be scaphoid and stools passed by rectum before an oral diet is permitted. Anorexia is often a problem after surgery. Because protein and vitamins are essential to wound healing, nutrition becomes a primary nursing consideration.

Nasogastric tubes are often used after surgery either for feedings (Levine tube) or for suctioning (Salem-Sump), depending on the need of the particular child. If gastric decompression is necessary, the Sump tube is connected to intermittent suction on a low setting. Occasionally, gravity drainage is used. When bowel function returns (as evidenced by decreased drainage through the tube, bowel sounds heard with a stethoscope, and the passage of flatus and stool), the tube is removed (usually after 24 hours).

Gastrostomy feedings are used to provide nourishment while bypassing the suture line, as in repair of the esophagus. The infant may begin oral feedings of clear fluids after four or five days and progresses to a full liquid diet as soon as the suture line heals, at which time the gastrostomy tube is removed. However, in some cases of extensive defects, multiple operations are necessary and the child must return home on gastrostomy feedings. In such instances, the mother must be instructed in the care and feeding of the child.

DISCHARGE

As with adults, preparing the child and his family for discharge from the hospital begins in the early stages of hospitalization, as soon as the child's condition allows. If the parents are rooming-in, they are already involved in their child's care, and discharge planning and teaching will be easier.

Any parent who must care for the child after discharge must be taught the proper technique required by the child's condition. The parent's involvement may range from simply keeping the child home from school for a few days, to caring for the child while he is in a spica cast, to helping the child to adapt to a lifelong condition such as diabetes. Obviously, the more complicated the home treatment and care, the more time is needed in the hospital for pre-discharge planning and teaching.

The most proficient teaching method is to involve the parents early and to let them care for the hospitalized child with your guidance and support. As they become skilled and confident, permit them to give care unassisted. This method helps insure a smooth transition to the home, although not having the nurse down the hall may cause some anxiety in even the most confident and capable parents. Give them a number to call (the hospital unit, you, or the physician) if they have any questions or concerns. If necessary, make the proper referrals to other agencies (e.g., Crippled Children's Clinic, home health services, and so forth).

If the child is to take medication home from the hospital, be sure it is labeled correctly and that the parents understand its use and side effects. Give them an appointment card, or tell them to call the physician or clinic (after whatever period of time is deemed appropriate by the physician) for an appointment. Stress the importance of this follow-up visit.

SUMMARY

Contemporary pediatric nursing focuses on the parent-child unit. Parents of the child work with the health team and are involved in decisions that affect the child's care. The anatomical, physiological, and behavioral differences between the child and the adult contribute to the uniqueness of pediatric nursing. Play and preparation for procedures are integral parts of a therapeutic nursing setting, and the child is given appropriate choices in all aspects of his care.

Bibliography

Ayer, A.H. Is Partnership with Parents Really Possible? *American Journal Maternal-Child Nursing* 3:107, 1978.

Bellack, J.P. Helping a Child Cope with the Stress of Injury. *American Journal of Nursing* 74:1491, 1974.

Calkin, J.D. Are Hospitalized Toddlers Adapting to the Experience as Well as We Think? *American Journal Maternal-Child Nursing* 4:18, 1979.

Chadwick, B.J., Pfledener, D., Ray, M.A. Maintaining the Hospitalized Child's Home Ties. *American Journal of Nursing* 78:1361, 1978.

Goldman, M., Sponseller, D., and Ream, B. A Play Program in a Community Hospital? *American Journal Maternal-Child Nursing* 3:42, 1978.

Hardgrove, C. and Rutledge, A. Parenting During Hospitalization. *American Journal of Nursing* 75:836, 1975.

Hill, C.J.S. The Mother on the Pediatric Ward: Insider or Outlawed? *Pediatric Nursing* 4:26, 1978.

Isler, C. The Fine Art of Handling a Hospitalized Child. *Registered Nurse* 41:41, 1978.

Jackson, P.B., Bradham, R.F., Burwell, H.K. Child Care in the Hospital—A Parent/Staff Partnership. *American Journal Maternal-Child Nursing* 3:104, 1978.

Jenkins, J.E. Personal Communication, Vice-President for Patient Care–Director of Nursing. LeBonheur Children's Medical Center. Memphis, Tenn., 1979.

Luciano, K. The Who, When, Where, What and How of Preparing Children for Surgery. *Nursing 74* 4:64, November, 1974.

McGuire, M., Shepherd, R., Greco, A. Hospitalized Children in Confinement. *Pediatric Nursing* 4:31, 1978.

Petrillo, M. and Sanger, S. *Emotional Care of the Hospitalized Child.* Philadelphia: J. B. Lippincott Co., 1972.

Roberts, F. *Review of Pediatric Nursing,* ed. 2. St. Louis: C.V. Mosby Co., 1978, pp. 1–7.

Shufer, S. Communicating with Young Children. *American Journal of Nursing* 77:1960, 1977.

Standards of Maternal-Child Health Nursing Practice. Kansas City, Missouri, American Nurses' Association, 1973.

Treolar, D.M. Ready, Set, No: Something is Missing From Pediatric Pre-op Preparation. *American Journal Maternal-Child Nursing* 3:50, 1978.

Whitson, B.J. The Puppet Treatment in Pediatrics. *American Journal of Nursing* 72:1612, 1972.

CHAPTER **3**

The Family in Stress

BEHAVIORAL OBJECTIVES

After studying this chapter you will be able to:

- Describe and offer examples of different types of family behavior patterns.
- Discuss stress, identifying adaptive and pathogenic stressors.
- Discuss what constitutes a crisis and the nursing intervention process.
- Explain autosomal recessive, autosomal dominant, and sex-linked inheritance, describing the inheritance patterns.
- Describe the home and neighborhood as physical environmental influences on the child.
- Identify the effects of socioeconomic class on nutrition, transportation, and health care.
- List different types of parents' emotions when their child has an acute illness. Describe seven behaviors that demonstrate these emotions.
- Describe the change in the parenting role during a child's acute illness and how this change affects parent and child.
- Describe common behaviors of children in acute care settings.
- Discuss how a child's chronic illness can jeopardize his family's well-being.
- Identify three behavior types commonly seen in children with chronic illnesses.
- Discuss the effects of fragmented services on the child with a chronic illness.
- Explain the stages of the grief process.
- Discuss the child's concept of death according to developmental stages.
- Describe positive ways of dealing with the child who doesn't know his diagnosis.
- Discuss ways of offering support to the parents and siblings of a child who is dying.
- Differentiate between the impact of a lingering death and that of a sudden, unanticipated death.
- Describe the sudden infant death syndrome (SIDS) and the importance of an autopsy on SIDS victims.
- Discuss nursing interventions for the family of a SIDS victim.
- Discuss acculturation, cultural diversity, cultural imposition, and biological diversity, explaining their interrelationship and implications for transcultural nursing.
- Discuss various health practices of the Native Americans, Hispanics, blacks, and Asian Americans, listing specific nursing actions for health promotion.
- Discuss parent-child bonding, identifying deviations from the normal bonding process.
- Describe the failure-to-thrive syndrome, identifying specific assessment informa-

tion and interventions for the parents and child.

- Define terms specific to the child abuse syndrome.
- Discuss the "World of Abnormal Rearing."
- Explain three factors that precipitate abuse.
- Describe common injuries seen in abused children.
- Discuss nursing interventions for the abusing family.

TERMS AND CONCEPTS

Stress
Young Family
Middle Age Family
Older Family
Family Behavior Patterns
Stressor
Crisis
Heredity
Chromosomes
Sex Chromosomes
Autosomes
Genes
Alleles
Homozygous
Heterozygous
Trisomy
Autosomal Recessive Inheritance
Autosomal Dominant Inheritance
Sex-Linked Inheritance
Environment
Acute Illness
Behaviors
Regression
Withdrawal
Aggression
Hysteria
Chronic Illness
Health Care System
Death
Grief
Denial
Anger
Bargaining
Depression
Acceptance
SIDS
Crib Death Syndrome
Apnea
Autopsy
Cultural Imposition
Parent-Child Bonding
Maternal Sensitive Period
Rooming-In
Entrainment
Failure-to-Thrive
Physical Abuse
Battering
Sexual Abuse
Emotional Abuse
Physical Neglect
Emotional Neglect
Abusogenic
World of Abnormal Rearing
Role Reversal
Wringer Injury
Eggshell Fracture

A group of individuals sharing common cultural values, economic resources, and a geographic setting, the family is the child rearing unit of society. Families differ in development, composition, and role behavior. Families are constantly exposed to stress. *Stress* is any demand that requires a response; the demand may be biological, social, or psychological. This chapter discusses families: their composition, roles, and tasks, as well as the nature and process of stress and nursing interventions that decrease stress and promote equilibrium. Specific physical stresses of genetic inheritance, the environment, and acute, chronic and terminal illness are discussed as are psychosocial stresses of cultural diversity and deviations in parent-child relationships. The focal point of this chapter is the family and how the nursing process can facilitate the family's adaptation to stress.

FAMILIES

Adults and children who live together, are related by blood, adoption, or marriage and share a particular socioeconomic status constitute a family. Individual family members and the group as a whole have needs, expectations, roles, and tasks to fulfill. The action of one individual affects all other family members, and the reactions of the family unit to an internal or external force depend on the characteristics of the family. The family develops and changes as new situations demand response.

In assessing family functioning, note the age of the family unit. *Young families,* comprising a unit for three years or less, are still settling into roles, tasks, and responsibilities. They have little experience with child care needs and child-rearing practices. Family values are in the formative stage, and the young family is receptive to health care education and guidance, frequently seeking direction from health personnel. The young family is especially vulnerable to heightened anxiety and excessive concern regarding child care practices and the stress of illness. The *middle age family* of four to ten years is less susceptible to outside opinions and has set standards of behavior and communication within the family unit. There is more economic stability and child rearing practices are more firmly established. The added stability of this family may promote complacence and a tendency to ignore potential and existing health problems, making the family less receptive to health education and guidance. The *older family* of ten to twenty years has definite patterns, values, and practices. Separation of family members, such as occurs when adolescents leave the home for college or marriage, can be extremely disruptive, and close attention is needed to assess family perception and reactions.

Regardless of economic, cultural or developmental characteristics, most families display similar behaviors when confronted with the hospitalization of a child. The following family descriptions are intended to identify common patterns of family interaction, not to stereotype or generalize family behavior. Behavior and attitudes are learned; they can be unlearned and changed. Time, patience, understanding, and concern are crucial to the initial establishment of a collaborative relationship between staff and the family in stress.

The Deceptive-Denying Family

This type of family offers little or false information to the child regarding the illness, forthcoming hospitalization, future treatments, and care. Parents may present a scheduled hospitalization as a weekend trip or visit to the city, maintaining that concealing the facts will decrease the child's awareness and fear. By withholding information from the child, parents facilitate their own denial of the realization of the illness. Parents frequently make impossible promises to the child about the outcome of treatment. The child's perceptions, fears, and anxieties are usually never expressed. If the staff members avoid interactions, family denial is supported in that silence reinforces the parents' perception that nothing is seriously wrong. Be alert to signs of parental deceit and denial. Talk to the child honestly, preparing him for procedures and answering his questions, being careful not to alienate the child from family members. Parents frequently change their attitude about giving false information, and may ask for help in explaining their behavior to the child. For parents to apologize while maintaining their child's respect is difficult. Aid parents in explaining to their child that they care and love him and that they felt withholding information was best, but now realize that it was a mistake.

Punitive-Depriving Family

Harsh discipline is a favored method of control, and children are made to submit to parental authority in the punitive-depriving family. For fear of spoiling them, the parents do not cuddle, hold, or comfort their children to any extent. These children are told repeatedly that they do nothing right. The child views illness as further punishment for bad behavior. Conditioned to rigid structure and punishment, the child may be confused by the concern and kindness of the staff. Parents may feel the care and attention constitutes needless overindulgence and permissiveness. The punitive-depriving family is difficult for most staff to work with because punitive behavior elicits feelings of anger and frustration from many people. Maintain a calm, concerned attitude in the hope that parents may permit and emulate such behavior toward the child. Discuss child rearing practices with the parents, offering developmentally appropriate methods of reward and punishment. For example, withdrawal of a favorite toy, television, the radio, and/or parental attention for a fifteen-minute period following inappropriate behavior is an alternate discipline to spanking or abusive language. Discuss, demonstrate, and plan with the parents and child a consistent form of discipline. Offer clear, simple information to the child and parents about treatments and procedures, encouraging the family to express their perceptions and anxieties.

The Family Whose Religious Beliefs Conflict with Medical Treatment

Certain religions prohibit specific medical procedures, for example, Jehovah's Witnesses believe that accepting blood transfusions is a violation of their faith. If parents agree to such treatments, they and their family members may be banned from the religious sect. Each family's religious beliefs should be acknowledged and respected. Parents are best persuaded when asked to consider the optimal health of their child. It is important to make parents aware of possible health consequences if the recommended treatment is not followed. If parents continue to reject recommended care, court action may be pursued.

The Superstitious Family

To the superstitious family, illness is a sign of God's displeasure, a part of one's fate, an omen of things to come. The superstitious family is suspicious, skeptical, and may pray to secret protectors for safety. The child may wear certain garments or jewelry, attributing protective power to them. If possible, permit the child to continue to wear the jewelry or affix the items to the pillow. When offering information and instructions to these families be clear and direct. Use simple, concrete language and brief explanations. It is preferable for one person to relate to this type of family to minimize the possibility of added fear and confusion.

The Economically and Intellectually Deprived Family

The family of poverty is usually present-oriented, having a fatalistic outlook on the future. Rigid family roles are maintained with limited verbal communication. Ignorance of basic physiology and health care practices is common. These families experience a high incidence of marital conflict and frequent interruptions in the family composition, such as parental absence or lengthy separations. Children usually behave impulsively, projecting blame onto others. Physical, frequently harsh, discipline is common. Middle-class communication patterns and the future-oriented outlook that predominates among health professionals are not appropriate for this type of family. An overpowering, judgmental approach is equally inappropriate since this method only reinforces parental behavior. Express concern and offer care in a consistent manner, avoiding lengthy explanations, and confusing terminology. Identify terms that the family understands and use illustrated material and written directions. Act as a role model to the parents, praising them for accomplishing tasks and using a consistent method of discipline.

The Overindulgent Family

Every whim and desire of the child of the overindulgent family is acknowledged and gratified. The child is placed on a pedestal and expected to fulfill all family dreams. A quick cure is sought for the child's illness, and the ability of the staff is under constant parental scrutiny. Assure the family of the staff's competence and abilities. With the family's cooperation, set a limit on the extent of the family's involvement during the child's hospitalization. The child of an overindulging family is usually demanding, and self indulgent. He may be anxious and confused as limits are set on previously unrestricted behaviors. Explain to the child firmly what behavior is acceptable in a hospital, being quick to acknowledge and praise pleasant behavior.

The Adaptive Family

The adaptive family is characterized by a trusting, harmonious parent-child relationship and consistent expectations and discipline. There is a warm, expressive relationship among family members that promotes communication, self-esteem, and positive coping behaviors. The child's feelings are acknowledged and accepted, and channels are provided for the release of emotions. The children of adaptive families tend to be creative and demonstrate appropriate play, academic skills, and task ability. The family successfully strives to maintain a supportive relationship, despite the anxiety of separation and illness.

Families often exhibit a combination of the traits described above, or they may shift from one behavior pattern to another. Being aware of family behavior patterns can promote individualized and effective nursing care approaches.

STRESS

Any stimulus that disturbs one's normal functioning constitutes stress. The *stressor* is the agent that produces stress at a given time. Cold, heat, mechanical trauma, chemicals, and pathogens are all examples of stressors. Stress responses may be nonspecific, affecting the whole body, or specific, affecting a specific area of tissue or a certain muscle group. Each stressor has its particular characteristics, and each places a demand for adaptation on the child and/or family group.

If the adaptation is beneficial and promotes health, the stress is positive; however, if the response is inappropriate, the stress may be harmful and produce illness. Allergies and inflammation are examples of pathologic responses to stress. Some responses to stress, such as heart activity, chemical secretions, and electrical activity, can be measured and recorded. Other less well-defined behaviors that indicate stress include an inability to sleep, eat, or concentrate.

Stress is not necessarily harmful, nor is it to be avoided or eliminated. Stress is inevitable, and adaptation is essential for life. The response to stress can be adaptive and health-promoting, as when stress is channeled constructively to complete a difficult task.

The hospitalized child and his or her family are frequently said to be in a state of *crisis*. A crisis is any occurrence that causes a temporary or permanent disruption in one's ability to function. Stress causes disequilibrium, which may result in a crisis.

Like stress, crisis need not be detrimental. New situations can elicit new behavior and a higher level of child and family functioning. Reaction to stress and crisis is individualized; no two children or families will react in the same way to any given situation.

In dealing with the family in crisis, the nurse's assessment necessarily begins with an acknowledgement of the crisis state. Psychosocial assessment then takes into account family strengths and weaknesses, coping mechanisms, and support systems (see ch. 2). The nursing process continues with planned interventions aimed at mobilizing the family's emotional resources. Express concern and support, allowing for cultural differences in the family's expression of emotion.

A primary nursing intervention for any family in crisis is the provision of information. Parental anxiety, guilt, and confusion can be reduced if parents understand the nature of the child's illness. Families need specific information about the course of the illness; present and future treatments and procedures; and expected changes in the child's functioning due to the regimen of medical and nursing care. Parents need to know when expected physiological and/or behavioral changes will begin, their duration, and management techniques. It is important to offer repeated explanation of care, using books, pamphlets, and other visual material. Anxiety hinders one's learning ability and parents who ask the same question several times are usually not slow learners or inattentive but rather extremely anxious and concerned. Remain calm, patient, and available to re-explain, acknowledging to parents that it is normal to need several explanations. Parents are learning to trust you; they need to be certain that you are willing to listen and guide them without condemnation or annoyance. Parents also need to be informed of services that can offer assistance during the crisis; for example, the social service department, therapists, community agencies, and special schools or workshops. Help parents assess their community's resources, and identify those that are appropriate for their immediate and long-term needs.

Providing direct care is one way parents can relieve their anxiety and feel that they are contributing to the child's comfort during the crisis. Promote care by demonstrating, allowing, and encouraging parents, siblings, and relatives to render emotional and physical care to the child.

When a family is in a crisis state, each member is under stress. Parents need assistance in explaining the ill child's condition to siblings. Each sibling needs an honest, direct answer. Inadequate explanations can lead to feelings of guilt because siblings may feel that they are somehow responsible, because of some misdeed or bad thought, for the ill child's sickness. Explanations to friends, relatives, and employees are equally important. Allowing the parents to role-play an explanation to you as a curious neighbor or worried relative can aid parents in choosing words that foster understanding. Parents need to be aware of the possible effects of their child's hospitalization on their marital relationships. Frequently, marriages are strengthened or weakened when a child is hospitalized. Parents may need to consider the time demand of each family member and to establish a schedule allowing periods for home and hospital involvement.

Evaluate the effects of the nursing interventions, revise plans, and offer guidance. The nursing goal is to restore the family to a precrisis state of functioning with positive changes in family behavior patterns.

HEREDITY

Human characteristics are transmitted from one generation to the next by sexual reproduction. The inherited traits are transmitted by *chromosomes*. There are 23 different kinds of paired chromosomes, thus there are 46 chromosomes in each human cell (Figure 3–1). One of each pair is contributed by each parent at conception. During the formation of ova and sperm the chromosomes separate so that each ovum or sperm receives only one of each type of chromosome. Thus, each ovum or sperm carries only 23 chromosomes instead of the full complement of 46 chromosomes. The union of a sperm and egg at conception restores the complete set, and all subsequent cells formed by the normal embryo contain 46 chromosomes.

Two of the chromosomes differ, according to the sex of the child, and are known as *sex chromosomes*. The other 44 chromosomes are termed *autosomes*. Sex chromosomes differ from one another in size; the larger is termed the X chromosome, and the smaller is called the Y chromosome. Females have two X chromosomes (XX) while males have one of each type (XY). Chromosomes can be visualized and studied by a process called *karyotyping*, a separation and staining technique used to closely examine chromosomes for added or deleted material. Chromosomes can be obtained for study before birth by a process called *amniocentesis*. A needle is inserted through the mother's abdomen and amniotic fluid is withdrawn to study the chromosomal make-up of the fetus. By this means certain chromosomal disorders can be diagnosed before birth.

Specific linear segments of chromosomes are termed *genes*. Genes exist in pairs, as do chromosomes. A minute change in the structure of a gene may occur and alter its function; thus alternate forms of the same gene may be found, and these different forms are called *alleles*. Many alleles may exist for a given gene, but only two of them occur in any person with a normal chromosome complement. Everyone inherits a pair of genes for each trait, but we each can inherit various alleles of that gene, and it is

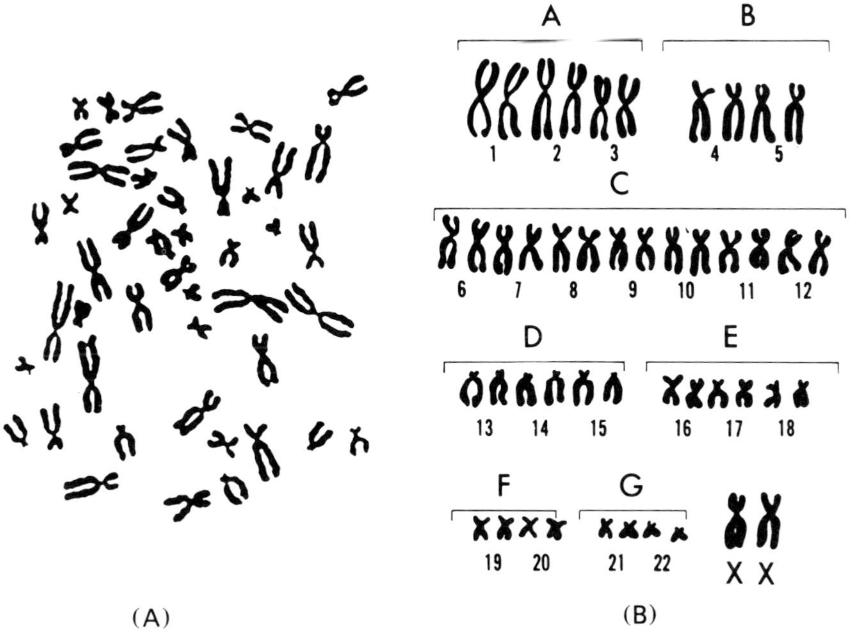

Figure 3–1. *Normal Human Chromosomes.* (A) *Scattered chromosomes as they appear within the cell nucleus.* (B) *Chromosomes arranged in pairs and labeled according to standard nomenclature. The two X chromosomes identify this person as a female. The male would have one X and one very small, dissimilar-looking Y.*

the expression of these alleles that produces the biological differences visible in all of us. If the alleles are identical, then the child is *homozygous* for that gene pair and for the trait that the two alleles determine. If the alleles are different, then the child is *heterozygous* for that particular characteristic. If a trait is determined by only one allele of the pair then the allele that is expressed in the child is *dominant,* and the other allele, which is present but not expressed, is *recessive.*

Changes in chromosomal composition are usually *numerical* or *structural*. If a malfunction occurs during the formation of ova and sperm, it is possible that both, or neither, members of a chromosome pair will be included. If an egg contains two similar chromosomes, when a third chromosome of that type is contributed by the fertilizing sperm, the resulting embryo will faithfully reproduce all three similar chromosomes and be *trisomic*. However, for each egg formed that received both members of a chromosome pair, another egg was formed that lacked that chromosome altogether. If this egg is fertilized, it will contain only one chromosome of that type, the one contributed by the sperm, and the resulting embryo is *monosomic*. Structural abnormalities of chromosomes usually arise from breaks, causing deletion of chromosomal material. If a broken chromosome is incorporated into another chromosome it is termed a *translocation.* Chromosome changes may be transmitted from parent to child; arise spontaneously due to an alteration in the duplication and/or division of chromosomal material; or result from environmental influences such as chemicals or x-irradiation.

Specific deviations from health are frequently inherited. Common inheritance patterns are *autosomal dominant, autosomal recessive,* and *sex-linked.* These patterns are illustrated and discussed in Figures 3–2, 3–3, and 3–4. (It should be emphasized that these patterns of heredity govern the transmission of normal and abnormal traits, not abnormalities only. However, for the purpose of this discussion, these terms will be explained with reference to pathology.) Disorders arising from these three inheritance patterns and the chapter in which each is further discussed are listed in Table 3–1.

Multigenetic Inheritance

Inherited conditions may also depend on the combined action of several alleles. For example, certain combinations of alleles will cause physical defects in the child. Multigenetically determined abnormalities include pyloric stenosis, cleft lip and/or palate (ch. 18), and meningomyelocele (ch. 27). In each of these conditions no specific allele is totally responsible.

Families of Children with Inherited Conditions

The family of a child with an inherited condition experiences a crisis. How the family reacts depends on many factors, e.g., the visibility and extent of the disorder, the effect the disorder will have on the child's present and future physical and mental functioning, and the need for future hospitalizations, economic expenditures, and repeated health agency visits. Family behavior patterns depend largely on the status of these variables. Families react to inherited conditions with feelings of loss, grief, and guilt. The parents need to mourn the perfect child they had anticipated. As the family grieves, they experience immense guilt and suffering, searching for answers to why the condition happened. Parents are also confronted with the grief and guilt of relatives and siblings of the affected child.

Nursing interventions for the family include assessing parental *feelings, perceptions,* and *reactions.* Identify strengths and initiate intervention to support and facilitate family acceptance. Assess the parents' *feelings* about the child's condition by asking what their initial reaction was when informed that the child had an inherited problem, and what they feel is the most difficult part about their child's condition. Assess the parents' *perceptions* about the child's condition by asking them to explain what is different about their child, what they have been told about the condition, and what they anticipate for the future. Assess parental *reactions* to the child by asking if the child is enjoyable and if they feel close to the child. Assess the family's attitudes toward one another and toward those outside the family. Ask the parents if they have told family and friends about the child's problem, and if so, what were their reactions, and how do they feel about the reactions? Have their feelings toward these people changed? If relationships are impaired, what further help do the parents need? Aid families in obtaining needed resources.

The family in crisis needs information, support, and guidance in getting appropriate resources. The principles of genetic in-

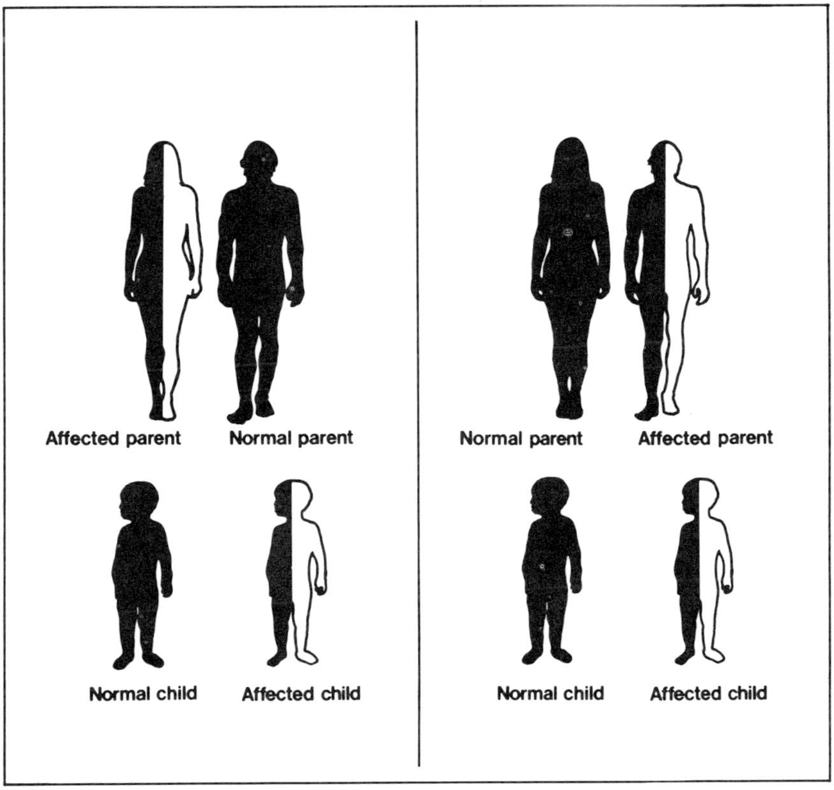

Figure 3–2. *Autosomal Dominant Inheritance is the manifestation of a characteristic determined by a single allele of an autosomal gene. The parent who is heterozygous for a given dominant condition will transmit either the dominant allele or the recessive allele at each conception. The probability of transmitting either allele is 50 percent. The probability of transmission remains the same for each conception; it never changes. If the other parent is homozygous for the normal recessive allele, then each child has a 50 percent chance of being heterozygous and having the condition and an equal chance of being homozygous and normal.*

heritance may be difficult for some families to understand. Chromosomes and alleles are intangible, invisible matter that can cause profound alterations. Be certain to use terms that are understood when explaining inheritance. For example, genes can be referred to as messages, transmitted from parent to child at conception, that determine body structure and function. Cells can be called packages in which the mes-

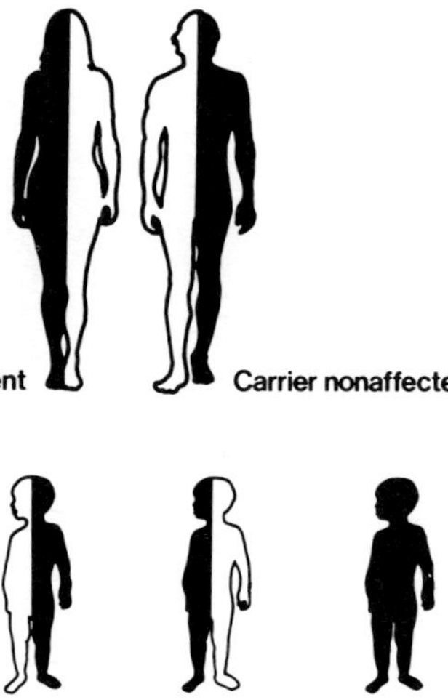

Figure 3–3. *Autosomal Recessive Inheritance is the manifestation of a characteristic determined by two abnormal alleles. Children who have inherited an autosomal recessive condition usually have parents who are normal for the disorder and have one abnormal allele and one normal partner allele; they are heterozygous and are commonly referred to as having a trait of the condition. Parents who are both heterozygous for a recessive condition have a 25 percent chance of passing their recessive gene to an offspring with each conception. The same (25 percent) chance exists of each parent passing the normal allele to an offspring and the child being normal for the condition. The greatest probability, 50 percent, is that one parent will pass an abnormal allele and one parent will pass a normal allele so that the child, like the parents, will be unaffected and heterozygous for the condition. It is frequently assumed that if a person has a recessive condition, then all of that person's offspring must also have the condition; this is not true. If a person with a recessive condition mates with a person who is heterozygous for the same condition, then each offspring has a 50 percent chance of inheriting a recessive allele from each parent and having the condition, and an equal chance of inheriting a recessive allele from the homozygous parent and a normal allele from the heterozygous parent; this child would be unaffected and heterozygous for the condition. If a person with a recessive condition mates with a person having two normal alleles for the condition, then each offspring will have heterozygous alleles for the condition; no other possibilities exist.*

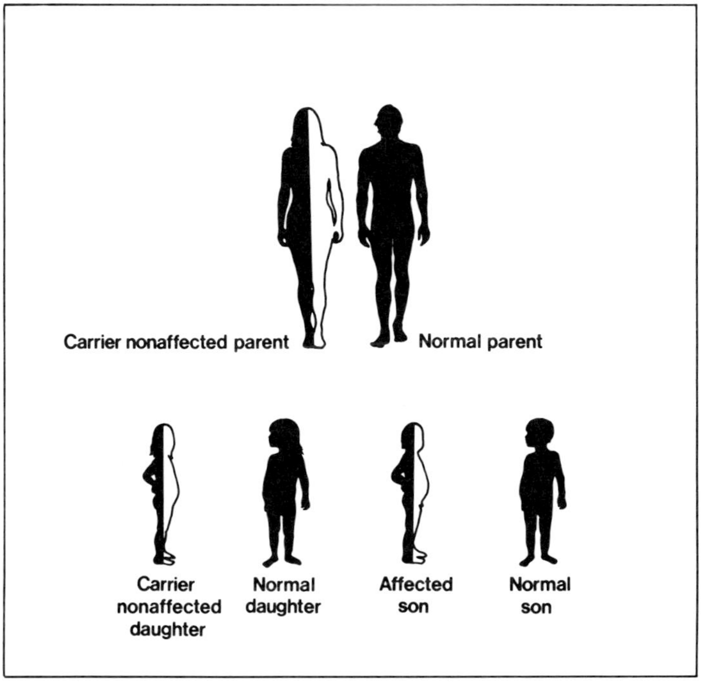

Figure 3–4. *Sex-linked inheritance is the manifestation of a characteristic determined by an abnormal allele carried on one sex chromosome. Since only one trait—hairy ears—is carried on the Y chromosome, the major sex-linked chromosomal disorders are carried on the X chromosome. Sex-linked disorders are labeled as X-linked recessive or X-linked dominant. If the sex-linked condition is recessive, the effects of the condition are produced only when no opposing allele exists on the other chromosome pair. Thus, males who have inherited an X-linked disorder will always demonstrate the disorder. The sisters of the same male who inherit the X-linked disorder will receive a second X that is usually a dominant allele and will therefore supress the recessive allele; these females will be carriers of the X-linked condition. Each male offspring of a female carrier has a 50 percent chance of receiving the abnormal X chromosome. Each daughter of the same carrier female has a 50 percent chance of receiving the abnormal X chromosome and being a carrier of the condition.*

Table 3–1. Inherited Disorders

Inheritance Pattern	*Disorder*	*Discussed In Chapter*
Autosomal Dominant	Diabetes Insipidus	19
	Muscular Dystrophy (certain types)	28
	Osteogenesis Imperfecta	28
	Spherocytosis	24
Autosomal Recessive	Adrenogenital Syndrome	19
	Tay-Sachs	11
	Deaf Mutism (certain types)	10
	Microcephaly	27
	Muscular Dystrophy (certain types)	28
	Phenylketonuria (PKU)	11
	Sickle Cell Anemia	24
	Thalassemia Major	24
	Cystic Fibrosis (CF)	23
Sex-Linked	Color Blindness	10
	Hemophilia	25
	Glucose-6-Phosphatase Deficiency	24

sages are carried. The use of illustrations and whatever other materials that can simplify the explanation is important in facilitating understanding and eliminating the fear and anxiety that arise from misunderstanding.

THE ENVIRONMENT

Environment is the world that surrounds a child wherever he goes, whatever he does. Environmental influences on health can be psychosocial, physical, or both.

As the earlier discussion of genetics makes clear, the potential of every person is limited by one's genetic makeup. The extent to which one can fulfill this potential is influenced by the environment, although the question of where heredity "stops" and environment "begins," or which factor is more important to the individual's development, is still unanswerable at this time. For example, would a small-for-age, undernourished child be larger if he were well nourished? A look at his parents' physical characteristics may not provide the answer; perhaps they, too, were malnourished as children.

A child's environment is usually shaped by his family's socioeconomic status. There are exceptions to this principle, such as the case of the rural family that is impoverished but grows its own food, but generally, the poor suffer environmental deficits that affect health.

The air surrounding the child is, of course, an important element of the environment. Significant characteristics of the air include the particles suspended in it and the level of noise carried by it. All air has such *pollutants,* but (to cite one example of an environment that is inherently less-than-optimal) an urban setting exposes the child to a higher level of pollution, hence a higher degree of environmental stress.

Epidemiologists have shown relationships between different pollutants and disease (e.g., cancer, respiratory and hormonal conditions). Middle- and upper-class families can remove some of the air's harmful matter through their homes' heating and cooling systems, which allow for filtered air in a closed house. However, the poor family may not even have screens on open windows and certainly not an air filtering system. Factors within the home may create further problems in the air (e.g., faulty heating systems, cigarette smoke, pesticides).

Air also carries the hazard of noise. Just as the poor family has few resources for reducing chemical air pollution, it also has difficulty in decreasing noise. Audiologists, professionals who study hearing, are now assessing the effects of noise on the hearing of infants and children. As more knowledge is accumulated, society as a whole must act to prevent hearing loss. You must consider noise as you plan for care in the acute setting, especially in a ward with several machines and many people. Noise pollution is an even more serious problem in the critical care units, where the noise level is higher because of respirators, monitors, and many busy people in a relatively small space.

The child's home and neighborhood, powerful environmental determinants of health, are dependent on the family's socioeconomic status. The effects of the neighborhood include availability of recreation areas, public transportation, shopping facilities, water supply, and protection from crime, roaming animals, air pollutants, and pests. Houses within a neighborhood are usually of similar construction, but individual homes may vary as to heating and cooling systems, type of paint on furniture and walls, toilet facilities, electrical wiring, play areas, and the dangers of open windows, steps, medicines and poisons, and pests. Families of the middle and upper classes can control their immediate environments. Being generally better educated, they are more likely to understand the relationship between health and environment, and they have the resources to create conditions that lead to a comfortable, efficient way of life. The family experiencing the stress of poverty is almost always under increased environmental stress and is at increased risk for illness.

The problem of adequate transportation for poor families is a major concern for health care professionals. The family that owns a car can obtain the necessities of life, including health care. The family that has access to adequate public transportation can also obtain the necessities but with the inconvenience of walking to, waiting for, and transferring within the transportation system. Understandably, there is little motivation to get a checkup if the person without transportation is not obviously ill. In the absence of assistance from a friend or relative who has a car, the person who is sick or immobile is forced to pay relatively exorbitant fees for the more convenient taxi, if he must rely on public transportation. Some neighborhoods provide health care consisting of basic screening, counseling, and early treatment services, but most people must travel for treatment of acute illnesses. Some neighborhoods also have some shopping facilities, but these are usually of the "convenience" type with much higher prices than the larger stores.

Food is another environmental factor that influences health. *Malnutrition* is a source of physical stress related to culture and the socioeconomic class of a family, although the problem transcends class boundaries. The middle- and upper-class diet is characterized by excessive cholesterol, salt, and sugar. Children eat large quantities of snack foods between or instead of meals. Their parents drive to the stores with the lowest prices, purchase large amounts of food, and have it readily accessible to children and adults as desired. The poor family has a very different set of nutrition problems. Money is scarce, and small amounts of food are bought with each trip to the store. The family cannot take advantage of quantity buying because of insufficient funds, inability to transport large purchases, and lack of storage and freezer space. Another major factor in the nutrition/money equation is a "live for today" value system: since there is no assurance of good things tomorrow, enjoy all good things to the fullest today. The illness, accident, and crime rates among the poor indicate that this is too often a logical way of living. We see a mother purchasing both junk food and expensive steaks the day her food stamps are issued, instead of buying large amounts of cheaper but nourishing items; the family is often hungry before the next issue of stamps. An additional problem for the economically deprived is the usual lack of knowledge of nutrition and economical meal planning. There are, of course, exceptional families of all classes who plan well-balanced diets.

The physical environment also provides transportation for disease-bearing *microorganisms* through air, water, humans, and animals. The microorganisms are passed more easily from person to person when the home is small and crowded, or from animal to person if the animal and pest populations are not controlled. The family with adequate income invests in space for each person; the family with inadequate income is forced to allot less space per person. Space is only one determinant in inhibiting contagious disease. For example, it may be very difficult to explain the need for immunizations to a lower-class mother whose infant is happy and healthy if she has no understanding of disease prevention.

It can be seen that environmental stress influences all aspects of health, and socioeconomic class is a determinant of one's environment. The upper and middle classes have the means to reach optimal health but do not always choose to do so; the lower class does not usually have resources to reach its potentials and accepts whatever is available at the time. These factors help explain why poor people are present in proportionately larger numbers in hospital populations, are sicker when they initially seek medical intervention, and are hospitalized for longer periods of time. Nurses in acute care settings must understand these class-related phenomena in order to plan nursing care realistically.

THE CHILD WITH AN ACUTE ILLNESS

The child with an *acute illness* creates a crisis in his family. The onset of an acute illness may be rapid and severe. Until parents have had experience in gauging the degree of an illness, deciding that medical assessment is needed, and obtaining appropriate medical care, each illness provokes anxiety. Parents of a first child seldom have enough knowledge for decision making about illness. Mothers frequently reject or do not have access to advice of older and experienced family members. Public schools do not include enough health care courses in their curricula, and the health care system does not generally provide this type of health education. Nurses in pediatricians' offices and emergency rooms describe numerous calls from young mothers who describe symptoms and ask if something is wrong with their children.

The infant with an acute illness causes his parents to agonize over whether to wake a physician in the middle of the night; memories are searched for earlier signs of the illness. Guilt is always present, often because parents blame themselves for their child's illness. They ask themselves why they did not call the physician earlier, why they did not see those early signs, and, in the case of accidents, why they did not prevent them. Fear is another common emotion: fear that the child will be hurt or will even die, fear that someone will blame them for the illness, fear that illness will put the family in debt. Other problems for parents of a hospitalized child include care of siblings at home, transportation to and from the hospital, need for facilities to room-in with the child. Parents experience a role change from child protector and care provider to helpless observer as the health care team takes over. This is distressing to the parents and confusing to the child. Guilt, fear, and concern about the home situation all compound the inevitable anxiety parents have during a child's acute illness.

Emotions are manifested by behavior. Common behavior of parents in emergency rooms, outpatient offices, and acute care units include:

Increased Activity Level. Parents often begin repetitious, purposeless activities (e.g., pacing, wringing hands, chain smoking, flipping pages in magazines, finger tapping).

Questioning. Parents ask many reasonable questions about treatments, prognosis, and length of hospital stay. These questions do not always have definite answers, so parents ask them again and again. When specific answers are given, parents may be too anxious to understand or remember, and more questions are necessary. Confirm that the parents understand each time you answer. Anticipate questions whenever possible.

Complaining. Even when the best possible care is provided, expect complaints from anxious parents. However, never regard these only as symptoms of anxiety; the complaints may be based on fact. Elicit details about the complaint: "You feel that Ms. N. was too rough with Jody? Tell me more about what happened."

Misunderstanding/Misrepresentation. Determining whether misunderstanding or misrepresentation has occurred is frequently difficult. Parents are naturally less calm during a crisis, and may pass their misconceptions on to the physician or another nurse. This occurrence must also be explored thoroughly in order to determine the facts.

Verbal Distress. Verbal behavior manifests stress through high-pitched, rapid, incoherent speech, quiet to noisy crying, and moans. This behavior often makes the nurse uncomfortable, but she must allow parents this expression of distress.

Withdrawal. Parents may withdraw from the situation because of real or imagined inadequacy in the acute care situation. Indications of withdrawal are apparent lack of interest in the child's condition, sitting or standing apart from the child and those working with him, and the failure to attempt to participate in his care or to console him. This parent, the nurse's patient as much as is the child, should be taken aside and provided with support. Giving the parent increasing responsibility according to ability to accept it will be therapeutic to parent and child.

Dependency. Parents rely on the nurse for decisions and assistance. Although this is desirable behavior, extremes occur when the child has a very long or terminal illness, when the parents have weak or nonexistent patterns of coping, or when the family lacks the resources (e.g., intelligence, money, energy) for taking part in the child's care. Whenever possible, the nurse should increase the parents' responsibility for the child's care. When this is not feasible, referral to the nurse specialists, hospital social worker, or appropriate community agency is in order.

Do not consider these behaviors to be directed at you, personally. They are parents' reactions to the stress of their child's illness. If you find yourself resenting a parent, try to find a solution to the problem using the nursing process. If this effort does not enable you to handle your inner conflict, ask for assistance from a person who does not share your feelings. When, occasionally, you find that you cannot resolve your dislike for a parent after a sincere effort, arrange for someone else to care for the parent and child.

The child who is acutely ill is in stress. He may not understand his discomfort and wonder why his parents do not meet his need for comfort as they have in the past. The child sees his parents change from being self-confident and authoritative to being fearful and uncertain; they cannot answer questions or make decisions for the child in the acute care setting. Hospital policy may force separation of the child and his parents. Only a caring and perceptive nurse can recognize parent-child needs and plan interventions.

The behaviors of hospitalized children may be similar to those of their parents; these are managed according to the child's age, stage of development, and the interaction of physical and emotional states. Types of behaviors commonly seen on the acute care unit include regression, withdrawal, aggression, and hysteria.

Regression is the occurrence of behaviors appropriate to an earlier age and stage of development. Although regression, if excessive and prolonged, may be abnormal, it usually serves to help the child adapt to his situation; the extra physical and emotional energy that was invested in his most recently acquired skills is rechanneled into the task of coping with the stress of hospitalization. Thus, you would expect the potty-trained toddler to start having accidents, the preschooler to use baby talk, and the school-age child to sob for his parents when they leave him. The child loses his most recently learned skill first, but even the older child may regress temporarily to infantile states if the stress is great. Explain this process to parents since they are often confused and embarrassed by the behaviors. Encourage them to permit regression while the child needs additional energy, and act as role model for the parents by accepting but not reinforcing regressive behaviors. As the child regains strength, work with his parents to reestablish the normal limits on behavior. The child may regress again when he gets home from the hospital, and parents need preparation for this occurrence before the child's discharge.

Withdrawal is the process of turning inward and/or away from others in order to protect oneself from outside threats. This, also, is adaptive behavior that provides extra energy for coping with stress, but severe withdrawal may be misinterpreted as "good" behavior by the nursing staff, since the child rarely requests assistance. The child may not talk to anyone, may turn his body away from people, cover his head with a sheet or pillow, and/or engage in excessive self-stimulation (e.g., masturbation, rocking, and head-banging). Making the parents feel welcome, important, and comfortable enables them to maintain their roles as the child's protectors. As much as possible, the child needs to be able to predict his schedule of daily activities, his treatments, his nurse, and to collaborate in decision making concerning his care. The more control the child has over himself and his environment, the more secure he feels. Do not try to force the child to interact with you; accept his behavior but talk to him, provide opportunities for brief conversation, and touch and/or hold him as he permits. Try reading a story or showing pictures with pauses for responses. A quiet congratulation to the child is appropriate when he is more open, but an overreaction may result in further withdrawal. Other children on the acute care unit can occasionally help. An infant who needs holding may interest the withdrawn ten-year-old girl, and the bored teenager may establish a warm relationship with a withdrawn preschooler. Peers may also involve the withdrawn child in games, hobbies, or watching television.

Aggression is an act of unprovoked hostility resulting from the child's inability to express his anxieties in more appropriate ways. A child may inflict pain on parents, nurses, and other children by hitting, biting, or throwing objects. He may try to hurt feelings through constant criticism or ridicule. Aggression can also be exhibited by offensive behaviors (e.g., bad language, voluntary loss of bowel control, and destruction of property).

Tommy, aged seven, had been a "good patient" on bed rest for several days. One morning, upon return from the linen closet, his nurse was shocked to discover that he had furiously marked all over the wall with a red crayon. He was lying quietly in bed, staring out the window.

Tell the child in no uncertain terms that he may not harm people or property. If he persists, separation from others is necessary. Whenever possible, give this child activities that expend energy, require the use of long muscles, and allow forceful contact with objects. Pounding toys, modeling clay, and jump ropes are appropriate tools for his play. Finger paints and water colors may provide an outlet for his aggression. Try to make friends with him by listening and talking to him, and by letting him make as many decisions as possible. Notice the child's ability to control an impulse and congratulate him. Do not reward disruptive behaviors by excessive attention. Take the child to a quiet place, but allow him to rejoin the group as quickly as possible.

Hysteria, for the purpose of this discussion, is an uncontrolled response to fear. The child screams, kicks, hits, bites, and turns his body to avoid treatments that he perceives as threatening (i.e., causing pain, bodily mutilation, or death). Hysteria can often be prevented by a careful explanation of all procedures before they are done, establishing trust between child and nurse. Tell the child that his control is helpful, but that another nurse will be available to assist his staying still, and that crying is okay. If the child becomes hysterical, give him a couple of minutes to regain composure, then restrain him and carry out the treatment as quickly as possible, since any hesitancy will increase his anxiety. Talk to him throughout the treatment to assure him of your concern for his feelings. When the child has quieted down, pull up a chair and discuss his behaviors with him. You might say to the six-year-old child, "The hospital is a scary place for little boys and girls. Sometimes I have to do things that hurt you, and that makes it scarier for you. I understand that you are afraid and that you cannot always be quiet and still when you are hurt. That's why we are here to help you be still, to let you cry when you need to, and a lot of other things to make you well. I will always let you know what I'm going to do *before* I do it." The child should be encouraged to reenact the procedure on his doll, puppet, nurse, or parent. Parents need explanations about the child's behaviors, since they may be embarrassed to the point of spanking their child if they do not understand.

There are many types of behaviors not discussed here. Some general rules for reacting to all children's and parents' behaviors can be put forth: be nonjudgmental, do not take attacks personally, search for underlying causes, keep communications open, and seek help from other team members when necessary.

THE CHILD WITH A CHRONIC ILLNESS

Chronic illnesses are long-term or even lifelong health problems, ranging from minor nuisances to major debilitating conditions. The child may be born with an anomaly that requires immediate intervention to save his life and leaves him with a disability. He may be born with an obvious inherited disorder, or the problem may not appear until later in childhood. A child may be afflicted with an acute illness (such as meningitis) with complications causing a wide variety of handicaps, especially mental retardation and decreased mobility. Yet another possibility, and a major cause of long-term disability and disfigurement, is accidental trauma.

Chronic illness has a tremendous impact on the physical and emotional development of the child. If the problem causes separation of the child from his parents, parent-child attachment is interrupted and impaired. When a defect is highly visible (e.g., cleft lip or large facial birth marks), all people see the anomaly and react before they can begin to look further at the child as a person. When mobility is decreased, almost every aspect of the child's development is delayed, since he learns much about himself and his environment through movement. A disorder that impairs one aspect of development can obviously affect a related ability. For example, if the child has a speech defect, he may also have impaired reading ability. If the child's body size is abnormally large or small, his self-image is frequently distorted. When his appearance is perfectly normal but any activity causes pain and/or fatigue, many people in his life may have little understanding of his dilemma.

Regardless of the problem, each child has tasks to accomplish according to his developmental stage, and success depends on positive interaction between the child and his family. The three behaviors most commonly seen in children with chronic illnesses are adaptation, aggression, and dependency. The adaptive child copes with his problem and directs his energies toward tasks he can complete with success; he may overachieve in these areas. He controls his illness rather than being controlled by the illness. The child who is aggressive feels hostility toward others and directs verbal and/or physical attacks against his siblings, peers, parents, and others. He may be passively aggressive by refusing to meet his parents' expectations or offensively aggressive, (e.g., having deliberate bowel movements in his pants). The dependent child makes few decisions for himself, resists separation from his parents, and avoids challenging situations at school or at play. He appears content with his sick role, and allows his parents to protect him from harm. All children demonstrate each of these behaviors occasionally. Note the predominant behaviors without stereotyping the child, and use this information in planning for his care.

The family of a child with a chronic problem is in stress. The resources of time, emotional and physical energy, space, and money are depleted. A good example of this concept is the child with obstructive pulmonary disease. The child requires medications and machinery to help him breathe, treatments (postural drainage) three to four times a day, special diet, and periodic visits to different types of specialists. The family members providing this intensive care may be the parents, grandparents, siblings, and others. Since the expense is astronomical, most families require financial assistance from governmental or voluntary agencies. The child's health maintenance can require full-time services of a single family member, usually the mother. Although the family often needs her income, her care of the child must take precedence. The whole family may lose time since vacations are limited or built around the child's disability. Caring for a child for years, day and night, and week after week, may drain all emotional and physical energy from the parents. Great sibling rivalry is a common consequence. Siblings in the family have difficulty getting their share of attention and often display behaviors that demand parental action. The family that must direct its resources to one member is placed in a high-risk category, since the members of many such families are often separated from each other by the pressures of caring for the ill child. Parents divorce, siblings are sent to live with relatives, or grandparents move in to help shoulder the work load. Some families have strong coping mechanisms, and they actually become a closer unit if resources and responsibilities are divided fairly and sufficiently. This family is still to be considered at risk as you assess and plan care for its members.

The child with a chronic illness is a child first. He is not a CP child; he is a child with cerebral palsy. He is not a diabetic or an asthmatic; he is a child with diabetes or asthma. If a child is labeled as an illness, he sees himself as ill, and he learns to use his illness as a manipulative mechanism.

Jason, who at age four had moderately severe asthma, was angry because his mother refused to give him a snack at 5 pm. He said in a sulking manner: "If you don't give me a cookie, I'll start coughing." Mrs. H. still refused, and his ensuing temper tantrum brought on a severe asthma attack, which did not respond to the usual medications. His mother quietly took him to the emergency room after calling the physician. The emergency room nurse gave him an injection of a bronchodilator. Jason tried this behavior once again three days later as his parents were leaving for a party; again he received the necessary emergency room treatment without blame or punishment from his parents. Upon returning home, his parents went on their way to the party. Jason never again used his illness to manipulate his parents.

Heather L., who at age seven had had many severe asthma attacks, was in the hospital. She had toys piled all over her bed and stacked around the room. Every few minutes, she demanded a different toy from her mother, who had to get up from her knitting each time. She ordered Mrs. L. to get her ginger ale, then, refusing to drink it, pushed it away. Soon she wanted another kind of drink. Mrs. L. lost patience and slapped Heather's leg. Heather began to cry and wheeze audibly. Mrs. L. quickly left the room to buy the drink that Heather asked for.

All children need to have limits set on their behaviors. If these limits have been established at home, support the parents' efforts to maintain them. If not, collaborate with the parents. Parents and children are usually relieved to have reasonable guidelines established. Limit the stimuli in the child's room. Have one toy visible and available for play. Use logic in responding to the child's requests; the child will learn that he will receive nothing for a while if he rejects the things just requested.

The term chronic illness now includes diseases that once were considered fatal. The parents never know which term actually applies to their child, and this unknown factor can interfere with parent-child relationships. Some chronic diseases will inevitably lead to death, but the family's total dedication to keeping the child alive can prolong life for many, many years until young adulthood. This child struggles with developmental tasks just as normal children do, even though he knows he may not grow up, get married, have a career, or have children.

The health care system is fragmented into many agencies. Each agency has its own eligibility criteria, fees, professionals, routines and services. No one agency can meet all the needs of these chronically ill children and their families, yet agencies frequently do not collaborate with one another on planning for care. All too often, mechanisms for reporting services among agencies are faulty or nonexistent. There are gaps and overlaps in care, with children shuttled from place to place without ever knowing why. Parents arrive at a clinic for an appointment only to learn the clinic does not meet that day. Waiting time for services can amount to hours, necessitating whole days for certain services that are required regularly. Elaborate arrangements may be necessary for transportation. Time, energy, and money are used for travel and for waiting time. Children frequently must be left in out-of-town hospitals for long-term treatment because the parents have work and child-care commitments at home. Frustration reaches an unbearable level. Fragmentation of health services occurs in all socioeconomic classes, but it is much worse for the impoverished and poorly educated. They are less able to coordinate their children's care or to complain about agency deficiencies. They may become resigned to the fact that continuity of quality care is not available and refuse to return for appointments. Some communities have made progress, but coordination of services remains a major problem in our society.

THE CHILD WITH A TERMINAL ILLNESS

The loss of a child is perhaps the most devastating experience a parent can face. Parental hopes and dreams for the child are left unfulfilled with his death. Earlier in this century, it was not unusual for at least one child in a family to die. With advances in medical knowledge, better nutrition, hygiene, and living standards, life expectancy has increased; the fact that childhood mortality is no longer inevitable makes it more difficult for parents to accept a fatal illness in a child.

Caring for the child and family experiencing a terminal illness is a challenging and rewarding task. There are no defined methods, no perfect words, no illustrated procedures. Each family is unique, and each child, an individual. It is necessary that you be aware of your own feelings and reactions as well as those of the family. You will feel sad, angry, depressed, joyful, and at times fatigued, and you will want to forget and deny the presence of the child and family who are experiencing the loss of a life. Nursing is only one part of you. Stresses from other parts of your life complicate your ability to deal with these emotions. Your own concept of death will influence your reaction to the child who is dying. Everyone working with dying patients needs the support of the health team, especially inexperienced team members such as nursing and medical students. Acknowledge your feelings and express them in an appropriate place. You may find that you can release your emotions in previously established ways. However, you may need the help of someone or something, such as a sad movie, a hilarious book, or a rigorous tennis match to help you deal with your feelings rather than evade them. This may be your first step toward self-assessment in relation to death. Self-awareness fosters objective care and concern for the child who is dying.

This section will discuss the child's perceptions of death; his reaction and his family's reaction to his terminal illness; the stages of grief, and appropriate nursing interventions.

How the Child Perceives Death

Generalizations regarding the child's concept of death at different ages are presented to facilitate care; however, remember that each child is unique, with his own special needs.

Death is not perceived as a reality by the child under five. His concern with death stems chiefly from the fear of separation from his parents. He does demonstrate a beginning interest in the phenomenon, however.

Brian, aged two and a half, spied a dead frog. He asked, "Mom, why that frog not hopping?" She answered that he was dead. Brian bent over to study the frog more closely. After a moment, he said, "Ribit, ribit." His mother responded, "No, Brian, the frog's dead. He can't say 'ribit, ribit' anymore." Brian looked at the frog for one long moment, turned, and walked away.

The preschooler has usually had some exposure to death. He may have seen violent deaths on television, or animals splattered on the highway. A significant person in his life may have died. The type of death he has experienced determines his developing concept of death. The violent deaths give rise to feelings of vulnerability and a fear of mutilation; beyond this, the child's concept of death is still vague and is associated with sleep, an absence of movement or light, and separation. He sees death as a reversible event, assuming the dead can return at his wish.

Kelly, aged three and a half, said while riding in the car, "Mom, that puppy don't like that car 'cause it runs him over dead." Her mother replied, "What do you think happens then?" Kelly answered, "The puppy barks at that car and bites it hard."

The early school-age child (five to nine) conceptualizes death as a separate person, or a dead person. It may be the "boogyman" or the "angel of death."

Amy, aged six, interrupted her mother's letter-writing, saying, "Momma, when I die, and God starts taking me up to heaven, I'm going to grab your hand and take you up there with me."

The child between five and nine years of age is aware that death is permanent but not that he himself will die. Toward the end of this period, however, he begins to realize that he and his loved ones will die. Anxiety arising from this realization is manifested by disturbance of sleep, excuses to be with parents after bedtime, and crying that the child himself cannot explain.

After age nine, the child realizes the fact that he, too, will die, but sees the death as far in the future.

The adolescent, striving for self-identity, is vulnerable to thoughts of death, since an increased awareness of one's individuality also heightens one's concern with death. At this stage of development, there is a concern for the future, for what one will be; the possible loss of this future through premature death deprives the adolescent of his future identity. He is by now aware that death is permanent and inevitable.

The Child Who Is Dying

The child who is dying is still living (Figure 3–5). He is a child first; his disease process is secondary. What the dying child needs most is open, honest communication. Usually, the child receives parental help and guidance in most new situations, and gains security, but on this loneliest of journeys, he is often confused and unsure of parental support. He is doing something neither he nor his parents have ever done; he is dying.

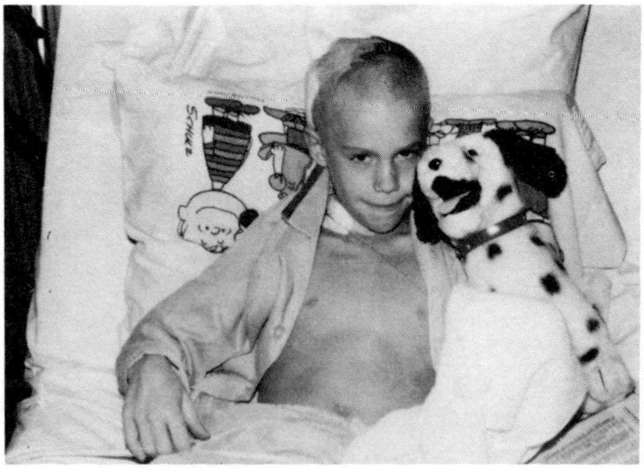

Figure 3–5. *A terminally ill child.*

Too often the child is victimized by a conspiracy of silence. His parents and/or physician may not want him to know how seriously ill he is because of their own unresolved conflict with death or because of their genuine belief that it is best that the child not know. Nurses often feel caught in a bind between the request not to tell and the child's haunting looks or actual questions regarding his condition. As a result, nurses often move the child to the far end of the hall, away from the nurse's station, in order that he may "rest," thereby avoiding the family, anxiety-provoking questions, and tearful scenes.

Even the youngest child will perceive changes in his relationships with significant people. Children are very perceptive and recognize anxiety in adults as well as adults' evasiveness about their condition. When his questions are met with silence, tears, or a change of subjects, the child may conclude that it is wrong to discuss his illness or that it is even more terrible than he had dreamed. He may believe that discussion of the subject will drive his family from him. Children often feel that illness is punishment for a real or imagined wrongdoing. This guilt fosters a sense of worthlessness.

Parents often attempt to bribe or spoil the child into playing the quiet game. They shower him with presents and attention and let discipline lag. This is a disruption of his normal routine. Because of the turmoil and insecurity of his internal environment, the child now needs, more than ever, a consistent, secure external environment. It is unfair to deprive him of this security; children who are pampered through a final illness feel lonely as well as unloved. The preschooler and adolescent are especially concerned with their body image and loss of appearance or function. In addition, the adolescent fluctuates between a sense of invulnerability and a sense of impending doom. His anxiety increases when people respond with withdrawal or excessive permissiveness.

Terminally ill children who have been allowed to discuss their illness and prognosis seem to experience less anxiety than do children who have not had this opportunity. Adults tend to think that, if the child has not been told, he does not *know* that his illness is fatal. However, even when not directly informed, terminally ill children have a conscious and/or subconscious preoccupation with death, expressed in fantasy, feelings of isolation, and loneliness. They show a greater overall anxiety than do chronically ill children and feel helpless to control or affect either their internal or external environment. Adults may be blinded to the child's anxiety because of their own fears and concerns and sense of helplessness.

John, aged eleven, was in the terminal stage of leukemia. A nursing student felt that John knew he was dying and was prepared to explore this with him. His physician, who deeply cared, felt that it was best not to tell him and forbade discussions of the illness with John. Later John drew himself lying in a box (Figure 3–6).

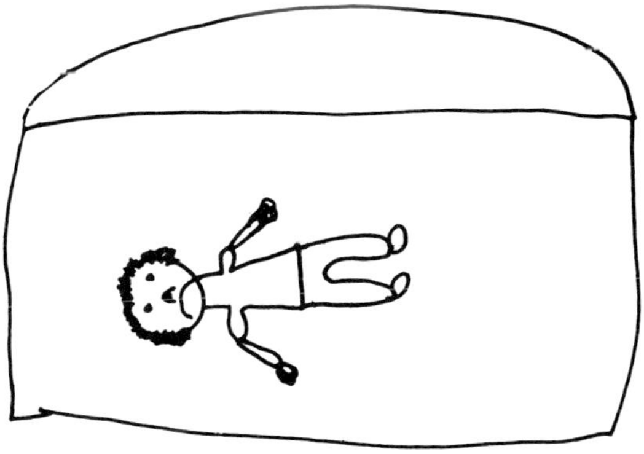

Figure 3–6. *A self-portrait by an eleven-year-old dying of leukemia.*

If the parent does not want the child to know, you should not *tell* him he is dying. Rather, you should assess the child's concern for his condition, using the nursing process, and convey this information to the parents. Often, they will realize their child's need to acknowledge the prognosis. Offer to assist them in talking with the child. You may say, "Would it be easier for you if I talk with him?" Don't push him, but if the child begins to test your reactions by toying with the subject, permit him to express himself through conversation, play, or drawings. If he wishes to pretend, avoid, or bargain, let him. Don't respond to the child's despair with false optimism by changing the subject with, "Oh, you look better today." The child can spot a phony and will realize that you, too, are playing the quiet game. If permitted to talk or express his fears nonverbally, as in drawings, the child will ultimately be able to deal with them. If he needs to cry or be depressed, it is better that he have supportive help than have to suffer his feelings in silence.

Try to determine the reason for the child's question, and answer honestly. If the child asks, "What does death feel like," ask him what he thinks it would feel like, or ask why he wants to know. He may be thinking of someone who died, or he may be wondering about himself. If he is in pain at the time, responding that "death doesn't hurt; the body just stops working" may confuse him, although the statement is basically true. It may be necessary to explain that although he is in pain at the present, death itself is not painful. Truth is essential. If he asks, "When am I going to die?" an honest reply is "I don't know when anyone will die." Answers to specific questions such as "Will I be home for Christmas?" may be answered with an indefinite but honest "I don't know; I hope so."

The child with a terminal illness has often had chemotherapy, radiation, and/or surgery. He suffers from both the side effects of the treatment and the disease. He has been subjected to numerous invasive procedures, for diagnosis and for treatment, each insulting to the integrity of body and spirit. He is in need of good physical care and comfort measures that decrease his suffering and contribute to his feeling of security and well-being. Specific nursing measures are discussed in preceding chapters.

Children who are terminally ill often possess a maturity beyond that of their siblings or parents. Their ups and downs, disappointments, and losses prepare them to face dying in a manner others find difficult to comprehend.

Parents of the Child with a Terminal Illness

During the diagnostic period, most parents fear the worst. With mass media carrying stories of children with leukemia and brain tumors, parents usually associate such diagnostic procedures as bone marrow studies and brain scans with serious illness. If they ask, "Do you think my child has cancer?" you may respond by asking what makes them think their child has cancer; this open-ended question allows them to express their fears. Telling them that you really do not know, but that the physician is running tests, is both honest and supportive.

Breaking the news to the parents should be a collaborative effort of the physician and the nurse. The physician may soon leave, and you will be the parents' immediate source of support. Take the initiative in calling other family support persons such as a clergyman or relatives, and give them the names of other parents who have gone through the experience and have volunteered to help.

How the parents cope with their child's diagnosis depends on how they have reacted to previous crises, their experiences with death, and the special meaning the child has for them. Assessment of the parents' response to past losses will yield clues to coping patterns they may employ in dealing with the prospect of their child's death. Families rarely go through the grief process as a collective unit. Assess each parent separately, remembering that they not only comprise a unit; they are two persons—and every person, including you, works through his or her grief in a highly personal way.

GRIEF

Grief is the natural reaction to a loss. It is a necessary and complex state of mourning. The five stages of the grieving process identified by Elisabeth Kübler-Ross are *denial, anger, bargaining, depression,* and *acceptance.* The family and child do not necessarily move directly through the grief process in an orderly fashion but may vacillate between the stages. Do not hurry the family or child through any stage or encourage them to "accept" the situation; meet them "where they are" and support them as they express their feelings of the moment. Not all clients or family members go through each stage of grief, and helping them to "reach acceptance" is not always the goal.

Denial—"No, Not Me"

Parental reaction to the diagnosis is usually one of shock and denial. The parents are unable to believe the diagnosis and may seek other opinions, especially if the child has not been seriously ill. This is a necessary step allowing time for assimilation of the tragic news they have received.

Do not attempt to hurry parents through this period of denial, since such an attempt would interfere with their coping behavior or destroy the mechanism that sustains them through the early part of their grief when they do not have a more effective mechanism to replace it.

Parents need privacy to work through their shock and disorientation. Hospitals are not known for their abounding space, and many do not have "screaming rooms." The diet kitchen, stairwell, or an unoccupied room, although a poor substitute, may be the only space available to provide privacy for the parents. The chapel is an obvious choice but a poor one, since the parents are likely to curse God as they express their anguish. Many parents find it difficult to curse God in a chapel. The nursing action at this point is to offer your physical presence to the parents. Touch is necessary for some, and proximity without physical contact may be appropriate for others; in any case, your presence, openness, and acceptance are vital.

Anger—"Why Me?"

As anger is experienced, the parents begin to ask, "Why my child?" "Why me?" "What have I done to deserve this?" There are no simple answers to these questions, and since the cause of the parents' anger, the child's fatal illness, cannot be removed, the anger is displaced on to someone or something in the external environment (e.g., God, the child himself, or the medical personnel). Most often, the nurse rather than the physician receives the brunt of this anger; parents often feel that if they show anger toward the physician he will "let" their child die. This anger is frequently expressed in the form of complaints. For example, the mother may complain because you were delayed in administering her child's medication when, in fact, you were not. Your first reaction is to get angry in return and to refuse to subject yourself to this unjustified abuse. Acknowledge your anger and the parents' angry behavior. Open acceptance of anger helps both parents and staff to work through feelings of hurt, helplessness, and confusion. Denial of anger only serves to stifle and prolong the grieving process. It may be helpful at this time to permit the mother to verbalize by saying "You seem to be angry. Would you like to talk about it?"

Parents need time away from the child to ventilate their anger and guilt, express fears, and question the "why" of it all. They may equate the child's disease and subsequent death as punishment and may blame themselves and each other. They need understanding and reassurance that they are not responsible for the child's illness (if, in fact, they are not). If the parents *are* responsible for the illness, their guilt will, of course, be much greater, and they may need professional help in order to deal with it.

Bargaining—"Just a Bit More Time"

In the bargaining stage of the grieving process, the fact of impending death is accepted, but the person (or family) bargains for more time. The bargaining is usually carried on with God (even if the person has never called on Him before); the parent asks for one more year, or month, or week of life. Often, the bargainer promises to attend church every Sunday or do a good deed every day, if only God will let the child live.

Depression—"Yes, Me"

As the parents move toward resolution, they mourn past losses, such as the death of a relative. They may be unable to talk about the sick child and may instead focus on previous grief.

As the reality of the situation strikes the parents, they may seem to regress in their grief work. They begin to cry a lot and may seem depressed. Actually, they are not losing ground; they have begun the painful process of realization and are experiencing anticipatory grief and are getting ready for death.

They may shower the child with presents and attention and may find it difficult to leave the child, even for a coffee break. The mother is usually the chief nurturing person and, as such, is usually more guilt-ridden. They should be taught and encouraged to participate in the child's care as long as they are able. This is important to the child, who may imagine people are avoiding him or thinking of him as already dead. If the child sees the parent participating in his care, his fear is decreased because he feels their support and senses that they understand and agree with what is being done for him.

Parents need a sympathetic listener to help them release many feelings that otherwise may be suppressed. They welcome your comment that "It is 'OK' to cry." Crying is a natural and beneficial outlet for grief and should be encouraged. Some men find it difficult to cry and need reassurance that crying is "OK." A gentle touch often creates the supportive bond that is so necessary to the parents during their struggle.

Offer to stay with the child or make arrangements for someone else to stay and encourage his mother or parents to take a break. Provisions should be made for a quiet area, away from the child's room, in which parents may have coffee and relax. The parents should feel confident that you will notify them of any change in the child's condition. Other parents are supportive at this time, and parents can learn from each other and profit from observing the others' coping behaviors. The common fear of "going to pieces" is greatly reduced by watching how others go through the experience. As the child moves from exacerbation to remission and back to exacerbation, parental grief goes through a cycle of hope (with remission) and back to despair and depression with exacerbation.

Acceptance—"It's True and It's OK"

The longer the stage of anticipatory grief, the easier it is to cope when death actually occurs. However, in prolonged dying, the family members often finish grieving before the actual death. They may think of the child as dead and begin to give away his toys and clothes and curtail their visits. When they do visit, they may spend time with other children on the unit, in effect, disengaging themselves from their child before the actual death. They may wish for the death, to alleviate suffering and end the ordeal. The family may reach this stage of acceptance before the staff and other relatives do, and these others may misinterpret the acceptance as callousness. The parents may become bewildered and feel guilty for having worked through their grief. You can convey understanding, acknowledging that death wishes towards the terminally ill are human and acceptable. A short coma during this time may be a blessing, since the family may not be able to deal with a conscious child after they have reached this stage of acceptance. Also, they can see that the child is no longer suffering and may actually seem to be in a peaceful state.

As with the other stages of grief, your physical presence and concern are most important during the final stages. You need not suppress feelings of loss. To cry is a natural response to loss. Crying with the parents and sharing your grief is acceptable and conveys to the family your concern and love for their child. However, never feel obliged to express feelings that are not felt; be honest.

If, for some reason, the parents were not with the child at the moment of death, they should be permitted to see his body and to hold him if they wish. (Viewing the body is an important step toward realization of the death.) Allow private time for the parents so that they may feel free to express their grief through crying (Fig. 3–7).

Siblings

Parents may need help in dealing with the siblings of the dying child. Their own behavior may prevent their detection of behavioral signs of distress in their other children. The child whose sibling has died suddenly is in a state of shock and disbelief just as his parents are.

Siblings should be told about the severity of the illness and gradually be informed of the child's impending death. Parents may try to protect them from this knowledge, but this deception only serves to heighten their anxiety. They should be permitted to visit the sick child and be included in the situation. Exclusion may make them feel hurt and jealous. Gradual adjustment will be easier than the sudden surprise that the sick child has died. This sudden reality may overwhelm their powers of coping, since children must cope with loss gradually.

The young child has no concept of finality; therefore, death wishes toward others are normal as is the wish for them to return. The child needs assurances when his wishes "come true." He can be told that although he sometimes may have "wished away" the child, his thoughts and wishes did not hurt the child or make him go away. Tell him everyone has these wishes at times. If the child feels that he sent the dead child away, he may believe that he can cause tragedies and may become afraid of himself. In the absence of accurate knowledge children create fantasies (such as that the mother threw the child away, or like a guppy, that she ate it) that can be more terrifying than the truth.

The natural mourning state of the parents will temporarily lessen the amount of attention they give to the surviving children. The parents may need help to be aware of this facet of their mourning. Young children need to be reassured that they have not lost their place in the family. They need an opportunity to question, to wonder, and to cry. They need to know that being sad and missing the dead child is a normal reaction. Physical closeness is important at this time. They should be hugged, rocked, and cuddled.

Parents should be encouraged to use correct terms, that is, "death," "died," "buried." Terms such as "passed on," while softening the blow for adults, only add to a child's confusion.

When the child is familiar with his parents' religious beliefs, death can be dis-

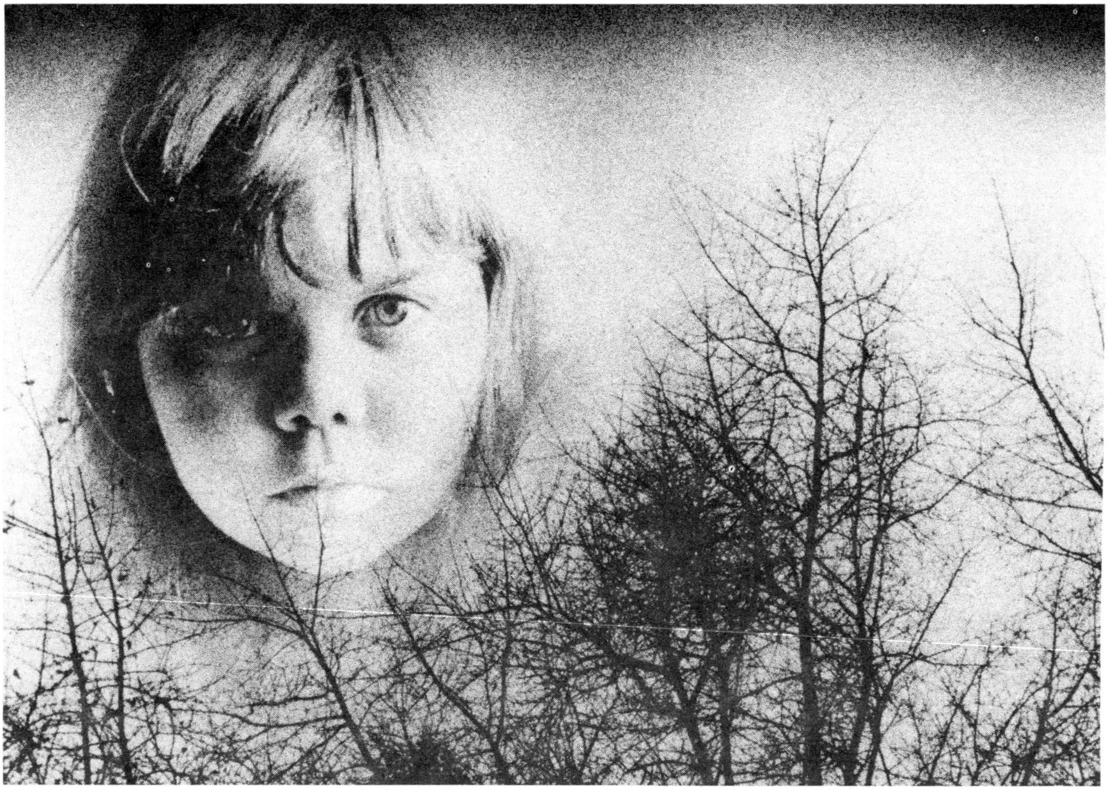

Figure 3–7. *Still mourning the death of her child, a mother reports, "I see her everywhere."*

cussed within the context of those beliefs, however, the child should never be told that "God wanted him" or "he was so good, God took him to live with Him." The child may feel that God may want *him* next, feel threatened by God, or hate and fear Him. He may also surmise that if God takes good children, there is no reason to be good. Parents don't have to explain everything. They may admit they don't know.

Death should not be likened to sleep or a long trip. Aside from being untruthful, these explanations can lead to sleep disturbances or adverse reactions to trips. Death should be explained in terms that the child can understand: "When you are dead and no longer alive, you cannot eat, sleep, run, or play. You cannot feel or be sad, angry, or happy."

The siblings should be permitted to attend the funeral services if they wish. However, they should be prepared for it beforehand, and someone should be available to take them home if necessary during the service. Emotional reactions expected of children should be explained to the parents. The child may not equate the sorrow he sees with separation from his sibling, and may ask when the dead child is coming home. Parents will have to remind him that death is final, that the dead child cannot return. Siblings may feel angry that the dead child left them behind and may have guilt feelings arising from magical thinking (see ch. 6). Children react differently to grief than do adults. They may feel deep pain and yet go out and play. This return to the familiar allows them time to assimilate and accept the horrible and the unfamiliar. Children handle trouble at their own pace and in their own way. Adults should allow children their retreat. This apparent indifference during the first few weeks serves as an adaptive mechanism and should be distinguished from persistent denial of the death.

SUDDEN UNANTICIPATED DEATH

Although most unanticipated sudden deaths in the hospital occur in the emergency room, there are times when a child on the unit dies suddenly. This may occur shortly after admission (e.g., from trauma or infection) or in a child who is hospitalized for a seemingly mild illness.

Parental reaction to this sudden death is usually different from the reaction to a lingering death. Parents look for a scapegoat, for someone or something to blame. They transfer their hate and anger to anyone around. Not surprisingly, most people tend to shy away from parents when they are in this stage. It is our job as nurses to accept this anger and help parents express it without feeling guilty.

The physician, rather than the nurse, clergyman, or social worker, should inform the parents of the death; otherwise, the parents may think no medical help was available to the child.

Some physicians sedate the family in order to prevent hysteria. This can be detrimental to the parents in that it prevents them from experiencing their grief and anguish and thus prolongs the grief process. Parents seem to have more questions and harbor more guilt if they are sedated throughout the ordeal. The truth won't actually hit them until all of the activity (funeral, relatives and friends visiting) stops, about one month later. The nurse should call the family four weeks after the death, and invite them back to the unit to visit once more and to ask questions. During these four weeks the emptiness has set in, and the same questions haunt the parents over and over. "Did he ask for me? Was he alone? Did he have pain? Did anyone hold his hand?" Answers to these questions make the death real for them.

SUDDEN INFANT DEATH SYNDROME

Sudden infant death syndrome (SIDS), or *crib death,* refers to the sudden death of an infant that is unexplainable by history, clinical picture, or autopsy. A *syndrome* is a cluster of symptoms and phenomena which when considered together constitute a specific condition. The term is especially useful when the exact cause of a condition is unknown. SIDS claims the life of 1 out of every 350 infants. In the United States, 8,000 to 10,000 infants die of SIDS each year. Sudden infant death syndrome is the leading cause of death of children between one week and one year of age and, statistically speaking, is second only to accidents as the greatest killer of children under the age of fifteen (although it rarely affects children over one year of age). It kills more children each year than cystic fibrosis, cancer, child abuse, and heart disease *combined.*

The victim of SIDS is usually between two and four months of age. The premature and/or low-birth-weight infant has a six times greater risk of SIDS. The incidence also increases with multiple births, in which the offspring are frequently of low birth weight. As newborns, SIDS infants usually have a lower Apgar score and more respiratory difficulties. Males are affected more often than females, but since this is true for most serious pediatric diseases, sex may not be a significant factor.

In the United States, the Native American is the most vulnerable to SIDS, with blacks, whites, and Orientals following, in that order. Lower socioeconomic status and inadequate prenatal care also correlate positively with a higher incidence of SIDS; therefore, the infant at greatest risk is one of a lower class minority group family.

The deaths usually occur in colder weather and are associated with upper respiratory or viral infections. Since most SIDS deaths occur between midnight and 9 am, many researchers conclude that the syndrome is related to a prolonged period of deep sleep, when metabolic processes are basically different. The most popular theory is that SIDS results from prolonged sleep *apnea* (a temporary cessation of breathing), usually associated with upper respiratory infections.

Postmortem studies often show signs of chronic hypoxemia, including abnormal thickening of the walls of the small arteries of the lungs and abnormal retention of brown fat around the adrenal glands. These findings are part of the characteristic pathologic picture of SIDS, which usually also includes intrathoracic petechiae on the lungs, pericardium, and thymus, minor inflammation of the respiratory tract, and pulmonary congestion and edema.

Typically, the SIDS victim is a healthy infant who is put to bed for the night and several hours later found dead. A call is put through for police or an ambulance and resuscitation efforts, however futile, are begun. Someone may ask, "Did you or anyone else hit the baby?" This question is often prompted by the detection of livor mortis, a condition in which dependent parts of the body turn blue after death due to pooling of blood. There may be a frantic trip to the emergency room, where the parents are not allowed to see their child again. A false diagnosis of pneumonia or suffocation may be given, and the parents sent home, alone in their grief and shock (Figure 3–8). Depending on the awareness and knowledge of medical personnel present, the parents may be told that SIDS was the cause of death, but this is often not the case.

If an *autopsy* is performed, the results may not be made available to the parents for weeks or months. Relatives and friends begin to question the parents' ability to care for the child. The parents are totally

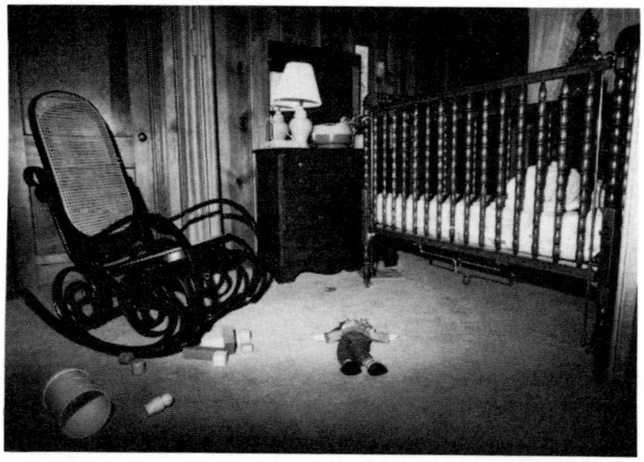

Figure 3–8. *In many cases of sudden infant death syndrome (SIDS) the parents return home after a frantic and futile trip to the emergency room, alone in their grief and shock.*

unprepared for this sudden shock. They react with intense guilt, blaming themselves and each other, and agonizing over the part they may have played in the death. Thoughtless comments coupled with a delayed autopsy report serve only to increase parental guilt and anguish. They wonder if the baby suffocated or choked and they blame themselves for not checking on him earlier.

If the death does appear to be a SIDS death, the parents need basic facts concerning SIDS. Tell the parents that:

- SIDS is neither predictable nor preventable.
- The baby did not suffocate, even though he may have been entangled in his blanket (even a young infant can turn his head to find an air space).
- The baby did not suffer; SIDS occurs instantaneously or in minutes.
- There is no danger to the rest of the family; SIDS is not contagious.

The National Sudden Infant Death Syndrome Foundation has local chapters in many large cities. Provide parents with information on the chapter in their area. This organization provides group support by helping parents realize that they are not unique in their crisis and that others have experienced the same feelings.

An autopsy should be performed on every SIDS victim. It confirms the diagnosis and offers an explanation to parents that aids in relieving guilt and self-accusations. The physician should explain the autopsy report to the parents as soon as the preliminaries are over.

It is helpful if the nurse (or another knowledgeable person—such as a social worker or the parent of another SIDS victim—who helped the parents through the initial period of shock, usually in the emergency room) contacts the family one week after the death and again after one month. The parents may need help in dealing with the siblings. Encourage parents to express their love and concern for their children without being overprotective.

The children themselves will need to feel secure about the integrity of the remaining family unit. They need ample love and close physical contact with their parents. Open lines of communication are most important because the siblings may have a great need to talk about the death. However, some children may not be able to verbalize their feelings. Instruct parents to explain to the siblings that nothing they did or thought made the baby die. They might say, "Wishes don't kill people. The baby died of a disease that only kills little babies and does not harm big boys and girls."

Parents of SIDS victims usually approach subsequent pregnancies with caution. They may need counseling from the nurse or from parents who have "been there" before. Children born later may suffer because of the parents' excessive anxiety over SIDS.

The parents may consider the subsequent child to be a replacement for the SIDS victim, and some go so far as to name the child after the dead infant. They tend to be overcautious with the child, especially when he has a cold, and may be overprotective to the point of hysteria.

The Packs lost an infant to SIDS two years ago. Baby Jeff is now two months old, and his mother keeps him in a portacrib which she moves from room to room as hse does her housework. Mrs. Pack cannot bear to leave Jeff's side even to permit him to nap or to enjoy an evening out with her husband.

TRANSCULTURAL NURSING

Each child is an individual different from every other child. Variations in body structure and size, skin, eyes, hair, beliefs, and perceptions contribute to individual uniqueness. The ability to identify cultural variation and to provide appropriate nursing interventions constitutes transcultural nursing.

Transcultural nursing is the study and application of the nursing process to varying cultural practices, values, and beliefs. Each child needs safety, comfort, stimulation, support, compassion, and health restoration, maintenance, and promotion. The meeting of these child health needs depends on an awareness and knowledge of individual cultural differences. *Cultural diversity* is the variation in values, beliefs, language, behavior, and physical characteristics of different cultural groups. Members of individual cultural groups tend toward *ethnocentrism,* the belief that one's own beliefs and values are more desirable than those of others. Ethnocentrism predisposes to *cultural imposition,* the tendency to impose one's values and beliefs on others, limiting consideration of their cultural beliefs. Cultural differences are inevitable, and they need not impede a meaningful relationship between child and family unit and nursing staff. An awareness of cultural variations and general behavioral differences can facilitate the nursing process and promote optimal health care delivery.

It is important to realize that individual children and groups of children vary culturally and biologically. *Biological variation* in muscle size and function, facial structure, and skin color are responses to past environmental influences. Present-day differences provide a historical account of our evolutionary past. Biological variation occurred over thousands of years, usually as an adaptive, health-promoting response to environmental stress. The black American, Hispanic Americans, Asian Americans, and Native Americans, are each minority groups of the American population. Major life styles, health practices, and unique nursing implications of each are presented for added awareness and knowledge.

Black Americans

Many black American families today do not represent a traditional matriarchal society; the parents work together in performing economic and nurturing functions. However, some blacks live in clustered matriarchal groups in which the grandmother is the central authority figure, and a young teenage mother may have returned to school, leaving her mother to rear her children. Fathers may be absent, and state and federal economic aid are the families' means of support. Extended family members are important to blacks, and children are especially valued, maintaining a close relationship to the parents. Home remedies are used to cure ills, and folk medicine, more religious than magical in origin, is still a strong force in most large black communities. Older women in the community are consulted for health advice; fear of hospitals and economic hardships frequently leads to the postponement of seeking medical care until the problem is serious.

The obvious difference in black Americans is skin color. *Melanin* is the pigment that gives skin its color. The more melanin, the darker the skin. In black persons, color is best assessed in the conjunctiva of the eye, the palms, and the nail beds. Since streaking and/or skin redness are not easily observed in the black child, evaluate pain, warmth, and tenderness as indicators of inflammation or infection. Special considerations are important for the child's hair. If the hair is to be washed, apply petroleum jelly while the hair is wet and comb or plait the hair before it dries. Food preference should be assessed.

Hispanic Americans

Mexican Americans are clustered primarily in the Southwest and are the largest minority group in the United States. They have clearly defined cultural values and behavioral patterns that are closely adhered to. The Mexican American family tends to be present-oriented, placing less value on material possessions than non-Hispanic white families do. The family is of primary importance in this culture; the self is second. Families are closely knit and are used to meeting their own needs; others are consulted only as a last resort. The family structure is typically patriarchal, and few decisions are made without the father present. A knowledge of Mexican American religious beliefs is central to an understanding of their health practices. Individual suffering and illness are signs of God's will and must be accepted and tolerated.

Puerto Ricans live in greatest numbers on the Northeast coast. Most families have an income below the poverty level, and Puerto Ricans as a whole have the least education of all minority groups. Families tend to be large, home-centered, and closely knit.

Most Puerto Ricans are Catholic, and religion is a major force that sustains the family unit. Infant mortality, parasitic diseases, malnutrition, and tuberculosis are prevalent health problems. Folk medicine is practiced widely, and the use of herbs and charms to cure ailments is common.

Although the language and religion of the Puerto Ricans are the same as those of Mexican-Americans, it is important to recognize the differences between the two groups and to tailor nursing care to meet specific needs. Of course, just as the two minorities are not "alike," neither are individuals within either group. As is true of any group, each client is an individual and must be treated accordingly.

Native Americans

Each Native American traces his ancestry to a tribe. Numerous tribes exist, each with its own culture and language. Attitudes and values vary greatly from tribe to tribe. An Apache has a totally different life style and value system than a Cherokee. Like each minority group, Native Americans are not all alike and they resent being considered so. The income of the average Native American family is one-half of the poverty level, the infant mortality rate is the highest in the United States, and death rates from common conditions, such as diarrhea and pneumonia, are extremely high. Family ties are strong, and the sharing of possessions is valued more highly than individual ownership. Native Americans believe that each living thing follows a birth-life-death process and that illness is one part of this natural life cycle. An important person in the Native American health practice is the medicine man. Remembering and acknowledging this cultural belief is extremely important. Indians are warm, quiet, cooperative people who may be erroneously perceived as passive and apathetic. When providing nursing care to the Native American child and family, be patient, provide privacy, and do not force conversation. The Native American patient may not maintain eye contact during a conversation because this is considered an invasion of privacy in some tribes. As with the Hispanic American, English is a second language for many Native Americans. Brochures in native languages that are heavily illustrated aid in health explanation and education.

Asian Americans

Asian Americans include people of Chinese, Japanese, Korean, and Vietnamese descent. The cultures of these groups tend to show a strong Chinese influence although each group has its own beliefs and values. Extended family relationships are important to the Asian American, and the family is usually patriarchal.

In Chinese culture, health is defined as a normal flow of energy, which is thought of as a balance of the forces of *yin* and *yang*. Yin is negative, cold, and female; yang is positive, warm, and male. An imbalance between yin and yang produces illness or disease. Traditional Chinese medical practices include the use of massage, spiritual healing, acupuncture, and meditation.

Each child is different. Each culture is different. The values and beliefs of a culture are maintained from one generation to the next through its child rearing practices. Most parents accept the way they raise their children as the best possible way. Acknowledge this fact, assessing verbal and nonverbal behavior to determine cultural difference and priorities. Individual behavior, family role behaviors, verbal and nonverbal responses, and amount and type of body contact all vary from one culture to another. Understanding cultural and biological variations will aid in developing a meaningful relationship with the child and his family and in planning appropriate nursing care.

PARENT CHILD-BONDING

Every woman approaches pregnancy differently, each with her own set of values, strengths, weaknesses, and degree of emotional maturity. She has a preconceived image of the baby she will bring into the world. How well the infant measures up to her image determines to some degree how fulfilled or disappointed she is with her baby. If a woman dreamed of a curly-haired little boy and is delivered of a bald-headed girl, the baby does not equal her preconceived image.

An infant's earliest bond will be an emotional attachment to one person, his caretaker, usually his mother. The quality and strength of this bond will influence the child's future attachments.

This section will discuss healthy *parent-child bonding*, including nursing actions necessary to foster this bonding process, alterations of bonding, and appropriate nursing interventions.

The Bonding Process

According to Klaus and Kennell, the infant is a *passive* recipient during the labor and delivery, and he becomes an *active* participant in the mother-infant bonding process after his birth. His sex, size, appearance, and activity level all influence his mother's response to him.

There is a period in the first few minutes and hours after birth termed the *maternal sensitive period* by Klaus and Kennell, that seems to foster parent-infant attachments.

Klaus and Kennell define an attachment as a unique relationship between two people that is specific and enduring. When parents are allowed a period of privacy and quiet with their newborn right after delivery, they tend to form an earlier and stronger bond with the baby. They exhibit more "parenting" behaviors, such as cuddling and talking to the infant. This also holds true for mothers and infants "rooming-in" after birth. *Rooming-in* refers to the practice of placing a neonate in the room with his mother for all or part of the day. As the mother assumes responsibility for the infant, she receives guidance and support from the nursing staff. This early contact significantly affects later mothering behavior, and thus tends to influence the child's development.

This initial period of "getting to know each other" is an interactive process in which both parents and infant send and receive stimuli that enhance the attachment. The parents must receive some response from the infant, such as eye or body movements, in order to form a close bond. For example, the mother strokes the infant's face, and the infant responds by turning to suckle at the breast, an act which is satisfying to them both. In most instances this bonding process takes place in the first few days of life and is strengthened by continued interaction.

Mothers want to see their infants' eyes and often say, "Open your eyes; open your eyes so I'll know you're in there." This eye-to-eye contact, which allows the mother to relate to the baby as a person, is an important aspect of the early bonding process. Mother and child are said to be in the *en face position* when the mother's face is in the same vertical position as that of her infant. The en face position can be observed as the mother holds her baby up to talk to him or turns her head to align her face with his as he nurses. The newborn can focus best at 12 inches and prefers the human face to other visual stimuli. The nursing position, then, with the mother's and infant's eyes about 12 inches apart, is ideal for providing continued eye-to-eye contact.

The infant's greater attraction to speech in the high-frequency range makes him more receptive to female than male voices. Mothers consistently use a high-pitched voice in speaking to their neonates but are unable to explain their reason for doing so. Nature has apparently provided a maternal instinct that ensures auditory stimulation that is attractive to the infant.

As the mother speaks to her infant, he responds with body movement, in effect moving in rhythm to her speech. This synchronized movement, termed *entrainment*, is rewarding for the mother and serves to enhance the parent-child bond. If the parents receive positive feedback from their newborn, their self-esteem is enhanced, which leads to feelings of being a "good parent." However, they may receive negative feedback from the infant as they attempt to care for him. They may interpret his crying, restlessness, and vomiting as signs of dissatisfaction with their care. This negative feedback precipitates an alteration or disruption in bonding.

The early bonding process is more difficult to foster in hospitals in which mothers and infants are separated shortly after birth with infants being brought to their mothers only for feeding at four-hour intervals. Mothers who are separated from their infants during the early newborn period (e.g., mothers of premature babies or babies with birth injuries) often find it difficult to care for the baby or to develop an emotional attachment to him (Figure 3–9).

The mother and her child may be separated for correction of minor problems, such as slight hyperbilirubinemia or mild respiratory disturbances, that are resolved before the mother and infant are discharged. The disturbance in the mother-child bonding process may last for the entire first year of life or throughout childhood. There is a significant relationship between early maternal-child separation and mothering disorders such as failure-to-thrive and child abuse. A disproportionate percentage of premature infants are later victims of failure-to-thrive and/or battering.

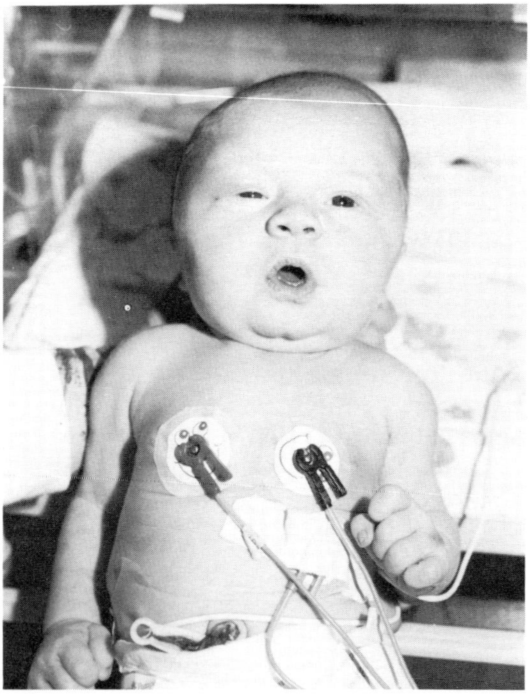

Figure 3–9. *This infant has possible birth injuries; note the edema around the face. Although he was full-term, he has been separated from his mother for observation in the neonatal intensive care unit.*

Medical personnel can do much to foster early parent-child bonding. Parents can be encouraged to participate as partners in the pregnancy and the birth of the baby, maintaining some control over the birth process. Immediately after birth, provide privacy for father-mother-newborn contact. A heatlamp is used to keep the naked infant warm. The administration of eye medications, such as silver nitrate, should be delayed for the first hour after birth to allow eye-to-eye contact between parents and child. Encourage rooming-in so that the mother can have responsibility for her infant. Provide assistance and morale-boosting as necessary. Make positive comments about the baby: "Look how alert he seems," or "What a healthy-looking baby!" Encourage father-sibling visitation to help cement the family bond (Figure 3–10).

FAILURE-TO-THRIVE

Failure-to-thrive (FTT) refers to a syndrome in which a child fails to grow and gain weight adequately. The child typically falls below the third percentile on standard

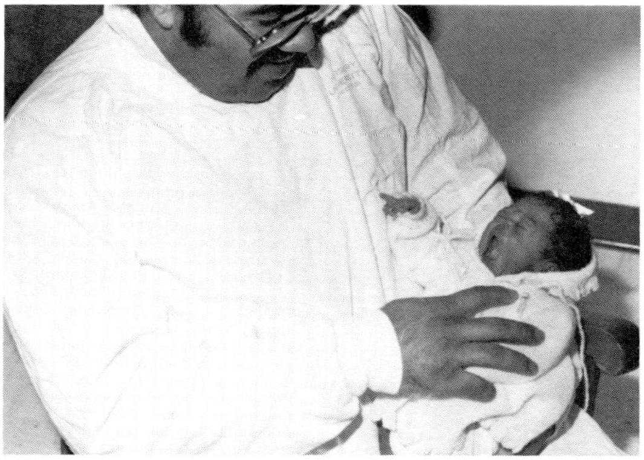

Figure 3–10. *Father-infant bonding.*

growth charts (see chapter 17 for an explanation of growth parameters). Failure to gain weight, developmental lags, and poor muscle tone may be present. There is no organic cause for these deviations. (FTT does exist secondarily to such organic disorders as cardiac and metabolic dysfunctions, but this discussion is limited to nonorganic FTT.)

Although FTT is attributable to a disturbed mother-infant relationship, often it is secondary to inadequate food intake due to the mother's difficulty in perceiving her child's needs accurately. The mother may truly love her baby, but due to a lack of education, she doesn't feed the child properly.

Jane was a spitter and Mrs. B., her mother, turned to a neighbor for advice. The neighbor advised Mrs. B., a college graduate, to dilute the formula. Mrs. B. did, but Jane kept spitting up. Mrs. B. kept diluting the formula. When Jane was admitted to the hospital with a diagnosis of failure-to-thrive, she was one year old and weighed nine pounds.

Barry J., aged three months, was admitted to the hospital weighing six pounds—four ounces less than his birth weight. When quizzed about Barry's eating habits, Mrs. J. stated that she gave Barry a bottle every time she ate. She couldn't understand why Barry was not getting fat. Mrs. B. ate two meals a day.

The mother-infant relationship is reciprocal. The mother's failure to provide adequate emotional care and, often, adequate nutrition, may result in a child who fails to gain weight. The child's failure to gain may be interpreted by the mother as rejection of her mothering efforts, and this interpretation naturally undermines her confidence. This lack of self-confidence is reflected in her care; thus, a pattern of interaction is established between mother and child.

Hufton and Oates found that families at risk for failure-to-thrive are often in a lower socioeconomic class, suffer from environmental deprivation, and exhibit marital instability. The child is usually the youngest family member, born within 18 months of a sibling.

Infants who are not gaining weight or who are losing weight should be hospitalized for evaluation and treatment. If physiological problems, such as congenital defects or infection are ruled out, and the history and physical examination points to FTT, further diagnostic testing may be delayed while proper emotional care and feeding are initiated. The child usually begins to gain weight on a regimen of adequate intake and nurturing. Parents should be encouraged to visit and participate in the infant's care.

Medical and nursing intervention begins with an assessment that includes health, developmental, and social history. It is important to note complications of pregnancy, delivery, and parental expectations of the child. Note infant feeding patterns and behaviors. Observe the mother as she prepares the formula (most FTT babies are not breast-fed) and feeds her infant. Does she use proper formula-to-water concentrations? Does she jerk the bottle in and out of the infant's mouth, or permit him to suck and rest? What supplemental foods does she give? Note the interaction between mother and child. Mothers of FTT infants usually exhibit very little positive, loving behaviors toward the infant. Does the mother talk, cuddle, and stroke the child? Does she prop the bottle and not hold and rock the baby for feedings? Assess the child's sleeping patterns: Where does the child sleep and what are his sleeping periods? Often the infant who fails to thrive does not sleep well. His sleep is fitful; he cries more than normal and is restless.

Nursing care of the family with an infant who fails to thrive is centered around fostering adequate mothering. This includes teaching specific nurturing techniques and offering assistance to solve problems that interfere with the nurturing process. The FTT infant should be fed on demand, not according to a clock schedule.

The infant's weight gain, although crucial and an important result of successful treatment, is not the only factor to be considered. Improvement in the mother-child relationship is also essential. This may be difficult to accomplish since FTT parents often do not visit their hospitalized infant. It may be beneficial for you to refer this family to your local public health facility for follow-up care.

The failure-to-thrive mother may not relate well to authority figures. She may feel threatened by the thought that the nurse is a more adequate caretaker than she. Be concerned with mother and child. Involve the family in planning and caring for the child. Teach the mother the nutritional requirements of her infant and help her with food and formula preparation. Discuss and demonstrate feeding techniques that are age-appropriate for her child (e.g., holding the tiny infant, or offering finger-foods to an eight-month-old). Encourage the mother to increase satisfying contact with her infant during feedings, such as talking, maintaining eye contact, laughing, stroking, and cuddling the child. Plan with the family to provide quiet, adequate nap times and a consistent nightly bedtime. Discuss and demonstrate ways of providing stimulation during feeding and bathing (e.g., cooing, talking, holding, and playing with the child). Praise the mother's positive parenting behaviors and share your observations of her child's responses to her mothering efforts (cooing, smiling, sleeping better, crying less).

In the event the mother is not available for participation in the child's care, the nurse should see that the person caring for the child gives him adequate "mothering." He needs plenty of "TLC" coupled with an adequate diet. A minimum number of caretakers is necessary for the child who fails to thrive to increase his chance of developing trust through consistent relationships.

Often, the FTT mother feels hostile toward her infant and will need help in dealing with these feelings. She may believe that close physical contact will "spoil" her baby. The FTT mother needs help in developing appropriate ways of handling her frustration. Permit her to verbalize her feelings about the infant. Explain that the infant communicates his needs through crying, and that this is his way of signaling to her that he is hungry, uncomfortable, or wants someone to play with him. Acknowledge that frustration and irritation are normal responses to an infant's prolonged crying. Help the mother to assess the baby for physical causes for the crying (hungry, wet, tired) and to eliminate these if possible. If the situation permits, encourage the mother to provide adequate rest for herself when the baby is sleeping, and to plan some time each day for herself. (This goal may be unrealistic if there are other small children in the home.) Tension within the family unit is often a problem. Discuss these problems with the parents and utilize other members of the health care team (social worker, clergyman, psychologist) to establish improved communication patterns within the family unit.

The Child Abuse Syndrome

The child abuse syndrome is a clinical condition in young children who have suffered serious and nonaccidental physical or emotional trauma or neglect at the hands of their parents or guardians. Physical trauma, probably the most critical aspect of child abuse, is not the only facet of the syndrome but is the most overt indicator of a dysfunctioning family unit and a disturbed parent-child relationship.

Physical abuse is defined as an instance of one or several episodes of physical harm inflicted on the child, usually as "discipline." *Battering,* or the battered child syndrome, is severe and repeated abuse, usually of a child under four years of age; it includes serious injuries to long bones, internal organs, and the central nervous system. *Sexual abuse* includes the exposure or fondling of the child's genitals and rape. *Emotional abuse* refers to continued demeaning of the child. *Neglect* is classified as either *physical* (i.e., the failure to provide adequate food, clothing, shelter, hygiene, or medical care) or *emotional* (the failure to nurture the child's sense of self). Emotional abuse or neglect almost always coexists with any of the other forms of abuse.

Abuse other than physical trauma may go unnoticed since it is less obvious, but all of these components of the child abuse syndrome may have serious and long-lasting effects on the developing child.

Approximately 10 percent of all children seen in emergency rooms for injuries are victims of the child abuse syndrome. Between 100,000 and 200,000 children are routinely abused by their parents with sticks, hot irons, cigarettes, and fists. The same number of children are sexually abused yearly, and nearly 700,000 are denied basic food, clothing, and shelter. Each year 2,000 children die of child abuse and neglect. These startling figures are probably underestimates, since many, if not most, cases of child abuse are not reported.

Child abuse does not discriminate; it occurs in families of every race, creed, and socioeconomic class. Steele asserts that less than 10 percent of abusing parents have a psychiatric disorder of such severity that the treatment of the abuse situation is impossible.

According to ten Bensel, roughly one third of abuse victims in this country are adolescents, one third are of school age, and one third are preschool-age children or younger. Most severe abuse, resulting in mental retardation or death, is perpetrated on children under the age of three; about 90 percent of deaths occur in children under one year of age.

The younger the child, the more biologically and emotionally vulnerable he is. The younger child lacks the options of the older child, that is, running away or dodging a blow. The child from birth to age two, and again from age thirteen to fifteen, is more difficult to care for and places extra stress on the parents with regard to their abilities to care for their children. This is one reason for the high incidence of the abuse of children in these age groups. Abuse in the form of excessive discipline is seen most often in the school-age child.

Kempe and Helfer identified three factors that are necessary in order for abuse to occur: an *abusogenic* adult (i.e., one who was probably abused as a child and who now tends to abuse his own child), an event seen as a crisis, and a "special" child. To understand the abusogenic parent, it is necessary to examine the environment of the abused child.

The Environment of the Abused Child

Helfer refers to the environment in which the abused child is reared as a "world of abnormal rearing" (WAR). The child has usually been in a suboptimal environment since conception. He may have been abused while in utero by physical blows to the mother's abdomen. Early bonding disturbances—inadequacies in feeding, holding, and caring for the infant—are characteristic.

Routine care times, such as when the baby is being bathed or diapered, are not enjoyable, playful periods of mother-infant interaction. The child's crying does not result in the relief of hunger or other basic needs. Rather, the mother responds negatively; for example, by slapping or ignoring the child. The child's crying is perceived by the mother as an unjustified intrusion.

Parents make impossible demands on the child; for example, they may expect the child to be potty-trained at nine months or to cook and serve meals at age four. The child is not permitted to express his feelings, to say he is angry, or to engage in normal childhood play. This misperception of the child's abilities is termed *role reversal.* The parents look to the child for gratification of their needs. If mother is depressed, the child must comfort her even though she rarely reciprocates. Gray and Kempe estimate that 75 percent of abused children actively "parent their parents." The child's failure to accomplish unreasonable goals not only makes his parents angry but also makes the child feel worthless. Failure to comply with parental expectations is viewed by the parents as stubbornness or meanness on the part of the child, behavior which they have a moral duty to correct; punishment is viewed as instructive.

The child is expected to be good. Discipline is inconsistent, and the child never knows what to expect. He may be laughed at for a certain behavior one day and slapped for it the next. The child quickly learns that his parents' moods determine their responses to him.

Emotional dependence is not permitted, nor is it actually possible; the infant quickly learns he cannot depend on others to satisfy his needs. However, independence is also forbidden. The demands for obedience, coupled with total disregard of the child's thoughts and feelings, inhibit the development of mature emotional responses and good judgment in the child.

The child's home is usually not a happy one. There is little laughter. The parents have few outside friends or interests. They fight verbally or physically. The child senses that the outside world is like his inside world, hostile and demanding.

The effects on children brought up in this world of abnormal rearing are profound. They lack basic trust, confidence, and self-worth. These deficits follow them into adulthood and parenthood, where they tend to perpetuate this WAR, the only world they have known.

The Abusing Parent

The abusing parent spent so much time as a child trying to meet his parents' needs that his own childhood needs had to be relinquished. As a result, he did not undergo the emotional development necessary for becoming an adequate parent, not having been loved and cared for and having learned neither to trust others nor to feel good about himself. The immaturity and dependence fostered by the child's WAR are ever-present and continuing problems. The abusive mother is often married to a man who, although he is often passive, sometimes physically abuses her. The abusive parent has a yearning for the love and security he never received as a child. He has a child in order to meet this need and during pregnancy often fantasizes that the baby will provide the love and comfort he missed. Lacking basic trust, the abusive parent is fearful of establishing and maintaining friendships, so he turns to the child for love and affection. The child, unable to comply with these demands, inevitably fails. This failure is seen as a punishable offense by the abusing parent.

The Precipitating Crisis

The crisis that precipitates an act of abuse by an abusogenic parent may not be considered a crisis by others. The event may be as minor as a spilled glass of milk or as major as the loss of a job. Nonetheless, it is an event that triggers an emotional and/or physical outburst at the child.

The Special Child

The abused child may not seem different or abnormal to others, but his abusing parent *perceives* him this way. The infant may not meet his parents' prenatal expectations. He is often the product of a difficult and complicated pregnancy, often delivered by cesarean section, and is frequently premature, necessitating separation from the mother after birth. He may have an obvious birth defect that necessitates the use of outside support systems for the parents. However, the child with mild central nervous system dysfunction is *not* seen as different by others and the parents are offerred no support in caring for him. If the child has a CNS dysfunction, he *will be* difficult to care for. He may be irritable and fussy, cry a lot, or be listless. The child offers little positive feedback to his parents. The abused child may actually invite punishment through provocative behavior; he may be expressing aggression or getting parental attention in the only way he knows.

Recognizing Child Abuse

Although specific laws vary, reporting suspected child abuse is mandatory in every state. Any person reporting in good faith, (i.e., not maliciously) is immune from litigation. A responsible person, such as a teacher, social worker, nurse, or physician, who fails to report a suspected case of child abuse is subject to a fine and/or imprisonment in some states.

Certain conditions are associated with child abuse and neglect. If a child presents with any of these conditions, child abuse should be considered a possible cause.

Inconsistent History

The classic sign of child abuse is a history that is inconsistent with the injury.

Melinda, aged twenty months, was brought to the emergency room by her mother, Mrs. J., who said that the child fell down the back steps. Melinda had a fractured femur and two cracked ribs. The nurse asked Mrs. J. how many steps Melinda fell down. "Three," answered the mother.

Each time the story is told it is changed a little; when not telling the truth, one soon forgets to whom one has told what. Because of this factor, different medical personnel gather different impressions of how the injury was sustained.

Lesions in Different Stages of Healing

Lesions in various stages of healing are indicative of recurrent trauma. New cuts may be superimposed on old scars. Bruises are characteristically seen in different stages of resolution; fresh bruises are purple or blue and progress to green and yellow with age. X-rays reveal unexpected fractures, also in various stages of healing. A full skeletal survey should be taken when a child has multiple skin lesions.

Instrument Imprints on the Skin

Instruments used in beating the child leave their imprint; scars in the shape of belt buckles, looped appliance cords, and coat hangers are common (Color Plate 1).

Characteristic Lesions

Cigarette burns, typical bruising patterns, and wringer injuries are commonly seen. *Wringer injuries,* evidenced by bruising and necrosis of the elbow, are caused by twisting the child's arm and compressing it against his back (Figure 3–11). Head injuries are the most frequent cause of death and irreversible cerebral damage in the abused child and are often caused by the "whip-lash syndrome" or "baby-shaking" when the adult shakes the baby violently. The skulls of small babies are very fragile and often show a typical *eggshell fracture* pattern. However, eggshell fractures are not limited to the infant; they may also be seen after a direct blow to the skull of the older child as well. Internal abdominal injuries are the second most common cause of death among abused children and should be suspected in a child with abdominal distress and scattered bruises and skin lesions.

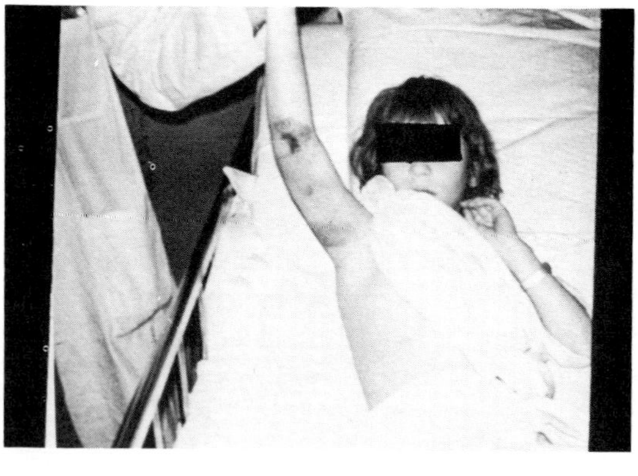

Figure 3–11. *Wringer injury; note the bruising and necrosis of the elbow.* (Courtesy, ten Bensel RW *The Battered Child Syndrome, Famous Teachings in Modern Medicine* New York, Medcom, Inc., 1971.)

Neglect

The abused child is frequently dirty and unkempt, and exhibits other signs of neglect, such as open sores and undernourishment (Color Plate 2).

Family History

Abusing parents often take the child to different hospitals or physicians, making detection more difficult. The family history may reveal abuse of other children in the family.

Parental Indifference

The parents may overreact or underreact to the child's injuries. Although they may voice concern, they are often vague and indifferent toward the child. They may indicate unrealistic expectations of him, saying, "he cries just to upset us," "he's clumsy" or "he's a mean kid." The parents may not visit the child during his hospitalization, or they may fail to show appropriate sympathy for the child. On the other hand, the parents may cling to the child, showing exaggerated concern for him.

Burns that Could Not Possibly be Self-inflicted

Many abused children have severe burns caused by immersion in scalding water (Figure 3–12).

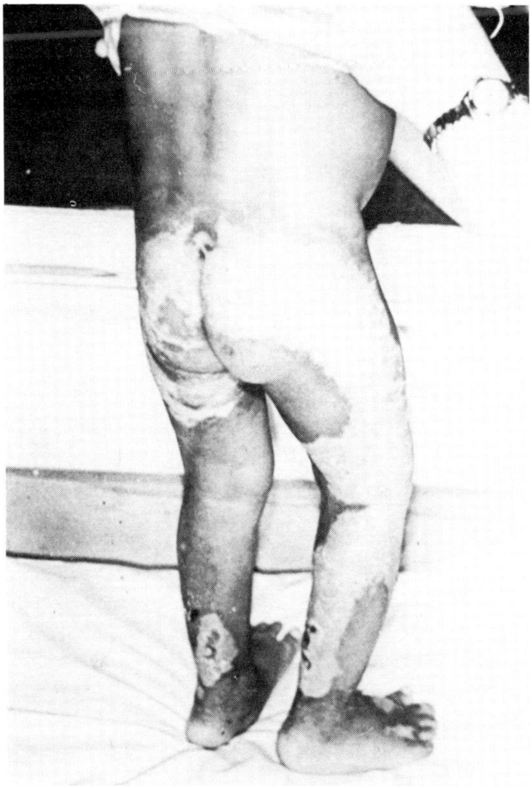

Figure 3–12. *Burns caused by hot liquid on the legs, perineum, and buttocks of a five-month-old girl.* (Courtesy, ten Bensel RW *The Battered Child Syndrome, Famous Teachings in Modern Medicine* New York, Medcom, Inc., 1971.)

The Child Himself

The victim may also provide clues to abuse, even though he rarely admits that his parents beat him. The abused child tends to be wary of contact with adults; he seldom cries and may react with apathy or hopelessness. He may submit passively to painful procedures or may show aggression and hostility in anxiety-provoking situations.

Treatment of Child Abuse

Treatment, concerned primarily with healing the child's injuries and preventing further trauma, often compounds the emotional problems of the abused child. The child is usually hospitalized and separated from his parents. He experiences a loss of the security and the parenting he has known—poor as it may be. The child may be involved in legal and emotional battles that lead to his ultimate removal from the family. It may be years before parental rights are legally severed. These are years of uncertainty as the child is shuttled between foster homes, with little or no opportunity to establish long-lasting and meaningful relationships. By the time legal arrangements are made final, the child is older and no longer an optimal candidate for adoption.

If child abuse or neglect is suspected, the child is usually hospitalized, even if the injury does not warrant hospitalization, unless an emergency shelter or foster home is available. The primary concern is the child's safety, and, without separating the child from the abusers through hospitalization or admission to a temporary shelter, it is difficult to diagnose the child and begin a treatment program with the family.

Ideally, the physician will tell the parents that he cannot determine how the child got hurt, but that he is concerned about it and would like to hospitalize the child, run some tests, and develop a plan of treatment. A nonjudgmental attitude is most important at this time. To accuse the family of abusing the child will only put them on the defensive; they will probably refuse to talk about it and may leave the hospital. These parents are threatened by their inability to keep from harming the child, and the external threat of legal or punitive reprisal only adds to their distress.

Further evidence of their fear of reprisal is manifested in their overconcern with the child. The parents may react with an unusual display of concern. For example, they may not leave the child's side (for fear he will "tell on" them). They may threaten the child with beatings upon his return home.

The mother of fourteen-month-old Becky acted overly concerned about Becky's health. The staff thought she was handling the situation well; however, Becky's mother was overheard to say, "When I get you home you're going to get a beating for being so bad."

In some cases it may be necessary to hospitalize the child without parental consent; this is legal in some states and requires a court order. There is a definite danger in returning the child home if the abusers are not helped to change their behavior. Parents Anonymous is a self-help group with over 800 local chapters. It offers support to abusers from parents who were or are abusers themselves.

Nursing Implications

Hospitalization is frightening to any child, but for the abused child it is even more so. He is used to reading cues from people around him in determining how to behave. The strangers (physicians, nurses, social worker) the child sees in the hospital do not give him the cues he is used to reading, and he is therefore unsure of how to act. This insecurity compounds the usual fears of hospitalization; that is, strange environment, painful procedures, and so on.

Almost all diagnostic and treatment procedures are stressful to the hospitalized child, but for the abused child, they may be overwhelming. If he has suffered a third-degree burn by submersion in hot water, for instance, a whirlpool bath for treatment may be terrifying. If the nurse's feelings make it impossible for her to care for the child and his family, she should acknowledge this fact and ask for another assignment.

Nursing interventions include establishing a trusting, helpful relationship with the parents, one devoid of condemnation. Involve the family in the care of the child, supporting the *strengths* of the parent-child relationship. Promote a sense of the parents' adequacy as parents by assessing their competencies. Build on things the parents do satisfactorily. Having the parents participate in the child's care reduces the trauma of his hospitalization. Even the abused child would rather have a bad mother than no mother at all.

Four-year-old Cathy was admitted to the unit with multiple bloody belt buckle marks. She was pale and weighed only 20 pounds. Her mother, the abuser, was jailed and could not visit Cathy in the hospital. In spite of the abuse, Cathy cried all night for her mother and would not be comforted by the staff.

As you work with the child and his family, demonstrate alternate ways of handling behaviors by role modeling, expressing feelings, and providing discipline. For example, if the child misbehaves, let the parents hear you tell him he cannot watch TV for that night.

Child abuse and neglect is a complex, pervasive problem that requires the concerted efforts of the entire health team. Physicians, nurses, and social workers are all necessary in the fight against the child abuse syndrome. The sad fact is that the health team usually enters the picture "after the fact," when abuse has already occurred. This fact points out the need for parenting classes in the community. We hold classes on expectant childbirth, but we neglect to follow up with classes on child rearing, dealing with the infant, the toddler, and so on. Until the prevention of child abuse and neglect is given as much attention as the treatment, battering and neglect will continue to plague our children.

(Note: For further information on child abuse and its prevention, contact the American Humane Association, Children's Division, 5351 S. Roslyn, Englewood, Colorado 80111.)

SUMMARY

Families differ in composition, role and behavior patterns, and cultural background, yet all experience physical and psychosocial stress. Stress, whether it is sudden and acute or predictable and chronic, demands a response from each family member and from the family as a unit. If the family can identify the sources of stress and use the appropriate resources to reduce the stress and the accompanying anxiety, the family's equilibrium is maintained; however, if the family does not have access to psychosocial, environmental, and economic support, family functioning is thwarted, and each family member will display anxiety-relieving behaviors that may range from physical assault (as in cases of abusing parents) to withdrawal and depression.

Helping families to cope with a crisis and to reestablish or maintain equilibrium requires the use of the nursing process to assess functions and roles within the family and to identify the coping behaviors of family members. By examining the behaviors of children and parents in the family, the nurse can ultimately implement a plan of nursing interventions that will reduce stress during the crisis period and help the family toward optimal functioning and health.

Bibliography

Anthony, E.J. and Koupernik, C. The Child in His Family, in *The Impact of Disease and Death,* vol. 2, New York, John Wiley & Sons, Inc., 1973.

Barnard, N.U. and Wolf, L. Psychosocial Failure to Thrive. *Nursing Clinics of North America* 8:557, 1973.

Barnell, L.M. Crisis Intervention: Partnership in Problem-Solving. *Nursing Clinics of North America* 9:5, 1974.

Beckwith, J.B. *The Sudden Infant Death Syndrome.* Rockville, Md., U.S. Department of Health, Education, and Welfare, Public Health Services Administration, 1977.

Bergman, A.B. Psychological Aspects of Sudden Unexpected Death in Infants and Children. *Pediatric Clinics of North America* 21:115, 1974.

Bergman, A.B. et al. Sudden Infant Death Syndrome, Proceedings of the Second International Conference on Causes of Sudden Death in Infants. Seattle, University of Washington Press, 1970.

Brink, P.J. *Transcultural Nursing: A Book of Readings.* Englewood Cliffs, N.J., Prentice-Hall, 1976.

Brown, M.S. Child Rearing in Cross Cultural Perspective. *Health Values: Achieving High Levels of Wellness* 1:77, 1977.

Burton, L. (ed). *Care of the Child facing Death.* London, Routledge and Kegan Paul, 1974.

Carter, F.M. *Psychosocial Nursing,* ed. 2. New York, Macmillan Co., 1976.

Chase, N.F. *A Child is Being Beaten.* New York, McGraw-Hill, 1976.

Clark, A.L. and Affonso, D.D. Infant Behavior and Maternal Attachment: Two Sides to the Coin. *American Journal Maternal-Child Nursing* 1:94, 1976.

Coombe, E.I. Tuning in on Stress Signals. *Journal of Nursing Education* 15:16, 1976.

Davit, L., Sameshima, Y., Davit, J. Suffering as Viewed in Six Different Cultures, *American Journal of Nursing* 76:1296, 1976.

DiFabio, S. Crisis: A Complex Process. *Nursing Clinics of North America* 9:47, 1974.

Freiberg, K.H. How Parents React When Their Child is Hospitalized. *American Journal of Nursing* 72:1270, 1972.

Friedman, A.S. and Friedman, D.B. Parenting: A Development Process. *Pediatric Annals* 6:564, 1977.

Furman, R.A. The Child's Reaction to Death in the Family, in Schoenberg, B. (ed). *Loss and Grief: Psychological Management in Medical Practice.* New York, Columbia University Press, 1970.

Gil, D.G. Unraveling Child Abuse. *American Journal of Orthopsychiatry* 45:346, 1975.

Glaser, H.H. Hospitals as an Environment for Children and Their Families. *Pediatric Annals* 1:10, 1972.

Goldfogel, L. Working with the Parent of a Dying Child. *American Journal of Nursing* 70:1675, 1970.

Gray, J. and Kempe, R. The Abused Child at Time of Injury, in Martin, H.P. (ed). *The Abused Child: A Multidisciplinary Approach to Developmental Issues and Treatment.* Cambridge, Mass., Ballinger Publishing Co., 1976.

Guilleminault, C. et al. Apneas during Sleep in Infants. Possible Relationship with Sudden Infant Death Syndrome. *Science* 190:677, 1975.

Gyulay, J. *The Dying Child.* New York, McGraw-Hill, 1978.

Hall, J.E. and Eaver, B. (eds). *Nursing of Families in Crisis.* Philadelphia, J.B. Lippincott Co., 1972.

Hardgrove, C.B. and Dawson, R.B. *Parents and Children in the Hospital: The Family's Role in Pediatrics.* Boston, Little, Brown and Co., 1972.

Hardgrove, C. and Warrick, L.M. How Shall We Tell the Children? *American Journal of Nursing* 74:448, 1974.

Harrison, L.L. Nursing Intervention with the Failure-to-Thrive Family. *American Journal Maternal-Child Nursing* 1:111, 1976.

Helfer, R.E. *Childhood Comes First.* Michigan, Ray E. Helfer, 1978.

Helfer, R.E. and Kempe, C.H., Child Abuse and Neglect: The Family and the Community Cambridge, Mass., Ballinger Publishing Co., 1976.

Helfer, R.E. and Kempe, C.H. *(eds). The Battered Child.* Chicago, University of Chicago Press, 1974.

Hufton, J.W. and Oates, R.K. Nonorganic Failure to Thrive: A Long-term Follow-up. *Pediatrics* 59:73, 1977.

James, V.L. and Wheeler, W.E. The Care by Parent Unit. *Pediatrics* 43:488, 1969.

Johnson, M. Folk Beliefs and Ethnocultural Behavior in Pediatrics: Medicine or Magic. *Nursing Clinics of North America* 12:77, 1977.

Kastenbaum, R. and Aisenberg, R. *The Psychology of Death.* New York, Springer Publishing Co., 1976.

Kavanaugh, R.E. Dealing Naturally with the Dying. *Nursing '76* 6:23, October 1976.

Kempe, C.H. and Heifer, R.E. *Helping the Battered Child and His Family.* Philadelphia, J.B. Lippincott Co., 1972.

Kennedy, J.C. The High-Risk Maternal-Infant Acquaintance Process. *Nursing Clinics of North America* 8:549, 1973.

Kennell, J., Voos, B., Klaus, M. Parent-Infant Bonding, in Helfer, R.E. and Kempe, C.H. (eds). *Child Abuse and Neglect: The Family and the Community* Cambridge, Mass., Ballinger Publishing Co., 1976.

Klaus, M.H. and Kennell, J.H. *Maternal-Infant*

Bonding. St. Louis, C.V. Mosby Co., 1976.

Klinzing, D.R. and Klinzing, D.G. *The Hospitalized Child* Englewood Cliffs, N.J. Prentice-Hall, 1977.

Kübler-Ross, E. *Coping with Death and Dying* (Cassettes) Ross Medical Ass.

———. *On Death and Dying*. New York, Macmillan Co., 1969.

———. A Letter on Dying, in *Dealing with Death and Dying*, Jenkintown, Pa., Intermed Communications, 1977, p. 8.

———. Personal Communication, 1979.

Kübler-Ross, E. and Goleman, D. The Child Will Always Be There, Real Love Doesn't Die. *Psychology Today*. 10:48, 1976.

Leaman, K. Recognizing and Helping the Abused Child. *Nursing '79* 9:64, 1979.

Leininger, M. Cultural Diversities of Health and Nursing Care. *Nursing Clinics of North America* 12:5, 1977.

———. *Transcultural Health Care Issues and Conditions*. F.A. Davis, Co., 1976.

Lidz, T. *The Person*, rev. ed. New York, Basic Books, 1976.

McKeel, N.L. Child Abuse Can Be Prevented. *American Journal of Nursing* 78:1478, 1978.

McKusick, V.A. *Human Genetics*. Englewood Cliffs, N.J., Prentice-Hall, 1964.

Mandell, F. and Wolfe, L.C. Sudden Infant Death Syndrome and Subsequent Pregnancy. *Pediatrics* 56:774, 1975.

Martin, H.P. (ed). *The Abused Child: A Multidisciplinary Approach to Developmental Issues and Treatment*. Cambridge, Mass., Ballinger Publishing Co., 1976.

Martinson, I.M. (ed). *Home Care for the Dying Child: Professional and Family Perspectives*. New York, Appleton-Century-Crofts, 1976.

Mead, M. Understanding Cultural Patterns. *Nursing Outlook* 4:260, 1956.

Miller, C. Working with Parents of High-Risk Children. *American Journal of Nursing* 78:1228, 1978.

Miller, P.G. and Ozga, J. Mommy, What Happens When I Die? *Nursing Digest* 2:77, 1974.

Naeye, R.L. et al. Sudden Infant Death Syndrome Temperament before Death. *Journal of Pediatrics* 88:511, 1976.

Nakushian, J.M. Restoring Parent's Equilibrium after Sudden Infant Death. *American Journal of Nursing* 76:1600, 1976.

Neill, K. and Kauffman, C. Care of the Hospitalized Child and His Family: Nursing Implications. *American Journal Maternal-Child Nursing* 1:117, 1976.

Newberger, E.H. and Hyde, J.N. Child-Abuse: Principles and Implications of Current Pediatric Practice. *Pediatric Clinics of North America* 22:695, 1975.

Nissen, C. The Case for Parent-Child Nursing. *RN* 32:80, 1969.

Nitowsky, H.M. Genetic Principles in Pediatrics, in Barnett, (ed). *Pediatrics*, ed. 16. New York, Appleton-Century-Crofts, 1977, p. 295.

Overfield, T. Biological Variation: Concepts from Physical Anthropology. *Nursing Clinics of North America* 12:19, 1977.

Patterson, K. and Pomeroy, M.R. Nursing Care Begins after Death When the Disease is Sudden Infant Death Syndrome. *Nursing '74* 4:85, 1974.

Petrillo, M. and Sanger, S. *Emotional Care of Hospitalized Children*. Philadelphia, J.B. Lippinocott Co., 1972.

Petrillo, M. and Sanger, S. *Emotional Care of the Hospitalized Children*. Philadelphia, J.B. Lippincott Co., 1972.

Primeaux, M. Caring for the American Indian Patient. *American Journal of Nursing* 77:91, 1977.

Prugh, D.G. et al. A Study of the Emotional Reactions of Children and Families to Hospitalization and Illness. *American Journal of Orthopsychiatry* 23:70, 1953.

Robertson, J. *Young Children in Hospitals*. London, Tavistock Institute of Human Relations, 1970.

Schowalter, J.E. Death and the Pediatric Nurse. *Journal of Thanatology* 1:81, 1971.

Selye, H. Further Thoughts on Stress without Distress. *Medical Times* 104:125, 1976.

———. Secret of Coping with Stress. *US News and World Report* 82:51, 1977.

———. Forty Years of Stress Research: Principal Remaining Problems and Misconceptions. *Canadian Medical Journal* 115:53, 1976.

———. *Stress Without Distress.* Philadelphia, J.B. Lippincott Co., 1977.

Sheer, B.L. Help for Parents in a Difficult Job—Broaching the Subject of Death. *American Journal Maternal-Child Nursing* 2:320, 1977.

Starbuck, G.W. The Recognition and Early Management of Child Abuse. *Pediatric Annals* 5:146, 1976.

Steele, B.F. *Working with Abusive Parents from a Psychiatric Point of View.* Washington, D.C., U.S. Department of Health, Education and Welfare, 1975.

Szybist, C. *The Subsequent Child.* New York, National Sudden Infant Death Syndrome Foundation.

ten Bensel, R.W. Personal Communication. Professor, School of Public Health, Minneapolis, University of Minnesota, 1979.

Tinkham, C.W. and Voorhies, E.F. *Community Health Nursing.* New York, Appleton-Century-Crofts, 1977.

Tseng, V.S., McDermott, J.F., Fukunaya, C.S. Family Diagnosis and Classification. *Journal of Child Psychiatry* 15:15, 1976.

Valdes-Dapens, M.A. The Sudden Infant Death Syndrome—Current Knowledge. *Florida's Health* 68:81, 1976.

Visintainer, M.A. and Walfer, J.A. Psychological Preparation for Surgical Pediatric Patients: The Effect on Children and Parents Stress Reponses and Adjustment. *Pediatrics* 56:187, 1975.

White, E.H. Giving Health Care to Minority Patients. *Nursing Clinics of North America* 12:27, 1977.

PART II

The Changing Child

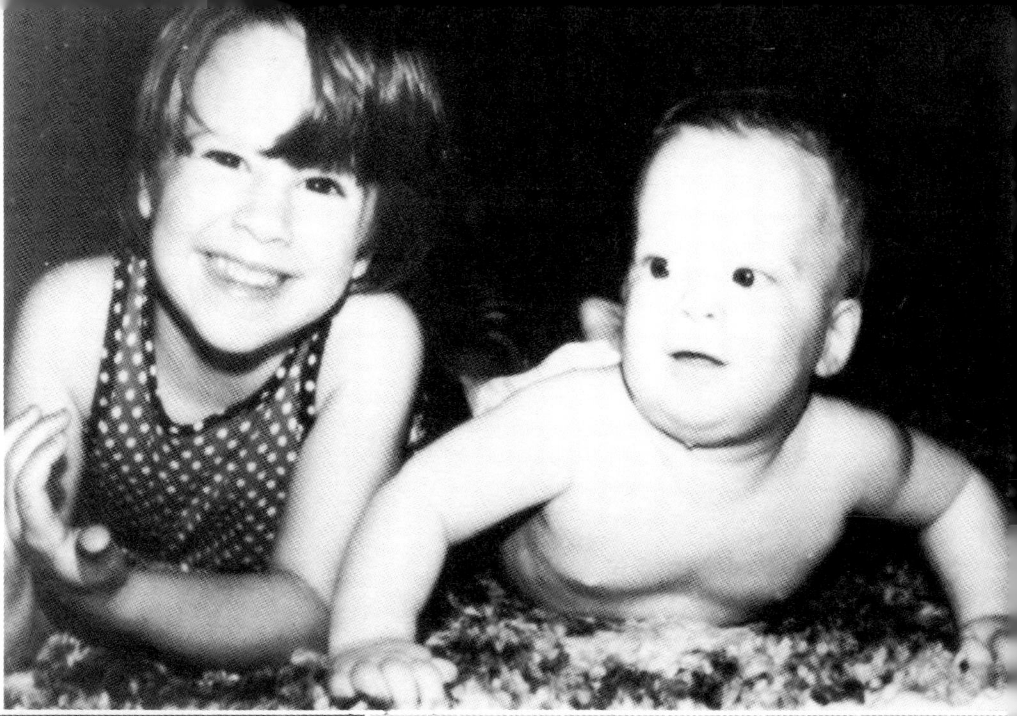
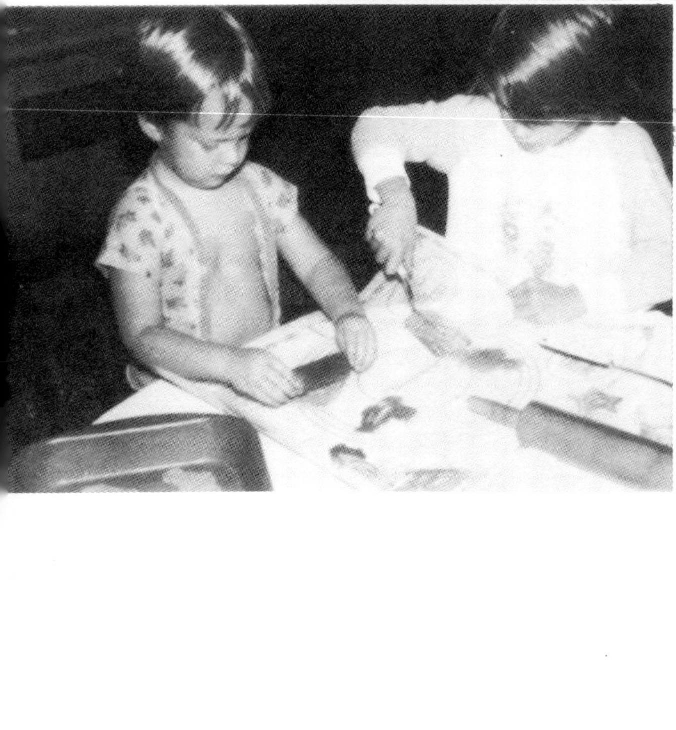
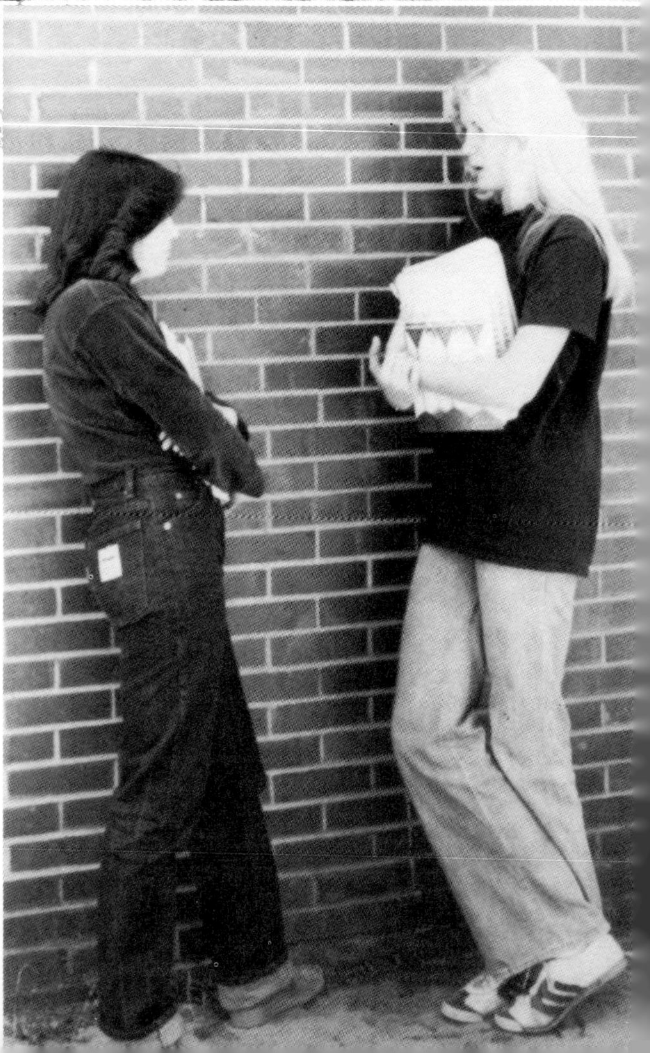

Introduction to Part II

Part II comprises chapters that deal with the developing child. Since each age and stage of development is different, you must have a basic understanding of each if you are to provide appropriate nursing care on the pediatric acute care unit. Parents will frequently ask your advice about their child's everyday problems or about parenting in general. They will listen to what you say and may go to great lengths to follow your instructions. Each chapter is divided into different aspects of development, but each aspect is so interrelated with the others that the divisions are, at best, artificial.

The child's development is governed by several principles. First, children progress through the same sequence of developmental tasks, but an individual child may do so at a rate different from the average. Occasionally, parents cannot remember the achievement of a specific task, such as crawling, but generally the child does sit, pull up, stand, walk, and so on in a predictable order. He may move so quickly that a stage goes unnoticed by his parents, or so slowly that no changes are noticed for a while. Second, development progresses from head to tail (*cephalocaudal* development) and from center of the body to the extremities because the nervous system matures along these routes. The infant, therefore, raises his head, then his shoulders, then sits, etc. He uses his upper arms, then his lower arms, then hands, and finally, the fingers. Third, movements advance from the simple and undifferentiated to the complex and specific. For example, the young infant can only close his fingers around an object. When he is older, he can use his thumb and an opposing finger to pick up small objects or to hold a pencil for scribbling and, later, for drawing pictures. Parenting, formal education, and nursing interventions must all be based on a working knowledge of these principles.

Probably the most popular screening tool for assessing the child's development is the Denver Developmental Screening Test (DDST), a standardized test used to identify the child who might have a developmental problem (Figure II–1). This tool is designed to assess the personal-social, fine motor-adaptive, gross motor, and language development of the child from birth to six years of age. The DDST is widely used by a variety of professional and nonprofessional health personnel, some of whom have had little or no preparation for administering the test. Unfortunately, this lack of adequately prepared testers has caused some decreased confidence in the test and its findings. It is very important for you to study the DDST manual and to view the films before attempting to administer the test. Once you acquire the ability to ad-

DENVER DEVELOPMENTAL SCREENING TEST

STO. = STOMACH
SIT = SITTING

PERCENT OF CHILDREN PASSING: 25, 50, 75, 90

May pass by report → R
Footnote No. - see back of form → 1
Test item

Date

Name

Birthdate

Hosp. No.

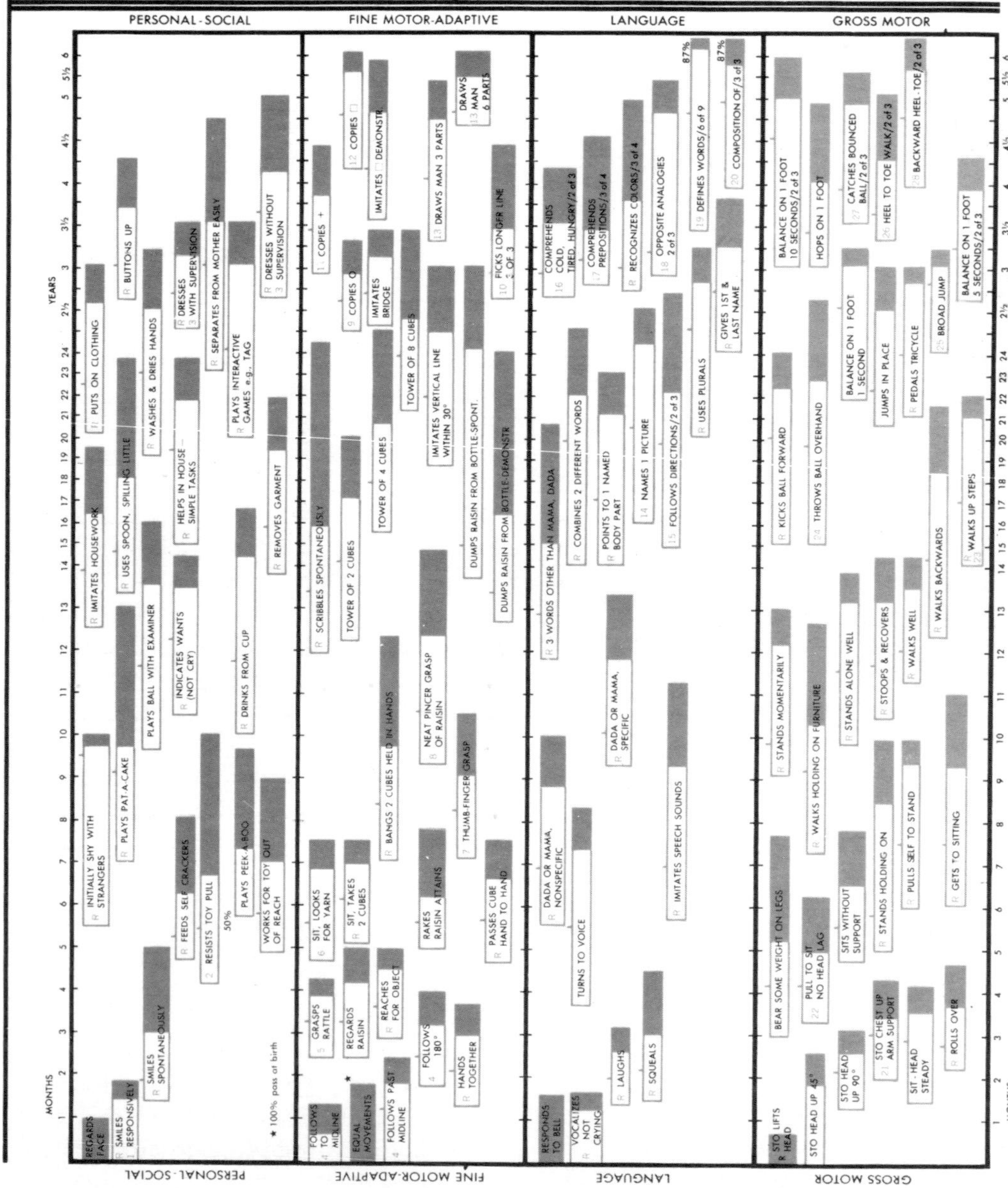

1. Try to get child to smile by smiling, talking or waving to him. Do not touch him.
2. When child is playing with toy, pull it away from him. Pass if he resists.
3. Child does not have to be able to tie shoes or button in the back.
4. Move yarn slowly in an arc from one side to the other, about 6" above child's face. Pass if eyes follow 90° to midline. (Past midline; 180°)
5. Pass if child grasps rattle when it is touched to the backs or tips of fingers.
6. Pass if child continues to look where yarn disappeared or tries to see where it went. Yarn should be dropped quickly from sight from tester's hand without arm movement.
7. Pass if child picks up raisin with any part of thumb and a finger.
8. Pass if child picks up raisin with the ends of thumb and index finger using an over hand approach.

9. Pass any enclosed form. Fail continuous round motions.

10. Which line is longer? (Not bigger.) Turn paper upside down and repeat. (3/3 or 5/6)

11. Pass any crossing lines.

12. Have child copy first. If failed, demonstrate

When giving items 9, 11 and 12, do not name the forms. Do not demonstrate 9 and 11.

13. When scoring, each pair (2 arms, 2 legs, etc.) counts as one part.
14. Point to picture and have child name it. (No credit is given for sounds only.)

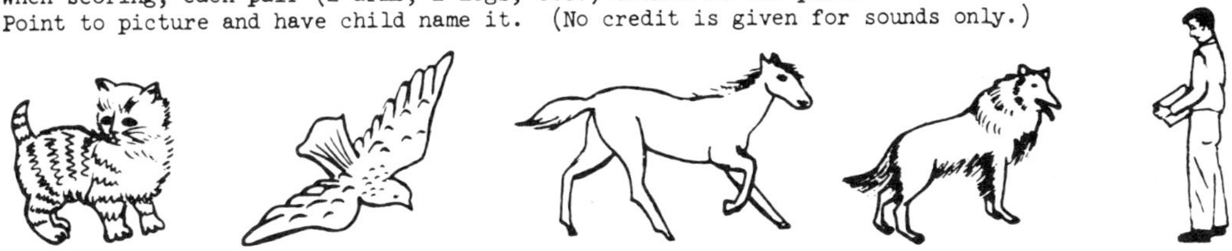

15. Tell child to: Give block to Mommie; put block on table; put block on floor. Pass 2 of 3. (Do not help child by pointing, moving head or eyes.)
16. Ask child: What do you do when you are cold? ..hungry? ..tired? Pass 2 of 3.
17. Tell child to: Put block on table; under table; in front of chair, behind chair. Pass 3 of 4. (Do not help child by pointing, moving head or eyes.)
18. Ask child: If fire is hot, ice is ?; Mother is a woman, Dad is a ?; a horse is big, a mouse is ?. Pass 2 of 3.
19. Ask child: What is a ball? ..lake? ..desk? ..house? ..banana? ..curtain? ..ceiling? ..hedge? ..pavement? Pass if defined in terms of use, shape, what it is made of or general category (such as banana is fruit, not just yellow). Pass 6 of 9.
20. Ask child: What is a spoon made of? ..a shoe made of? ..a door made of? (No other objects may be substituted.) Pass 3 of 3.
21. When placed on stomach, child lifts chest off table with support of forearms and/or hands.
22. When child is on back, grasp his hands and pull him to sitting. Pass if head does not hang back.
23. Child may use wall or rail only, not person. May not crawl.
24. Child must throw ball overhand 3 feet to within arm's reach of tester.
25. Child must perform standing broad jump over width of test sheet. (8-1/2 inches)
26. Tell child to walk forward, heel within 1 inch of toe. Tester may demonstrate. Child must walk 4 consecutive steps, 2 out of 3 trials.
27. Bounce ball to child who should stand 3 feet away from tester. Child must catch ball with hands, not arms, 2 out of 3 trials.
28. Tell child to walk backward, toe within 1 inch of heel. Tester may demonstrate. Child must walk 4 consecutive steps, 2 out of 3 trials.

DATE AND BEHAVIORAL OBSERVATIONS (how child feels at time of test, relation to tester, attention span, verbal behavior, self-confidence, etc,):

minister the DDST correctly, you will be able to determine the child's need for further evaluation. The acute care unit is not a good place to administer the DDST because the child is under tremendous stress, but it is occasionally useful to have an idea of the child's developmental level at the time of his hospitalization.

Throughout Part II, parenting guides for all aspects of development are based on first recognizing *cues* that the child is ready for change and the use of *gradualism, consistency,* and *flexibility* to encourage the change. Parents who have either an academic background in development or much experience with children may have no trouble identifying signs of readiness for change. Often, however, parents must be told about the cues that indicate that their child is ready to give up his pacifier, to begin potty training, or to discuss death, and so forth. Gradualism is important in that it gives the child an opportunity to become familiar with the "new" before he gives up the "old and familiar," whether it is changing to a new bed or to the routine of going to the potty. Consistency in parental limits, routines, and expectations makes the child feel safe; he is secure in the knowledge that these decisions are firm, so he is able to direct his energies toward the tasks at hand: playing, learning, exploring, creating, and so on. Without consistency, the child is confused and wastes time and effort trying to make decisions about what is safe to do. Flexibility in parenting shows the child that any rule, routine, or expectation may be changed to meet certain unusual needs. Parents may need to remove a restriction because it is no longer necessary, as in the case of allowing a child to walk up and down stairs alone when he demonstrates skill in doing so; the parent must be consistent yet flexible, according to need.

EMOTIONAL DEVELOPMENT

The child's emotional development progresses through the stages described by Erik Erikson, whose summarizing terms describing both positive and negative resolutions of emotional conflicts is helpful in understanding the child's behavior. The following list, giving potential outcomes of each stage, will provide the framework for each chapter in Part II.

Infancy: Trust *vs.* Mistrust

Toddlerhood: Autonomy *vs.* Shame and Doubt

Preschool: Initiative *vs.* Guilt

School Age: Industry *vs.* Inferiority

Adolescence: Identity *vs.* Role Diffusion

The importance of the family, school, and peers is discussed in relation to each stage of emotional development, and ways to promote positive outcomes are given.

COGNITIVE DEVELOPMENT

Cognition (i.e., "knowing") develops in the logical manner psychologist Jean Piaget observed in his own children. Piaget labeled the stages *sensorimotor* (birth to two years), *preoperational* (two to seven years), the stage of *concrete operations* (seven to eleven years), and the stage of *formal operations* (eleven years and older). These divisions of cognitive development do not correspond exactly to the stages of development discussed in each chapter of Part

II; nevertheless, Piaget's concepts will be incorporated into each chapter's discussion of cognitive development.

LANGUAGE DEVELOPMENT

The development of language is so closely related to cognition that the two faculties progress together. Language is also related to physical factors such as sex, hearing, vision, and the structure of the speaking apparatus, and to such psychosocial factors as socioeconomic class, number of siblings, birth order, and number of languages spoken in the home. The Denver Development Screening Test can serve to identify the child who needs further evaluation by a speech pathologist (see Table II–1). The Denver Articulation Screening Test (DASE) may be used to detect articulation abnormalities during the preschool period.

GROWTH AND PHYSICAL CHANGES

Growth in the child occurs in predictable spurts that usually form a relatively smooth curve if plotted on a graph. Growth charts show a variety of percentiles for such measurements as weight and height that allows a comparison between the individual child's growth and that of other children his age. Since physical stature is highly

Table II–1. Normal Speech and Language Development

Age	*Speech*	*Language*
1 month	Throaty sounds	
2 months	Vowel sounds ("eh"), coos	
2½ months	Squeals	
3 months	Babbles, initial vowels	
4 months	Guttural sounds ("ah," "goo")	
7 months	Imitates speech sounds	
10 months		"Dada" or "Mama" nonspecifically.
12 months		One word other than Mama or Dada.
13 months		Three words.
15–18 months	Jargon (language of his own)	Six words.
21–24 months		2- to 3-word phrases.
2 years	Vowels uttered correctly	Approximately 270 words; uses pronouns.
3 years	Some degree of hesitancy and uncertainty common	Approximately 900 words; intelligible 4-word phrases.
4 years		Approximately 1540 words; intelligible 5-word phrases or sentences.
6 years		Approximately 2560 words; intelligible 6- or 7-word sentences.
7–8 years	Adult proficiency	

Reproduced, with permission, from Kempe, C.H., Silver, H.K., O'Brien, D. (ed). *Current Pediatric Diagnosis & Treatment,* ed. 5. Copyright 1978 by Lange Medical Publications, Los Altos, California, *Ch. 2. Growth & Development.*

valued in our society, parents often need the reassurance that their child's increase in size is appropriate for his age, even if he has grown very little (see Figures II–2—II–5). An individual child may grow to more or less than the average size for his age but may still show normal gains in relation to his previous measurements. When a child is above the 95th percentile (i.e., when more than 95 percent of all children his age are not as heavy and/or tall as he) or below the 5th percentile (95 percent of all children his age are heavier and/or taller than he), he needs medical evaluation.

Body systems mature continuously but at different rates. This accounts for the fact that changes in body proportions, vital signs, blood pressure, vision, whole blood components, immunity, and genitalia are not necessarily parallel at each developmental stage. Tables II–2—II–4 show normal values for various physiological changes that occur with age.

MOTOR DEVELOPMENT

Motor development is dependent on not only the neurological and musculoskeletal systems but also on opportunities for practice by the child. Even the very basic task of learning to walk can be hastened by allowing the infant freedom to pull up and hold on to furniture, holding his hand while he walks, and praising his attempts to take a step forward. Motor development is related to emotional development in that the child must feel safe to run, jump, and climb and have the desire to try out these skills while risking failure. Movement is also related to cognitive development, especially during infancy when moving largely *is* knowing.

Once the child can perform a task, he repeats it time and time again until it is mastered, often losing interest in other activities. He then turns his attention to a new task. This is true of all skills, but especially of motor development. The infant pulls up on furniture and walks around and around the table, having no other purpose than to walk; the school-age child shuffles cards over and over until he is satisfied with his ability. Improvement with practice gives the child the incentive to achieve a still greater degree of skill.

Parents, nurses, educators, and others who work with the child should facilitate motor play by providing a safe environment, space, time, appropriate materials, and, of course, approval. They must know the child's ability, keeping in mind that development proceeds from head to tail, from the center of the body to the extremeties, and from the general to the specific. The infant is engrossed with learning to move his whole body, while the school-age child is more interested in perfecting specific movements; the toddler is happy with scribbling but the preschooler wants to draw a picture. Knowledge of each age and stage of development will guide you in counseling parents and in providing adequate motor play for the hospitalized child.

NUTRITION

To the average parent, food is love. This feeling may lead them to overfeed their baby, child, or adolescent (or each other, for that matter), or, optimally, to balance the diet carefully. Eating patterns are determined by culture, family preference, economics, peer influence, emotional state, hormonal levels, and many other factors. The child's age and developmental stage af-

BOYS: BIRTH TO 36 MONTHS
PHYSICAL GROWTH
NCHS PERCENTILES*

NAME ____________ RECORD # ____________

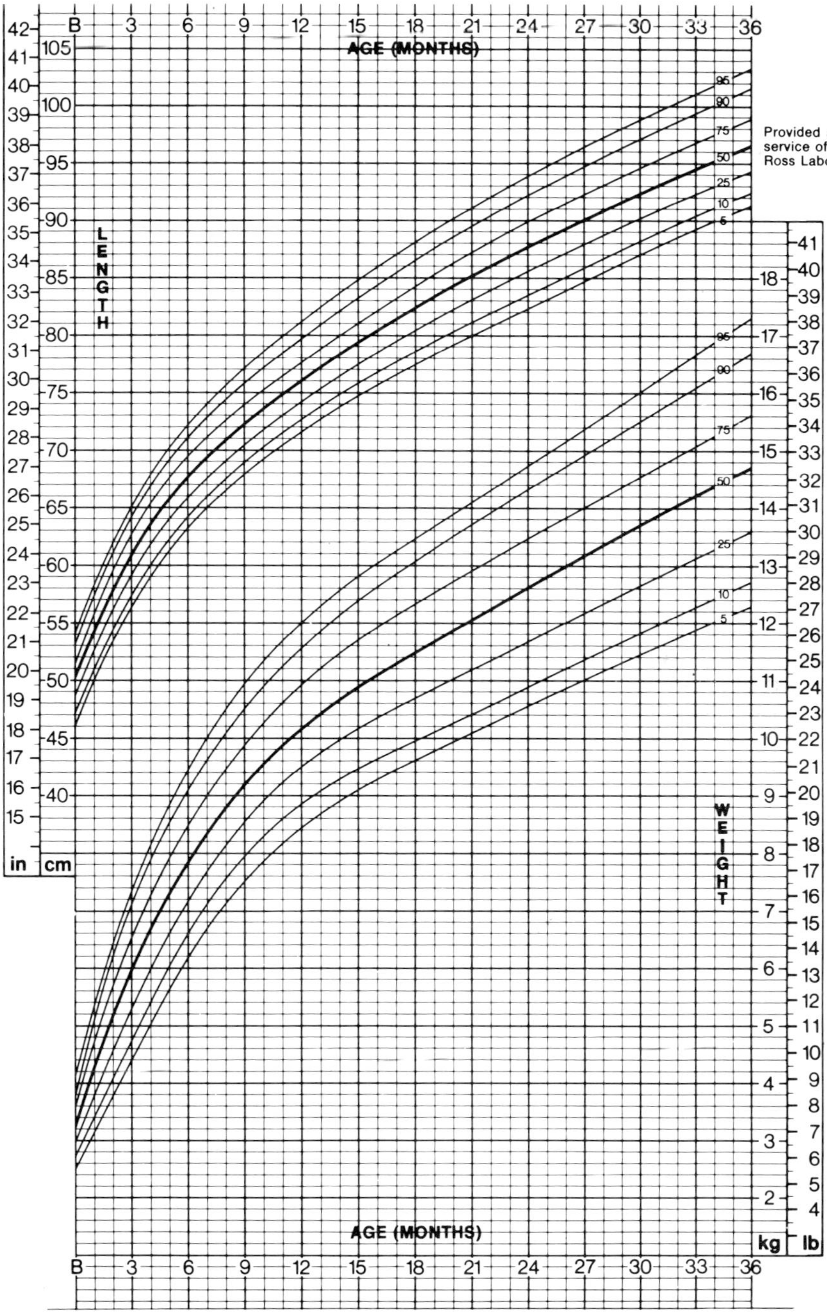

Provided as a service of Ross Laboratories

GIRLS: BIRTH TO 36 MONTHS
PHYSICAL GROWTH
NCHS PERCENTILES*

NAME ______________________ RECORD # ____________

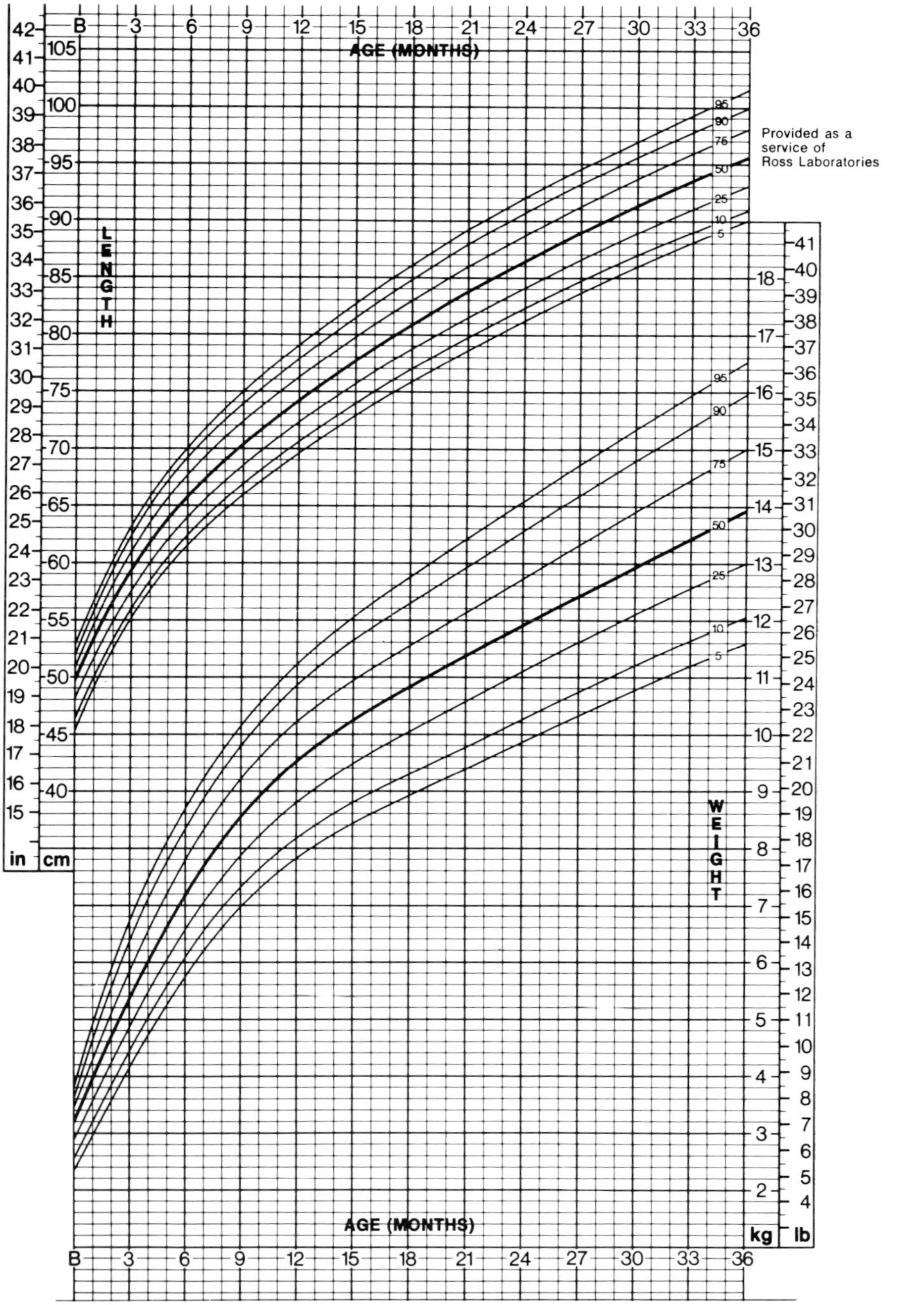

BOYS: PREPUBESCENT
PHYSICAL GROWTH
NCHS PERCENTILES*

NAME ____________________ RECORD # ____________

DATE	AGE	STATURE	WEIGHT

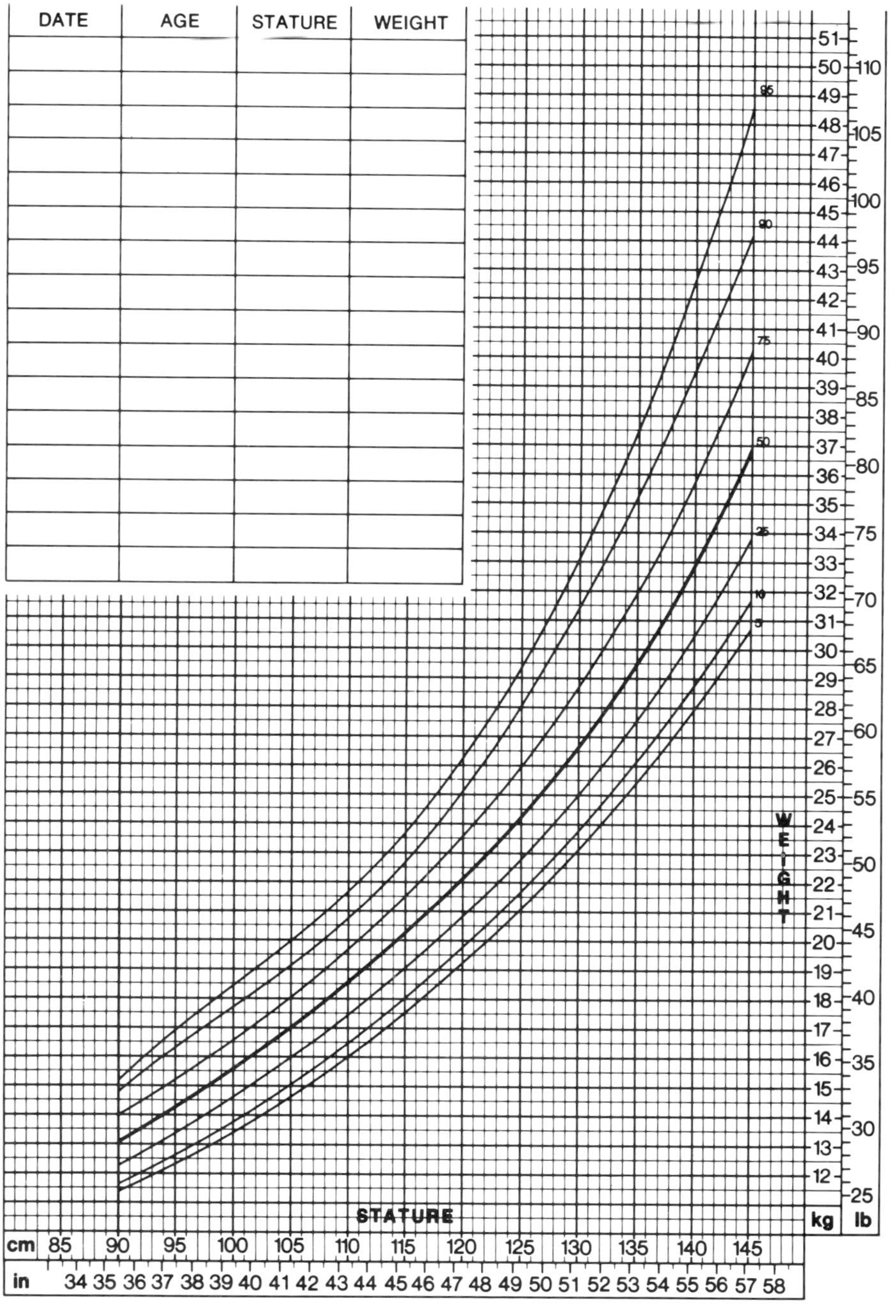

GIRLS: PREPUBESCENT
PHYSICAL GROWTH
NCHS PERCENTILES*

NAME ______________________ RECORD # ____________

DATE	AGE	STATURE	WEIGHT

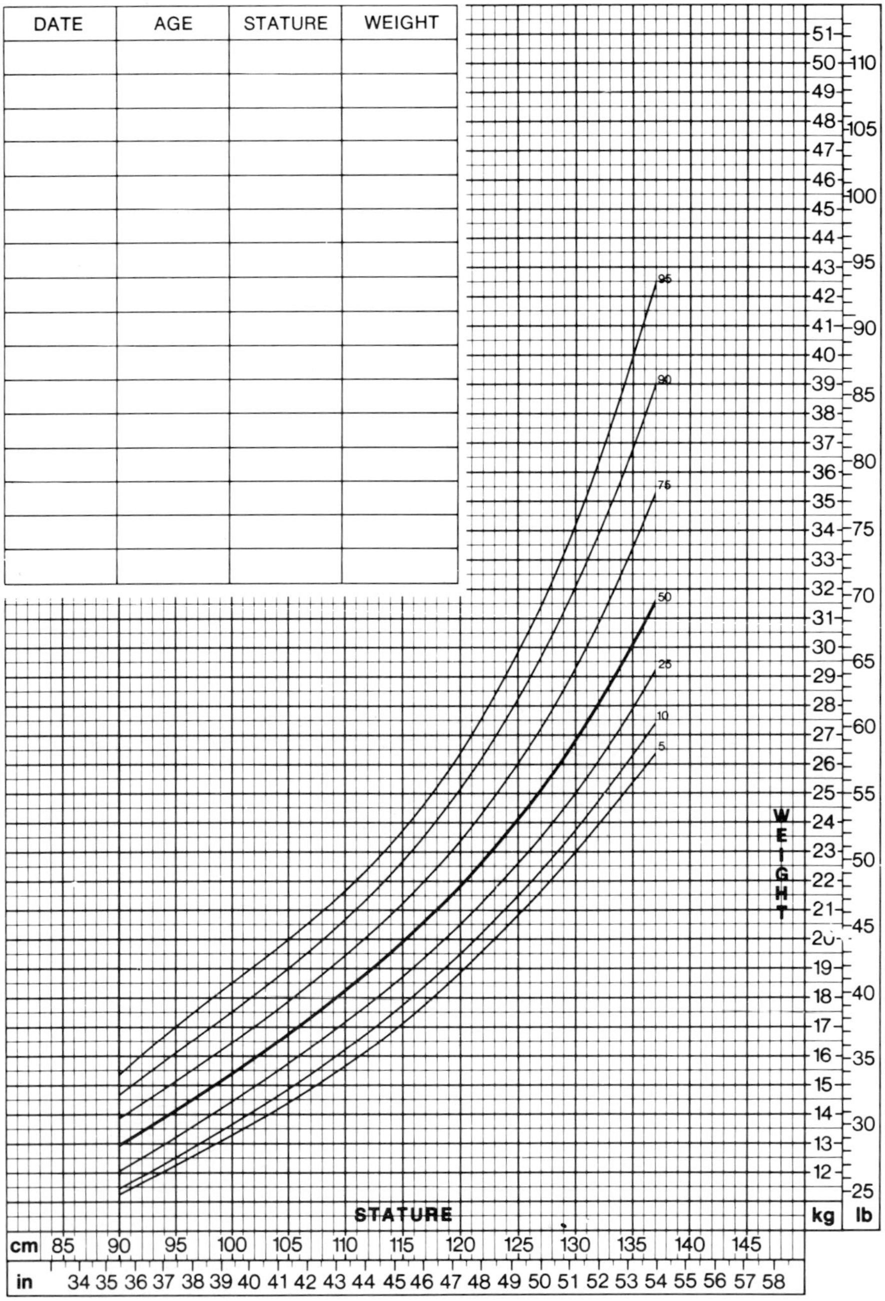

Table II–2. Normal Blood Pressure: Newborn to Age Fourteen

Ages	*$\overline{M}$ Systolic	$\overline{M}$ Diastolic
Newborn	80 ± 16	46 ± 16
6–12 months	89 ± 29	60 ± 10
1 year	96 ± 30	66 ± 25
2 years	99 ± 25	64 ± 25
3 years	100 ± 25	67 ± 23
4 years	99 ± 20	65 ± 20
5–6 years	94 ± 14	55 ± 9
6–7 years	100 ± 15	56 ± 9
7–8 years	102 ± 15	56 ± 8
8–9 years	105 ± 16	57 ± 9
9–10 years	107 ± 16	57 ± 9
10–11 years	111 ± 17	58 ± 10
11–12 years	113 ± 18	59 ± 10
12–13 years	115 ± 19	59 ± 10
13–14 years	118 ± 19	60 ± 10

* $\overline{M}$ = mean

Adapted from Haggerty, R.J., Maroney, M.W., and Nadas, A.S. Essential Hypertension in Infancy and Childhood, *American of Dis. Child* 92:535,1956, Copyright AMA.

fect the type of food he can eat, his appetite, his food preferences, his table manners, and nutritional requirements. An understanding of development is necessary for planning adequate nutrition and maintaining a pleasant dining environment. Table II–5 shows nutritional requirements according to age.

DAILY ROUTINES

Routines are important for the child because they enable him to predict the course of a day, giving him a sense of security. Rigid routines restrict exploration, creativity, and the development of self-discipline; nonexistent or inconsistent routines confuse the child and waste his energy as he tries to make decisions about what to do. Obviously, a balance of flexibility and consistency are as important as routines. Daily routines change drastically with the child's age and stage of development. Their importance to the child changes, too; for example, the very young infant usually does not care when he gets his bath, but the toddler often needs his bath to be part of his bedtime routine. Parents frequently find that new schedules and rituals evolve almost automatically as the child eats new foods, has greater coordination, goes to school, and so on. The child himself makes the decision to begin a new way of doing things. However, some parents may have difficulty in allowing change in their child and may maintain routines that are inappropriate for the child's needs and abilities. they also may enforce restrictions on the child's activities before he can easily adapt to them. As with all parenting, gradual changes according to the child's readiness are best for establishing new routines.

COMMON PROBLEMS

As the child passes through each stage of development, he is likely to have several problems that are typical in children of that stage. The problems are often normal changes that require little or no treatment. You may be tempted to answer a concerned parent's question about a common developmental problem according to common sense or according to your own parents' solution, but you should avoid giving advice without supporting data.

Ms. H., a pediatric nurse specialist, was waiting in Dr. T.'s office when she overheard Ms. P., the office nurse, counsel a parent about a common problem. Ms. H., amazed to hear the incorrect but

Table II–3. Average Ranges of Vital Signs, Boys and Girls to Age Eighteen

Age Range (years)	*Pulse Rate per Minute*		*Respiratory Rate per Minute*		*Mean Body Temperature (°C)*	
	Boys	*Girls*	*Boys*	*Girls*	*Boys*	*Girls*
0–1	132–138	123–129	30–32	29–31	37.3(99.1F)R*	37.3(44.1F)R
1–2	103–107	102–106	25–27	26–28	37.3(99.1F)R	37.2(98.9F)R
2–3	92–94	92–94	24–26	25	37.2(99.0F)R	37.1(98.8F)R
3–4	86–88	88–90	24	24	37.2(98.9F)R	37.0(98.7F)R
4–5	83–85	83–85	23	22	37.0(98.6F)	36.9(98.5F)
5–6	78–80	78–80	22	21	36.9(98.5F)	36.9(98.5F)
6–7	75–77	76–78	21	21	36.9(98.4F)	36.9(98.5F)
7–8	74–76	75–77	20	20	36.8(98.3F)	36.9(98.4F)
8–9	72–74	72–74	20	20	36.8(98.3F)	36.8(98.3F)
9–10	69–71	69–71	19	19	36.7(98.1F)	36.8(98.2F)
10–11	66–68	68–70	19	19	36.7(98.0F)	36.8(98.2F)
11–12	66–68	68–70	19	19	36.7(98.0F)	36.7(98.1F)
12–13	65–67	68–70	19	19	36.6(97.8F)	36.7(98.0F)
13–14	64–66	67–69	19	18	36.5(97.7F)	36.6(97.9F)
14–15	61–63	65–67	18	18	36.4(97.6F)	36.6(97.9F)
15–16	60–62	64–66	17	18	36.3(97.4F)	36.6(97.9F)
16–17	60–62	65–67	17	16–18	36.2(97.3F)	36.6(97.9F)
17–18	59–61	63–67	15–17	16–18	36.2(97.2F)	36.6(97.9F)

*R = rectal temperature.

Adapted from Iliff, A. and Lee, V.A. Pulse Rate, Respiratory Rate, and Body Temperature of Children Between 2 Months and 18 Years. *Child Development* 23:237, 1952.

seemingly logical information offered, was in no position to contradict her. Later, Ms. H asked Dr. T. his opinion, and he offered entirely different solutions from those of the office nurse. The next day Ms. H. sent Dr. T. a set of parent "handouts" based on developmental knowledge with ways to handle common problems. The doctor selected some handouts for the office nurses to use as guides in telephone counseling and made copies to give to parents as needed.

Once you have acquired a knowledge of growth and development, you will be able to formulate solutions to problems without concrete guides. This is also true for parents as they struggle to decide whether to call for help or to handle the situation alone. They are much more able to make appropriate judgments when they have knowledge of their child's age and stage of development.

ACCIDENTS

Accidents are responsible for more deaths in children than any other cause. Certain accidents are more common to each developmental stage than to others: The infant, who is immobile, does not accidentally ingest medicines, as does the toddler; the preschooler on a riding toy is hit by an automobile more often than the toddler, who is usually supervised more closely. The child may be hurt or killed because his par-

Table II–4. Normal Values for Hemoglobins and Hematocrits, Various Ages

	Hemoglobin g/100 ml	*Hematocrits ml/100 ml*
1st day	14–24	54±10
2nd day	15–23	
1 week	13–23	51
2 weeks	15–20	
1 month	11–17	40
2 months	11–14	
3 months	10–13	35
6 months	10.5–14.5	35
1 year	11–15	36
2 years	12–15	37
5 years	12.5–15	37
8–12 years	13–15.5	40
Men	13–18	40–54
Women	11–16	37–47

Adapted from Kempe, C., Henry, Silver, Henry K., O'Brien, Donough: *Current Pediatric Diagnosis and Treatment*, ed. 3. Los Altos, Calif., Lange Medical Publications, 1974.

ents did not know of potential dangers common to their child's age. The child may have an accident because his family is temporarily upset (by a death in the family or a move to another city) or permanently in a state of chaos, leaving the child responsible for his own safety. Regardless of careful adult supervision, the child will inevitably have many accidents. Of course, deaths occur too, usually in freak situations that cause tremendous guilt in parents, siblings, and other survivors.

SIGNS OF ILLNESS

Body systems change in size and function with age, affecting the overall response to illness. The infant and young child have more serious reactions to infection because the immune system is immature, and structures are positioned close enough to allow

Table II–5. Nutritional Requirements According to Age

Age Group	*Infant 9–12 months small servings*	*Toddler 1–2*	*Preschool 3–5*	*School 6–12*	*Adolescent 13–18*
Milk	2 cups/day	2 cups	2 cups	2–3 cups	3–4 cups
Meat	2–3 tablespoons	1–2 servings	1–2 servings	1–2 servings	2 or more servings
Vegetables	4 tablespoons	2 servings besides potatoes, include one dark green leafy or yellow vegetable			
Fruits	4 tablespoons twice a day one citrus	2 servings a day, 1 should be citrus			
Bread/Cereal	4 small servings	2 servings	2–3 servings	3–4 servings	4 or more servings
Calories	100–120 cal/kg	1300	1600	2300	Girls 2500 Boys 3000
Protein	4–6 gm/kg	1.8 gm/kg	1.6 gm/kg	1.5 gm/kg	1.3 gm/kg

Adapted from Fleck, H. *Introduction to Nutrition*, ed. 3. New York. Macmillan, 1976.

rapid spread to adjacent structures. The child's other systems also are not as effective in coping with illness as are the adult's. While the sensitivity of the young child's respiratory and gastrointestinal tracts privides obvious indicators of illness, the larger, older child may not show signs of distress as quickly or at all. The signs of illness in children are the same for all ages, but the character and degree of the indicators vary as the child grows older. This information is helpful to parents who may have little knowledge of such problems as fever, vomiting, and diarrhea in infants and small children, although they understand the significance of these same problems when they themselves are afflicted.

HOSPITALIZATION

The child who is hospitalized for whatever reason is under tremendous stress (sec ch. 3). Just as what is appropriate in parenting, routines, play, and so forth is determined by the child's stage of development, so is nursing care. You must first learn the facts and principles of growth and development; you can then plan the child's care accordingly. You should not be willing to accept hospital rules that are contrary to the needs of the child, such as sending parents home at night, using rectal thermometers for every child under six years of age, and keeping every child in his crib. You have the responsibility of incorporating your knowledge of the principles of growth and development into hospital routines. The tasks of admission, support, preparation for procedures, administration of treatments, provision for play, and planning for discharge are very different for each age and stage. Parents will immediately recognize your knowledge when you allow them to hold their toddler as you take measurements or when you carefully allow privacy as the modest adolescent changes clothes. The child will feel less stress as you anticipate his needs. The application of the principles of growth and development to pediatric nursing care results in a less traumatic (perhaps even positive) experience for both parent and child, and knowing that you have fostered such an experience will be a source of considerable satisfaction to you, the nurse.

CHAPTER 4

The Infant

BEHAVIORAL OBJECTIVES

After studying this chapter you will be able to:

- Describe the infant's emotional development in relation to trust and mistrust.
- Discuss the implications of stranger and separation anxieties in parenting and nursing care.
- Identify methods of stimulating cognitive and language development during infancy.
- Describe physical and motor changes that occur during each quarter of the first year of life.
- Discuss infant nutrition in relation to breast and bottle feeding, introduction of solid foods, and eating with the family.
- List daily activities for the infant.
- Identify appropriate play activities and materials for the infant.
- Identify common problems and accidents that occur during infancy. Give preventive and treatment measures for each.
- Describe signs of illness in the infant.
- Discuss nursing care of the infant and his parents during hospitalization.

TERMS AND CONCEPTS

Trust
Mistrust
Stranger anxiety
Separation anxiety
Peek-a-boo
Sensorimotor stage
Object permanence
Receptive language
Productive language
Cruise
Crawl
Creep
Motor play
Colic
Erythema toxicum neonatorum
Milia
Miliaria
Cradle cap
Constipation
Regurgitation
Genital adhesions
Laryngeal stridor

Nursing care of the infant is best provided by the parents, with the nurse playing a supportive and educational role. There are exceptions, of course, such as those procedures requiring highly technical skills. Generally, however, the nurse cannot and should not attempt to assume the parenting role. Every infant has daily rhythms and preferences known only to the parents.

EMOTIONAL DEVELOPMENT

The infant's emotional development is best discussed as a part of the development of *trust*, which was identified by Erik Erikson as a key factor in the infant's development. The growth of trust is the key interactional process that occurs between the infant and his parents (Figure 4–1). During fetal life, the infant has no wants except perhaps to change position or to suck. Labor and delivery usually create the first stress in the neonate. Later, when physiological needs appear and then somehow disappear regularly, the infant begins to change. His newborn cry is replaced by several cries with different meanings: "I need something right now"; "I need to wind down—just wait this one out"; "I'm moderately uncomfortable—try rocking me." Each time a discomfort occurs, a form, making soft, pleasant sounds, appears close to the infant's face. Often, the form and warmth and rocking and a full stomach all "happen" at the same time. As the infant learns that his needs will be met, he associates the face (or faces) and voice with a sense of trust. This early security is the basis for living the rest of his life.

The younger infant has no understanding of, or capacity for, giving, yet he must re-

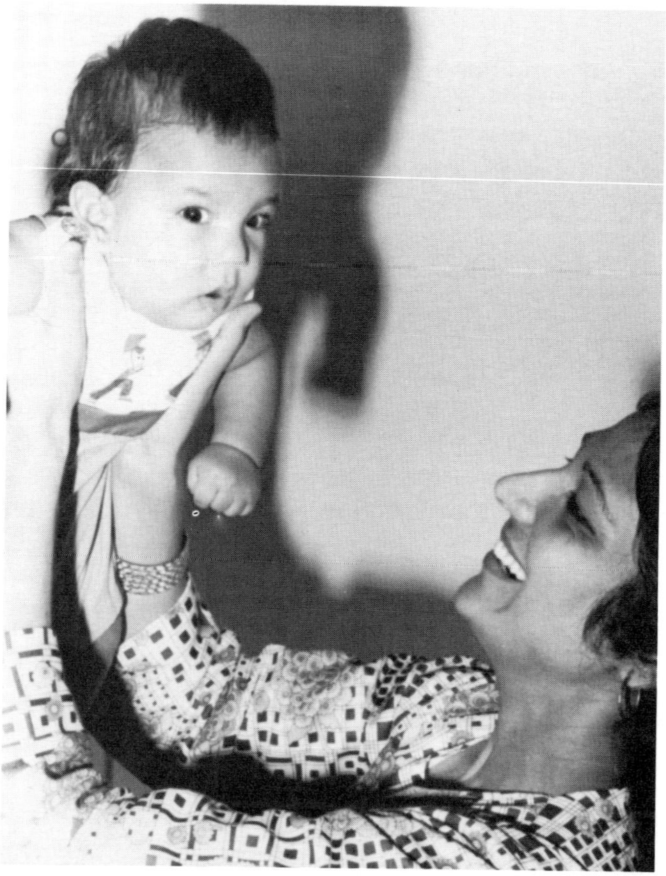

Figure 4–1. *The infant develops a sense of trust.*

ward his parents regularly if they are to meet his physical and emotional needs continuously. Simply going to sleep after a diaper change or a feeding is a gift to his parent, signifying their success and freeing up their time for other things. The infant's obviously curious look at his parent's face is a reward for the long and loving gazes at the infant's face, and cooing is tremendous compensation for the cheery chatter accompanying most child care tasks. A real prize for the parent is the infant's broad smile when the familiar face appears. With each reward, the parent perceives the infant as being "better" than other infants. These normal developmental changes act as potent inducements for parents to continue with previous methods of care and to try new ideas, as well as to provide the rocking, cuddling, and talking that promote the infant's emotional development.

Inevitably, the infant will be faced with a want that is not satisfied quickly enough: a pain is not relieved during illness or the bottle is not warmed during a trip. If the infant's needs are routinely met so that he develops trust, and if the frustration is not too great, he will learn to wait for short, then longer, periods before protesting loudly. The infant, however, may have to learn to live with unmet needs. He may simply give up attempts at communicating distress and turn to himself for gratification. He may receive relief so inconsistently that he begins to sense that he can never depend on his parents. Infants who are cared for inconsistantly lack trust and develop a sense of *mistrust* as a basis for living the rest of their lives.

It seems easy enough to meet an infant's needs. When he cries, his parents must change his diaper, feed him, rock him, keep him warm, or put him to sleep. The family of a first-born infant, however, is typically young, mobile, and lacking in child care experience, adequate funds, and family support. For the first time in her life, the mother may have to stay home with the baby instead of working at a stimulating job. She may arrange for day care yet feel guilty, even if her income is absolutely necessary for survival. She is usually dependent on her husband, family, and friends to provide her with company and news of the "outside" during her child's early infancy. She must resist the urge to demand that her husband focus on her needs as soon as he walks in the door in the evening. The husband is often striving for success in his work; he simply does not have the opportunity for frequent contact with the infant, so he is not as closely bonded to the child. Exceptions are increasing, of course, but the fact remains that most mothers stay home for at least several weeks after the birth, and fathers do not. The father must balance his drive to succeed at work, his desire to participate in hobbies and sports, and his need to support his wife with the need to get to know his baby. He may be jealous of the infant, who demands so much of the mother's energy and time. Both parents must face increased financial requirements. Resentment between husband and wife will occur in the most stable family, even if only transiently. The adaptive family uses its resources to meet the needs of each member, and from this it follows that the adults must make some sacrifices in order to raise a contented newcomer.

The unstable, chaotic family is unable to cope with the many stresses of a helpless newborn and his many needs. For such a family, much energy is spent on the survival of the adult members, and the infant is less likely to develop a strong sense of trust. Occasionally, however, a nurturing adult will consistently provide care even in the worst possible family situation, resulting in the infant's development of trust in spite of the disorder of the family unit.

The infant is born with traits that have profound effects on his parents and others who care for him. Most parents wish for a pretty baby who eats and sleeps with no problems and who stops crying when his needs are removed. Fortunately, most babies meet these expectations except for occasional periods of being inconsolable. There are some newborns, however, who do not sleep much, even in the newborn nursery. Such an infant squirms around in the bassinet until the sides stop him. He may crane his neck over the side, seemingly curious about his environment. These characteristics will thrill outgoing, energetic parents who cope with the baby's long wakeful periods by putting him in a backpack (or a "tummy pouch") and exposing him to their active world. Conversely, the parents who are shy and retiring may become exhausted by simply watching their child's continuous movement. They may try every trick they know to make him sleep, including stuffing him with food, holding a pacifier in his mouth, rocking him for hours, or warming his crib with a heating pad. None of these tactics works, of course, and the parents become more and more frustrated. Imagine how different the two interactional patterns are! One infant is rewarding and rewarded while the other is frustrating and frustrated. The same is true of the sleepy, docile baby who prefers not to do much of anything, and who becomes active later than others his age. Parents who are easygoing may find this infant perfect and may allow him to move at his own pace. Aggressive parents may be disappointed by an infant who doesn't lift his head or lock his knees in a standing position remarkably early. All emotional development is the product of an interaction between the child and those who care for him, and this interaction is obviously affected by the parents' personalities as much as by the child's.

The infant begins to smile and coo at the face he sees over and over. Almost any smiling face with a gentle voice will make him smile until, one day, a strange face brings about a frown or even a cry—a sign of *stranger anxiety*. After the middle of the first year, the infant develops a stronger memory and recognizes new faces as being unfamiliar. The closer the contact with one nurturing person, the earlier and more intense the onset of stranger anxiety, but the phenomenon will usually occur eventually, regardless of how close the infant is to one person. A strange face is better tolerated if the infant's familiar person is nearby. The infant's grandmother can no longer pay an occasional visit and expect the baby to cuddle happily in her arms. The father must make a real effort to spend time with the infant daily in order to avoid the "stranger" reaction. A night out can be a miserable experience during this stage. Parents are faced with leaving their crying infant with a sitter, and, with each call home, they may hear crying in the background. It seems logical to many parents that "slipping out" while the baby plays will prevent the crying spells, but he will cry even more when he finally meets the unfamiliar caretaker. Although stranger anxiety is a normal developmental phenomenon, it can be distressing to the whole family, and parents need preparation for the event before it occurs.

Separation anxiety begins to emerge

around the end of the first year as stranger anxiety subsides a little. The infant is developing an awareness that he is a separate being from his mother, and when she is gone this realization is frightening. He does all he can to prevent separation: crawling from room to room (including the bathroom, of course), clinging to legs or neck when she is about to leave, and screaming for her as she walks out the door. This, too, is normal behavior that parents must expect.

Adam, ten and a half months old, had always played happily in his playpen while his mother went outside briefly to empty the garbage, sweep the porch, or get the mail. One day, when she told him she would be right back, he began to cry and soon he refused to get in the playpen at all. One of the reasons was his need to go with her from room to room. After trial and error, his mother saved all outdoor chores until Adam could be with her, and he tolerated being in his playpen as long as she was in sight. She used the playpen only for safety and kept it in the room where she was working whenever possible.

Explain to parents that stranger and separation anxieties coexist for a while, and that the parents should try to have something very familiar and special for the infant to cling to (i.e., a "security object") during periods of separation. If possible, parents should leave the infant either with a person or in a place that he will recognize. The game of *peek-a-boo* helps the infant learn that a person "out of sight" is not necessarily gone forever. *Always* strongly encourage the parents to say good-bye to the infant before separation. He will learn that good-byes are followed by a distressing need, but also that he will never have to worry that his parents will disappear without warning. He also will develop a sense that they will always return.

COGNITIVE DEVELOPMENT

The infant's intellectual capacity develops as time passes. Because we think verbally whether or not we verbalize our thoughts, the infant's lack of vocabulary requires that he use his perceptions and his mobility to organize a view of the world. At this stage, the infant's cognitive development is said to be in what Piaget calls the *sensorimotor* period. At first, stimuli cause involuntary reactions through reflexes: loud noises elicit the Moro reflex, a touch on the face elicits the rooting reflex, and a stroke on the sole of the foot elicits the Babinski reflex, (see Table 4–1).

In a few weeks after birth, the infant seems to take control of his reflexes and refines them, making them more efficient. He gets to the nipple faster and sucks harder, but he continues to suck for sucking's sake after he is full. He repeats the same, seemingly nonproductive actions over and over again. He opens and closes his hands, moves his arms, and moves his fists to his mouth. At about four months, the infant starts repeating some of the same actions to prolong interesting results, such as toys jumping with each kick in the crib. From around seven to ten months, the infant makes major progress in "knowing." He begins to understand that objects can exist even when they are not in view, a concept that Piaget calls *object permanence;* he will look for an object that "disappears." At the same time, he uses those actions that he repeated over and over (first for no reason, later to prolong interesting effects) to solve a simple problem. The formerly purposeless hitting and kicking is now used to move an object that covers a toy.

At the end of infancy, experimentation and novelty seem to assume priority in

Table 4–1. **Reflexes during Infancy**

Reflex	*Appearance*	*Disappearance*
Cough	Birth	Remains
Moro	Birth	4–7 months
Stepping	2–3 days	3–4 months
Palmar grasping	Birth	5–6 months; replaced by voluntary control
Sucking	Birth	Throughout infancy, especially during sleep; decreases 3–5 months
Rooting	2 days	3–4 months while awake; 9–12 months during sleep
Tonic neck reflex	2–3 months	6 months
Babinski	Birth	1 year

cognitive development. The infant uses trial-and-error to solve a simple problem, but he is not satisfied with the solution; he is interested in trying new and different methods to accomplish the same results. Practicing a new method is just as enjoyable as success in problem solving. Infant behavior progresses from being predominantly reflexive to being purposeful, inventive, and/or investigative.

Parents play a major role in the infant's cognitive development. Simply allowing him to expore his environment while staying near to provide security, they contribute essential ingredients for learning. Whatever the home environment, it is filled with many sights, sounds, and smells that can be safely experienced through the infant's repeated touching, shaking, biting, and tasting. Of course, many play/learning materials can be bought or improvised for additional sensory stimulation. Parents can also foster cognitive development by talking to, touching, carrying, and rocking their infant. Each of these acts provides different learning experiences because they provide many sensations. Interactions with parents (or even a bouncing ball, for that matter) teach the infant that his world responds to his movements, voice, and facial expressions.

LANGUAGE DEVELOPMENT

Very early, even soon after birth, the infant discriminates types of sounds and prefers the human voice. He listens carefully, and in a few months develops *receptive* (understood) *language* before he can produce words with meaning. Crying, of course, is the first vocalization. At about two to three months of age, the infant coos and "talks back" in response to a smiling face to prolong this enjoyable stimulus. (The smiling face is usually talking, but sound is not necessary; deaf babies also coo responsively.) Babbling, a mixture of sounds resembling syllables, occurs during the middle of the first year. Later, the infant doubles syllables such as "da" and "ma" to form *mama* and *dada*, creating such a pleasurable reaction from parents that the infant perceives these sounds as meaningful. By the end of the first year, the infant's *productive* (spoken) *language* consists of two or three words.

Activities that accelerate the mastery of speech include talking to the infant face-to-face, rewarding his vocalizations with smiles and more talking, and identifying common objects by name (e.g., cup, car, ball) each time they are seen. Many parents do not know that talking to a baby is worth the effort. Young mothers may even feel foolish about talking to their infants. However, if you talk to the infant frequently and cheerily, the mother may do the same. Comment on her wisdom if she follows your example. Be sure to discuss the value of verbal stimulation if your assessment indicates a lack of understanding or interest on the mother's part.

GROWTH AND PHYSICAL CHANGES

The size of the newborn varies with sex, race, socioeconomic class, family traits, and fetal health. On the average, boys are larger than girls at birth. White babies in this country are heavier than those of other races.

The limits of growth are genetically determined, but the child's growth may be hampered by illness or environmental deficits. The intrauterine environment may have been lacking in oxygen or essential nutrients, or it may have infected the fetus, either of which conditions can affect birth weight. Once the healthy baby is born, his growth should follow a predictable curve if he is well nourished and cared for (see Figures II–2 to II–5).

The infant's growth assures the parents that the infant's needs are being met, that they are successful as parents, and that no disease is in progress. Unfortunately, some parents feel that any kind of growth is good, and "the more, the better." They may proudly point out how fat the child is, and many people, including nurses, may reinforce this feeling of pride in such an "accomplishment."

Mrs. E., a nursing assistant in the well-baby clinic, had a very matronly appearance. She weighed at least 200 pounds and had a tremendous bosom. She weighed each infant and exclaimed with delight over each fat baby. The smaller babies were also welcomed and hoisted onto that big bosom, but a frown of concern creased Mrs. H.'s face. This initial assessment made a real impact on each mother.

Length is also highly valued, generally more so in boy babies. Above-average length in the girl baby may cause some concern.

"Oh, well," Jodie's mother said, sighing long and loud as she discussed her daughter's length, "I just hope flat shoes are in style when she's a teenager. I don't really mind her being tall, but I was terribly self-conscious during that time, and I wish I could make it easier for her. I still cringe when I tower over pretty, petite girls. Of course, she can always be a model." Jodie's mother sighed again. The nurse noted that this mother's own self-image required further assessment and probable intervention to improve Jodie's chances of accepting her height.

Today's weight-conscious middle class has begun to move away from the "fat, healthy baby" ideal. Many parents want to know how to prevent obesity through nutritional planning.

Two mothers were talking in a pediatrician's office. One was describing her son's enormous increase in weight, which required that he wore clothes made for an eighteen-month-old although he was only seven months old. The other mother snapped, "Fat babies make fat adults."

Always assess the family's feelings about weight, height, growth, food, and how these feelings affect the parents' love for the child in planning counseling.

Proportion

The newborn's head is so large that it comprises 25 percent of the total body length as compared to 10 percent of the adult's total body length. The trunk is close to 50 percent of the total, and the legs make up the rest of the length. The whole body grows rapidly during the first year, but the legs grow at a faster rate than the other parts. The one-year-old still has short legs and looks top-heavy.

Weight

Normal birth weight ranges from 2,500 to 4,300 grams (4.5 to 9.5 pounds) the average being about 3,400 grams (7.5 pounds). The newborn loses up to 10 percent of his birth weight immediately after birth but regains the loss and increases his weight rapidly. He usually doubles his birth weight at around five months and triples it around twelve months. When weighing the infant, undress him to avoid errors due to clothing weight.

Length

Normal length at birth ranges from 47.5 to 53.7 centimeters (19 to 21.5 inches); the average is about 50 centimeters (20 inches). The infant's length usually increases to about 150 percent of his birth length by the end of one year; for one-year-olds, average length is about 66 centimeters (30 inches).

Head Circumference

The average head circumference is 34 to 35 centimeters (13.5 to 14 inches). The newborn whose head measurement deviates more than 2 centimeters from the average may have an abnormal skull or brain, or he may simply have a large-but-normal head. In such cases, a doctor's assessment is necessary in order to identify an anomaly. The head grows rapidly during the first year because the brain is growing and it, too, increases in size predictably. Measure head circumference with a cloth or paper measuring tape around the middle of the forehead and across the most prominent part of the occipital bone in the back; this is the greatest circumference of the head.

Fontanelles (soft spots between the skull bones) and *sutures* (lines where the skull bones meet) allow for growth. Premature closure of the fontanelles and fusing of the sutures result in a small skull that does not allow for brain growth. The posterior fontanelle closes several weeks after birth but the anterior fontanelle closes anytime from the end of the first year until eighteen or nineteen months of age. Bulging fonanelles and/or separated sutures usually indicate intracranial pressure. When recording abnormal head measurements, include a description of the fontanelles, noting any bulging above or sinking below the cranial bones. Asymmetry of the head may indicate a skull anomaly or simply a preference for sleeping on one side, and it may affect the total head measurement. The physician should be alerted in cases of asymmetry.

Chest Circumference

The chest circumference, which is slightly less than that of the head at birth, increases rapidly after birth. It is measured by placing the tape around the chest at the nipple level. Deformities of the chest, including asymmetry barreling and protrusions, may affect the circumference and should be noted along with the measurement.

Teeth

Normally, the infant is born with no teeth. Around four to five months of age, hand-to-mouth activity increases and drooling begins. Most parents will quickly explain that the poor baby is teething, and that any crankiness, low-grade fever, or diarrhea result from his sore gums. Sometimes the parents are right, and cool teething rings or even topical anesthetics are necessary for relief. The infant definitely will want to chew on any available object. The eruption of the central incisors (usually between six and nine months of age) seldom causes discomfort. Because the appearance of teeth mark developmental progress, parents usually are delighted, and, when teeth erupt earlier than expected, they may think the infant is "advanced." By the end of the first year, the child usually has his lower and upper central and lateral incisors, a total of eight teeth. If no teeth erupt by age one, a dentist should be consulted.

Hearing

The infant is born with hearing apparatus in perfect working order. Once the fluid has drained from the external canal and the middle ear, his hearing is as acute as it will be in his lifetime. He is accustomed to a noisy environment in his mother's uterus and then in the newborn nursery, so it is logical that he can tolerate noise at home. If allowed to, he can block out disturbing noises and go to sleep.

Vision

The newborn can focus well at a point a few inches from his face but not at closer or farther points. The lenses of his eyes cannot accommodate (adjust) well enough to focus at varying distances. He can follow a bright, large object from side to side if it moves slowly. By the end of the first year, his visual acuity approaches 20/100 (approximately 20 percent of the normal adult's acuity), and his accommodation enables him to see objects at different distances.

Vital Signs

The newborn's heart rate is very rapid, 120 to 140 beats a minute, and slows very little by one year of age. Always count the infant's heart rate by listening with a stethescope. Respiratory rates range at birth from 30 to 80 breaths per minute; at one year of age, from 20 to 40 breaths per minute. Respirations can be counted by watching the chest or abdomen rise rhythmically or by listening with a stethoscope (see the Skills Manual.) The infant's temperature is slightly higher than the adult norm (see ch. 15).

Blood Pressure

The newborn's blood pressure averages about 80/46, but it increases to approximately 96/66 by one year of age. The "flush" technique gives only an average of systolic and diastolic pressures. Amplifying devices allow the pulse to be easily heard without a stethoscope as the cuff pressure is lowered. Systolic and diastolic pressures can be measured with a properly fitted cuff (see the Skills Manual).

Hemoglobin and Hematocrit

The newborn has unusually high hemoglobin (hgb) and hematocrit (hct) values that drop rapidly during the first days of life (see chapter 21). Hemoglobin concentration is approximately 19 gm/100 ml of blood in the newborn and approximately 12 gm/100 ml of blood in the one-year-old; hematocrit values are approximately 58 ml/100 ml of blood in the newborn and 39 ml/100 ml of blood in the one-year-old. These laboratory values generally are used to assess the child's nutritional status during routine, well-baby visits to the physician or nurse practitioner.

MOTOR DEVELOPMENT

Motor development progresses with cephalocaudal (head-to-tail) maturation of the nervous system and development from the trunk to the extremities. The infant spends much of his time in motor play which increases his muscle strength and tone.

First Quarter (Birth to Three Months)

In the first three months of life, reflexes, which are easily elicited during the first month of life, account for much of the newborn's movements. He sucks, roots, jerks, and spreads his limbs in response to external stimuli. Other activity seems to be random but progresses to repetitive acts (as discussed earlier under "Cognitive Development"). The newborn may be able to lift his head when prone and crawl forward but he usually does not lift his head or turn it from side to side. His head requires support while he is being held in a vertical position. Soon, however, he can lift his head and shoulders (Figure 4–2), and by the end of the first quarter he can hold his head erect and steady while upright. Reflexes weaken significantly during this period as the infant gains more ability in directing his own movements.

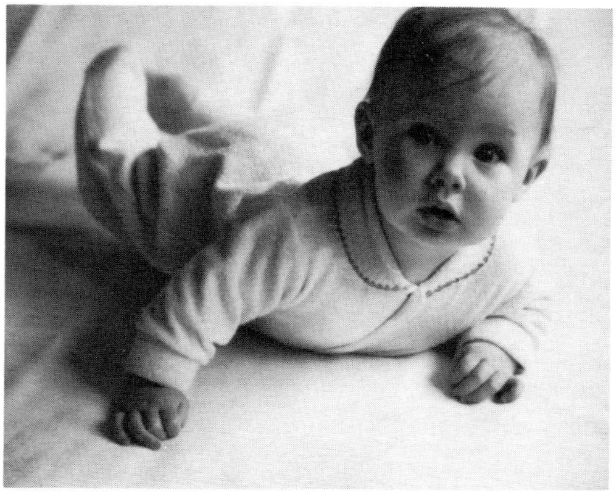

Figure 4–2. *By the end of the first three months, the infant can lift his head and shoulders.*

Second Quarter (Four to Six Months)

In the second quarter, the infant progresses to using his arms, shoulders, and legs to turn over. If pulled to a sitting position, he holds his head in line with his back, allowing no lag. He may be able to sit momentarily without support, but he cannot get to a sitting position alone (Figure 4–3). He may lock his knees and support most of his body weight when balanced by someone. He kicks his legs over and over again, learning more about what his legs can do and strengthening them for walking. He begins to grope for and grasp objects, which he moves to his mouth with perfection.

Third Quarter (Seven to Nine Months)

During the third quarter, the infant can get to the sitting position and stay there until he decides to move. He pulls up on furniture (Figure 4–4) and may *cruise,* that is, walk around his crib or sofa while holding on. He usually begins to *crawl* (abdomen dragging the floor) and *creep* (up on all four extremeties in coordinated movement). He develops an efficient thumb-finger grasp. He can transfer objects from one hand to the other easily and bang two objects together, enjoying the sound it produces. He

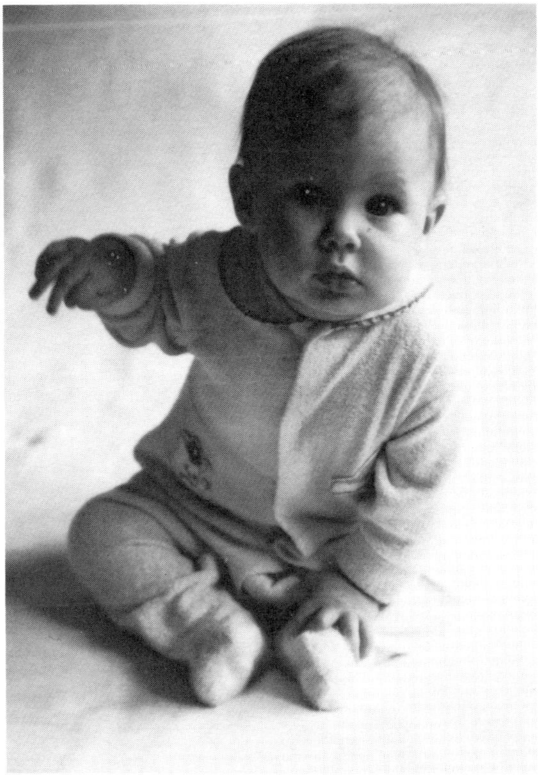

Figure 4–3. *At four months, the infant can sit unaided for a moment.*

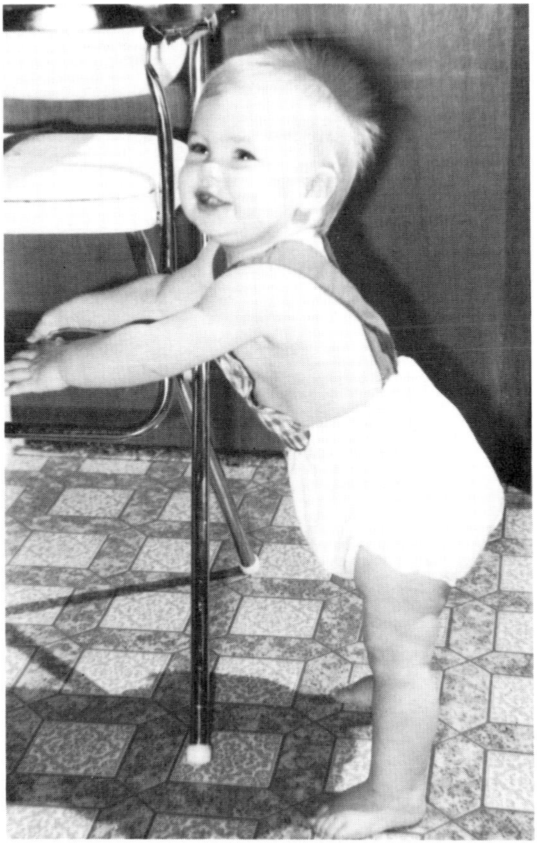

Figure 4–4. *At ten months, the infant can pull up.*

shows a preference for his right or left hand. He can hold his own bottle (often tempting his parents to put him to bed with his bottle, unfortunately).

Fourth Quarter (Ten to Twelve Months)

In the fourth quarter, the infant practices cruising and creeping (Figure 4–5). He changes easiily from lying to sitting to standing. He usually can walk when holding someone's hand, stand alone for a minute or so, and even take a step or two before falling. He enjoys climbing onto furniture, boxes, and up stairs on all fours. He refines his grasp and develops a pincer (thumb-and-forefinger) grasp for small objects, including food. He should be able to use a cup and perhaps even a spoon if he is permitted and encouraged to try with plenty of help.

Thirteen to Fifteen Months

By thirteen to fifteen months, the infant usually progresses from taking a few unsteady steps to confident walking and sometimes even running. He walks for walking's sake, first always forward, then backward. His feet are placed far apart, helping him to balance but giving him a

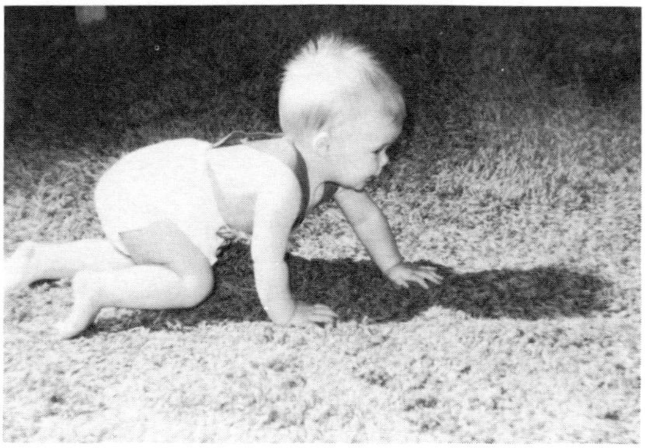

Figure 4–5. *Creeping at twelve months.*

"waddling" walk. He is able to perform the more delicate task of scribbling and stacking two blocks. The child at this age may actually be more toddler than infant, but he still is a "baby."

NUTRITION

The new mother must decide whether to bottle-feed or breast-feed her baby, although she may have made this decision in advance. If she is even slightly doubtful, present the advantages and disadvantages of each, and let her make the decision. Encourage the mother to consult the father in making the decision. Whichever method is selected, support the mother's efforts by providing information and approval.

Breast-feeding was once the only way to nourish the newborn (Figure 4–6). If the mother was unable to breast-feed, a wet-nurse was called in to feed the infant until he was old enough to tolerate other forms of milk. The popularity of breast-feeding declined with the introduction of infant formula except among lower-class mothers who could not afford formula. The use of formula became associated with wealth and status, and poor mothers gave up breast-feeding as soon as they could afford to. Currently, the practice of breast-feeding is widely recognized as beneficial to baby and mother, and many educated families now advocate this form of feeding. Hopefully, other mothers will follow this example. Success with breast-feeding is often a result of sympathetic, knowledgeable care and advice during the mother's hospitalization, usually shortly after she gives birth.

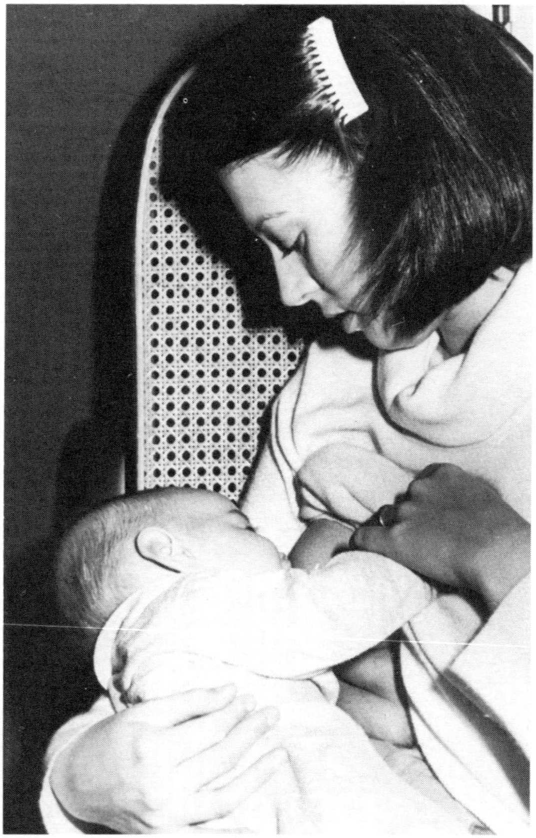

Figure 4–6. *Breast-feeding.*

There are several advantages to breast-feeding, but most of them do not constitute major differences except with regard to protection from infection and allergy. Human milk contains an abundance of immunoglobulins that provide at least partial immunity from a variety of infections. Since the gastrointestinal tract and part of the respiratory tract are coated with these immunoglobulins, the breast-fed infant seldom has gastroenteritis (inflammation of the stomach and intestines), and has fewer respiratory infections. Breast milk almost never results in an allergic reaction or constipation in the infant, whereas formula frequently does. Breast milk has a protein molecule that is easily digested by the infant, but protein in formula can also be digested with little trouble if the infant is normal. Breast milk has more carbohydrate and fat content, which supports body functions, supplies nutrients for neurological development, and saves protein for tissue building. Infant formulas have nearly the same proportion of fats and carbohydrates, and nourish the child sufficiently. Some mothers feel that breast-feeding is much more convenient, since the milk is always sterile, it is the right temperature, is readily available, and contains the right proportions of nutrients. Other mothers feel that bottle-feeding is less trouble since bottles can be prepared in advance, someone else can feed the baby, the mother knows exactly how much the infant drunk, and she does not have to be concerned about her own nutritional and fluid intake affecting her baby's milk. Some fathers advocate breast-feeding, while others do not. Always consider these pros and cons when helping a mother make such an important decision.

In his first few months, the infant needs approximately 110 calories per kilogram (50 calories per pound) every 24 hours. This amounts to 150 milliliters of formula or breast milk per kilogram (2.5 ounces per pound). The gastrointestinal tract can digest a variety of foods early in life, but these are not necessary for satisfactory growth, and most nutritionists recommend that the infant receive only formula or breast milk during the first few months. All recommended vitamins are added to commercially prepared formula and secreted in breast milk if the mother continues to take vitamins prescribed prenatally. The newborn's iron, which was stored for future use, is depleted by around four or five months, so iron must be replaced at that time. Iron-fortified formula and cereals, iron-rich foods, or iron supplement can meet this need.

Solid foods usually are introduced to the infant before six months of age. Each new food is offered one at a time in increasing amounts for three to five days so that any allergies that might develop can be identified. Feeding the infant new food without mixing it with other food allows him to experience different tastes and textures. Combining all foods with cereal, fruit, and/or sugar deprives him of variety. Either plain cereal or green leafy vegetables may be given as first solids to avoid early introduction to sweets. The solid food, pureed and strained, needs to be diluted with formula at first for easy swallowing, but the infant can soon manage thicker consistencies. He usually sticks out his tongue when fed, but this is a normal reaction to anything put in his mouth. Some mothers think this is the infant's way of expressing dislike, but this motion disappears quickly as the child learns to eat more efficiently. The infant will occasionally push food away or refuse to open his mouth; accept this and offer other foods, or simply wait for the next meal. Many families prepare infant foods from unseasoned family foods, using a blender. Commercially prepared baby foods are expensive but satisfactory, except for mixed dinners, which have relatively little protein and much carbohydrate content.

As soon as the baby can sit in a high chair (around the middle of his first year), he should be seated at the table during the family's mealtime if he is awake. This is the perfect opportunity to enhance social skills, including the sharing of food and the use of eating utensils. The infant can be encouraged to try his parents' food and to begin learning to drink from a glass and use a spoon. Increasing the child's intake from the family table also makes weaning from the bottle or breast much easier. He simply does not need as much milk from the breast or bottle. If milk is used to pacify the infant during any and all stress, he may reject all solids and develop *milk anemia,* an iron deficiency anemia (see Ch. 24). If he is allowed to take his bottle to bed, milk left in his mouth can cause severe tooth decay. If he enjoys a bottle or breast and has none of these problems, and if parents approve, there is probably no good reason for weaning. Since our society generally frowns on the mother who delays weaning beyond the first year, however, she may welcome the nurse's approval if she wishes to postpone weaning.

Lt. and Mrs. G. had three children in three years. The lieutenant had very short tours of duty, requiring five moves during that time. Mrs. G. kept all three children on a bottle for convenience. There was no danger of spilling while cleaning, staying in motels, and riding in the car. The children were allowed to drink from a cup at the table only. Mrs. G. received much criticism from her parents and neighbors, but she disregarded it totally. Once they settled down for an extended tour, the children were allowed to throw their bottles away for good.

Mrs. R. breast-fed Glen for a year. Each time he fussed, she offered the breast for comfort. Toward the end of the first year, instead of switching to a cup, she gave him a bottle, which he kept nearby all day and took to bed for naps and at night. At two years of age he had many cavities and mild anemia. His bottle was his security object. He soon learned to ask not only for a "bottle" but also requested a specific color. When Mrs. R. tried to take the bottle away when Glen was three, he started waking up at night and demanding his bottle, which he promptly got. The pediatrician finally referred the parents to a parenting group since he felt totally frustrated after years of advising them about proper nutrition.

DAILY ROUTINES

Routines are necessary for ordering the life of an infant and his family. Routines that provide structure but allow flexibility for individual needs give family members freedom to enjoy life and each other with some predictability. If parents never know when their infant will take a nap, for example, they cannot plan time for themselves.

Routines evolve from the tasks to be accomplished—infant care, housekeeping, preparation of meals, or full-time jobs for both parents. The infant adapts to routines gradually, accepting gentle coaxing to wait a few minutes for the next feeding, or to lie in bed awake a little long so that he'll start sleeping through the night. Routines change as the infant gives cues that he can tolerate a certain amount of frustration or that he's bored with the same activities.

Sleeping

The newborn remains in a sleeping or semiconscious state between 16 and 20 hours per day. Wakeful periods increase during the day and decrease in the night until the infant sleeps through the night, usually by four months of age. By six months, the infant may sleep ten hours at night and take three naps a day. At the end of the first year, he usually sleeps 10 to 12 hours at night and takes one long nap or two short naps during the day. The older infant often begins to wake up during the night again. This interruption of sleep may be due to the child's memory of his parents coupled with separation anxiety in the form of dreams. A pat on the back may be sufficient reassurance and comfort. He often puts himself back to sleep if allowed to. Some parents simply take the infant to bed with them for a while, a period of togetherness. This practice is strongly discouraged by many health professionals, but numerous healthy, happy families find it a satisfactory solution to the problem.

Eating

At first the newborn wants small amounts of breast milk or formula frequently, perhaps as often as every one or two hours. The breast-fed newborn must suck frequently to build up his milk supply. The formula-fed newborn is satisfied longer because he can drink more formula from a bottle and the milk molecule requires a longer period for digestion. Gradually he increases his intake of breast milk or formula but decreases the number of feedings as his stomach enlarges. When solids are introduced, they are usually offered once a day, then twice a day, and finally three times a day, at approximately the same times as family mealtimes. The six- to eight-month-old infant usually has three meals a day and three or four bottles or breast-feedings. Juice and water provide additional fluids. By the end of the first year, the infant can eat most meals with the family. With help, he can easily drink from a cup and occasionally use a spoon for soft foods.

Bathing

Most new parents are anxious about bathing their newborn; his body lacks tone, his head is heavy, the fontanelles are still noticeable, and the umbilical stump is still there. Until the stump drops off, the normal infant should be sponged daily with a little soap and warm water, and then rinsed with a cloth. The stump should be swabbed with alcohol three times a day as long as it remains attached.

Once the stump sloughs off, the infant can be bathed in a basin, in about 2 inches of water. Most babies enjoy lying in water, although the mother may elicit the Moro reflex when lowering the infant into the basin, and the child may cry. A towel should be placed on the bottom of the basin to prevent slipping, and the end of the towel should be doubled to make a pillow, which elevates the child's head. This last measure keeps the baby's face away from the water, although he will learn to avoid getting splashed as he turns his head from side to side.

One method of bathing that works very well is to soap the baby's body, including folds, crevices, and scalp, before placing him in the basin to rinse. Special attention should be given to the eyes, nose, ears, and genitalia. (See Skills Manual.)

As the baby becomes accustomed to the bath, he typically begins to enjoy it as a form of play, kicking and splashing, and enjoying the freedom from clothes. When he is able to sit up, his pleasure can be enhanced by floating toys. The bath also makes a great change of pace when the infant is cranky.

It must be stressed that the baby must *never* be left alone in the tub, not even for an instant; the danger of drowning or falling is too great.

Day Care

It will be recalled that the infant develops trust when his needs are regularly met by a nurturing person, and he develops stranger and separation anxieties during the last half of his first year. This knowledge should guide parents in determining the time for the mother (or the father) to go back to work, and the best type of day care for the child. Many other factors influence this decision, of course, such as any physical problems of the infant, method of feeding, financial needs of the family, career goals of the parents, and available day care facilities.

The most important requirement for any type of infant care is the presence of one person who will provide most of the care and support the development of trust. This person can adequately care for only a few children at a time. She (or he) may be an employee at a child care center, may offer services in her own home, or may go to the child's home. She must enjoy holding, rocking, feeding, and talking to babies to provide a soft, nurturing touch. She needs to inform the parents of their infant's nutritional intake, his bowel movements, and his activities and behavior frequently in order to provide for continuity of care and to assure the parents that she is aware of changes. The person needs to be flexible in planning for care and must avoid setting rigid eating, sleeping, or other schedules for the child. She needs to take the infant outdoors each day, when weather permits, for a change of scenery and the benefits of sunshine and fresh air.

The facility must have space for sleeping, eating, and moving around, and it must be thoroughly and regularly cleaned. Toys, equipment, and activities must be appropriate for the child's level of development, and, above all, they must be safe. Eating utensils for each infant should be kept separately, although each child will undoubtedly be exposed to the illnesses of the others.

If day care is begun before the appearance of stranger and separation anxieties, the infant may adapt more easily to new faces and surroundings. Later, when these anxieties develop, the infant will be familiar with his environment and his day care worker. At first, he may cry and resist being left in someone else's care, since these anxieties are part of normal cognitive development, but recognizing the environment and caring person will be helpful. If the child is abnormally susceptible to infections, he probably cannot tolerate being with several children. His parents simply must stay home with him or provide for individualized care. Parents may be able to work different shifts when absolutely necessary. They may hire someone to come into their home and share the expenses with other parents who bring their child there, also. A day care mother who keeps one or two children in addition to her own often proves to be satisfactory for the infant.

Parents who leave their infant to be cared for by others usually have separation anxiety themselves. If at all possible, a parent should stay home with the infant for a few months after birth in order to meet the needs of both infant and parent, and to promote bonding. The mother or father who routinely gets up for nighttime feedings and goes to work during the day often is too exhausted to enjoy caring for the baby. Parents who take turns and divide chores often adapt better to the responsibilities of caring for a baby. In single-parent homes, returning to work is often a necessity that creates much stress and leaves little or no time and energy for relaxed parent-baby activities. The career woman usually feels guilty about leaving her infant to go to a job she finds more stimulating than child care. Each person must weigh the pros and cons of this issue and decide what is best for the family. The infant will fare no better at home with a resentful mother than in a day care situation; he may actually receive much more nurturing from the joint efforts of a personally fulfilled mother and another person who takes care of him during the day.

PLAY

Play, from an infant's earliest days, is an important part of his learning, and its changing nature is most delightful to observe. Play is closely related to cognitive, emotional, and physical development; thus, how the infant plays is an important measure of progress in these areas. Play is the infant's most important way of learning. Although it may appear that the infant is totally dependent on his parents for play, what was once thought to be random motor activity has been recognized as motor play. The infant can entertain himself simply by moving. With the emergence of each new motor skill, the infant works to perfect it with practice. There seems to be a drive to master a task before progressing to the next.

Parents have a significant role in infant play. Keeping their faces close to the infant's clearly is an important source of stimulation. Stroking, rocking, and bathing provide a variety of stimuli. The infant soon begins to respond with movements and smiling. He finds novelty interesting and will concentrate on perceiving that which is new. For example, he will stop sucking to listen to a vacuum cleaner, and later he will begin to reach out in an effort to touch an object. Play then becomes an exploring process. Parents can provide many stimuli: different textures to feel, new foods to feel and taste, new places to see other than the nursery. Face-to-face contact remains an important source of stimulation, but the infant's horizons are expanding; he needs big, bright objects and squeaking rubber toys. His recognition of them is a sign of his cognitive development, just as is his ability to grasp them and bring them to his mouth. Although parents should avoid overstimulation (as by providing too many toys in the play area), a variety of new objects, sights, and textures gives the infant interesting means of learning.

Paul, aged 5 months, accompanied his parents on a visit to an old friend's home. His mother spread his blanket on a soft, furry, rug and put him down to play. In two minutes he had inched his way off the blanket onto the rug. He buried his fingers and face in the fur. He laughed out loud; his whole body moved with excitement. He laughed and laughed and rubbed his face back and forth in the fur. (He also was drooling quite a bit, and, although the friend was delighted to see him having a good time, she grimaced as each mouthful of saliva slid into the fur.)

When a baby begins to sit up and to crawl, new equipment is needed. For instance, a playpen often is necessary, and he now can sit in a high chair or spring from the floor in a jumper chair. Crawling helps an infant's coordination, so walkers should not be used too early or too much; they are better for the older baby who lacks the strength and coordination to move from place to place. Once he can crawl, the infant's play becomes a mobilized exploration of his world: he pulls up on tables and chairs, crawls into cabinets, end tables, and any other appealing space. Boxes are great favorites with the crawling baby, and parents can provide some that are big enough to be crawled into and examined. Water play in the bath is enjoyed, especially by infants who can sit up; they can feel and taste the water (and the soap!), splash it, make a loud noise with it, blow bubbles into it—in other words, he can stimulate all five senses during his bath. He develops a powerful attraction to the outdoors; he is interested in moving about and traveling, either in a stroller, a car, or his parent's arms. He enjoys bouncing on someone's lap. A breeze makes him stop to take in the sensation. Again, novelty is the key to the infant's interest.

Play is actually the infant's work. He learns by experiencing movement and stimulation of his senses. Parents can further support this process by providing a variety of play materials and a safe environment and, of course, by being nearby to give him a sense of security.

COMMON PROBLEMS AND NURSING INTERVENTIONS

Colic

The baby's cry is a potent stimulus for action for the average parents; they will try almost anything to prevent or stop his crying. When the healthy infant cries, meeting his needs for foods, warmth, and touch will usually quiet him. He may not cease crying until his parents pace the floor with him on their shoulders or bounce him rhythmically. When the infant cries for no obvious reason and nothing seems to help, parents first suspect an illness and take the child to the doctor, who may find a problem but more often finds nothing. The physician may try changing the formula or giving sedatives, but often the baby continues to cry.

Under such circumstances, the crying is labeled *colic,* paroxysmal crying that often occurs at about the same time each day during the first few months of life. The crying probably is caused by an immature neurological system. Only the unusually tolerant parent can cope with such crying without becoming so tense that the baby cries more. Any one of the "cures" passed down for generations may seem to help briefly but probably only the passage of two to three months will bring permanent relief.

Jimmy, aged four weeks, had been a cranky baby since birth, but he suddenly began to cry every night from 5 to 9 PM. He screamed so loudly that his parents were sure that he had appendicitis. Since the pediatrician found no physical problems, he reassured them that their baby was fine.

The next two and a half months were a nightmare. The parents passed Jimmy back and forth to each other and paced the floor. They became wild with worry and called in both grandmothers. They, too, passed the baby back and forth, but nothing helped. The grandmothers blamed the parents. The parents blamed the doctor. The baby cried even more. The doctor blamed the parents and grandparents for making the baby tense. A public health nurse assessed the home situation and recommended that these distraught parents go the the beach and let the grandmothers take over. Then everyone blamed the public health nurse for her obvious stupidity.

When Jimmy was three and a half months old he cried less. At four months he cried only when he needed something but he remained a cranky baby. No one could understand what happened to make Jimmy stop crying.

Parents require a tremendous amount of support when their baby has colic. The mother, often very bitter about having to stay home with a screaming baby, needs to get away if possible. Occasionally, the physician will admit the infant to the hospital to run "tests" while the parents rest.

Rashes

Several types of rash are common in infancy. During the newborn period most rashes come and go with no symptoms whatsoever. *Erythema toxicum neonatorum*, a blotchy, red, raised rash with a pale center, appears soon after birth and disappears about a week later. This rash is a common reason for visits to emergency rooms or pediatricians' offices. If pustules form, the physician usually cultures the lesion to rule out infectious disease.

Milia are tiny papules filled with sebum (skin oil) and debris. Neither this nor erythema toxicum requires treatment, but parents need reassurance that their newborn baby has no skin problem. The other common skin condition of the newborn, *miliaria* (commonly called "prickly heat"), appears when the sweat ducts cannot empty sweat as it is produced. Treatment consists of control of the environmental temperature to prevent the production of sweat. Parents often overdress their baby and overheat the room to prevent chilling because the child's feet are cool to the touch. The parents don't know that cool feet result form the normal immature circulation of infancy and not from lowered body temperature. An explanation to the parents is important here.

Diaper rash appears in the diaper area initially, but it can spread up the infant's back and abdomen and down his thighs. The average healthy infant develops diaper rash only transiently when his diaper is not changed regularly for some unusual reason. More frequent diaper changes and a careful cleansing of the area followed by application of petroleum jelly usually clears the rash. The child whose skin is especially sensitive may require more frequent diaper changes, application of medicated ointments, and special soaks and/or boiling of diapers.It should also be noted that the fat, sweaty child has an increased chance of diaper rashes because urine and feces seep into the deep folds and irritate the skin along with the sweat already there. Disposable diapers can have advantages and disadvantages. If the infant's cloth diaper remains irritating even after soaking and careful washing, disposable diapers may be the answer to his problem. If, however, the infant's skin is irritated by the plastic covering that holds urine close to the body, or by the deodorant in the absorbent material, cloth diapers must be used. Exposure to air is always good for diaper rash, but many parents refuse to take a chance on cribs smeared with feces and walls wet with urine. Heat lamps with 20-watt bulbs can promote healing, but the danger of burning is ever-present; unless the infant is entirely too young to sit or pull up, he must be restrained for protection. Diarrhea can result in a rash and skin breakdown of the diaper area.

Nursing care should include frequent diaper changes, careful cleansing with soap and water after bowel movements and with water after urination, application out of a protective ointment with medication for infection or inflammation as needed, and removal of irritating substances such as residual urine, deodorants, or soaps in diapers.

If diaper rash is caused by parental neglect, a team approach that includes home nursing and social services is necessary.

Simple explanation is not enough, since a lack of resources (time, energy, money, motivation) to provide adequate care is usually the underlying problem.

The family may need financial assistance to buy cloth diapers and transportation to get the diapers laundered. The infant in these unfortunate conditions usually has a persistent rash until he develops bladder control.

Cradle Cap

Cradle cap, seborrheic dermatitis of the scalp (and occasionally, the eyebrows and eyelids), appears as yellow, greasy scales and flakes, often accompanied by inflammation of underlying tissue. A rash may develop when the flakes fall on the infant's forehead, cheeks, nose and shoulders. Because cradle cap resembles very dry skin, mothers may try to remedy the situation by applying layers of oil and by avoiding shampoos; this, of course, makes the problem worse. Some parents are afraid to wash the infant's scalp because of the previously mentioned fears associated with bathing, i.e., dropping the child or damaging the fontanelles. These concerns can be eliminated or at least diminished with sufficient practice in bathing the baby before leaving the maternity unit of the hospital.

Mild cradle cap will disappear with routine shampooing every other day. Moderate cradle cap is first softened with baby or mineral oil, loosened with a soft brush, and shampooed with a mild soap. Persistent, extensive cradle cap requires softening and loosening, shampooing with a medicated soap, and application of a corticosteroid lotion or cream to decrease inflammation and oozing. Cleansing of the affected area should be firm enough to remove flakes and scales but gentle enough not to break the inflammed tissue below. The infant with severe cradle cap usually has seborrheic dermatitis in other parts of the body, especially in body folds. This uncommon appearance of the condition in parts other than the scalp may require considerably more treatment.

Constipation

Constipation has many definitions, but probably the most useful one is hard stools that cause pain during elimination. Infrequent bowel movement is usually mentioned in definitions, but if the stools are hard and passage is painful, the condition should be treated as constipation. Although increasing the infant's fluid intake with water or juices usually is sufficient to soften stools, adding corn syrup to the child's formula may be necessary. If the infant is taking solid foods well, an addition or increase of such foods as prunes and vegetables may help. The older infant will have fewer problems as he begins to eat table foods with his family, provided they regularly eat a well-balanced diet. If none of these remedies works, the infant should be examined to rule out bowel anomalies. Advise parents not to give laxatives or enemas to infants without medical advice, since these can cause abdominal cramps and diarrhea. If laxatives and enemas are given frequently, the bowel loses its ability to move feces through the anus on its own. When an infant experiences discomfort with each bowel movement, time after time, he may learn to hold feces in, causing further constipation. This will definitely make toilet training stressful for parents and child during toddlerhood. Assess the infant's bowel habits carefully and instruct parents how to prevent and treat constipation after collaborating with the physician.

Chronic Diarrhea

This brief discussion is not meant to include a study of severe cases of diarrhea (see ch. 18), but instead is limited to mention of the loose and frequent stools that may follow an infection and/or fever. This mild diarrhea may be the result of a sensitive gastrointestinal tract, or it may occur for no obvious reason. Although the child seems happy and is growing well, the loose, messy stools continue and can cause a great deal of anxiety in the parents. They are often unable to adopt a wait-and-see attitude and will press their pediatrician to begin tests or even to hospitalize the child; on occasion, an infection or congenital problem is found, but most cases clear up by themselves with time and, perhaps, some restrictions in diet. Encourage the parents to discuss their frustrations about this nuisance and, if test findings were normal, reassure the parents of this in hopes of helping them to tolerate the problem.

Regurgitation

Regurgitation is a spilling over or rolling out of food from the stomach. It is not to be confused with vomiting, which occurs with force. Babies who regularly spit up their milk frequently cause their parents a lot of anxiety. Even though these infants thrive and continue to gain weight, their parents may feel that something must be wrong. Regurgitation is usually the result of immaturity in the sphincter that separates the esophagus and stomach, and will correct itself as the infants grows; occasionally, it is due to overfeeding. Solid foods do not spill over as easily, and, as the infant begins to walk, gravity helps to hold the food down, so again this is a problem that will disappear in time. Emphasize this to the parents in your explanation.

Genital Adhesions

The genitalia of both male and female infants need special care to prevent *adhesions,* the joining of parts to each other. The vaginal orifice should be cleansed after each bowel movement and during baths to prevent the fusing of tissue, which can close the vagina entirely. This condition, of course, requires surgical correction. In boy babies, the foreskin, or the remnants of the foreskin following complete healing of circumcision, should be washed gently but thoroughly during each bath. If this is not done, the foreskin may adhere to the glans, and surgery may be necessary to separate the parts. Many new parents are not aware of these preventive measures and need to be shown what to do.

Thumb-Sucking and Pacifier Use

The infant is born with a sucking reflex, elicited by placing any object in his mouth. The reflex is strong at birth, begins to fade by the third month, and is nearly gone by the fifth month. During this period, the infant usually enjoys a pacifier. As the sucking reflex fades, the child will smile in response to a smiling face and drop his pacifier; this is a cue that he needs less sucking, and parents should be advised to heed the cue.

Some parents unwittingly reinforce the sucking reflex by putting a pacifier into the child's mouth whenever he is upset or bored, seldom providing human contact, a new environment, or the opportunity to sleep or to simply move and look around. Under these circumstances, sucking becomes associated with security, the need for which remains intense until two years of age.

Thumb-sucking is of course quite common; the infant may suck his thumb as early as when he is in the newborn nursery, much to the dismay of his parents, who may envision the expense of the braces that the child will surely need.

Often the infant will stop sucking his thumb when the sucking reflex is gone, or later in childhood, when he can occupy his hands in other ways. Harsh measures, such as taping the thumb, applying wire braces to the arms, or coating the thumb with a bitter-tasting substance, will upset the child and are therefore undesirable. The best solution to the problem is to ignore it, since undue attention will simply reinforce the thumb-sucking.

Congenital Laryngeal Stridor

Congenital laryngeal stridor is caused by a narrowing of the larynx and results in a crowing sound with each breath, but rarely requires therapy. It usually disappears by the first birthday. You may have a difficult time convincing parents that their child is well and thriving because of the constant noise that accompanies his breathing. Because the infant has to make a somewhat greater effort to breathe, especially when he tries to eat, he may tire quickly. He may stop sucking for a while in order to breathe, then begin again; feeding therefore takes longer and requires patience. If upper respiratory infections occur, the crowing will be even more pronounced; such infections must therefore be treated promptly.

ACCIDENTS

Accidents are a major cause of death at all ages, even during infancy, when parents can more easily control their baby's environment. Most daily routines are potentially dangerous: bath times, diaper changing, sleeping, and eating. Awareness of the possibility of accidents is the key to prevention. A chaotic family situation sets up a high-risk environment for the baby; lack of child development knowledge, absence of household rules, inadequate storage places for medicines and toxic agents contribute to the greater possibility of an accident.

While it is certainly easier to protect an infant who cannot yet turn over, this stage does not last long, and soon the baby develops new skills that increase his mobility. When he can reach for things, care must be taken to keep unsafe objects out of reach—no plastic bags, no sharp objects or open safety pins (or closed ones, for that matter), no tubes of medicine. Toys should be chosen with safety in mind, especially with an eye to parts that can be bitten off and swallowed, such as buttons or cotton bunny tails. A baby who can pull up in his crib puts most of his weight on the crib's side; an insecurely locked crib, or a broken one, can cause falls that can result in head injuries or broken bones. Even a few inches of water can drown an infant left in a bath for the little time it takes to answer a phone or door. As the infant learns to crawl and to explore his world, there is a greater chance of his coming into contact with unsafe objects; for example, he will pull on electrical cords and even bite them. As he begins to climb on things, the incidence of falls increases. From the earliest days of an infant's life, auto safety should be a great concern to the parents; infant seats should always be used and strapped to the car seats. Strollers and high chairs present the possibility of broken femurs because infants not strapped in simply stand up and fall forward, snapping the bone against the front bar.

Preventive measures, such as those mentioned above, should be used in the home to decrease the likelihood of accidents. However, accidents will inevitably happen, sometimes as a result of negligence, sometimes not. An infant's accident is always traumatic for his parents because they will feel enormous guilt as well as anxiety, as was discussed in ch. 3. Often the best thing you can do is listen to the parents. Ideally, once the initial shock has passed and, more important, after a good nurse-parent relationship has been established, the situation will provide an occasion to teach preventive measures. An empathic approach is essential in dealing with parents whose infant has had an accident despite the parents' awareness of preventive measures, so you must identify your own feelings regarding the accident before attempting to help the parents; if you feel very critical of them, you may need assistance from another nurse who can be supportive.

SIGNS OF ILLNESS

When new parents are faced with the questions "Is my baby sick?" and "Should I call the doctor?" there is no absolute formula for answering these questions, but some guidelines can be provided. Parents can consider their infant's appearance, eating and elimination patterns, activity level, and vital signs in the decision-making process. Marked and/or persistent changes in any area of functioning are more likely to indicate illness than a few minor changes, which can result from normal variations.

The infant who is ill often has sunken eyes, grayish skin, and a limp body. His skin may lack turgor, his eyes may be glazed, and his lips may be red. He may have a sad, tired look on his face, or he may have an apprehensive look, with eyes wide open. The infant usually displays a similar appearance with each illness so that his parents learn to recognize the early changes that no one else would notice.

A change in eating habits may come and go for no apparent reason, but it is often the first sign of illness in the infant. When offered a nipple, he may fuss or cry, turn his head back and forth, or simply refuse to suck. The more his mother tries to get him to suck, the fussier or more exhausted he becomes. He will often regurgitate or vomit his milk, regardless of the location of the disease process in the body. This lack of appetite seriously affects the infant's fluid and nutritional intake.

Deviations in elimination may change in response to pathology of the excreting organ or of any part of the body. Most infants will occasionally have bowel movements which are too firm or soft due to the previous day's meals or activities. Urinary output will change according to fluid intake, body temperature, and activity level. Persistent, increasing, or marked changes in elimination are reasons for medical attention.

Activity levels are usually fairly consistent in the infant, and a change in his daily pattern may indicate impending illness. The infant is often irritable and may refuse to sleep, or he may drop off to sleep and wake up, still irritable. He may sleep far more than usual. Extreme lethargy or irritability is frequently a sign of a problem that requires immediate attention.

The measurement of vital signs, including temperature, heart rates, and respiratory rates, can be helpful in determining the presence of illness. After the neonatal period, body temperature rises rapidly in response to illness, but normal temperature can be quickly restored with medication and cooling treatments (see ch. 15). A rapid increase in temperature may cause generalized convulsions (*febrile seizure*). The infant's respirations are usually smooth and regular. An alteration in rate and character of respiration during infancy is an important sign of illness since many diseases can easily obstruct the infant's tiny airways and decrease his supply of oxygen quickly. His heart rate, already twice that of the normal adult, usually increases with the stress of illness and, particularly, with elevations in body temperature.

HOSPITALIZATION

Hospitalization of a child is almost always a family crisis. When the child is an infant, his size and helplessness seem to increase parent anxiety. The parents have been accustomed to meeting the child's needs themselves; they now require the help of a team of people in a hospital. Any stress on the infant is felt by the parents because they are so interdependent. The older child develops inner resources to tolerate trauma of all types, but the infant has no resources of his own; his resources are those of his parents.

Nursing Interventions

If the child must be hospitalized, admission to an acute care unit is a crucial step in establishing a trusting nurse-parent relationship. Greet the parents and child with a smile. Express sincere sympathy to them about their sick baby and about their emotions and feelings of exhaustion. Tell them that they are welcome on the unit, that you will value their help in caring for their infant.

The young infant may be perfectly happy to have you pick him up for initial assessments, but if he is older than about six months of age, he will view you as a stranger. Encourage parents' active participation in weighing and measuring their infant. Leave the infant in his mother's arms while taking vital signs. Try to avoid separation of parents and baby during admission since being apart will definitely increase the parents' distress.

Most pediatric acute care units have initial assessment tools designed for different ages and stages of development (see ch. 2). Much of the tools are concerned with the child's developmental status, daily routines, and preferences. Do not attempt to obtain this information until the parents have had a chance to "tell their story" about the present illness; this is a compelling need in most parents. You will be able to pick up clues about their anxiety, need for sleep, misconceptions about the illness, feelings about their physician and the emergency room staff, and so on. Listen carefully to this story, then elicit details if necessary. Explain before you begin to get other data that you will use this information to plan for their baby's care and that you will let other nurses know about the child.

As you interview parents, you will find that they have many questions. Be sure to set aside time to answer their questions and to orient them to the unit. They will want to know if they can take their infant out of the crib to let him crawl on the floor, if they can bring baby food prepared at home, or if there is any possibility of ensuring privacy during breast-feeding. They may want to know if they can room-in with their infant, or if they can go home periodically. Explain the infant's need for their presence, but reassure them that he will receive care while they are gone.

Hospitalization disrupts the established lifestyle of parents and infant alike. Try to follow home schedules and routines as much as possible; do not make major changes, such as weaning or taking away a night bottle. This can be physically upsetting to the baby and emotionally upsetting to parents.

Dr. W. was outraged when he found that his ten-month-old surgery patient was fed nothing but milk and had developed anemia as a consequence. The doctor instructed the nurses to take the bottle away and to start feeding the child meat. He ordered an iron injection. The baby cried for his bottle for three days and refused to eat anything. His mother sat passively some distance from his bed for one day, then left for home. When she was called to pick him up after his surgery, she hid his bottle in her purse so that she could comfort him on the way home.

Try to convince the physician who orders a major change to reconsider. Offer logical alternatives, including gradual change and suitable substitutes. (The nurse always has the option of refusing to carry out an order which she feels is detrimental to the child's well-being.)

Polly was twelve months old when she was placed in traction for a broken femur. She was being breast-fed three times a day at the time of the accident. At first, her mother tried leaning on the crib, letting a nipple dangle in Polly's mouth. When someone walked in unannounced, she was caught in a most awkward position. A nursing student was horrified to see this sight, so she made a "Knock Before Entering" sign and helped the mother to climb into the crib and lie down with her baby to nurse without disturbing the traction.

The young infant can tolerate the presence of strangers and separation from his parents fairly well. Once stranger anxiety appears, the infant will have a very difficult time with the many strangers who come and go in a hospital day. If a parent is near, he can tolerate the new faces to some extent. If, however, he is faced with a stranger when his parent is not at hand, he may be terrified and may scream or simply withdraw. If no familiar person can stay with the infant, a grandmotherly volunteer who visits regularly may be able to establish a relationship with him by talking to him, holding and rocking him. Try to keep the infant close to someone, even if he has to sit in an infant seat or jumper chair in the nurses' station. This is not always realistic, of course, and occasionally an infant will have to remain alone in his crib with a few safe toys. Music provides some entertainment for the baby, and he can entertain himself adequately with motor skills and his senses for a while.

Parents need places to eat, sleep, bathe, eliminate, and smoke. This is particularly true for parents of infants who need them nearby at all times. Not all hospitals provide the necessary facilities, but a willing nursing staff can usually meet all of these needs with some creativity. Parents are truly impressed with nursing efforts to make them feel at home. This caring on the part of nurses strengthens the trusting relationship that is so necessary for parent teaching.

Preparation for Procedures

The infant can rarely be prepared for any procedures because he simply cannot comprehend what will happen to him, regardless of the techniques used. In the case of the older infant (six months or more), if he will return from surgery with a type of bandage or restraint, apply it (or something similar) the night before. Nurse and parents can wear a mask and take it off in front of him, playing peek-a-boo in the process. Parents need a complete explanation of any procedure performed on their baby. They are interested in the type of procedure, the desired outcome, and the infant's behavior afterwards, but they also are intensely concerned about what the baby will perceive while in surgery. Who will hold him if he cries? Will he be cold? After all, this is often the very first time that the infant has been relinquished to a stranger. Some progressive hospitals allow parents to stay with their baby until he is anesthetized, to help wake him in the recovery room, to assist with x-rays and scans, to stay by his side during lumbar punctures, and so forth. Not all parents can tolerate such situations, but many can if they receive proper nursing support.

Discharge Planning

Planning for discharge of the infant begins with admission and continues throughout hospitalization. By informing parents of all activities, you can minimize disruption in the parent-infant relationship, although most infants will show some changes in eating, sleeping, and crying during hospitalization. The child will resist any separation from his mother. Getting back into home routines requires patience and a gradual reestablishment of schedules. Explain to parents that behavioral changes inevitably occur but their presence in the hospital helps to keep these to a minimum.

While parents are in the hospital with their infant, encourage them to participate actively in any procedure that must be continued at home. Before the infant goes home, parents must assume full responsibility for his care so they will not be overwhelmed when no nurse is near. Give all instructions for home care in writing, along with the time of the next appointment at the clinic or physician's office. Be sure the parents know how to obtain assistance before the follow-up appointment if it is necessary.

SUMMARY

The infant whose emotional and physical needs are consistently met develops a sense of trust; if his needs are not met or attended to irregularly, he begins to sense that he cannot depend on his parents and develops a sense of mistrust. Around the middle of the first year of life, the infant distinguishes between the smiling face he sees so often (usually that of his mother) and new faces, and registers stranger anxiety by frowning or crying. Toward the end of the first year, separation anxiety emerges as the infant begins to sense that he is a being separate from his mother.

The infant is said to be in the sensorimotor period of cognitive development, during which moving his body and using his senses constitute play and are most important ways of learning about the world around him and his relationship to it. With his parents' prompting, he learns to understand several words, although he can say only a few. The infant's physical growth is very rapid during the first year but slows considerably toward the end of the period.

The infant and his parents must develop a schedule of daily routines that is tolerable to all concerned. The establishment of routines not only facilitates the regular performance of daily tasks of infant care but builds the foundation of a sense of orderliness in the infant's mind, and fosters in him a gradual tolerance for minor frustrations. As this tolerance, along with a readiness for new activities, manifests itself, the infant's parents can institute new routines.

Common problems of infants include colic, rashes, cradle cap, constipation, diarrhea, regurgitation, and congenital laryngeal stridor. Accidents increase as the child's motor skills improve. Parents must maintain a watchful eye and the awareness that the infant's ability to move about, reach, and grasp will make it necessary for them to assess constantly the potential for danger in everyday situations and objects.

The hospitalized infant, of course, is fearful of the strange faces, experiences, and routines that he is subjected to. His parents should be involved in his care to the fullest degree possible and should be instructed in whatever post-hospitalization care is necessary before they return home with their child.

CHAPTER **5**

The Toddler

BEHAVIORAL OBJECTIVES

After studying this chapter you will be able to:

- Discuss the toddler's emotional development in relation to autonomy, shame, and doubt.
- Describe the toddler's transition from the sensorimotor to the preoperational stage, and discuss the concept of egocentrism.
- Discuss the toddler's language development, ways to stimulate language development, and reasons for language delays in the toddler.
- Describe physical and motor changes that occur during toddlerhood.
- Discuss nutrition in relation to food requirements and developing autonomy in the toddler.
- List daily activities for the toddler and discuss the importance of routines.
- Identify appropriate play activities and materials for the toddler.
- Identify common problems and accidents that occur during toddlerhood. Name preventive and treatment measures for each.
- Describe signs of illness in the toddler.
- Discuss nursing care of the toddler and his parents during hospitalization.
- Discuss how prolonged separation from his parents affects the toddler.

TERMS AND CONCEPTS

Autonomy
Shame and doubt
Negativism
Temper tantrums
Gradualism
Self-awareness
Self-control
Security object
Preoperational stage
Egocentrism
Primary teeth
Sphincters
Parallel play
Protest
Despair
Denial

The toddler, despite his displays of independence, has an urgent need for continued contact with and support from his parents. He ventures only as far from them as the distance from which he can easily return to them. Nursing of the toddler is based on the knowledge that his feelings of security are dependent on the presence of and contact with his parents. Except in the case of highly technical procedures, parents should provide most of the toddler's care unless they are emotionally or physically exhausted. When they are unable to care for their child, the nurse's goal is to help them recover their parenting abilities.

EMOTIONAL DEVELOPMENT

The infant is so much a part of his mother (or mother-surrogate) that he feels that they are the same being or, at the very least, that he is an extension of her. As the child enters and progresses through toddlerhood (the period between one and two and a half years of age), he acquires a sense of self, separate both physically and emotionally from all others. Attaining a sense of independence, that is, *autonomy* (as Erikson calls it), is a major task for him. He must develop an awareness of his body as being his own and the ability to exercise some control over his impulses if he is to be autonomous. He must learn that he can do things "his" way successfully. These aspects of toddlerhood are closely related and interdependent. For example, the toddler must recognize his feces and urine as *his* before he can control their elimination. Parents have the enormous task of encouraging these many changes at once. If they approve of the child's progress (even when registering approval is inconvenient or downright irritating), the toddler learns that he is worthwhile. Although this period can be fascinating and delightful it will be very trying for most families, especially those who do not understand why their child is now very different from the lovable and easygoing baby he once was. Parents may react to each new step with disapproval and exasperation and may criticize the toddler for the time and effort he demands. The child judges himself by his parents' actions to him; if the responses are negative, the child comes to believe he is "bad." In this case, he develops not a sense of autonomy but one of *shame and doubt.*

Negativism is an obvious sign of developing autonomy. It is simply a device by which the toddler separates himself from his parents, and it takes many forms. The constant "no!" from a two-year-old can mean various things; in some instances, "no" can even mean "OK." The child does not *mean* "no," but feels he must say it. "No" also can mean "not right now," or "never!" or "I want to do something else that I don't know the words for," or even, "I'm sleepy." Other forms of negativism can be seen in the toddler-gone-limp when picked up against his will, or the toddler who eludes his mother in stores. The *temper tantrum* (see the later section on common problems), which may include kicking, biting, scratching, and crying for up to an hour or so, is another sign that the toddler sees himself as an individual whose will can differ from that of his parent. "Me do" are frequently heard words, especially when it is time to be dressed or fed.

The parents who understand this stage of childhood will know that their child needs to explore and will encourage the child within certain limits that are usually imposed by a combination of the need for safety and the parents' own needs. Then, as the toddler ventures away from the parents and returns to them for support and praise, he develops self-confidence and a sense of security that will aid him in trying new tasks (Figure 5–1). Praise for the accomplishment of a task should be gentle and not overwhelming, since excessive

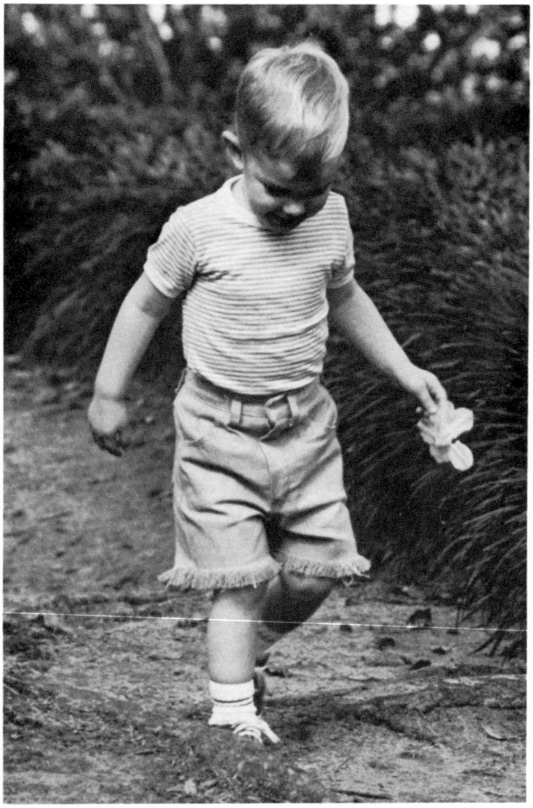

Figure 5–1. *The toddler develops self-confidence as he ventures a short distance from his parents.*

praise can imply that a later failure in the same task constitutes an enormous shortcoming. Parents should avoid using praise as manipulation and should use it in a moderate, genuine way, giving the child a sense of self-worth. The pride the parents feel as they watch their child master each task will be reflected in the child's self-concept—he can be proud of himself. This same positive self-concept can be enhanced by the sensitive adult in other ways: parents can "save face" for their toddler who has an "accident" by calling it just that and forgiving him instantly. Toddlers who struggle for independence will usually accept a compromise: "You put on your coat, but I'll do your boots." Ignoring a toddler's verbal rejection of an order helps to avoid a power struggle.

Gradualism in imposing and removing limits is the ideal approach to the changing child. The toddler himself will give *cues* as to what he is and isn't ready for, and these cues will have to be reassessed periodically to determine the amount of freedom permissible as time passes.

Self-awareness is a major component of autonomy, and is closely related to safety and the high incidence of accidents. The toddler's awareness of himself is growing rapidly but is still not complete. Still developing the ability to distinguish between his own body and objects outside of it, he might try to pick up a blanket he is standing on, and, unaware of the distance between himself and another object, such as the floor, he may fall from a chair or bed as he attempts to step or slide down. He doesn't realize that his body can be an obstacle to television viewing when he stands in front of it, even when his big brother pushes him out of the way. He has difficulty in identifying parts of his body he cannot see or touch, such as his back. The young toddler is not aware of his soiled diapers, and is unable to describe the location of a pain with any accuracy. A favorite game of toddlers is "name the body part"; they want to know what each part is called. They will ask about specific parts of the genitals, and parents can either answer truthfully or sabotage learning by calling them "privates," "down there" or nothing at all. Acceptance and approval from the parent set the tone for the toddler's self-appraisal, and he quickly learns their attitudes toward the body and his curiosity about his own body.

Another significant component of the toddler's autonomy is *self-control*. He begins to see himself as a person among other people, and with proper direction he will move toward a degree of self-control. Discipline should be aimed at gradually developing the child's self-control, the ultimate goal being to make parental control unnecessary. The motivating force behind the change to self-control must be a sense of pride and self-esteem, not the fear of authority.

Self-control is a complex task that is accomplished with the guidance of the toddler's parents, who must incorporate the gradual imposition of limits and routines, flexibility that arises from awareness of the child's cues, and a loving approach. The toddler's gradual development of self-control can be readily observed. First he sees a forbidden object, grabs it without concern, and is reproached by his parent. Later, he walks to the object, says "no" to himself, but grabs it anyway. Still later he will say "no," hold his hands behind his back to help resist the temptation, and soon move to an acceptable object or activity. He may not be able to control himself each time, but consistent reminders after he has had a chance to control himself will strengthen his self-discipline. Although the child seems to begin to recognize that certain behavior is unsafe or forbidden, and he acts accordingly, he must never be trusted to heed safety precautions. He is not yet capable of maintaining the degree of control necessary for safety.

The development of autonomy is a difficult task for the toddler. He continues to experience acute stranger and separation anxieties during the first few months of toddlerhood, and later develops an increasing tolerance for strangers and of separation from his mother. He needs the security of something familiar when he is in a strange situation or with strange people. The presence of a familiar person is ideal during separation anxiety, but a special object will help. The object, usually associated with sleep habits, maybe a satin-edged blanket, a stuffed animal, or, unfortunately, a bottle of milk. This *security object* is to be preserved at all costs during major changes such as illness, birth of a sibling, or a move.

Jason's grandmother had given him a foam rubber Humpty Dumpty when he was an infant. It soon became his faithful companion in his bed and on trips to the nursery. When he was twenty months old, his parents prepared to move out of the country. When the movers were gone and the house was empty, Jason's parents realized that "Baby" had been packed. Jason's father had to go to the warehouse to search box after box until it was found. Fortunately, the warehouseman understood perfectly why Jason could not possibly go to Panama without "Baby."

Parents need to stop and assess their family as the child's toddlerhood draws to a close. They can take pride in the toddler's accomplishments and the ways in which they made this stage of his life a positive and exciting one. The growing family can settle down now, but a new stage of the child's development is coming, complete with new challenges and achievements.

COGNITIVE DEVELOPMENT

The cognitive development of the toddler is a continuation of the process begun in infancy. Toddlerhood is an active age, full of experimentation, trial and error, and use of insight. The toddler completes the sensorimotor stage of cognitive development and begins what Piaget calls the *preoperational stage,* which lasts until early school age. The toddler has built a collection of memories by now—the sum of his cognitive development in infancy; he can distinguish himself from other objects in his environment, and he understands that these objects exist even when he cannot see them. His previous successes in solving simple problems—how to crawl to a desired object or place, or to reach for and grasp something he wants—are building blocks for attempting more difficult tasks. He can remember solutions that worked before and apply them to similar situations. He uses his memory to help him recall what his parents do and imitates their actions. During this preoperational stage of trying new skills, the toddler needs routines to give him the security necessary to support his experimentation. He must know what to expect; parents who provide routines and limits, along with freedom, will foster the child's cognitive development.

During the second year of life, the toddler can invent new ways to solve problems and control his environment. These solutions evolve not from trial-and-error experimentation, but from the use of intelligence to achieve results. The toddler can figure things out, that is, he can picture actions in his mind, discard the ineffective ways of dealing with a situation, and choose or invent his plan of action. This is a dual process of representation (the use of mental imagery) and invention.

Skipper, aged fifteen months, eyed the Christmas tree on top of the desk for several days. One day his mother walked into the room to find drawers pulled out like stair steps, and Skipper on top of the desk picking the glass balls off the tree and throwing them down into the different drawers.

The toddler learns to associate the components of a certain routine with one another and feels that these associated actions should "stay together." He becomes upset when a part of the whole seems to be out of place.

Andy, aged two, has his bath, drinks a glass of water, brushes his teeth, listens to a story, rocks with his father, puts his teddy bear on his pillow, climbs in the bed, says his prayers, kisses his mother and father, and puts his head on the pillow. His mother covers him with a blanket, turns on the night light and turns off the overhead light. On the night of his parents' big party of the year, they tried to put Andy to bed without a bath. He began to whine, then scream, as he pulled his mother toward the bathroom door.

John, aged twenty-two months, had been in the pool quite a bit in his short life. His parents took him to a rocky beach where shoes were an absolute necessity, even in the water. When he sat down to take off his shoes his mother tried to explain that he must have his shoes on. He began to cry, so she allowed him to take them off. He stood in one spot most of the day rather than wear his shoes in the water, which simply "was not *done!*"

The toddler begins to use words, first to symbolize objects, and, later, to describe events of the past or present.

Ben, aged twenty months, called his cuts and scrapes "boo-boos." When he fell down and scraped his hand, he cried long and loud, "Boo-boo! Boo-boo!" After he had played quietly and happily for a while, he noticed the hurt and he cried "Boo-boo!" again. His father came home several hours later and Ben reenacted the event complete with crying and the single word "Boo-boo!"

He also uses objects as symbols, as when he pretends that a block is a car or a broom handle is a horse. Each symbol has one meaning for one object. The use of symbols, especially words, can help the toddler to realize even more that objects continue to exist even when they are not in sight (i.e., he grasps the concept of object permanence).

He can now easily bring objects to mind by saying the words for them. The toddler often lies in his crib saying his favorite words over and over for the fun of practicing language, and to remind himself that important objects, including people, will be there when he wakes up.

The toddler is *egocentric,* and thus he can understand what he experiences only in relation to his own desires and previous experiences; he cannot understand that other points of view exist.

Jim, aged twenty-two months, saw a chicken beneath the house. His grandmother, who was grossly obese, was unable to lower herself enough to see what interested him. He asked, "What's that?" several times, and she answered, "I can't see." Since Jim could see the chicken perfectly, he assumed that she could too; he simply could not understand why she would not answer his question. Fortunately, the chicken soon clucked, and Jim's grandmother taught him a new word.

Brooks, aged eighteen months, hit Ellen, aged two, because she took his truck away from him. She began to cry, startling him. He ran to the farthest corner of the room (with his truck) and watched her cry. He had no reason to cry, so why was she crying? From his point of view, all was well.

Egocentrism prevents the toddler from being logical. Since explanation cannot change his point of view, parents must resort to firm, consistent limits on undesirable and unsafe behavior, and must also try to be tolerant.

LANGUAGE DEVELOPMENT

During the first six to eight months of toddlerhood, the child can use a few words meaningfully but he loses interest in learning new ones while he directs his energy toward learning to walk and run. Once this is accomplished, usually soon after 18 months of age, the parents delight in listening as he says one new word after another each day. His first words are nouns that first serve as whole sentences. "Ball" can mean "Let's play ball," "The ball is outside," or "Will Daddy play ball?" He uses words to express his wants, his recognition of objects, and his awareness of himself. His receptive vocabulary continues to exceed his productive one, often causing great frustration arising from his inability to make his thoughts known. Parents can stimulate his language development by talking to him throughout the day, naming new objects for him, and speaking plainly (no baby talk), face to face, so that he can imitate them. As in other developmental tasks, parents can set an approving tone for exploration and experimentation in language.

Delayed speech development can result from many causes. Lack of language stimulation, which may occur in a chaotic family or a too-busy professional family, may be the reason for inadequate speech development. Mental illness or retardation, and physical defects such as cerebral palsy or hearing loss are other problems that affect speech. Because of a personal communication system, twins develop normal speech more slowly. The youngest of several children, whose siblings anticipate his every need, has no need to talk, and actually enjoys the attention from not talking. The reason for language delay may be very obvious, but in some cases assessment by a speech pathologist may be necessary.

GROWTH AND PHYSICAL CHANGES

The child's growth slows so much by one year of age that it seems to stop abruptly.

Most parents become very concerned because the child also decreases his intake of food (see the later section on nutrition). Actually, he continues to grow, following a fairly smooth upward curve. Parents are so relieved when they learn their child's size is still normal that they are more than willing to accept changed eating patterns.

Proportion

A toddler's trunk is still large in proportion to the rest of his body when compared with the older child or the adult, but during his second year, both head and trunk growth slow down while the arms and legs begin to lengthen. The child's abdomen will protrude until the abdominal muscles are strong enough to support it, and since he is swaybacked his stomach continues to poke out until the end of the preschool years (Figure 5–2). As he first begins to walk, his legs may bow a little, and with a double diaper between his legs, he waddles somewhat like a duck.

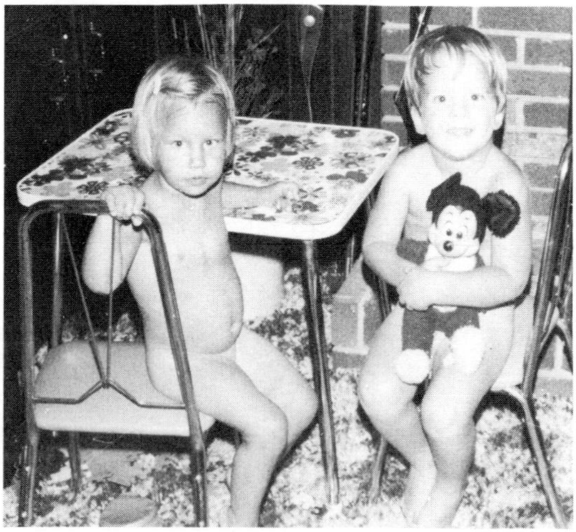

Figure 5–2. *The toddler has a protuberant abdomen. Note the security object.*

Weight

Although an infant triples his birth weight during the first year, his next year will show only a gain of the birthweight again, usually between seven or eight pounds. In other words, the toddler should have quadrupled his birth weight at age two. Height and weight should be considered together to assess weight gain. The young toddler is usually weighed on an infant scale, while the older toddler may be able to stand confidently on an adult scale if someone holds his hand until he feels balanced. He is usually very unwilling to part with his clothes, so lightweight clothing is often left on after removal of coats, sweaters, and shoes.

Height

Increase in height during a child's second year also slows considerably. By his second birthday, the toddler doubles his birth height and reaches approximately half of his adult height. The toddler's height is measured by standing him against a wall chart with his feet flat on the floor and face straight ahead. Extend a ruler or other straight object from the top of his head to the chart. This method is better than using a measuring board on which the negativistic toddler must be stretched against his will.

Head and Chest Circumference

A toddler's head circumference should continue to be measured until his second birthday, although head growth during this second year also occurs at a much slower rate. The anterior fontanelles should be closed by eighteen or nineteen months. At one year, the toddler's head and chest are approximately the same circumference. By two years, his chest is growing much faster than his head.

Teeth

The toddler gains several new teeth between his first and second year. About half of all two-year-olds have the complete set of 20 *primary teeth* (also called baby teeth or deciduous teeth). The toddler should be taught toothbrushing in the second year, to keep his teeth clean and healthy, of course, but also to establish a routine to be continued for life. He has no understanding of germs and will use this brush on anything or anyone, so his parents should wash the brush thoroughly before each use. Some pedodontists, (children's dentists) prefer to see the two and a half-year-old simply to establish a good relationship before actual care and treatment begin at age three.

Other Health Measurements

The toddler's pulse and respiration are somewhat slower than they were in infancy. Pulses usually range between 90–100 beats per minute, and respiration is usually around 25 breaths per minute. His blood pressure increases, averaging 95/65 during this stage. His hemoglobin and hematocrit increase after a low in infancy and reach a plateau at about age two that lasts throughout the preschool period. The average hemoglobin is 11–12 gm/100 ml of whole blood, and the average hematocrit is 33–35 ml/100 ml of whole blood.

MOTOR DEVELOPMENT

The toddler spends much of his time engaged in activities that strengthen his muscles and refine his coordination. He enjoys learning new motor skills, practicing them until they are mastered, and then moving on to something new.

Eighteen Months

The young toddler can walk well and can often run, pulling a toy behind him. He can walk upstairs but not downstairs. He will push stools, chairs, or a small table to a cabinet, and climb from the furniture to get to a desired object, or he may climb simply for the sake of climbing. He likes to use his pincer grasp to put small objects through an opening and to stack two or three blocks, which he promptly knocks down. He uses this ability to put many things in his mouth and, occasionally, in his ears, nose, and so on. He can use a spoon and cup but spills food and drinks regularly. He enjoys scribbling with a pencil or crayon but has little interest in the picture he has produced. He uses his small or large muscles not only to accomplish tasks but also simply to have fun.

Twenty-four Months

The toddler at this age is almost "little boy" or "little girl" instead of "baby" but he still has some infant-like ways. He can walk up and down stairs, he can jump, and he may be able to pedal a riding toy if it is the right size. He climbs almost any place within his home, so locked cabinet are now necessary for poisons of all kinds. The toddler stacks blocks for the fun of stacking, and he happily smashes his building again and again. He draws with pencils and crayons, but he'd rather finger paint, using the large muscles in his arms instead of the small ones in his fingers. His fine coordination is developing steadily, however, enabling him to feed himself with only occasional spills. He can slip on some of his clothing by himself. He continues running, jumping, and climbing to experience the sensation of motion.

Thirty Months

This is a transitional period for the child. His judgment is developing, but not enough to protect him from danger. He enjoys putting puzzles together and fitting objects into the proper spot, but he may take on a project so difficult that he becomes frustrated. He knows from experience that he can perform many motor skills, but he does not know the limits of his ability.

NUTRITION

As the child enters his second year and becomes a toddler, his growth rate slows considerably, as has been mentioned. He needs and wants less food but he still needs 1200–1300 calories a day. With his new sense of autonomy, he wants to decide what he will eat. Since he is feeding himself, he can push undesired food away. He can also climb off a booster chair or try desperately to climb out of his high chair. Naturally, this causes concern for parents if they do not understand that their child, who used to eat so much, is no longer an infant but a normal toddler.

During the second year, the toddler gains several more teeth, so he can now eat most table foods without gastrointestinal upsets because he can chew more thoroughly. He is not ready for nuts, chocolate, spicy foods, or excessive fats, however. He prefers tablespoon-size servings on his own plate and usually rejects mixed foods such as casseroles. He continues to enjoy finger foods, but he now views the use of a spoon as an enjoyable challenge. Parents can take advantage of their toddler's naturally adventurous nature to introduce a variety of foods from the table or from their plates at a restaurant.

The toddler usually does not drink from a bottle, and parents may have a difficult time ensuring adequate fluid intake. The child needs approximately 16 ounces of milk a day, which can be given with his meals. Water should be offered twice between every meal and at bedtime. Once during the day he should receive a cup of juice containing Vitamin C. The toddler often becomes constipated because of a decrease in fluid intake during this period (see the later section on common problems). A drink of water is usually welcomed after a play period, a fall, or a nap, even though the child definitely prefers something sweet.

DAILY ROUTINES

As has been mentioned, routines give the toddler a feeling of security about the present and the future: he knows what to expect. Routines do not have to be rigid to be effective, but a daily plan that is followed more or less closely will meet emotional and physical needs, and will allow some time for parents to meet their own needs.

Sleeping

The toddler generally sleeps for approximately two hours during his afternoon nap and twelve hours at night. He may try to give up his afternoon nap at the end of toddlerhood if he requires less than the average amount of sleep. When he is put to sleep at 1 P.M.., he cries, talks to himself, and/or plays alone until it is time to get up. He may stay in his crib for two hours, fall asleep at 3 P.M.. and not awaken until 5 P.M.. He will then not be ready for a night's sleep until 10 P.M.. Although the parents may be tired of having their active toddler around, he cannot go to sleep after such a late nap.

The toddler often perceives sleep as separation from his parents and from "the action" outside his bedroom door. He will use all his negativistic tricks to prolong contact with his parents. Routines help in getting a child to bed; they remove some of the impulse to rebel if it becomes an accepted fact that, after his bath, he will hear a story, say his prayers, have a few quiet minutes with a parent, and then go to sleep. As with the infant, the toddler may wake up during the night and need contact with his parents. He may be able to put himself back to sleep if given the opportunity. Some parents feel comfortable with his climbing into bed with them or lying on a blanket on the floor next to them. Others go to the child's bed to provide comfort and stay there until he is able to go back to sleep.

Eating

The toddler eats three meals a day, usually with his family, sharing their food and company. He needs mid-morning and mid-afternoon snacks to prevent irritability due to lowered blood glucose levels. Suitable snacks include fresh fruits, fresh vegetables, meats, cheeses, and eggs. Bedtime snacks should be avoided, since residual food in teeth will cause tooth decay.

Mealtime with a toddler can be outright chaos, or it can be pleasant for the whole family. First, the child should be moderately hungry and not sleepy. A glass of milk or a cookie given to pacify him while dinner cooks will inevitably kill his appetite. He needs a high chair, a plastic cup and plate, and a spoon that fits his grip. An inexpensive tablecloth under his high chair will catch most food dropped, thrown, and spilled. Parents can then roll the plastic up and shake it outside. The toddler should be allowed to eat with his fingers or spoon and hold his own half-filled cup (Figure 5–3). Often he much prefers eating from his parents' plates or their forks. Gradually, limits can be imposed on inappropriate behavior such as throwing food. Parents should forgive the child for spilling food but should gently disapprove of it to encourage caution with liquids. Once the child is finished eating, he is ready to be away from food and the confines of his chair. He will be able to tolerate longer waits as he gets older, but he usually needs to move onto something more interesting during toddlerhood.

Bathing

A toddler loves water play and baths, and there is generally no problem in establishing the bath as a daily routine. Shampooing, however, presents difficulties. A toddler does not always enjoy having his hair washed; he may feel afraid with his eyes

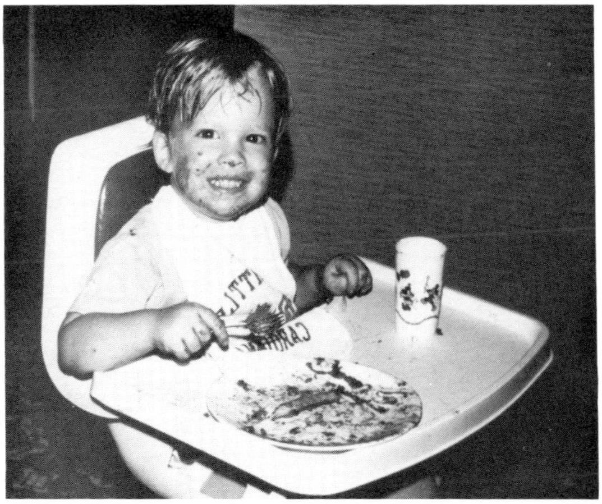

Figure 5–3. *Using his own plastic plate and cup, this child feeds himself.*

closed and with water in his face, and he will fear getting soap or shampoo in his eyes. Parents can try various approaches to shampoos; some children prefer to be shampooed in the shower, or in the kitchen sink, lying on the cabinet and letting the head fall back into a parent's hands; the water then runs down the back of the child's head and not into his face. Shampooing is an essential routine, so parents must use care to make it a pleasant one.

Toilet Training

Control of elimination is a major developmental task of toddlerhood. As with all parenting, cues and gradualism are keys to success. Cues, or signs of readiness, include the ability of the child to walk confidently, his awareness that he has a wet or soiled diaper, and the capability to hold urine for two hours. These signs indicate that the child is ready to learn to control his anal and bladder *sphincters* (which relax during elimination). Training can begin as soon as the signs mentioned above appear, at about 18 months, but progress is usually slow. Waiting a while after the appearance of these signs may speed up the whole process. Parents can heighten the toddler's awareness of bathrooms, toilets, toilet tissue, feces, and urine before training is begun. Feces in his diapers should be pointed out, dumped in the toilet, and flushed with his help. He should be encouraged to watch his parents and siblings as they sit on or stand at the toilet. It helps if the child has words for "urine" and "feces"; using the correct (or, at least, the same) terms will increase his awareness that he is the same as other family members. (Most families have pet terms for elimination, and these are fine if the toddler is taught the correct terms simultaneously or soon after.)

The next step in toilet training is the acquisition of a comfortable potty-chair that allows the toddler to rest his feet on the floor. He should be seated on his potty-chair at about the time he usually has a bowel movement, or soon after a nap if his diaper is still dry. Parents should avoid restraints and forms of entertainment to entice the child to perform the task at hand; the toddler will resist being strapped in and will forget why he is there. A ten-minute sit on the potty is long enough—a longer period is too similar to punishment and the child's legs may go to sleep. Gentle rewards will reinforce success in using the potty. When he uses the potty occasionally, he is ready for thick underpants. After a few weeks or months, he will enjoy being clean and dry. This sounds easy, but it is not. The toddler may refuse to eliminate at scheduled times because of his strong negativistic tendency, or may have bowel movements while he naps. He may have a small tear in his anal mucosa, or constipation due to inadequate fluid intake. Parents may not have the ability to be consistent, regardless of their attempts, and the toddler needs routines in order to acquire self-control. Most three-year-olds have daytime bladder and bowel control, and most five-year-olds have nighttime control. Accidents will continue to occur throughout preschool and early school age. It is very important for parents to avoid scolding the child for lapses in training; scolding shames the toddler when he has a genuine "accident," and it rewards him with a parent manipulation tool when he is actually being negative. Any major change in the toddler's life, such as a move, a separation of his parents, or a new sibling, will usually result in regression and the need for renewed toilet training.

Play School and Day Care

The toddler is plagued with stranger and separation anxieties, so attending any type of child care center is often very traumatic; he may even have difficulty in staying with a neighbor. It is probably best for the young toddler to remain with a "day care family" until this anxiety stage has passed. If at all possible, his parents should avoid initiating full-time day care until the resolution of these anxieties. If he must go to a day care center, he will need to visit the center with a parent to become familiar with the environment before being left there alone. He will definitely need his security object during this stressful time. As soon as he becomes a part of established routines, he will feel safer and begin to explore and enjoy the setting, although he may still cry when he is dropped off in the morning.

Allie K., aged two, went to a day care center daily. Mrs. K. had spent months trying to decide whether or not to go to work while her husband was out of the country for a year. The center seemed warm, friendly, and clean; the people who ran the center spoke of normal development, flexibility, and parent involvement. The other children appeared to be happy. However, each morning, Allie cried pitifully as they drove into the center's driveway, and clung to her mother's neck until she was pulled away by one of the women at the center. Mrs. K. cried all the way to work. As Mrs. K. described the situation (Allie is now getting ready for the first grade) she shook her head sadly. "It was great getting back to work, but I really paid a big price. I can still hear her crying. In the afternoon, she would cry again briefly when she saw me again. In a few weeks, she hopped out of the car to play in the morning and even resisted going home in the afternoon occasionally."

PLAY

As a toddler develops emotionally, cognitively, and physically, his play begins to change, too. His ability to run, jump, and climb allows him more freedom to explore his world and himself. He is able to use some imagination in choosing how he will play now, since objects can symbolize a variety of "real-life" things, and he can imitate the adult world as he sees it. Toddler play has more significance than the mere distraction it provides the child; he practices figuring out how to accomplish a goal and can test the practicality of his decision.

Motor play teaches the child what he can do in and with his environment. He needs space and large objects to exercise his large muscles. A large plastic box, sturdy enough to hold his weight, is fun to stand on, lean against, or climb into. Big balls are fun to push and kick. Small objects that fit together provide exercise for the small muscles. The toddler enjoys scribbling, painting with a brush or his fingers, splashing in water, and pushing a riding toy. Such activities improve muscular development and coordination, stimulate the senses, and teach the child about the world around him.

Play, too, is a socialization process; it necessitates the first attempts at getting along with peers. *Parallel play,* a type of play in which the toddler plays happily beside another with almost no interaction, is typical (Figure 5–4). The toddler has not yet learned to share things; no amount of shame or force will make him want to share his toys. The toddler also continues to play with his parents, and he is thus exposed to more ideas, more words, and more actions that he imitates, winning the approval of his parents.

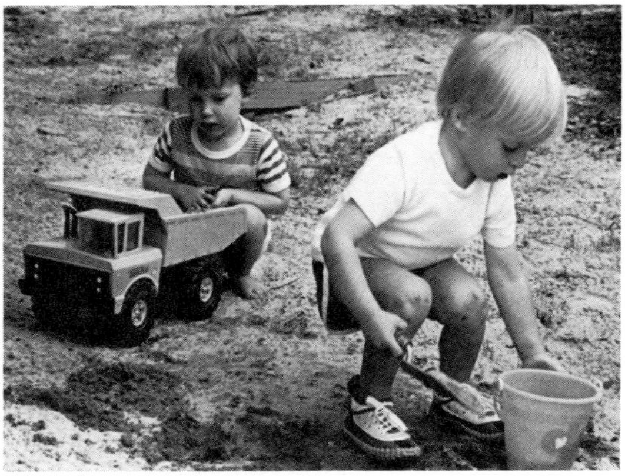

Figure 5–4. *Toddlers play beside each other but not with each other in parallel play.*

COMMON PROBLEMS AND NURSING INTERVENTIONS

The toddler's parents often call toddlerhood itself a "common problem." it is filled with the problems of eating, sleeping, toilet training, and so on which have been discussed. The following are other matters that concern parents as they struggle to cope with this stage of their child's development.

Constipation

The toddler no longer drinks from a bottle, so a decreased fluid intake may go unnoticed. His choice of food may not include sufficient bulk. He is being potty-trained, and he may hold feces (rather than comply with his parents' wishes) until they are hard and dry. Once the child is constipated, a glycerin suppository may be necessary for relief. Having a suppository inserted is a very upsetting procedure for many toddlers and preventive measures are far more desirable. To prevent constipation, increase fluid and bulk intake but hold milk intake to 16 ounces; offer natural laxatives such as wheat bran, cooked prunes, and raw fruit and vegetables. If these efforts do not promote soft, painless stools, the child should have medical attention. Occasionally, an anomaly of the bowel will cause constipation, which, in such cases, usually begins at birth, not during toddlerhood; examination and/or x-ray will help determine the cause.

Temper Tantrums

When a toddler is overcome with feelings of anger, frustration, and/or negativism, he may become so upset that he loses control completely. He screams, kicks, hits, and bites, and throws objects in a frenzy that he cannot stop. He becomes so overwrought by these powerful emotions that only the most appealing of diversions—or the quiet of exhausted sleep—can alleviate the tantrum. Spanking heightens the child's feelings of helplessness and may prolong the tantrum; bribing him with candy or toys simply rewards the behavior. Some of the more effective ways of dealing with tantrums include putting the child in the tub, where he can splash out his anger, giving him a drink of water or washing his face with a cool cloth to divert his attention, or removing him from play areas and placing him in a quiet room. Diversions of this sort should not be viewed as bribes, for they allow the child the chance to control his behavior.

Of course, parents have emotions too, and the tantrum may occur when the parents themselves are under stress. The parents cannot be expected to react in a calm, rational manner if, for example, the child is screaming and kicking while relatives are visiting. If the parents occasionally slap the toddler's hand or yell at him, the tantrum may last longer but the child will survive.

Parents should be advised to forgive themselves under such circumstances and try for a more logical response next time. However, if they consistently respond with anger and punishment, they need counseling in handling their child's outbursts.

Accidental Poisoning

The toddler explores his world through his senses, so he naturally puts objects that interest him in his mouth in order to taste them. Because he is now able to climb, he has access to many places that were beyond his reach when he was younger. It is no wonder that the toddler is the frequent victim of the accidental ingestion of harmful substances. Staying one step ahead of the child's development is essential to prevention; for example, the child's parents should keep medications in a locked box *before* the child demonstrates the ability to reach the medicine cabinet. All harmful substances (including cleaning products, petroleum distillates, insecticides, poisonous plants, and alcohol) should be stored in a place that is not only beyond the child's present reach but that is likely to be beyond his reach even when the child is older. Chemicals of all kinds should be kept in their original containers; if, for example, kerosene is stored in a Coca-Cola bottle, the child may take several gulps before he realizes that something is wrong.

If the child has ingested a harmful substance, the goal is usually to remove as much of it as possible from the stomach. The most effective means of emptying the stomach is to induce vomiting; this should be done in all cases of accidental poisoning, except those involving caustics and hydrocarbons. The administration of 15 to 30 ml of syrup of ipecac, orally, followed by at least one large (240-ml, or 8-oz) glass of water, usually induces vomiting; the dose may be repeated 15 minutes later if necessary. Ipecac can be given at home before taking the child to the emergency room, and a small amount of it should be kept on hand in homes with children. The original container for the substance, any remaining amount of the substance itself, and any vomitus should be taken to the emergency room.

Caustics, such as lye, should be removed by gastric lavage, since vomiting would cause further trauma to the mouth and esophagus. Large amount of hydrocarbons are also lavaged, while small amounts are permitted to remain in the stomach. Activated charcoal, which binds most poisons that are not removed by induced vomiting, should be given promptly; mix 15 to 30 ml of the charcoal with 240 ml of water. Activated charcoal also binds ipecac and should therefore not be given when it is desirable to induce vomiting.

Common Cold

Toddlerhood is plagued by a marked increase in the incidence of common colds. Whereas the infant generally is not exposed to many different people in different places, the toddler often is. He goes with his parents to more places away from home and may attend nursery school. With each new cold or other infection, the child's body produces antibodies that fight the same causative microorganisms in the future. Parents may become very upset about frequent colds and related sore throats, ear infections, and "runny noses," and may question the usefulness of repeated courses of antibiotics; they may demand that their child's tonsils be removed because they have heard stories of remarkable improvement after a tonsillectomy. Occasionally, other measures are indicated, but usually the toddler and parents must tolerate these frequent illnesses until early school age, when the toddler's body can resist infection more effectively.

Sibling Rivalry

The toddler has a great need for "sameness" in his life; a new sibling brings with him new and different sights, sounds, smells, and routines, and alters the older child's relationships with significant people, especially his mother. Things are not the same at all. The toddler's idea of what his family "should be" is based on his previous experience, and he knows that a strange baby "should not" be there! It is natural for him to attempt to bring the situation back to normal by disposing of the intruder, or to release his anxiety in the form of aggressive behavior, such as hitting the baby, sitting on him too, poking him with his finger, and so on (Figure 5–5).

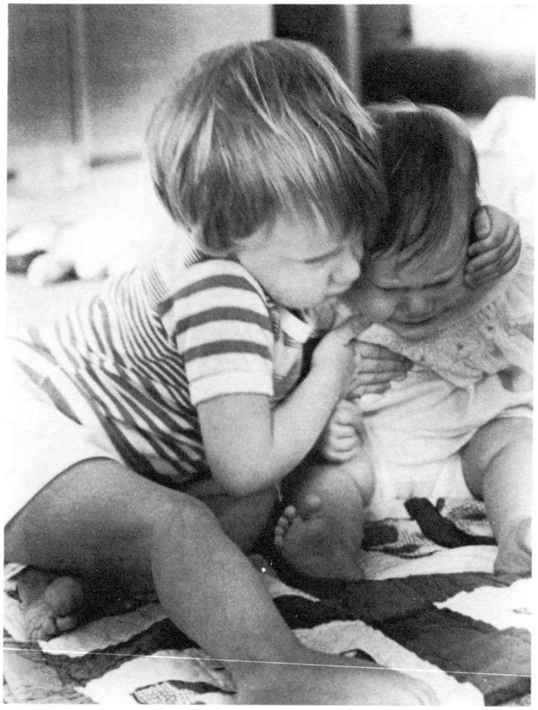

Figure 5–5. *Sibling rivalry may take the form of overly forceful displays of "affection."*

Mark, aged two, had always been a happy, easy-going child. His mother had provided a calm and loving family environment most of the time. When Jenny was born, Mark's grandmother came to stay and gave him lots of attention and affection. A week later, the grandmother went home, and Mark suddenly realized that things were not right. When Jenny was being breast-fed, Mark first cried for his mother to put her down and then insisted on being held in her other arm. He climbed into Jenny's bassinet and lay flat over her, scaring their father who was alone with them. Mark started whining, having temper tantrums and hitting Jenny on the head. He could not be left alone with her for a minute.

Giving the older child special attention while the baby sleeps can help him adjust somewhat, and involving him in baby care makes him feel that he is a part of his "new" family. The child should be encouraged to maintain his own important routines to restore his sense of security. He must not hurt his new sibling and limits on overt agression must be firm and consistent. Gradually, he will learn to control the impulse to hurt the baby just as he controls the impulse to turn the knobs on the television. Parents should avoid overreacting to hostile acts because the child will use the same acts to manipulate his parents. This is much easier said than done, of course. The mother who actually has two "babies" is often too exhausted to be patient and kind when her toddler slaps the sleeping baby's face. In time, the baby and new routines will become familiar and tolerable to the toddler.

ACCIDENTS

Accidents are the leading cause of death during toddlerhood and are responsible for many life-long disabilities. Toddlerhood is a period of exploration and curiosity, and a toddler will use his new skills of walking and climbing to reach things that appeal to him (Figure 5–6). Objects that were once out of his reach may suddenly become accessible. Because toddlers love being outside and running beyond their parents' reach, they are exposed to the danger of traffic on the streets or the family car in the driveway. The toddler begins to use riding toys of all sorts, and, unfortunately, he sees only that which is in his direct line of vision. He is interested in different colors and tastes; he finds opening bottles, jars, and boxes a challenge to be met, and he has no way of knowing if the contents are safe or harmful.

Parents must supervise their toddler constantly; *he cannot be trusted to heed safety precautions.* Consistency in imposing safety rules is of utmost importance.

Colleen, aged two, never rode in a car without being safely strapped in her seat. When her parents took a six-hour trip, she became restless several times. Her mother read her a story and played name games. They stopped for a drink and a walk every one or two hours. Colleen took her regular nap sitting up.

Bill, aged two, had always ridden in his car seat. His parents took a long trip, and when Bill started squirming in his seat, he was allowed to play in the back seat without protective seat belts. For several weeks after that trip Bill protested violently when forced to get into his car seat.

Parents must restrain their own behavior since the toddler will imitate them. They must be constantly aware of all dangers, including their own temptation to ease restrictions "just once." In some families, the parents are barely aware of the hazards their child is exposed to; under such circumstances, accidents are bound to occur more frequently.

Dottie, aged two, lived with her mother and three siblings in a two-room apartment. Her mother filled the toilet with caustic cleaning fluid and went next door for a visit. Dottie found a cup and dipped it into the toilet for a drink as she always did when she was thirsty. She has now spent 12 months on the pediatric unit undergoing numerous procedures to reconstruct her esophagus.

The most knowledgeable, caring parents will not be able to create a perfect balance between freedom and restraint at all times. Sometimes the toddler will get cuts, scrapes, bruises or even broken bones when he is adequately supervised in a "toddler-proof" environment. When accidents happen, the parents may be overwhelmed with guilt, even after the most freakish accident. Be sure to discuss their feelings at length, and allow plenty of time for listening to them. Telling them that all children have accidents does *not* usually make them feel better.

SIGNS AND SYMPTOMS OF ILLNESS

The toddler is much like the infant in that he cannot clearly explain where he feels pain or what happened. However, his parents know his reactions better by the time the child has reached toddlerhood, and they feel more comfortable about determining the need for medical attention. As the child's contacts with other people and places increase, so does the incidence of minor illnesses.

The healthy toddler's face reflects his interest in the world. The sick child loses his drive to explore all around him, and his

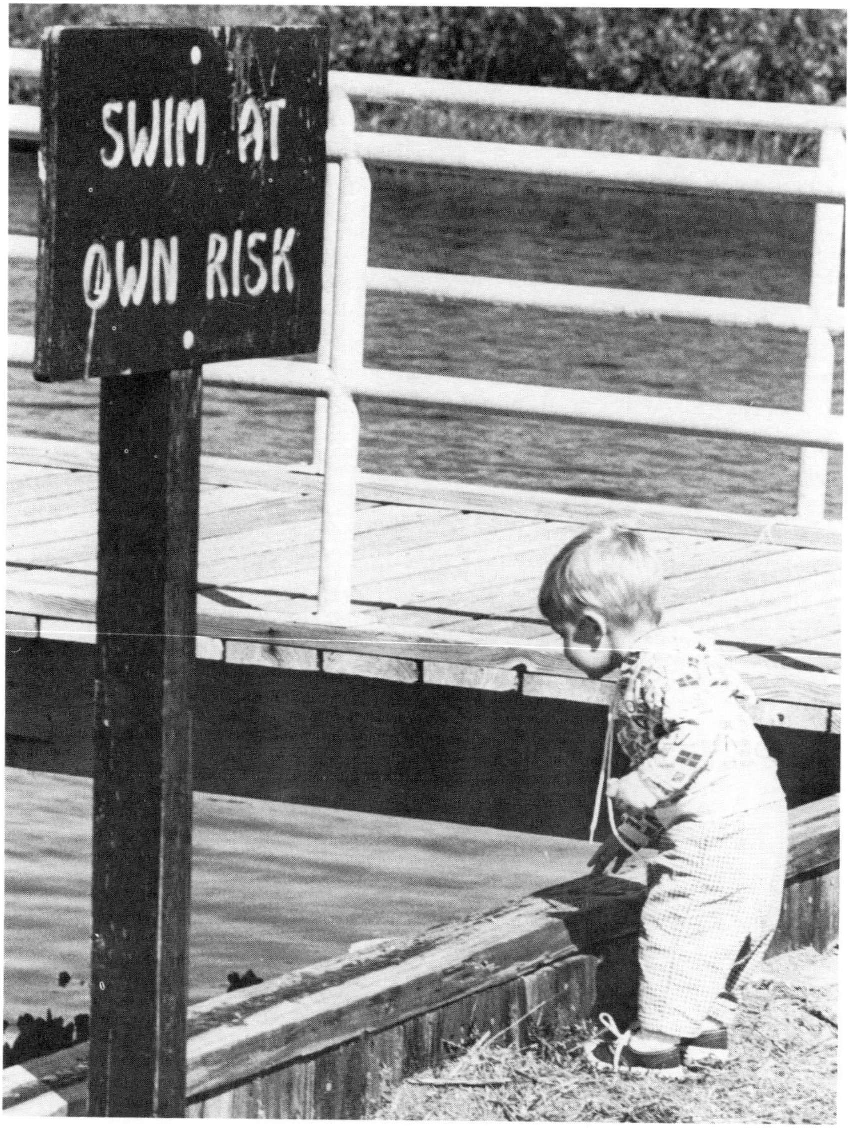

Figure 5–6. *The combination of curiosity and increased mobility places the toddler at risk for accidents.*

face has a flat, disinterested look. His eyes become sunken, and his skin becomes loose and dry with dehydration, regardless of the underlying pathology. His overall color is pale or gray, and dark circles form under his eyes.

The toddler decreases his total food intake in relation to his body weight because he is growing less rapidly. He may refuse to eat simply to be negativistic, but a decrease in appetite may be an early sign of illness, and parents may not be able to make the distinction between illness and normal toddler behavior. If there are no other signs of illness, a decrease or absence of appetite is probably a normal variation in the child's routines. A continued pattern of limited intake or a sudden change may be cause for concern.

The toddler's developing control of his bladder and bowel causes changes in his usual elimination patterns. As has been mentioned, the child often becomes temporarily constipated. His bowel may react to spicy, fried, and very sweet foods by producing loose stools. Parents (and sometimes professionals) cannot always determine whether these alterations are early indications of illness. Major changes, such as large, frequent liquid stools from a child who normally has one bowel movement a day, usually indicate a pathologic process (see ch. 18). Urinary frequency and output are difficult to assess while the child is still in diapers, but once he is in training pants, deviations in urination patterns are obvious. The toddler indicates that he is having pain with voiding by holding his or her genitals and crying. He may use his favorite word for "hurt." Unless the urethral opening is irritated, painful voiding usually indicates a need for medical attention.

The toddler's routines can become disrupted by his negativism and, since he no longer falls asleep easily at bedtime, he may sleep at unusual times of the day.

Linda, aged two, went to the carnival and had a great time. When she got home she was too excited to go to sleep for a while. She was irritable when she woke up early the next morning. Because she refused to eat breakfast and cried for no reason, her mother began to suspect an illness. Linda fell asleep at 9:20 A.M.. on a pillow in the den, and her mother became alarmed. She felt Linda's forehead to check for fever but found none. At lunchtime Linda's mother was relieved when a refreshed Linda woke up ready to eat.

Major changes in activity levels, such as extreme restlessness or lethargy, are often indications of acute illness.

The toddler is still much like an infant, but his body systems can tolerate the stress of illness without quite as much response. His temperature, pulse, and respirations continue to react to many illnesses with marked upward and downward swings. As he gets older, these changes in vital signs become less sudden and less dramatic. Fever can still develop suddenly, however; the toddler can be actively playing at 3 A.M. and have a temperature of 104° by 5A.M. A high fever in a toddler is not always a sign of serious illness, since the child's body may overreact to common illnesses. Febrile seizures, still occurring at this age, are caused by this rapid appearance of high temperature. Antipyretic treatments and medications can decrease fevers significantly and often quickly.

HOSPITALIZATION

The toddler and his parents have all the problems with hospitalization that the infant has, and more. It is a crisis for the family, but it may be an even greater crisis for the child because of his acute separation anxiety. The strangeness of the hospital and its staff disrupts the sameness and routines that are so essential to the child's feeling of security (Figure 5–7). Fortunately, most hospitals welcome his parents, who are so necessary for his adaptation. The progress made in developing body awareness, self-discipline, language, and toilet training usually comes to a halt with hospitalization; in fact, regression is to be expected as was discussed in chapter 3. A distinct series of reactions has been observed in toddlers who are separated from their parents because of institutionalization. The child first *protests* loudly and will not accept comfort from anyone. Next he gives up entirely, succumbing to *despair*. Later, he often develops a superficial relationship with anyone who walks into his room, but he rejects his mother when she comes. This stage, called *denial*, is often mistaken for satisfactory adjustment (Fig. 5–8).

These difficulties are minimized or non-

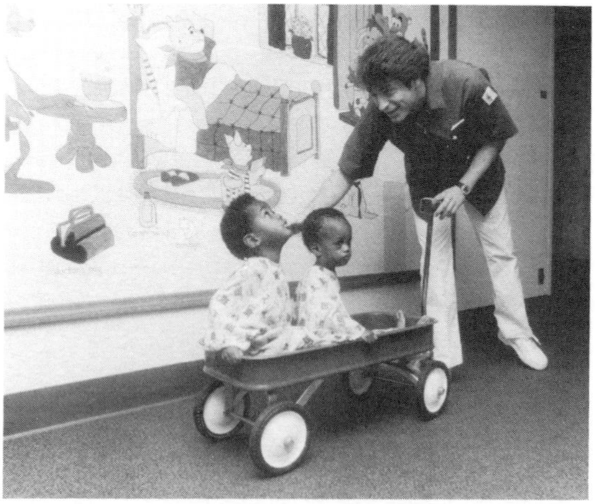

Figure 5–7. *The strangeness of the hospital environment is reflected in the faces of these children.*

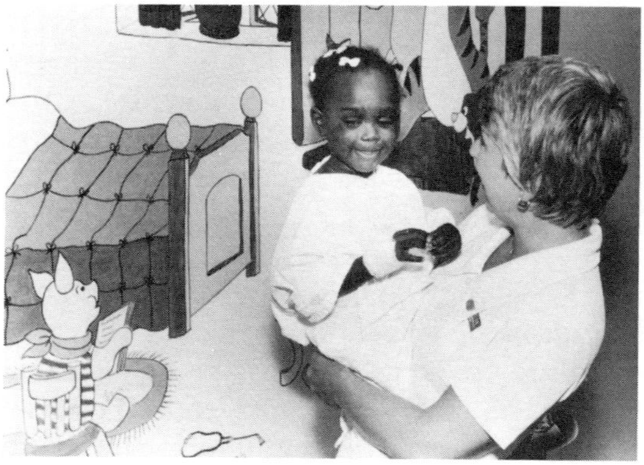

Figure 5–8. *The nurse should give extra attention to the child whose parents cannot room-in.*

existent when parents room-in with their toddler, and most hospitals welcome rooming-in. Your role, therefore, is not only to care for their child, but also to support the parents enough for them to maintain parent roles.

Nursing Interventions

The considerations and interventions relating to the admission of the toddler to the hospital are very similar to those that pertain to the infant. It still is very important to greet the parents with a smile, to let them give their account of their child's illness, and to provide information they will need during their stay in the hospital. Whenever possible, physical assessments should be made while the parent holds the child.

The toddler's hospitalization, as opposed to the infant's, requires that the nurse has a more detailed knowledge of the child's daily routines. It is not enough to know that the toddler eats table foods; each family has a group of favorite foods and rituals that the toddler has grown to expect. He may be accustomed to having his own plate, spoon, and cup, small hamburgers to be eaten with the fingers, and peeled apples. The ritualistic toddler simply does not adapt readily to eating different food in his crib from several glass bowls. If a parent is always present, he or she may automatically make some changes, such as peeling the apple, putting small portions of food on one plate, or holding the child in the lap while he feeds himself from the bedside table. Part of admission procedure is not only to record the toddler's routines in detail but also to encourage the parents to continue as many of these routines as possible during hospitalization; they may feel the need for express permission to do so, since the hospital is such an awesome place, creating an intense fear of breaking the rules. Parents are usually greatly relieved to find that you are interested in providing "sameness" for their child, especially if they must leave him without a familiar person. Assessing his individual routines may reveal the need for counseling, but admission is certainly no time to tell the parents to change their child rearing habits.

If the toddler has a security object, it should accompany him on all trips to different areas of the hospital. He needs to hold it when anesthesia is administered and when he is awakened in the recovery room. Always label these special items with the child's name and room number before he leaves the unit. When the object must be removed for a while, tell the child he will get it back as soon as possible and make sure that he does. He may not understand completely, but he may come to associate you with the same relief that is provided by the object. Watch for these objects as you change linens—too many have gone to the laundry and have never returned. The parents already know the importance of the security object, but they may not bring it because it is dirty or ragged. Encourage them to send for it or bring it to their child as soon as possible.

Generally, it is best not to initiate new routines in the hospital unless parents are directly involved with the process. Nurses who start changes in the child's daily living habits are telling parents, in effect, that their parenting is inadequate. For example, toilet training the toddler in the hospital on a comfortable potty-chair may not prepare him at all for balancing on the adult toilet seat at home if a potty chair is not available. He may learn to control his elimination, but he may be terrified by the height of the seat, requiring a much longer time to adapt to his family's facilities. The same principle holds true for eating and sleeping habits. Allowing a toddler to make a huge mess while eating when his parents greatly value neatness can cause family (not to mention nurse-parent) friction when the child gets home. It is much better to explain the need for his messiness as he learns; then simply allow parents to accept or reject your suggestions. Generally, the toddler is not in a hospital long enough to establish new routines, but when he is, family lifestyle and parents' wishes must be major considerations if a smooth transition back to home life is to be made.

The toddler's body boundaries, as he perceives them, include his clothing. Stripping him of his clothes is fear-provoking since part of his "body" has been removed. To stick something into his body violates the boundaries, yet every hospitalized toddler experiences many such ordeals. Reasoning, explaining, and demonstrating seldom help the toddler to maintain or regain self-control; it is therefore necessary to restrain him adequately and perform the procedure quickly. Replace his clothes immediately, hand him to his parent if possible, and stay close for a few minutes. It is important for the toddler to see you as more than someone who hurts him and then disappears.

Self-control takes a great deal of energy, and the toddler simply does not have energy to spare during hospitalization. Expect regression in areas requiring self-control, such as toilet training, eating, sleeping, and separation from parents. Parents are usually embarrassed when their child has a bowel movement in his pants when they had assured the nurse that he was trained; the toddler who seldom has temper tantrums may suddenly start kicking, screaming, and hitting his mother because she refuses to give him the ice cream on his tray before he eats his lunch. Regardless of the area of self-control, the child usually loses the skill acquired most recently: if he had just begun to urinate in the potty but long ago developed bowel control, he probably will wet his pants but still have bowel movements on the potty. Reassure parents that this regression is perfectly normal. Gentle guidance from parents will help the child feel safe and increase his self-control as he becomes more familiar with the hospital environment and routines.

Preparation for Procedures

The toddler can benefit somewhat from carefully planned preparation for procedures. Dress rehearsals give him the opportunity to experience some aspects of the procedure. Playing peek-a-boo from behind a mask teaches him that real people (hopefully, with smiles) exist behind the paper. Practice in breathing through a rubber mask (or whatever is used), with the child's mother included, may decrease some of his fear when the real event occurs.

Ted, aged two, was prepared by a nurse anesthetist for surgery. An extra digit was to be removed from his hand. Ted, his mother, and the nurse all dressed in O.R. garb, including masks. He was frightened when his mother covered her face with a mask but was completely relieved after a few peek-a-boo's. He refused to breathe through the black rubber mask until his mother tried it, and all three took turns breathing over and over. The nurse left clothes, cloth masks, and rubber mask with Ted's mother for further practice. The nurse anesthetist was surprised when her two-year-old patient willingly took deep breaths from the black mask the next day.

The toddler may show no response to your efforts to prepare him for a procedure. However, although he usually is unable to maintain total self-control, your efforts will not only benefit the child but will also strengthen his parents' trust in you. Preparing the toddler will build parents' confidence in you and this confidence will be transmitted to the child.

Discharge

The toddler's transition from hospital to home is usually more difficult than that of the infant. Even when his parents room-in, his routines are significantly disrupted during hospitalization. Prepare parents for behavioral changes and recommend a gradual but firm reestablishment of limits. Reestablishing routines is more difficult when the stay is longer than a few days and/or more traumatic in terms of pain and separation from parents. Most parents feel that just taking the child back to his own bed, high chair, and bathtub will minimize behavior problems, but they should be advised that the process of "getting back to normal" usually requires patience, consistency, and time.

As with the infant, the toddler's parents

must learn procedures by doing them, first with the assistance and support of a nurse, and finally at home, alone. The process of increasing the parents' independence and confidence in these procedures is usually very difficult, regardless of their ages, resources, educational background, and so on. Rooming-in with their child and practicing skills with the nurse's reinforcement definitely helps the family cope with homecoming. Always arrange for a home health referral if you feel that assistance will be needed at home.

SUMMARY

The toddler develops a sense of autonomy as he separates from his mother, often through negativistic acts. He learns much about himself, including how to control his impulses. If his parents show disapproval of his developments, a sense of shame and doubt results. The child explores and experiments with his environment as he enters the preoperational stage of cognitive development. He can see only from his point of view. He develops increased productive language after he has learned to walk and run with proficiency. His growth is slow but steady during this period, and his appetite decreases accordingly. He gains several new teeth and can chew most foods, but he usually selects a few favorites.

Routine is very important in guiding the child toward adaptation to the restrictions of everyday family and social life. He must learn to control his bowel and bladder during this stage; this task requires a gradual imposition of expectations from parents. Accidents are the leading cause of death in toddlers; the toddler is unaware of the potential dangers of most circumstances. Common problems include constipation, temper tantrums, common colds, and sibling rivalry. The onset of illness continues to be relatively abrupt, but the toddler's body can tolerate illness with a less dramatic reaction than an infant.

Hospitalization is very traumatic to the toddler; aside from the traumas of procedures, hospitalization imposes a disruption of routines and gives rise to stranger and separation anxiety. Parents should stay with their toddler at all times if possible. Nursing care must be directed at both the parents and child.

CHAPTER **6**

The Preschooler

BEHAVIORAL OBJECTIVES

After studying this chapter you will be able to:

- Describe the preschooler's emotional development with reference to initiative and guilt.
- Identify typical fears of the preschooler and his ways of coping with them.
- Discuss the preschooler's cognitive and language development.
- Describe physical and motor changes that occur during each year of the preschool period.
- Discuss the nutrition of the preschooler in relation to food requirements and developmental status.
- Describe daily activities, including preschool and kindergarten, that comprise the child's routines.
- Determine types of play, including projective play techniques, for the well and the ill child.
- Identify common problems and accidents of preschoolers and give preventive and treatment measures.
- Describe the signs of illness in the preschooler.
- Discuss nursing care of the child and his parents during hospitalization. Relate the child's egocentrism to all aspects of nursing care.

TERMS AND CONCEPTS

Initiative
Guilt
Magical thinking
Imaginary friends
Sex identification
Concept formation
Concrete experiences
Fluency
Pedodontist
Dramatic play
Projective activity
Nightmares
Masturbation
Nocturnal enuresis

The preschooler derives his sense of security largely from his parents' presence, but when he is hospitalized, he is able to tolerate and even enjoy nursing care that takes his level of development into consideration. The parents of the preschool-age child should be encouraged by the nurse to continue their parenting routines and to assume responsibility for selected procedures. The nurse can strengthen her relationship with the preschooler by presenting herself as the parents' friend and slowly building her own relationship with the child. The child is usually most comfortable in new experiences if his parents are within sight and reach, but the knowledge that they are nearby may be enough when he undergoes familiar routines. The preschooler gradually overcomes his fear of strangers and strange situations and will ultimately cooperate and participate with the nurse in some daily routines, play, and various procedures. Regardless of the degree of the nurse's success in interacting with the child, most parents will (and should) remain the major source of the child's strength; therefore, supporting their efforts is a nursing priority throughout the child's hospitalization.

EMOTIONAL DEVELOPMENT

The preschool years between toddlerhood and school age, from approximately three to six years of age, are truly fascinating ones, full of the preschooler's questioning, exploring, and developing more self-control and self-awareness, including a sense of sexual identity. The preschooler couples autonomy with some responsibility, delays gratification increasingly, and uses creative thinking to solve many of his own crises. He "takes a chance" by trying something new and a little frightening, and he learns that he indeed can accomplish new tasks, giving him what Erikson calls a sense of *initiative*. He has a developing conscience that is usually rather rigid. This conscience, if too controlling, can give the child what Erikson refers to as a sense of *guilt,* which results from the fear that his actions may not win the approval of significant others.

The preschooler learns by exploring, questioning, and sampling new parts of his world. His constant "whys" can become a nuisance to the most patient parent. His intrusiveness into new situations can be annoying and/or dangerous, but he learns that, with initiative, he can gain new knowledge and skills. These rewards inevitably tempt him to seek out more interesting unknowns.

The preschooler not only finds his surroundings fascinating, he wants to know more about himself. He picks his nose, rolls his testes, spits, sticks his finger in his ears and rectum, and pulls his eyelids down. As he explores himslf, he develops a fairly rigid image of his body boundaries. Anything that breaks these boundaries is perceived as threatening unless the child has had enough nontraumatic experiences with that particular situation to overcome his fears. If the boundaries are broken by injections, cuts, or surgery, the faster the insult is closed, the better. Bleeding is a definite sign of "openness" and "brokenness".

Britt, three and a half, fell down on the pavement and hurt his knee. It hurt and he cried for a minute or two. He had stopped crying by the time his mother got him to the bathroom where she took off his pants. When Britt saw blood trickling down his leg, he began wailing as though he had just fallen down. He continued to sob periodically until the blood was gone, and the insult was safely closed with a bandage.

A major aspect of the preschooler's emotional development is coping with anxiety that arises from fear and guilt. Fears and guilt are not completely negative aspects of life; they keep the child's behavior within limits, providing safety. His conscience develops partly from the anticipation of parental disapproval. Extreme guilt and fear during this critical period, however, may lead to excessive anxiety throughout life. An understanding of why such apprehension appears during this time enables parents to help their preschooler deal with his feelings and avoid the extreme. They need to know that the child's horizons are much wider; by this stage, the child may have experienced separation from his parents when he attends a preschool, a separation that may be difficult to endure. He now knows that his parents cannot protect him at all times. As he watches more television, he learns that there is much to fear, and his everyday life verifies this; he sees animals splattered on the highway, other children limping with deformities, and his own finger cut and bleeding. Another cause of fear is that the preschooler's parents may unwittingly imbue him with their own fears.

Sally has three boys. As a child she was terrified of thunder. When her husband was away for months at a time, she gathered their sons into her bedroom "to take care of them" during thunderstorms. When her husband returned home, he was shocked to find that their three boys panicked at any rumbling noise.

These are illogical years of *magical thinking,* when a preschooler believes that his wishes can cause events to happen, and this belief leaves him susceptible to fear and guilt. For instance, in the course of normal sibling rivalry, the child may wish his baby brother to be dead; if something happens to the infant, the preschooler blames himself. A children's afternoon television show deals with this when its main character assures children that scary, bad wishes don't necessarily come true.

The preschooler develops typical ways to handle the anxiety that plagues his life. He often develops an *imaginary friend* who may be one or both of two types: the big, hairy monster who is actually warm, loving, and obedient, or the friend who accepts blame for all the guilt-producing wrongdoings. Ordering around monsters helps to overcome fears of uncontrollable forces in life. Blaming mistakes and transgressions on someone else relieves some guilt in the child. This is delightfully described in A.A. Milne's poem about Christopher Robin and Pooh.

The Friend

There are lots and lots of people
Who are always asking things,
Like Dates and Pounds and ounces
And the names of funny Kings,
The answer's either Sixpence
Or A Hundred Inches Long,
And I know they'll think me silly
If I get the answer wrong.

So Pooh and I go whispering
And Pooh looks very bright,
And says, "Well, I say sixpence,
But I don't suppose I'm right."
And then it doesn't matter
What the answer ought to be,
'Cos if he's right, I'm Right.
But if he's wrong, it isn't Me.*

Play, too, strengthens the child's sense of his ability to control fearful aspects of his environment; for instance, he may pretend to be a nurse or doctor—thus, *he* is giving the orders and taking charge. Unfortunately, some parents see this type of fantasizing as lying when it is actually a sign of the child's struggle to rid himself of guilt and, of course, to avoid punishment.

Routines, which are very important during toddlerhood, continue to help the preschooler deal with anxiety. He does not have to decide whether an act is right or wrong if he has performed it many times since infancy. When he or his parents no longer wish him to continue a certain routine, anxiety will appear as he makes the change. Gradual change helps him to become familiar with the new before he has to give up the old, thereby reducing his fear of the unknown.

The preschooler expresses his fears in numerous ways. A common manifestation is the appearance of nightmares (see common problems) in which conscious or suppressed concerns of the day emerge during the night as dreams. The child suddenly refuses to go outside to play with a certain child or toy; he may beg not to go to fairs, circuses, or parades because he is afraid of getting lost or being hurt by the elephant. He often delays bedtime with several requests for water, trips to the bathroom, or complaints of a stomachache. He may become quieter than usual or he may regress to earlier stages of development when he did not have to assume any responsibility for his own safety. He may show renewed dependence on thumbsucking and security objects. The normal preschooler will demonstrate some of these behaviors during times of stress, but most of the time, he will take chances on the unexplored aspects of his world through exploration, questioning, and play. Parents can provide considerable support for their child by looking for signs of anxiety, questioning the child, and listening carefully to him. Parents should praise the preschooler for trying new things, not just succeeding in them. They can increase a child's sense of security by setting limits within which new activities are permitted and by giving him room to explore. There is nothing wrong with parental interventions that reduce fear, such as leaving on a "night-light" if the child is afraid of the dark.

Preschoolers must accomplish the task of *sex identification*, incorporating one sexual identity or the other into the self-image. The little boy develops a noticeable attraction to his mother and jealousy toward his father. The little girl becomes "Daddy's girl" and is jealous of her mother. The child sees his parents in a variety of situations, which may include sexual intercourse, and takes note of love, respect, and admiration, or the lack of these, in the parents' interactions. By the end of the preschool period, the child usually resolves the conflict by identifying with the parent of the same sex. During this stage, the child has a heightened awareness of his or her genitals; he or she manipulates them in order to feel the pleasurable sensations and comfort the manipulation brings. The male child may want to press his genitals hard against his mother's leg or waist. He often explores beneath playmate's underwear to see what is there. He asks himself and his parents how he came about, and how babies get into and out of the swollen abdomen of a pregnant woman. No wonder the preschooler is periodically overwhelmed—so many facts and feelings present themselves that he cannot cope with them all at once.

Parents are of monumental importance in shaping the child's sexuality. Hopefully, by the end of toddlerhood, he will have learned the correct names for genitalia and will have been made to feel that these parts are acceptable to the family. He does learn, however, that something is "wrong" with the genitals because he has been told he must not handle, show, or use them in public. Conflicting messages confuse the preschooler, but he obligingly starts hiding his bottom, sneaking peeks at other's hidden parts, and, of course, feeling guilty. Parents can only explain that his body is clean and good, but that most people do not want to see genitals or buttocks or the act of elimination in public. They should allow the child to look at their own naked bodies and discuss the differences in children and adults in relation to size, breasts, hair, and so on. The preschool girl and boy need to know that boys have penises, and that girls have vaginas and uteruses, very special parts of their bodies that cannot be seen. When the preschooler begins to cling to the parents of the opposite sex, both parents should continue to demonstrate open love for each other and include the child as part of a threesome. Both parents must maintain authority with the child; it is especially important that the parent of the same sex, with whom the child will have begun to identify, be seen as a positive figure. When the child begins to ask questions about reproduction, the parents should not attempt an answer until they know what the child already thinks; what he already knows; what he really wants to know; and why he is asking. With this information in mind, parents can provide answers that are direct but simple enough for the child to understand. Since the child cannot handle large amounts of information at one time, he may concentrate on one aspect that is especially significant to him.

Al, aged four, was living with his parents in a country that provided a series on human reproduction on public television. One day his mother came home to find him sobbing in the sitter's arms. He ran to her and cried, "I don't want to put my penis in girls' "china's" to make babies, Mama. It might hurt or get caught."

Parents who respond to their preschooler's questions about sexuality and reproduction with simplicity, enthusiasm, and interest give the child positive cues and minimize his guilt and fear. Parents can use various approaches to sex education, such as reading books together, viewing the birth of a pet, and feeling a baby's kick through the mother's abdomen, but these experiences should be combined with explanations and reexplanations during the preschool period.

Parents may state emphatically that their child has no interest in his or others' genitals, or in reproduction. Perhaps this phenomenon can occur, but it is highly unlikely; the normal preschooler wonders about his world too much to ignore such a fascinating segment of everyday life.

Mrs. H. was six months pregnant when she brought her four-year-old, Sean, to the nurse practitioner for his health assessment. She described how her pregnancy had come at the perfect time to begin sex education. She, her husband, and Sean lay in bed together waiting to feel the baby kick on Saturday mornings. They had pictures to show the special canal that lets the baby out. Each time Sean's mother answered one question, he asked another. In time he developed a fairly good understanding of human reproduction.

Mrs. S. was eight months pregnant when she brought her four-year-old daughter Marti to the nurse practitioner for her yearly health assessment. The nurse, after hearing that Mrs. S. had a master's degree in early childhood education, assumed that Marti had learned much about human reproduction in the last few months and stated so. Marti's mother responded, "She has shown no interest whatsoever, so why should I force sex education on a sweet, innocent little girl? I told her that Mommy's tummy is fat and that satisfied her. She knows we are going to the hospital to get a baby soon, though." The nurse never established a trusting relationship with Mrs. S. but did give her reading material on the normal development of children Marti's age. Mrs. S. soon requested that Marti's records be transferred to a nearby health facility.

COGNITIVE DEVELOPMENT

The preschool period of the child's life falls within Piaget's preoperational stage of cognitive development, which is begun in toddlerhood. The young preschooler uses symbols and insight in his everyday world of play and problem-solving. Since he is egocentric, he cannot see from another point of view, be it another's opinion or physical vantage point. He must rely on his perceptions of previous experiences to sort out facts, events, sensations, and so on. Unfortunately, his perceptions are often distorted by his fears, fantasies, and personal viewpoint. He misses much of what happens around him because he focuses (or *centers*, in Piaget's terminology) on only one thing at a time. As the preschooler gains more information about his world, develops the ability to cope with more than one thing at a time, and becomes less egocentric, he thinks more logically. The developmental task of *concept formation* is begun in infancy and continued during toddlerhood, but understanding of the concepts of time, space, number, class, and causality are begun during the preschool period. These concepts can barely be grasped in the early part of this period.

John, aged two and a half, was trying to describe to his uncle his trip to the fair, which had occurred a week earlier. At first he explained that he left his house after lunch. He then told his uncle that he went "one day tomorrow." He knew that he was not using the right words, but he did not know how to express past tense correctly. When his frustration became obvious, his mother said, "Last week, John." He agreed heartily, saying "Yeah, last week."

Early concept formation is dependent on the child's *concrete experiences*. An example of this is seen in the story of "The Three Bears." The preschooler has an immature concept of quantity and comparison; the story bridges this gap by using Papa Bear, Mama Bear, and Baby Bear to represent big, medium, and little. The child can easily understand relative quantities and sizes of porridge, bowls, chairs, and beds as long as they are joined with the Papa, Mama, and Baby concepts. Because he lacks the concrete experience to understand the concepts, the story would have little meaning to him if the concepts were not linked to the characters. Later, the preschooler understands the concepts of larger and smaller and does not require such obvious connections.

The process of cognitive development depends on the preschooler's experiences, real and imaginary. Parents can support this process by answering the child's questions, demonstrating ways to accomplish tasks, encouraging different forms of play, and allowing his active participation in many activities. They need to set limits so that the child will feel free to explore and to imagine. He will soon be able to organize information about himself and his world in a logical fashion.

LANGUAGE DEVELOPMENT

Although a preschooler will know approximately 2,500 words by six years of age, his favorite words invariably will be questioning ones: "why," "what," "when," "how." In language as in other aspects of his life, he imitates the adult world, including what his parents say to each other and to him. He also imitates his playmates, his kindergarten teacher, and television characters. He uses language to verbalize his fantasies and to spin long tales full of imaginary people and places. He participates, too, in family conversations and can recount many details of his day's events.

The preschooler knows many words, asks many questions, and surprises his parents with his understanding of some aspects of life, but he is still not ready for complex discussions, answers, or instructions. He needs to have instructions and explanations repeated, and even then he may not fully comprehend what is said. He usually knows only one meaning of a word, and when another meaning is intended, he is completely confused. He interprets words literally, so when someone uses an idiom like "hit the road," he does not understand.

The child first shows an awareness of language rules during toddlerhood. He continues to learn rules of language as a preschooler but becomes confused. Having observed that plurals of words are usually formed by adding an "s," the preschooler may say "leafs" for *leaves* and "childs" for *children*; because the past tense is usually created by adding "ed," he may say "hitted" instead of *hit* and "seed" for *saw*. By the end of the preschool period, the child has learned several exceptions, but he has many more to learn during school age.

During this period, the child thinks much faster than he can speak. He stumbles over words, repeats some as he tries to think of the next one, and simply cannot get the word out because he has forgotten what he intended to say. Parents call this "stuttering" and often try to correct the problem by having the child repeat the word until it is said correctly, or by saying the word themselves. This makes the child unduly aware of the problem and creates anxiety, which decreases the regularity of word flow, or *fluency*. Parents should ignore this problem; if it does not improve after several months, or if the parents are noticeably concerned, the child should have a speech evaluation and any necessary therapy by a qualified speech pathologist.

The preschooler enjoys using "bad" words, not only for the pleasure of breaking a rule but also for the shock effect on others. He develops a "toilet tongue," i.e., he uses several words related to elimination. He knows that words related to the bathroom should not be used in public, so he saves them either for when adults are not listening or when he wants to get their undivided attention. Parents' overreacting to a socially unacceptable word imprints it in the child's mind forever, ready for use when needed to upset or embarrass them. It is therefore best to ignore the use of such words and to bear in mind another possibility, namely, that the child does not understand the meaning of "bad" words, and is using them quite innocently.

Laura mispronounced the word "truck" so that the "tr" sounded more like "f." This mispronunciation delighted her mischievous ten-year-old cousin, who asked her to repeat it time and time again, laughing harder each time. Laura was soon asking everyone on the family beach trip. "Do you want a truck," mortifying her parents. They were wise to ignore this, however. The cousin was given the choice of pretending not to hear Laura's "truck" or sitting in his room alone (for the rest of his life). He chose the former.

Occasionally, parents must tell the child that a word simply is not used in their family. If the family provides other outlets for frustration and the child has little need to upset his parents, the child will learn when and when not to use certain words.

The family plays a major role in the preschooler's language development. Listening to and commenting on what he has to say is as important as speaking to him directly, clearly, and simply. The child learns that his fantasies, stories, and feelings are interesting, and this success stimulates him to develop more creativity and function in language.

Tommy, aged three, had had a difficult life with his natural parents. His new foster parents startled him when they stopped what they were doing, looked directly at him, and listened when he spoke to them. At first he was so uneasy and shy when their eyes were on him that he stopped talking and covered his face or hung his head. Later, he could tolerate hearing his own voice in an otherwise silent room, and finally he began to enjoy carrying on a brief conversation with these caring people.

GROWTH AND PHYSICAL CHANGES

Body Proportions

The pattern of growth is slow and steady in the preschooler but his proportions change remarkably. Although both his chest and head continue to enlarge, his chest grows more rapidly. His arms and legs are longer in proportion to his trunk. His abdomen becomes flatter as he loses his swaybacked appearance, contributing to his slimmer, taller profile.

Height

The child will average a gain in height of approximately 7 centimeters (2.75 inches) a year during this period. This relatively slow growth may concern parents, who often request vitamins for the child. The parents can be reassured if you plot the child's height on a standardized growth chart and show how his growth follows a normal curve. The preschooler's height can be measured by having him stand barefoot on the floor, against a growth chart. A straight object should be placed on the top of his head, perpendicular to the chart, for accuracy. Some scales have a built-in metal bar that touches the top of the head to measure height.

Weight

The preschooler has an average weight gain of approximately 2 kilograms (4.5 pounds) a year. This slow weight gain, coupled with an increase in height, gives the child a very thin appearance. His arms and legs are long and skinny, and his ribs protrude beneath his skin. This is normal, however, and standardized charts will again be a source of reassurance for parents. The child ususally removes only his socks, shoes, and outer clothing for routine weight assessment.

Teeth

The average preschooler neither gains nor loses any teeth. Occasionally, he will lose a tooth during the later portion of this period, but he will seldom gain a permanent tooth. He should go to the dentist for his first exam no later than three years of age and continue to brush after meals with a fluoride toothpaste.

Hearing

The normal preschooler has very acute hearing. If he has a cold or an allergy, he may develop a temporary hearing loss due to the accumulation of fluid in his middle ear. This problem often resolves itself without treatment but may require medical intervention. Most preschoolers can have their hearing tested with an audiometer.

Vision

The young preschooler should have a visual acuity of 20/40, and by the end of this period, his acuity is usually 20/20, but 20/30 is acceptable. His eyes should be aligned; any imbalance is reason for referral.

Other Health Measurements

The preschooler's heart rate, slowing somewhat during this period, is usually 90 to 100 beats per minute. His respiratory rate, also slowing, averages 20 to 30 respirations per minute. His temperature may be slightly higher than the adult normal of 37.0° C (98.6° F). His blood pressure rises steadily from infancy to the average readings of 100 systolic and 65 diastolic pressures by about three years of age. Both the systolic and diastolic pressures drop several points until they rise again in early school age (i.e., six- or seven-years-old).

The preschooler seems to be such a picky eater that parents and professionals alike are concerned about adequate nutrition. Hemoglobin and hematocrit measurments are useful indicators of overall nutrition and, specifically, of iron intake. The normal hemaglobin values are 11.5 to 12.5 g/100 ml during early preschool and 12 to 13 g/100 ml during late preschool. The normal hematocrit values are 37 to 41 ml/100 ml of whole blood for the younger preschooler and 34 to 40 ml/100 ml for the older preschooler.

MOTOR DEVELOPMENT

The preschooler spends much time at motor play. He makes rapid progress in fine and gross motor coordination, often surprising his parents with his abilities.

Three-Year-Olds

The child of this age continues to practice gross motor skills, which include walking easily up and down stairs, running at full speed, climbing on outdoor climbing equipment, and jumping from place to place. He enjoys drawing, coloring, and painting for the fun of hand-eye coordination and the production of colors and shapes. He can use scissors only with difficulty, but he wants to have a pair for his use. He needs equipment designed for safety because he is unaware of potential dangers.

Four-Year-Olds

The child now has no problems with the basic gross motor skills of running, jumping, and climbing, so he begins to experiment with these activities. He may feel confident enought to jump across a ditch or to hang by his legs from monkey bars. After he has mastered the art of pedaling, he often can ride a bicycle without training wheels if it is small enough for his body.

The child refines his small muscle activities to some degree; his pictures often have recognizable shapes, and his skill with scissors improves (although he still only cuts around large objects). As he tries to imitate his parents' activities, such as cake decorating and sewing, he is satisfied with any likeness. He becomes more aware of potential danger and avoids it increasingly, but materials and activities still must be safe if the preschooler is to play freely.

Five-Year-Olds

An empty kindergarten room tells you much about the motor development of the five-year-old child. Small chairs are placed around low tables; five names printed in large letters are taped to the table, one in front of each chair. A large, empty space covered with soft carpet is the area where children inevitably play marching and dancing games or sit and listen to brief stories. In one corner, there are easels with primary color paints and large paint brushes. The floor is covered with clear plastic. Another corner holds a mock kitchen complete with stove, sink, dishes, mop, broom, aprons, and so on. A child-length mirror stands there also. A big clown face with an open mouth is always ready for the bean bag to be thrown either from close or distant range. The shelves hold rounded scissors, unlined and lined paper, colored paper, fat crayons, pencils, and paste. The walls have bright pictures and letters. The children's papers show that some write their names quite well while others must have the teacher write their names. Outdoor equipment includes a jungle gym, three swinging tires, a traditional swing set, a balance beam, and large, soft balls for kicking. Obviously, the five-year-old continues to practice fine and gross motor coordination as a part of his everyday play and learning. Opportunity plays a big part in the development of motor skills at this age: a deprived child might easily learn to ride bicycles, swim, dance, and draw, if only he had the equipment and instruction.

NUTRITION

The young preschooler's nutritional needs are similar to those of the toddler. He is not growing rapidly, so his appetite remains limited. As he grows older and his activities require more energy, his caloric need increases from 1,300 calories to 1,800 to 2,000 calories per day. He often selects a favorite food, such as peanut butter, and wants nothing else for a while. He likes to choose what and how much he will eat, so sensitive parents take this into account when planning and preparing meals. The average preschooler prefers finger foods, such as raw vegetables, quartered sandwiches, cubes of meat or cheese, and slices of fruit. He enjoys many mildly flavored, plain foods but generally dislikes vegetables. Since he does not care for extremely cold or hot foods, he waits until ice cream is soft and hot corn is cool. Foods that have an unusual consistency, such as thick mashed potatoes, may be rejected because they are different and therefore not good. The child does like very sweet foods and popular fast foods, such as hamburgers, french fries, pizza, and fried fish, but these can irritate his gastrointestinal tract and take the place of more nutritional meals. These problem foods should seldom be included in the child's diet (see eating).

DAILY ROUTINES

Sleep

The preschooler often gives up his nap during this period and may compensate somewhat by lengthening his nighttime sleep. A rest in the middle of the day is a good idea in case he needs extra sleep. He may avoid going to sleep at night if he has frequent or terrifying nightmares, and he may need to sleep with or near someone for reassurance.

Finally, Peggy, aged seven, Anne, aged five, and Paul, aged three were to have bedrooms of their own. Thrilled with the idea, they made elaborate plans about decorating, having friends over to spend the night, shutting out the rest of the world. Their mother looked forward to less bickering and fighting over possession of toys. The first night in the new home surprised everyone. Paul was the first to wander to Peggy's bed. Later, Anne joined them in the single bed. After two months in the new house, Anne occasionally slept with her sister, and Paul slept there almost every night. Sometimes Peggy would leave the two younger siblings in her bed to climb in with her parents. This process of musical beds seemed to disturb no one.

Eating

The preschool child requires only enough food to support his activity and metabolic levels and his relatively slow growth. He can eat all family foods during regular mealtimes, but he does not enjoy new or mixed foods as a rule. He needs protein and/or fruit for midmorning and midafternoon snacks to prevent the irritability that accompanies decreased blood glucose between meals. Parents often try to increase or improve their child's overall food intake by bribing him with desserts to eat his vegetables, forcing him to sit at the table until his food is eaten, or withholding all between-meal foods. The use of these tactics may result in a tense, unhappy dining atmosphere. Offering the child one small helping of each food (including a small dessert, if part of the meal) and his usual snack between meals without threats, bribes, or scoldings helps to keep mealtime pleasant.

The child will learn some table manners simply by imitating his parents, and he can be gently reminded of other manners. Generally, however, the preschooler cannot hold his fork and knife perfectly, balance a napkin on his lap if his feet dangle above the floor, or serve himself without spilling. He cannot understand why others are upset when he chews with his mouth open (perhaps a mirror would help). Establishing a few rules at a time helps the child accept limitations on his behavior at the table. Lots of talking, laughter, and interest in one another will help him to adapt to family expectations during mealtimes.

Bathing

During the preschool period, the child can usually bathe most of his body. He may need some help with his back, ears, face, and genitals. It is safe for him to play in the tub alone for short periods of time as long as someone is within hearing distance. He often will use this time to explore his whole body and to engage in masturbation. He enjoys water play with floating objects and squirting toys. He would like to have bubble baths, but the soap may cause vaginitis in little girls and various skin disorders in both sexes. Careful rinsing can prevent some of the problems, but the child may have to do without the bubbles altogether. Standing in the tub, rough play, and getting out of the tub alone should not be allowed.

Dental Hygiene

The preschooler can brush his own teeth, but his parents need to complete the task by brushing his molars and surfaces he cannot reach. He should brush his teeth after meals with a fluoride toothpaste to prevent decay. *Pedodontists* (children's dentists) recommend that parents floss their child's teeth once a day to remove debris between close surfaces. Toothbrushing should be established as an important health routine. The child should visit the dentist every six months starting at age two and a half or three.

Nursery Schools and Day Care

The preschooler enjoys play with other children, creative activities, games that have rules and winners, trips to exciting places and events, and warm contact with adults other than his parents. The nursery school can provide all these benefits if it is well planned, with the child as its focus. Some parents do not feel that their child needs nursery school experience, however, since they offer the same assets in his daily life. Many of the various centers have planned programs in the mornings and play in the afternoon. Parents often utilize this type of "extended care" while they work at full-time jobs. Some child care services (and some baby sitting agencies) offer television and "free play" instead of learning activities and should be avoided.

The preschooler may not be ready for participation in a daily, all-day program. If he has been separated from his mother only for brief periods, he may need to try nursery school two or three mornings a week for a year and then increase his total attendance. Public kindergarten is increasingly available to five-year-olds in this country, and nursery school attendance is a good way to prepare for this new step. Occasionally, the preschooler cannot adjust to an organized learning/play environment. The problem may lie with the child (fear of separation from his parents, lack of self-control in his activities with others, excessive shyness and withdrawal, etc.), or the facility itself may be at fault: incompetent teachers, too many children, and inadequate facilities. Parents must evaluate the child and the center to decide whether or not to remove the child. They may need the help of a child behavior specialist, or simply a good listener, to make the decision. Occasionally, the child needs another year at home to mature, but the parents should ensure that the child is engaged in activities with other children in order to prepare him for public kindergarten. When parents feel confident and enthusiastic about a developmentally sound nursery school experience, their child usually shares their feelings.

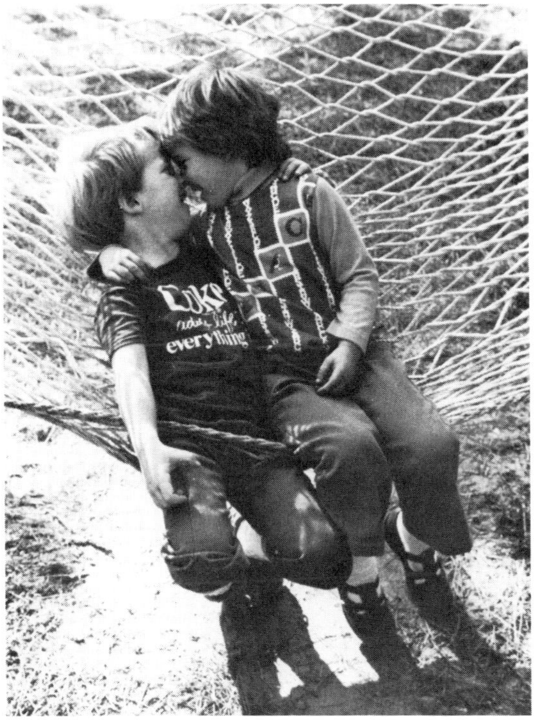

Figure 6–1. *These prescoolers obviously enjoy sharing a hammock.*

Play

As toddlerhood ends, the child's play changes in many ways. At age three, the preschooler becomes much more sociable and begins to seek friends, and he is willing to share with them (Figure 6–1). He is able to communicate with other children as his language development continues. The preschooler's ability to imitate and to use symbols allow him to have lively imaginary games with other children his age. His increasing desire to play with friends eases him into brief separations from his parents. By the fourth year, he is ready for groups and group games. *Dramatic play,* in which the child acts out scenes from the adult world that he has seen and enlivens them with imaginary friends and situations (in which he often appears important and in charge), is a favorite form of play for the preschooler. He projects his feelings and experiences into these dramatic sessions.

Nina, aged three, was an unhappy child. Her mother, separated from her father, had a full-time job but had difficulty in providing the bare necessities for the two of them. Her mother was tired and irritable at the end of each day, criticizng Nina for all she did. A neighbor frequently overheard Nina spanking her doll and saying, "You bad baby! Can't you do anything right? What is wrong with you? You know better than that!"

Jim, aged five, had received many injections during his hospitalization. He could not get over the trauma of one before someone gave him another. The pediatric nurse specialist explained to Jim's mother Jim's need to continue acting out his painful experience until he would be able to move on to happier play. When he got home, his mother gave him a syringe with a needle so he could stick a doll (which he fashioned into a nurse) until he tired of it. Jim's mother always supervised his needle play to ensure Jim's safety. A week later, Jim no longer enjoyed this form of play for long periods, although he continued to enjoy it from time to time.

Dramatic play demonstrates the evolution of the preschooler's sex identification. At first, both boys and girls imitate both parents; soon afterward, boys play "Daddy" and girls play "Mommy." The preschooler's play also gives evidence of the child's curiosity about what his parents do when they go off to work; unless the parent's occupation is one the child has seen portrayed on television, the child is not likely to have much understanding of what constitutes "work."

Johnny, aged four, was the only boy in a group of five children. He naturally played the father who went off to work. The girls took turns being mother, teacher, baby. Johnny was very dissatisfied as he sat in his corner "at work," unable to figure out what his father did. He decided that he might as well try being a mother for a while, although this was not his idea of a proper role for a boy.

The child's dramatic play is one *projective activity* that is useful both to parents and to nurses. Having the child draw pictures is another, and it allows not only an expression of feelings but the opportunity to perfect motor and creative skills.

Lucy, aged five and a half, drew a picture of her family. Her sister Amy, 22 months older, had always stolen the family spotlight with naughty behavior coupled with remarkable intelligence. When Lucy was asked to draw a picture of her family, Amy was drawn considerably larger than the other family members (Figure 6–2).

Puppets are an enjoyable vehicle for dramatic play and an especially productive projective activity. The child not only acts out a part but also can speak for the puppet, revealings that might otherwise remain hidden.

Margie, aged five, was recently admitted to a children's home because her mother was hospitalized with severe alcoholism. Margie's physical examina-

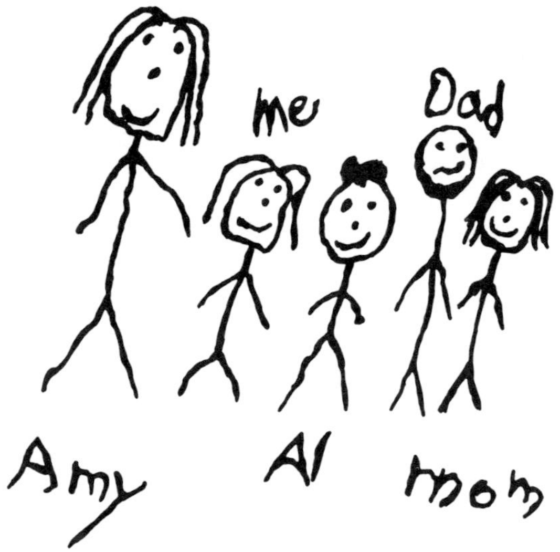

Figure 6–2. *The child who drew this picture sees her sister Amy as the dominant member of the family.*

tion revealed a urinary problem that required immediate surgery. When the nurse specialist brought in the bag of puppets for Margie to play with as part of her preparation for surgery, Margie selected a "Mama" puppet to be part of her "show," although she knew that Mama would not be there the next morning to send her off to the operating room. The nurse said nothing but began the show. Margie played with the Mama puppet, kissing the "Margie" puppet good-bye over and over while the nurse sat by, simply watching. Margie finally put the Mama puppet aside and selected a "Housemother" puppet and a "Nurse" puppet.

These projective activities will reveal different aspects of the child's development as well as aspects of his immediate situation. Parents need to provide opportunities for the child to express his anxiety so that they can reassure him, and give him more freedom to explore and clarify his misconceptions.

The preschooler continues motor play, but it is now more goal-directed. He runs less for the sake of running, but he now climbs on monkey bars for the sake of climbing, coordinating many movements at once. He learns the thrill of heights—seeing farther away, feeling the breeze in his face, looking at people below—while keeping safety in mind and controlling his fear. He enjoys using fine motor skills as in drawing and painting. He is not a perfectionist, so any likeness of the intended image is fine with him. The response, "What a nice picture! Tell me about it," is much better than "What is it?" He enjoys building play "houses" with blocks that stack or fit together, or with sheets and sofa cushions, incorporating motor skills, imagination, and imitation in his play. Toys that require no imagination or motor skills are essentially useless to the preschooler, except perhaps for the visual stimulus they provide.

The child needs a balance of play with adults, with other children, and by himself. A variety of play experiences exposes him to new ideas, words, and games, and he quickly learns that he can entertain himself. The child should be limited to one or two toys at a time to avoid overstimulation and subsequent boredom. Most preschoolers enjoy playschools or kindergartens that provide opportunities for play with other children, an adult other than his parents, and, often, new and different materials.

COMMON PROBLEMS

Nightmares

The preschooler's vivid imagination and his fears account for nightmares as he sleeps. The younger child perceives these dreams as real events and continues to be afraid of dream images after he awakens. He should be told that he had a dream, which is not real. He will not accept this explanation because he is unconvinced that perceiving something in a dream is different from seeing while awake. Getting him up to look out the window, under the bed, in the closet, and down the hallway may relieve some anxiety, but he will not be able to understand the differences between dreams and reality until he has heard numerous explanations and has developed some awareness of imagination as such.

Lights help the child deal with his fears, but some parents refuse to leave lights burning during the night. They are afraid that leaving the lights on is a form of "babying" the child; there is no basis in this fear and parents should be so advised. Lights themselves can be frightening if they cast soft shadows throughout the room; experimenting with different types of lights may be necessary. If the child can see around the room after a nightmare, he may learn more quickly that images during dreams do not, in reality, exist. He may need human contact. Depending on the family, he can be comforted by joining siblings or parents in bed, or on a blanket beside their bed, or by his parents' staying with him until he is ready to sleep again. As he gets older, he will be able to stay asleep after his bad dreams and tell about them the next morning. If the child is frequently, unconsolably terrified after a dream, some professional advice should probably be sought in case there is some underlying emotional problem.

Masturbation

The preschool-age child is developing a sexual identity and an awareness of sexuality. He has increased interest in his genitals and the sensations he feels there. Boys enjoy experimenting with their penises to make them "big," "up and down," "hard," and so on. Girls, although they cannot observe such obvious physiological reactions to *masturbation*, also gain much pleasure by manipulating their clitorises. The child may wish to masturbate during quiet times when his hands are unoccupied; he will often manipulate his genitals when his clothes are off during his bath or at bedtime, and when he is in a stressful situation such as hospitalization. This is normal behavior that does not cause a weak mind and body, hair on the palm, blindness, and so forth; though few people now believe these old wives' tales.

The preschooler already knows his parents' attitude about touching his genitals. He learned this in infancy and toddlerhood from their reactions to his explorations of his body.

Stewart was three years old when he came home from a foreign country and saw his paternal grandparents for the first time. His mother was very open and positive about bodies, sexuality, and reproduction; his father tolerated this attitude with some reservations. Stewart had on pajamas and no underwear when he went downstairs to say goodnight. His grandmother spied his penis barely showing through the little fly and jumped nervously to close it. Stewart appeared puzzled only for a moment, but his father, obviously embarrassed, ordered his son upstairs to put on his underwear.

When the child is not allowed to learn about his body, he usually will continue to masturbate, but he will feel guilty, although the feelings of guilt may cause him to suppress his desire to the extent of not masturbating at all. When the child is permitted and encouraged to explore and experiment with his body and its sensations, he may need some controls to avoid offending others. Parents can respond to this problem by explaining that masturbation is normal and acceptable, but that it is a private activity to be postponed until one is alone. They must then provide for some privacy. The child should know that some people disapprove of masturbation altogether, since he will inevitably learn this through exposure to other children and adults.

Excessive masturbation is frequently a sign of an emotional disorder. If the child usually prefers masturbation to nonsexual play by himself and with other children, he and his parents need the assistance of a child behavior specialist. The child may also indulge in such other forms of self-stimulation as head-banging and rocking. However, the child who masturbates excessively may simply be lonely, bored, or frustrated, and an increase in activities appropriate for his developmental needs (e.g., active and creative play) may decrease his need to turn inward for pleasure.

Fantasies

The preschooler's point of view is influenced by his imagination, fears, and memories of earlier perceptions. When he tells tall tales, conjures up imaginery friends, or makes up a story to explain an accident, he is not deliberately "lying"—he is expressing himself through fantasies. Parents can acknowledge these yarns for what they are, saying, "What a nice story," "It's fun to have a pretend playmate," or "We all have accidents."

Parents should avoid asking the child if he committed a wrongdoing if they are sure he did. It is preferable to say, for example, "I can tell that you ate the cookies by the crumbs in your bed"; this confronts the child with the issue at hand and does not invite him to lie. Parents should set a good example for the child by not lying themselves; if "white lies" are necessary to make someone else feel good, the child needs an explanation of why.

Bedwetting

The child usually stays dry through the night by three years of age, but bedwetting is not considered abnormal until age five when it is termed *nocturnal enuresis*. Waking up most mornings with a dry diaper is a sign of readiness to sleep in training pants. If the child shows no sign of readiness, he can either continue to use diapers for a while or wet the bed. Some authorities feel that the child should sleep peacefully through the night in a diaper rather than be wet and cold. Others feel that the child will never be motivated to keep dry if permitted to sleep with a diaper. Nighttime control is related to both physical and psychological competence; each child's problem must be viewed in light of both factors. If the neurological system cannot competently control the child's sphincters, then diapers may be best for a while. If the child seems to respond to rewards, trying a gold star on a calendar for each dry night might work. Once the child is out of nighttime diapers, he may be highly insulted by even the suggestion that they be used again. Parents are so anxious to solve the problem that they may restrict all fluids after 5:00 PM or take the child to the bathroom to urinate in the middle of the night. These approaches do not work but they do, however, make the thirsty child feel punished and the exhausted parent feel irate and resentful. Time and patience are the two factors most likely to end the problem.

ACCIDENTS

Accidents are the leading cause of death in preschool-age children, as well as in toddlers. Hazards of the preschool stage include many of those of infancy and toddlerhood, although the preschooler has more motor skills and enough self-control to be trusted with more freedom. His motor skills are often more advanced, however, than his judgment, and accidents inevitably occur. He climbs trees only to find that he cannot get down; he tries to jump across a ditch but falls into the water because he misjudged the distance to the other side. He can learn, remember, and frequently heed safety rules, but new and interesting situations tempt him to ignore them for a while. The preschooler can assume some responsibility for his own safety only when his parents are aware of his limitations and set limits accordingly.

The preschooler, as has been mentioned, is egocentric; he cannot look at his environment from several different angles, only from his own. He cannot possibly recognize all potential dangers because he has not experienced the results. When he has had a burn, fall, or cut, he usually remembers the surrounding circumstances and avoids them. He learns symbols for danger and, although he does not understand, he often heeds these symbols.

Chris, aged three, was in perpetual motion on the nursery school playground. He was running very fast when the teacher spied a freshly dug hole in his path. "Chris!" she yelled. He stopped in his tracks, frightened by the tone of her voice. He did not know what was wrong, but he sensed danger.

The preschooler's fears of bodily harm often keep him safe when he suspects danger; in fact, these fears may be so overwhelming that he will take no chances on exploring the new and exciting. As he moves through this period, he begins to classify different objects and events as dangerous. For example, the toddler learns "hot" when his food is hot enough to burn his mouth. The word "hot," a symbol for things that burn, can be used to describe the stove, the hot water faucet, and the outdoor grill. Soon the preschooler classes many things as "hot" and avoids them. He still gets burned, however, because he does not know that exhaust pipes are hot, that fires spread, or that water may turn hot after it runs cold for a while.

Motor vehicle accidents cause the most accidental deaths in the preschooler. These accidents occur when the child rides various toys in the street, crosses the street, plays behind a parked car, rides without a seat belt, and so on. His egocentrism explains much of his vulnerability to motor vehicle accidents. Picture the child standing between two parked cars: He can see parked cars on each side of him and a narrow stretch of street in front. Since there is no danger from his point of view, he feels that he is safe to run across the street. He does not know that a car can move very quickly down the street from either side and may not be able to stop in time to avoid him. The preschooler can learn to stop and look both ways before stepping into the street, but he simply is too young to take full responsibility for his safety on streets. He can buckle his own seat belt, but, since he cannot imagine being thrown out of a car during a collision, he often will need a firm reminder.

Parents of preschoolers can teach safety by consistently enforcing rules for all family members including themselves. They need to explain "why" to the preschooler repeatedly until he can understand the reason for the rule. The child needs to explore his environment, so rules should allow freedom within the limits of safety. This balance can be achieved most of the time if parents have an awareness of their child's egocentricism and immature concept formation.

SIGNS AND SYMPTOMS OF ILLNESS

The preschooler is developing a more competent immune system with each illness he endures. His body can resist some microorganisms entirely and can minimize the effects of others through antigen-antibody responses. His body is larger and his organs are farther apart, so infection does not spread quite as rapidly as before. He still has many infections, especially when he enters a nursery school or kindergarten. The preschool child can express the pain he feels and approximately where the pain is, but he cannot accurately describe the pain as to duration, frequency, or intensity. He usually cannot differentiate between nausea and stomach pain.

Parents are less upset by illness by the time the child reaches preschool age. They know more about fevers, activity levels, medicines, and ways to get medical help. They often know that many illnesses go away untreated and that waiting a day is worth a try except with severe illness. They still are anxious during their child's illness, however, and need support and repeated explanations.

The preschooler continues to have high fevers with many illnesses, but these generally do not rise quite as rapidly or as high as before. Occasionally, a child will become rather ill before his parents are aware of it because of this change in temperature reaction. He is less susceptible to febrile seizures than the infant and toddler, but these may occur, especially if he has already had several in the past.

The preschooler may not go out to play on a pretty day, may turn down a visit with a friend, or take a nap at an unusual time. His sleep may be restless, or he may wake up frequently during the night. These problems alert parents to the fact that all is not well with their child. As with all extreme signs and symptoms of illness, marked lethargy or restlessness indicates a need for immediate medical attention.

The preschooler has fairly regular patterns of elimination. His parents usually know his routines, especially for bowel movements, because he needs help in wiping clean. Parents also tend to notice frequency of urination in relation to watching television shows and movies, going shopping, and taking trips. Moderate changes in elimination, such as several fairly loose bowel movements in a day, may indicate the onset of an illness or simply an intestinal reaction to an overload of food or excitement. The same is true with urination: increased frequency of voiding may be due to increased liquid intake or a urinary tract infection. A burning sensation that accompanies urination can be caused by irritation around the urethral opening, or again, a urinary tract infection (see ch. 31). A "wait and see" attitude is appropriate for early changes, unless, of course, the child has a history of some related disease.

The preschooler, "picky" about his choice of food, often seems to eat very little. Parents are frequently concerned about this small intake, thinking that the child is ill; they may want the child's blood tested for reassurance. A decreased appetite is, indeed, an early sign of many illnesses, and deciding whether or not a slow change in eating warrants medical attention is a difficult task. The physician usually will perform some laboratory tests to reassure the parents and to rule out diseases.

The preschooler's vital signs change noticeably with acute illness, but show less change than those of younger children. His body systems can now maintain homeostasis more effectively during illness. Since his respiratory tree is larger, he can tolerate some alterations due to illness without noticeable difficulty in breathing. Respiratory character and rate continue to be sensitive indicators of many types of illness. The child's pulse increases with fever, causing tachycardia with high fever.

The preschooler develops the same "sick" appearance as he did during infancy and toddlerhood. His face may look droopy and sad, or he may be taut with anxiety. His eyes look sunken and his skin is dry and loose if he is dehydrated. His skin becomes pale if it is normally light, or grayish if it is normally dark. Appearance may be so subtle an indicator of illness that only parents can recognize a change, or so obvious that any observer knows the child is ill.

HOSPITALIZATION

The preschooler bases his expectations of the unknown on his previous experiences, whatever they are. If his grandfather recently went to the hospital and died there, the child may very well expect to die if he, too, must be hospitalized. If his only experience has been with his new baby brother's birth there, he may think that he will also get a baby on the trip. If he has only seen the hospital on television, he may have visions of people gasping noisily through masks as murderers try to cut off the oxygen, emergency rooms bustling with one crisis after another, or doctors and nurses engaged in nonmedical affairs. He uses fantasies to fill in gaps in experience or understanding, thus confusing his concept of hospitalization even more. His immature concept formation often distorts his expectations and perceptions. His developing sense of self-control is a source of pride, hence a loss of self-control can be all the more humiliating. The preschooler, still highly susceptible to separation anxiety, needs his parents during most of his hospitalization, but he may feel secure enough to go to the playroom or to allow his parents to eat a meal by themselves. If he is without his parents most of the time, he goes through stages of grief and may reject them when they visit, or cling to them in hopes of keeping them there with him. Security objects can provide a source of comfort and security, and his command of language and use of play help him cope with the stresses of hospitalization.

Admission

The admission of the preschooler is an important first step in hospitalization. Your interest in the parents' story behind the hospitalization, including the reason for admission, their child's habits, and their present level of energy (or exhaustion), tells them that you are aware of their needs and stresses and that your care will be based on this knowledge. In addition to the usual admitting information, the nurse must obtain an account of previous experiences with hospitalization, other illnesses, and recent deaths in the family; be sure to question the child as well as the parents. Admission is not the time for an in-depth assessment of this information, since the parents will be anxious and usually unable to give a complete account. Further information can be added to the child's nursing care plan later. Be sure to give parents information about hospital routines and facilities as well as what to expect in the way of care for their child.

The preschooler is afraid of intrusive procedures but, unfortunately, admission includes a minimum of a venipuncture, temperature assessment, and disrobing for weighing. If the child is very ill, he may require intravenous fluids, multiple injections, and various forms of oxygen therapy. Whenever possible, prepare the child for these procedures and perform them quickly and confidently; bandage any breaks in the skin and permit the child to replace his clothes as soon as possible. Parents can usually take their own child's temperature, height, and weight with your assistance. If the child has had satisfactory experiences with a nurse in the past, he often will be happy to let you perform these procedures with a parent nearby. He is delighted when he controls his fears enough to cooperate with you.

Preparation for Procedures

The first step in preparing the child for a procedure is to find out what he already knows and thinks. Various projective techniques, such as drawing pictures, telling stories, and giving puppet shows, will help the child express himself when he cannot say what he thinks or feels. After you know his expectations, these same techniques can be used to prepare him for procedures (Figure 6–3). If he can project himself as a puppet and act out a role, the puppet show is an excellent way to expose him to much of the procedure (see ch. 2). When he repeats the show, you can quickly see areas of misunderstanding, predominant fears, and the need for more specific information. Most preschoolers enjoy puppet shows immensely, and, of course, parents learn much about what their child will experience. The parents will also be grateful that you know their child's stage of development and use appropriate teaching tools.

Because the child naturally enjoys dramatic play, "dress rehearsals" are a good way to prepare him for procedures. This provides concrete experience with the procedures without pain or discomfort. He can try on masks, bandages, or casts so that they will not be foreign to him when the time arrives. Parents and various professionals can join in the rehearsal.

Other Nursing Interventions

The preschool child is developing self-control; when he loses this control and screams, kicks, and fights before a painful procedure, he usually feels very guilty and ashamed about his behavior (Figure 6–4). His parents may be embarrassed and/or angry because of his outbursts. Explain to the child that his actions are understandable, but give special attention to the fact that the preschooler's self-control is rela-

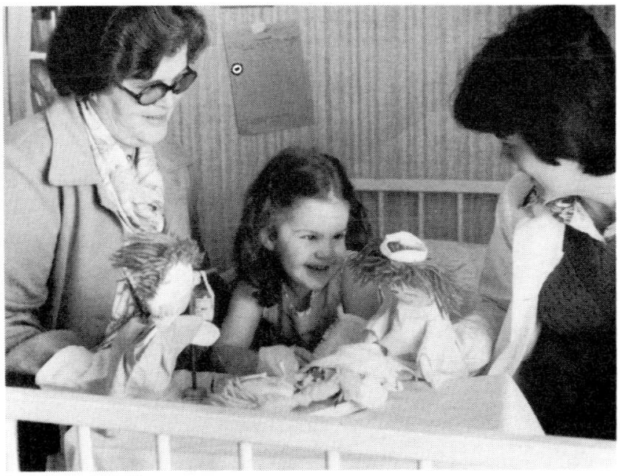

Figure 6–3. *The puppet show is an excellent way to prepare the child for surgery.*

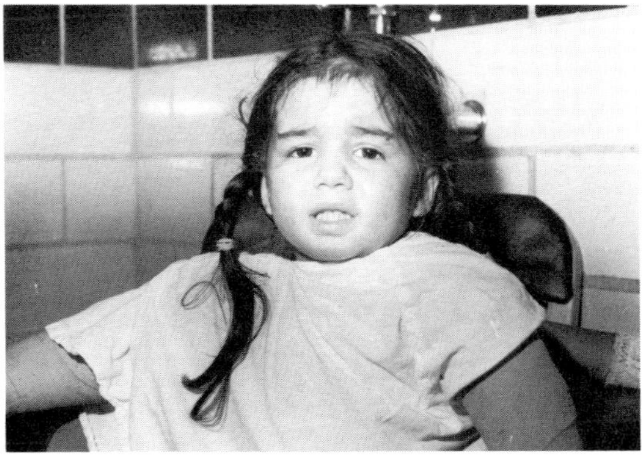

Figure 6–4. *The child is in pain and is struggling to maintain control.*

tively new and a temporary loss is therefore particularly upsetting. The parents need reassurance that acceptance of his behavior as normal will help him regain self-control. Do not ask the child to be a "big boy" or "big girl" by not crying during a painful procedure; the preschooler releases tension by crying. Do not give him excessive rewards because he resists crying; he may want to cry next time, and if he is "great" when he does not cry, he may feel "awful" when he does cry. Quiet congratulations are an appropriate reward for his struggle for self-control whether he is successful or not.

Play is a critical part of nursing interventions for the preschooler. He is imaginative, imitative, and dramatic. He enjoys fine and gross motor play. He likes to try new things, but he has fears that often inhibit him. Dramatic play can be used not only to prepare him for procedures but also to help him resolve the hostilities and fears that occur during hospitalization. He needs doctor and nurse garb, dolls, masks, syringes, needles, bandages, and anything else representing the pain, fear, and anxiety that inevitably occur (Figure 6–5). He may stick the nurse doll, or he may play the doctor who hurts the child doll. He can draw or paint pictures that reflect his feelings, although you may be unable to identify the characters. Once the preschooler is better able to handle his emotions related to hospitalization, he progresses to normal play, including games, imitation of adults in daily life, and various creative activities (Figure 6–6).

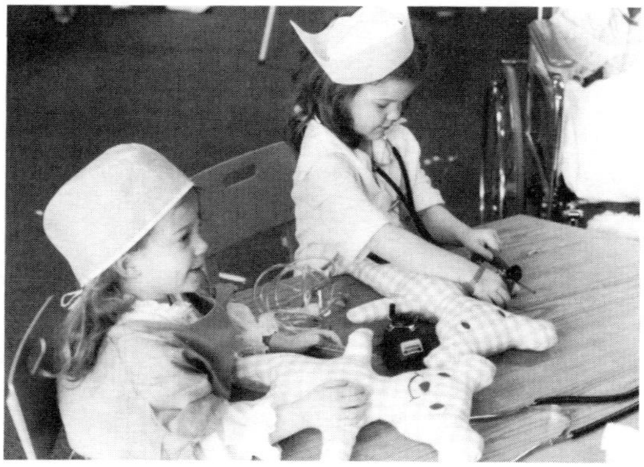

Figure 6–5. *In dramatic play, these hospitalized children act out doctor and nurse roles.*

The preschooler has an immature concept of time, so he needs help to keep track of hours and days. Mealtimes, playtimes, a special television show, or a visit from a parent can help orient him to the hours of the day. Marking days off on a calendar helps him to see that time is passing. He does not usually understand how long he must endure hospitalization if he must stay longer than a day or two without a "countdown" device. Unfortunately, hospital stays are influenced by many factors, and length cannot be accurately predicted. The child, therefore, is often overwhelmed with what seems to be an interminable stay in the hospital.

Regression occurs frequently in the hospitalized child. If the stay is long and stressful, the likelihood and severity of regression are increased. The preschooler may use baby talk, wet the bed, whine, cry, and have temper tantrums although he has long ago developed more appropriate behavior for his age. He loses the developmental skills that were most recently acquired, so bedwetting is a very frequent regressive reaction to hospitalization. The parents should be told that he will make progress in these areas if gentle but consistent limits are set when he feels better. Carefully assess regression of the child before you plan your care: you may need to accept the infantile behavior openly, or you may need to ignore it. If the child begins to wet the bed, should you put diapers on him or not? The child may be-

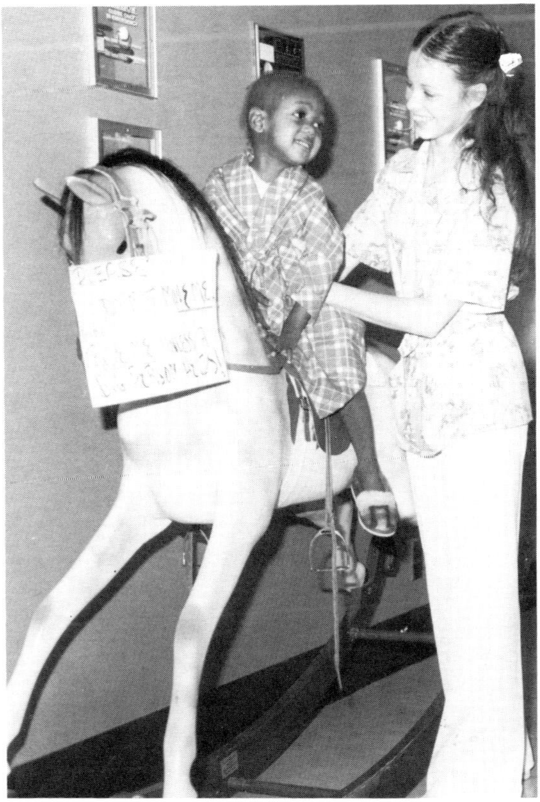

Figure 6–6. *This rocking horse stays busy much of the time.*

come highly insulted or humiliated. Another child may be so upset with a wet bed that diapers would be a welcome relief as he tries to sleep. The preschooler usually can express his wishes on the matter, so involve him and his parents in making the decision.

Discharge

The preschooler's usual post-hospitalization behavioral changes include bedwetting, nightmares, poor eating patterns, various attempts to prevent going to bed at night and other situations that separate him from his parents, and, sometimes, the need to act out the procedures he underwent (Figure 6–7). These changes occur less frequently if the parents were rooming-in, but they do occur. As with younger children, the preschooler's parents can assume responsibility for treatments at home more easily if they room-in with the child, practicing procedures with support of nurses.

SUMMARY

The preschooler wants to try new and interesting experiences, but since he is afraid

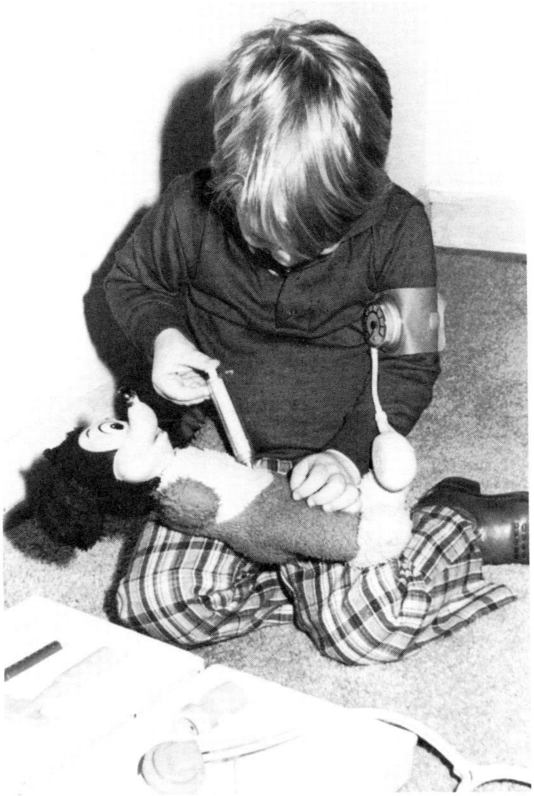

Figure 6–7. *The preschooler may need to act out hospital procedures after he returns home.*

of real and imagined threats, he sometimes shies away from exploration. His understanding of his environment is increasing, but he fills gaps with illogical explanations that may truly confuse the issue or provoke other fears. As he learns more about his world and develops a less egocentric point of view, his thinking becomes more logical. He usually identifies with the same-sex parent after resolving an earlier attraction to the parent of the opposite sex. His growth is slow during this period, and he neither gains nor loses any teeth. His neurological system matures, and his fine and gross movements become more refined.

Common problems include nightmares, sibling rivalry, masturbation, fantasies, and bedwetting. Accidents kill more preschoolers than any other cause of death. The child has numerous infections as he is exposed to new microorganisms, but his body begins to develop a more effective immune system. Hospitalization is generally a frightening experience; the preschooler's perception of the hospital is greatly influenced by television, previous visits, and family members' descriptions. The child may regress by losing general control during painful procedures, losing bladder and bowel control, and so on. He needs his parents' support throughout his stay. Play, especially the puppet show, is an effective tool for explaining procedures for learning more about the child's fears and expectations. Most preschoolers regress in some areas of daily living after hospitalization, particularly in relation to sleep disturbances.

CHAPTER **7**

The School-Age Child

BEHAVIORAL OBJECTIVES

After studying this chapter you will be able to:

- Describe the school-age child's emotional development with reference to industry and inferiority.
- Discuss the concrete operations stage of cognitive development.
- Describe the school-age child's language development as it relates to cognitive development.
- Identify physical and motor changes that occur during school age.
- Discuss the nutrition of the school-age child in relation to food requirements and developmental status.
- Describe daily activities, including school attendance, that comprise the child's routines.
- Identify appropriate types of play for the well and the ill school-age child.
- Identify common problems and accidents of the school-age child and give preventive and treatment measures.
- Describe signs and symptoms of illness in the school-age child.
- Discuss nursing care of the school-age child and his parents during hospitalization.

TERMS AND CONCEPTS

Industry
Inferiority
Death anxiety
Concrete operations
Mainstreamed
School phobia
Immanent justice
Functional disorders

The school-age child is accustomed to meeting new adults and going to new places, but he is still frightened and insecure in the hospital. He continues to need his parents, especially during traumatic procedures, when he is likely to regress. Nursing care should be directed equally to the child and his parents now that the child can take much responsibility for his own care.

EMOTIONAL DEVELOPMENT

The child entering the school-age period, the years between 6 and 12 years of age, must direct his efforts toward developing a sense of what Erikson calls *industry* while learning to relate to peers and adults outside his family and coping with the pressures of formal education. If the child's earlier emotional development has been satisfactory, he has developed trust in others and himself, autonomy in much of his work, play, and thought, and enough initiative to try new tasks (Figure 7–1). He also developed a sexual identity, considerable self-control, and some understanding of other's feelings and opinions. If previous stages of emotional development have been unsatisfactory, personality disorders often emerge as the child faces the new tasks of school age.

The child's sense of industry results from setting out to accomplish a task and completing it to his satisfaction. A six-year-old may be happy with his airplane model even if it is streaked with glue but the ten-year-old is upset if his model is marred in the slightest. The child begins to judge his work by standards that may have come from previous achievements or from expectations of an older brother or sister, from his peers, his parents, or his teachers. When standards are derived from another person's accomplishments, they may be impossible to live up to, as with the younger child who strives to produce on the same level as his older sibling.

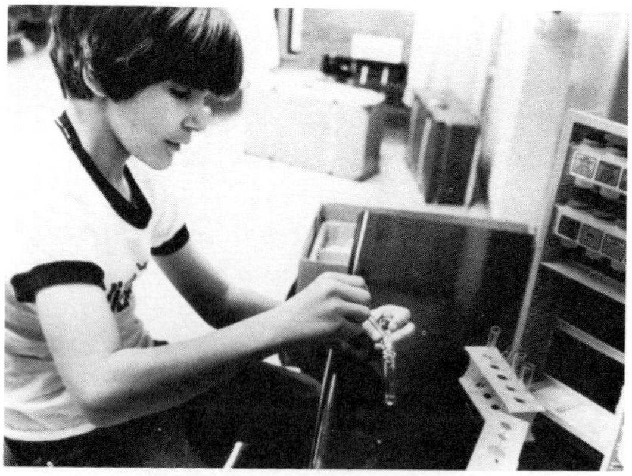

Figure 7–1. *A school-age child performs a chemistry experiment.*

Jason, six years old, and Skipper, nine years old, could sketch remarkably well for their ages. Their art teacher congratulated them frequently for the progress they made and praised their creations. Jason, however, could easily see that his work was not as good as Skipper's. Telling Jason that his sketches were outstanding for his age was fruitless. Giving the two boys very different tasks did not work either. Jason soon was too busy to go to art lessons. He stopped drawing altogether for a while (his parents waited with silent concern) but began again the next year in school, where standards were geared to his age. His poster for the book fair won second place in his classroom.

When standards are based on the expectations of others, the average or above-average child has a much better chance of success, whether he is at home, school, or a community center. The child who does not have at least average motor, cognitive, and social skills often is unable to meet the expectations of significant others. Repeated lack of success in the school-age child (or a person of any age, for that matter) results in a sense of *inferiority,* which is opposed to *industry* in Erikson's terms. The child who develops a sense of inferiority loses his sense of initiative and stops trying to achieve. He turns his efforts to other achievements which, unfortunately, may include excessive daydreaming, getting attention with noisy behavior at school, or stealing simply for the sake of stealing.

The child compares not only his achievements but also his belongings, his family, and his body with those of others. This phenomenon is closely related to his developing sense of identity, which will intensify during adolescence. He surveys his hair, physique, clothes, toys, family car, his parents' appearance, and so forth. He is self-critical to the extent that he is very unhappy if any of these aspects do not measure up to those of others. If his emotional development has been satisfactory, he will learn to tolerate the fact that he is superior in some ways, average in others, and inferior in still others. The child may strive for extremes, trying to be superior at everything or at nothing, and he and his parents need professional help in alleviating the problem. By the end of this period (i.e., around age 12), the average child should be able to assess his strengths and weaknesses without an overwhelming feeling of inferiority.

Timmy, aged nine, has four older brothers, all of whom excel in athletics. Timmy had a severe foot deformity at birth that required several operations and left him with a noticeable limp. Timmy participates in organized sports and enjoys them, but he seldom scores or makes spectacular plays. When he was in the first grade, his teacher commented to him that he read exceptionally well. His parents noted that he brought home a different book to read every night and that he read newspapers and magazines; he was soon reading on a fourth-grade level. Now he not only reads on a high-school level, but writes interesting stories, one of which was published in a children's magazine.

Parents can support their child's development of a sense of industry in several important ways. By showing enthusiasm for their own household and professional work, they shape their child's attitude toward accomplishment. The provision of materials, such as paper, glue, paints, fabrics, thread, scraps of wood, nails, hammer, and so on, allows the child to be creative and productive. He particularly enjoys collecting stamps, insects, and personal "junk," and needs space for these collections. Assigning regular household chores gives him a feeling of belonging and responsibility. Whatever task is assigned to him, it must be within his capabilities if it is to afford both challenge and success. Selecting appropriate activities is often very difficult for parents who have unrealistic expectations of their child. Many parents are unaware of the pressures they place on their child to continue family traditions or to fulfill their own dreams.

Richard's father, Mr. F, was never allowed to participate in sports as a child, so he joined at least one athletic team every season and played tennis at every opportunity. Richard, nervous when he joined teams, kept his hands in his pockets most of the time. He dreaded the games, during which his eyes sought his father's inevitable smiles and frowns. After the game, Mr. R criticized Richard's every move but closed the lecture with, "It's only a game, son. It makes no differences how many points you make or if the team wins, as long as you have a good time." Mr. R was shocked when the coach stated that Richard seemed under a lot of stress during the games and hinted that the father-son relationship could be the cause.

The high expectations of parents are not always detrimental to the able child's developing sense of industry, since they can encourage the child to achieve. Conversely, when parents anticipate little or no accomplishment from their child, the child usually will make their implicit predictions come true.

The school-age child is increasingly subjected to the opinions of important people outside his family, such as teachers and peers. He is less egocentric than a preschooler, and he has some regard, however limited, for another's point of view. This broader viewpoint causes trouble. He questions his parents' beliefs about religion, politics, and parenting. Parents may feel threatened when their own child not only questions their beliefs but also challenges them. He generally adopts the family's traditions except when he has the need to rebel.

Peers become increasingly important to the school-age child. Whereas the preschooler delighted in interactive games with other children but remained very much a product of his family, the school-age child is influenced by his peers in his play, dress, hobbies, and language.

Lucy, aged nine, had a new pair of jeans with flared legs that made her feel superbly attired. Her older, much admired cousin took one look and said, "Are you still wearing flared legs? Straight legs are 'in' now." Lucy's face fell, but she managed to wear the jeans for an hour before she took them off and sadly folded them to put them away. Her mother gnashed her teeth as she stitched up the sides to convert the new jeans to straight legs.

Peers form groups according to similarities including socioeconomic class, religion, intellect, race, athletic ability, and sex. Generally, the sexes separate during the school-age period. Being in a group provides tremendous security during this stage. The groups have strict rules that are usually unwritten but are occasionally listed. Exclusion from the group is a terribly painful experience, and most members abide by the regulations unless several defectors form another group at one time.

Clark, aged eight, was tall and agile. The neighborhood gang was playing football when Toby, a child with a heart defect, asked to join. He was tiny and somewhat uncoordinated for his six years. Clark was unhappy that Toby had been allowed to play and caught every ball intended for the newcomer. The group decided that Clark was not doing his part to let Toby have a good time and ostracized him. They did not talk to him, throw the ball to him, or include him in the huddles. Clark finally ran home sobbing hysterically to his mother, who simply listened. She did not need to point out the "moral" of this sad story to him.

The child must learn his role in relation to his peers and to children older and younger than he. He learns the role not from parents or teachers but from interacting with other children in a group that is free to restructure itself as new children and new goals present themselves. The young child carefully watches the older children, preparing to participate when permitted. Eventually, the group will need another player, and he will be allowed to join the game. This exciting but frightening first step is followed by a gain in confidence and full acceptance as a group member. Now the younger children watch *him*, but soon he tires of "baby" games and begins to think about the activities he will participate in when he is older.

Parents sometimes decrease their physical contact with their child during this period, because he is supposedly "too old"; on the contrary, his need for skin-to-skin contact is as great as ever.

Coach H, 6 feet 4 inches tall, seemed to be a giant to the boys (aged seven to ten) on his basketball team. When he first began coaching this age group, he was a little uncomfortable when they held onto his legs, slipped their hands under his shirt, patted his head, and threw an arm around his neck when he sat beside them. Later, he began to respond to this obvious "skin need" and hugged, touched, patted, and held the children. Now he does not even realize that the boys hang on to him or that he is using touch to communicate. His own sons, who are on the team, receive considerably more physical contact at home also.

A backrub or some other form of warm physical contact at bedtime may encourage the child to express his fears and joys of the day. He usually will talk more freely about his death anxiety, which surfaces now that he understands the finality of death.

Angie P., aged nine, was sitting close to her mother on the sofa in the nurse practitioner's office. They were talking about sleep, and Mrs. P. stated that Angie had no sleep problems. The nurse explained that the school-age child often develops a death anxiety that causes sleeplessness, followed by different tactics to stay near a parent until sleep overcomes him. Angie nodded her head vigorously and said, "I feel that way lots! I get a funny feeling in my stomach." Mrs. P. was surprised and a little upset to learn that she had not helped Angie with this aspect of development.

Talking with an older sibling can also be very comforting to the child who has begun to think about death. Discussions of the family's religious beliefs will give the child further direction in his thinking about life and death. Bedtime stirs thoughts of death because the atmosphere of quiet, dark, and separation from people and action is quite similar to the child's concept of death.

The child has definite ideas about sex by the time he is ready to go to school. He may have already learned much about reproduction from his parents, books, television, and events, such as the birth of puppies, or he may have acquired only a bit of information, and this may be distorted by guilt.

Diane was six years old when a teenage boy in the neighborhood talked her into lying down in the closet with him and pulling her panties off. When he tried to penetrate her vagina, first with his finger and then with his penis while he talked gently to her, she cried and told him it hurt. Frightened, he stood and ran away. Diane cried because of the guilt she felt. She did not really understand what had happened or why she felt as she did, but she knew the experience was bad and unmentionable. She told no one, of course.

If parents have already begun teaching the child about sex in response to the child's questions of the preschool period, continuing the process is fairly easy. The child's sex education should be complete by the time hormones begin to change his body and emotional upheavals occur. He needs to know about reproductive development, not only of his own sex but also that of the opposite sex. Although he should be taught that human reproduction is a fascinating scientific phenomenon, a purely mechanical explanation is inadequate. The child needs to relate sex to love, joy, physical excitement, and satisfaction. If he does not know that intercourse is intensely pleasurable, he often assumes that it is performed simply for the sake of reproduction. Why else would a man put his penis in a woman's vagina, or a woman tolerate such an act? Discussing the positive and negative aspects of sexual activity—physical satisfaction, a closer relationship with a partner, babies, abortions, venereal disease—helps the child to draw many accurate conclusions. Parents, at this point, can state their expectations regarding sexual behavior in relation to the family, religion, and society. The school-age child cannot possibly learn all about sex in one or even several sessions, and he will forget many facts he learns.

Parenting may become difficult during this period as the child is increasingly influenced by peers, teachers, other adults, and television. As was mentioned, the child may disagree with his parents' point of view, resulting in parent-child conflict. Although he has often learned from earlier stages that his parents will eventually meet his needs if he waits long enough, when he is older and bigger, his parents may suddenly want him to take responsibility for his school work, household chores, and maintaining schedules. When the child does not accept responsibility for himself (especially at school), parents are embarrassed and/or angry. They may belittle or punish him, attend parenting courses, read child rearing books, or seek various sources for counseling. Punishment and shaming simply do not work to change a child's behavior except in the immediate situation. Most experts on parenting offer the same advice: keep communications open by listening to what the child has to say; avoid criticism and, instead, explain why certain behavior is unacceptable; give the child choices whenever possible; never ask a child to lie when you already know he has done something wrong; let him accept consequences for his successes, failures, and mistakes; ignore irritating behavior, and it will often disappear; give the child lots of praise; and, finally, show affection by hugging, holding, patting, stroking, and kissing. The overall principles of gradualism, flexibility, consistency, sensitivity to developmental cues are still very important in dealing with the school-age child. If these methods of parenting were not employed during early childhood, the family often needs information and support if they wish to change established patterns. Be aware of community resources for referral of parents with child rearing problems.

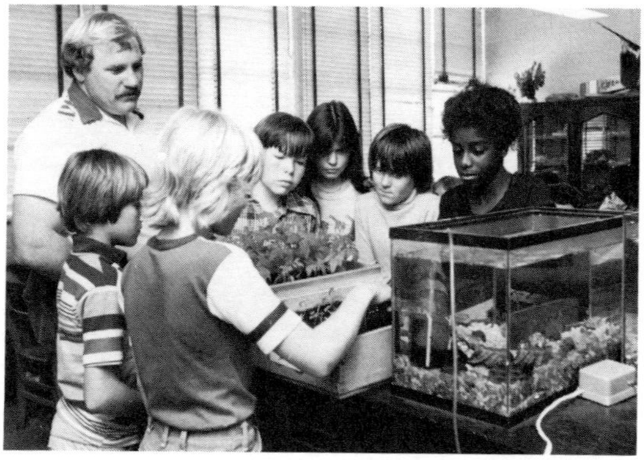

Figure 7–2. *The school-age child learns through concrete experience.*

COGNITIVE DEVELOPMENT

Most of the school-age period coincides with what Piaget calls the stage of *concrete operations*. The child at this stage is capable of relatively logical thinking since he is able to think conceptually, and is less egocentric. His logic is limited, however, to real (as opposed to abstract) people, objects, and events (hence "concrete"). (See Figure 7–2.) He organizes facts about the real world, employing them as needed to solve individual problems. He cannot engage in purely hypothetical reasoning. He would have a difficult task, indeed, if he had to understand, say, subtraction after no more than a verbal explanation. The school-age child's capacity for logical, concrete thinking has tremendous significance to parents, teachers, and, of course, nurses.

The child of school age can understand several related steps to accomplish a task or solve a problem, and can proceed in a logical, orderly manner until completion. He is capable of reversible thought and can follow a line of reasoning from start to finish and back to start again. He recognizes that a quantity of liquid remains the same regardless of the size of the container it is poured into.

Joe, aged four and a half and Jim, aged seven, were in the kitchen painting. They watched their mother mix exactly one cup of water with each of two colors and pour the mixtures into jars of different sizes and shapes. Joe expressed concern that there was not enough red paint in the big jar. Jim retorted, "Joe, you dummy! Didn't you see Mom pour the same amount of paint in each jar? Just the *jars* are different!" Joe was not at all convinced, but he remained silent.

The child can also arrange objects in order according to length, width, or quantity. He can categorize according to specific characteristics, enabling him to enjoy collection hobbies. Because the child may progress at a rate different from the average, his level of readiness is of utmost importance in introducing cognitive tasks, whether at home or at school. Success in learning (at whatever level) is absolutely essential for the satisfactory development of a sense of industry.

LANGUAGE DEVELOPMENT

The most remarkable aspect of the preschooler's language development is that he learns to understand and speak sentences. The school-age child steadily increases his vocabulary and is able to use more complex sentence structures by the proper placement of parts of speech. He uses new grammatical patterns, including the passive voice, or varies the use of older patterns. Since the school-age child can produce all the sounds in the English language, the child who articulates incorrectly should be referred for speech and hearing evaluation.

The language of the school-age child reveals his emotional and cognitive development. Words related to production, achievement, and logic are abundant. He uses words to be critical of others or to express childhood humor; he enjoys rhymes, riddles, and chants. Rhymes and riddles provide an opportunity for laughter, creative and logical thinking, and a method for "getting even" with a force he cannot overtly attack, such as a teacher at school.

Glory, glory hallelujah,
Teacher hit me with a ruler;
Met her at the bank with a U.S. Army tank,
And she ain't no teacher anymore.

The school-age child uses language for problem-solving. He labels objects and events, storing and recalling them for later use. He solves difficult problems more quickly when he uses language in his solutions. However, the young school-age (six- to eight years old) child, whose reasoning is concrete, has difficulty with purely verbal explanations and reasoning without an opportunity to experience some aspects of the event through his senses. As he progresses to the end of school age, he learns through actual experiences and develops more facility in hypothetical and verbal reasoning.

GROWTH AND PHYSICAL CHANGES

Growth is slow and steady until a sudden increase called the prepubertal growth spurt. Girls began this growth spurt at about nine years of age; boys begin at about eleven years. Many organs approach maturity in size and function during the school-age period, so the child can eat, sleep, and fight infection much as the adult can. A notable exception is the development of reproductive organs and secondary sex characteristics, which usually occurs after this period.

Proportion

The school-age child seems thin to his parents because an increase in height precedes an increase in weight. The child often seems to "shoot up" and then to "fill out." His arms and legs grow faster than his trunk, and his head grows very little, giving him more adult-like proportions (Figure 7–3).

Height

The child gains about 5 centimeters (over 2 inches) each year. This growth is steady,

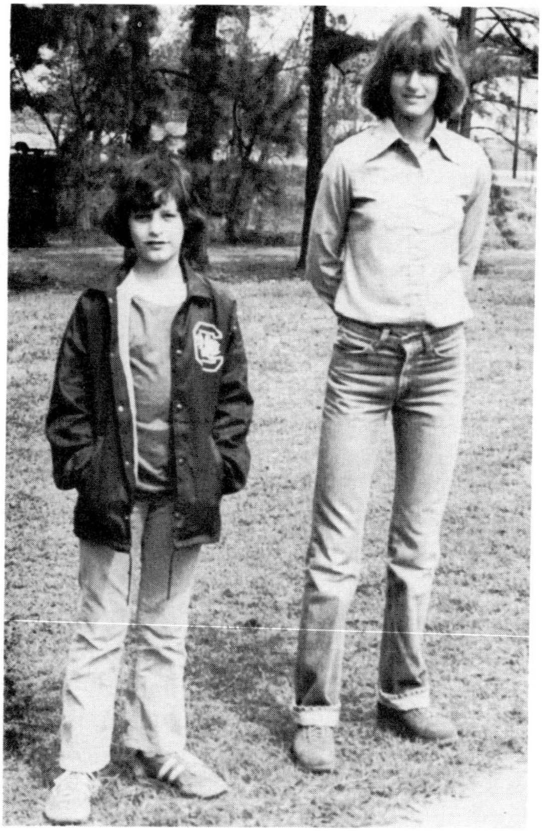

Figure 7–3. *Both of these girls are eleven years old.*

since it is relatively unaffected by such changes in lifestyle as nutrition. (Severe malnutrition, stress, and trauma can, however, stunt the child's skeletal growth.) The average child is near 135 centimeters (5 feet) when his growth spurt begins. Skeletal x-rays during this stage can provide an accurate estimate of adult height because ossification of the long bones occurs at a predictable rate.

Weight

Weight gain averages 3 kilograms (6.6 pounds) per year during school age, but increases are slower during the early years than during the later ones. The child gains a significant amount of weight during the prepubertal growth spurt, and this may cause the school-age girl to feel "fat." An excess of snacks or the junk foods advertised on television may also influence weight in the older school-age child. By the end of these years, the average weight is 37 to 41 kilograms (81 to 90 poungs).

Hearing and Vision

Hearing should remain acute in the normal child during school age, but visual problems frequently develop in the child, and school vision testing programs are very important; an unrecognized or uncorrected vision deficit can result in a learning handicap. The school-age child's visual acuity should be 20/20, although many screening programs do not recommend further evaluation for the child under eight years of age if acuity is as good as 20/30.

Other Health Measurements

The body temperature of the school-age child is slightly above the adult average. Pulse continues to slow throughout the period until it is 67 to 90 beats per minute; respirations also decrease to about 19 per minute. Blood pressure averages 110/60 at the end of the period. Hemoglobin and hematocrit values reach 14 gms/100 ml and 40 ml/100ml; respectively.

Teeth

Primary teeth begin to loosen when their roots are resorbed, usually around six years of age. The lower central incisors are usually the first to go, with all primary teeth gone by the twelfth year. The first permanent teeth to emerge are molars, followed by upper and lower central incisors that replace the primary teeth. Only the second and third molars remain to erupt after this period.

MOTOR DEVELOPMENT

If given the opportunity, the average school-age child will choose many activities that require precision movements. He also will choose tasks that require fine motor coordination if he has the necessary material and instruction; this eagerness to use motor skills is closely related to the child's developing sense of industry and to his relationships with other children. The young school-age child is much less able to control his gross and fine muscles than the older child, but an interest in the same kind of activities is common to all school-age children.

Gross Motor Development

The first-grader plays kickball because he only has to kick and run; little strategy or precision movement are required by the game. He continues to try out skills such as hanging by his knees upside down on a jungle gym, jumping over obstacles, and climbing trees (Figure 7–4).

Boys and girls often form separate groups for play, but they will quickly join forces when necessary for a game. In addition to the pleasure of competition in ball games, hopscotch, gymnastics, skating, and swimming, the school-age child enjoys the opportunity these same activities afford to improve his previous record. The child's modes of transportation—walking, running, and bicycle riding—also provide the opportunity to develop gross motor skills.

Opportunity is a major factor in gross motor development. If the neighborhood has no trees for climbing, water for swimming, or fields for playing ball, the child may grow up without learning these common skills. He may develop, instead, "street" games that are dangerous to the child and others, or he may simply stay inside and watch television, do his homework, watch more television, and go to bed. If, by age ten or eleven, the child has not already acquired the ability to "hold his own" in at least some athletic endeavors, he often develops a sense of inferiority and dares not try anything new.

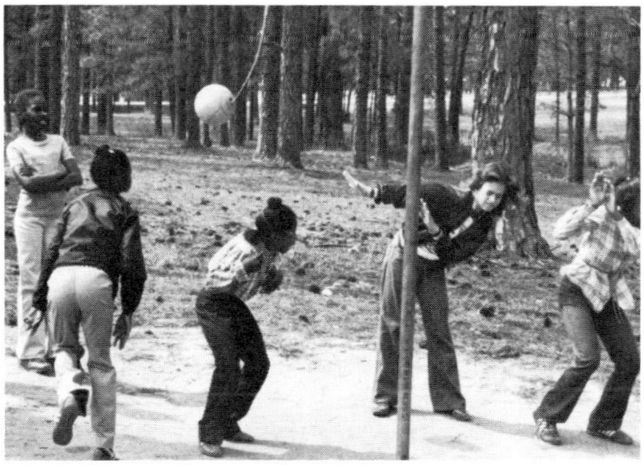

Figure 7–4. *These girls are enjoying a game that involves gross muscle activity.*

Sig, aged ten, wanted to play basketball so badly that he worked for six weeks to bring up his grades. As soon as he brought home his much-improved report card, his mother put him in the car to register him for basketball. The man at the recreation center firmly but kindly stated that the registration period had ended. Sig made it to the car before he started wailing, "I'll be too old next year! All the other boys have played a year already, and I'll never be ably to play!" His mother instantly thought of all the things she should have done to get him on a team. She felt guilty throughout the basketball season, suspecting that he might be right about not being able to play for the first time at age eleven. His father also felt guilty about the situation, so he frequently practiced dribbling, shooting, and passing with his son at home. The next year Sig joined the team although he was reluctant to do so because he lacked experience. He sat on the bench most of the time, but he played enough to gain enough confidence to want to play again the next season.

Fine Motor Coordination

The child's fine motor coordination increases remarkably during the school-age period. His brain matures in that each side becomes more specialized in many functions, such as speech and motor skills. The normal child shows a preference for either the right or left side, usually during early school age. He is able to write increasingly well and can begin cursive writing at about the second grade (Figure 7–5). He enjoys drawing, painting, and building with all types of materials.

Electronic games in which the child must coordinate mental and manual reactions are enormously popular with the school-age child. Hobbies, such as mounting collections of insects, performing chemistry experiments, or making jewelry, require precision placement of parts. Playing musical instruments also gives the child the opportunity to develop his fine motor coordination.

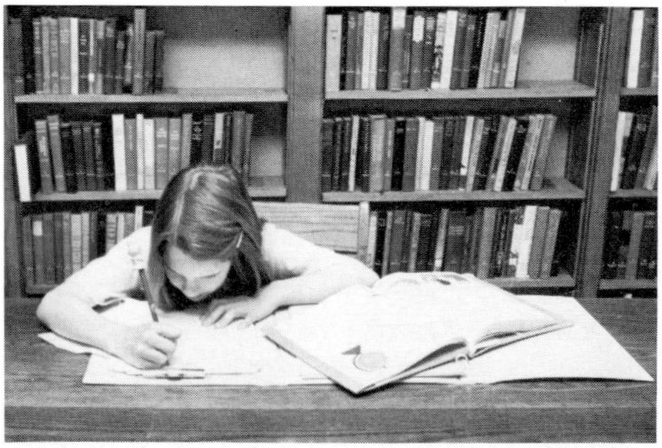

Figure 7–5. *By second grade, the child is ready to learn cursive writing.*

The child's ability to direct his fine muscles accounts for an important part of his overall self-concept. He compares the product of his efforts with those of his peers, siblings, and significant adults. Occasionally, he can enjoy a quiet activity alone and compete only with his own previous record, which gives him an opportunity to perform with little pressure. If he has stimulating and rewarding experiences during the school years, he will continue to develop his motor skills along with self-confidance.

NUTRITION

As was mentioned earlier, the school-age child generally grows slowly but steadily, so his nutritional requirements increase smoothly until his growth spurt begins. His average daily intake contains approximately 2,200 to 2,400 calories until it increases by 400 more calories to support prepubescent growth. The child's appetite usually improves as he participates in more strenuous activities, such as basketball, bike riding, cleaning windows, and mowing lawns, and as he is exposed to new foods at school and at friends' homes. If his parents were tolerant of his "poor appetite" during the toddler and preschool stages, then he probably will not refuse to eat for the sake of getting attention during the school-age period; he will learn to enjoy a variety of tastes and textures. If, however, the dinner table has been the scene of a struggle to make the child eat everything on his plate, he often will continue to resist his parents' demands.

Parents frequently seek advice from books, newspapers, relatives, neighbors, and professionals about how to ensure proper nutrition for their child. Guidelines for the preschool child continue to be appropriate during school age: the child must eat most of each meal before he is offered second helpings or between-meal snacks; parents must avoid forcing him to eat anything, depriving him of a favorite food as punishment, or using desserts as rewards for eating something he dislikes. Parents should set good examples since the child almost invariably will imitate their habits. Knowing that the school-age child will want snacks, parents can help to maintain good nutrition by having only fruit, vegetables, and meat snacks available. The child often has access to a neighborhood store where he buys soft drinks and candy, but this is less of a problem if he has already eaten a turkey sandwich or an apple after school. If the child is to be enrolled in a day care program, parents should select a facility that provides fruit and protein snacks rather than sweets in their after-school programs.

In families in which both parents work, the child can help prepare meals, or prepare them himself. Cold bran cereal with milk, grilled cheese sandwiches, and orange juice comprise a nutritious breakfast that he can make for the whole family. He can perform many other kitchen duties with the supervision and help of his parents. Creating a special dish, such as a casserole, is a challenge that often tempts the child to sample foods that he has avoided or disliked. Preparing food is another accomplishment that can enhance his developing sense of industry.

Hot, nutritious, inexpensive lunches are available to almost every public school child, and many school meal programs now include breakfast. Unfortunately, the meals are often poorly prepared; dietitians report that a tremendous amount of food is thrown away each day, and some schools now offer a selection of popular foods such as hamburgers, hot dogs, tacos, and so on. This practice has sparked much controversy since some health professionals feel that the child should be exposed to a variety of foods if he is to learn good nutritional habits. Be that as it may, meals at school probably have little impact on the child's overall eating patterns, which are usually established at home.

The school-age child learns about food from books, significant adults, other children and, of course, television. If proper nutrition is presented to him as a science, without any judgemental implications, he may be able to apply the facts to his own eating habits.

Chip, aged nine, was studying nutrition in school with a teacher who avoided labeling foods "good" or "bad." She simply presented the consequences of eating an unbalanced diet. At about the same time, a television special stressed negative effect of too much sugar in a child's diet. Chip began to take note of his sugar intake and soon stopped asking for a second dessert or sweet snacks. He switched to noncarbonated drinks after athletic events. His mother, pleased to see the change in him, wondered why he suddenly began to change his eating habits after years of hearing her lecture him about proper nutrition.

The nurse who is teaching nutrition to hospitalized children should similarly avoid *should's* and *ought's*; discussing nutrition without reference to "right" and "wrong" implies that you trust the child to make a wise decision on his own.

DAILY ROUTINES

The school-age child engages in so many extracurricular activities that he may seem to have no routine at all. The family often must eat early or late to accommodate a schedule that includes Boy Scout meetings and dancing lessons, or they may have to plan a whole weekend around a swim meet. Nonetheless, the school-age child still benefits from routines in that they ensure regular meals, adequate sleep, and proper hygiene, as well as the security that comes from "sameness."

Sleeping

The child's sleep requirement ranges from 10 to 12 hours for the younger school-age child and from 8 to 10 hours for the older child. Parents must monitor the child's overall sleep habits, but a rigid regulation of bedtime hours may result in considerable conflict. Giving the child some responsibility for seeing to it that he gets enough sleep can be an effective solution to the problem.

Tim, aged eight, never seemed to require much sleep. He gave up all naps by two years of age and slept no more than 10 hours a night as a preschooler. When he started school, he resisted going to bed each night for months. Finally, his parents decided to allow him to regulate his own sleep on a trial basis. They agreed that they would say nothing about his sleep if he would be in his room by 9 P.M. and if he would arrive at the breakfast table on time (using his own alarm clock). The first few days were a struggle for Tim, and for his parents, who tried not to remark on his droopy eyes. Tim now sleeps seven to nine hours a night, which seems to be adequate for him.

When siblings share bedrooms, nighttime rules may be necessary to ensure sufficient sleep for each child. In very large, poor and/or disorganized families, each member remains wherever he happens to fall asleep, including sofas and floors. In many homes, the child frequently watches television late into the night and misses school the next day because he is too sleepy to get up. As with other ages and stages of development, the school-age child usually needs some restrictions on his behavior in order to ensure a productive routine.

Bathing

Taking a bath is usually a part of the school-age-child's bedtime routine. The child may rather watch television and procrastinate when it coms to bathing, but a sure remedy for this problem is to allow him to select his own bath time with the understanding that he must be in his bed or bedroom by bedtime. If he does not accept the responsibility, parents can require that he finish his bath before television or play. He may need reminders about hard-to-reach areas such as his back and areas he tends to forget such as his neck. The genitals require special attention, since secretions can accumulate and cause irritation and/or infection.

The child may become modest during the school years, even before any pubescent body changes occur. This modesty usually occurs as a consequence of the child's developing awareness of sexuality, regardless of how open and honest his parents have been in relation to sex. He demands privacy in the bathroom or in the bedroom while he dresses. He also begins to respect the privacy of others. Large families who live in cramped quarters cannot provide privacy for their members, so the child in such a family either develops a disregard for his own privacy, or he may dress in a closet, or he simply endures the lack of privacy. If taking showers at school or camp causes acute anxiety for the modest child, he may have a problem that requires the assistance of a behavior specialist.

Eating

The school-age child needs three meals a day and an after-school snack. If the family as a whole has a well-balanced diet, the child will almost always be adequately nourished. The meals need not all be hot; peanut butter sandwiches and raw vegetables, for example, comprise an excellent lunch. A planned time for each meal, even when the child prepares his own sandwich on the weekend, will probably limit random snacking. The child's after-school activities may disrupt meal schedules, especially when there are other siblings participating in other planned activities. Too often, parents who are driving their children from place to place stop at a fast food drive-in window and buy junk food to eat in the car.

The school-age child is ready to learn some table manners. It should be emphasized to the child that manners arise from a consideration for others, and that this consideration is more important than the rules of etiquette themselves. An awareness of development is important here: the younger child cannot keep his elbows at his sides while cutting with knife and fork but the older child can. Table etiquette does not interest the school-age child as a rule; that comes in pubescence and adolescence.

Dental Hygiene

The school-age child can take a lot of responsibility for his dental hygiene. He should brush all tooth surfaces with a soft brush after every meal, floss every night, and visit his dentist every six months for cleaning and a flouride treatment. In many disadvantaged families, the child does not have a toothbrush and has never seen dental floss, not because these items are too costly but because the family is unconcerned with preventive health care. Such children develop multiple cavities in their permanent teeth, leading to pain and infection that can result in systemic disease. If and when the child finally sees the dentist, his teeth are often so decayed that they must be extracted.

Frequently, parents do insist on the child's brushing in the morning and at night, but not on nightly flossing, which may require their assistance, especially during early school age. The child seldom brushes his teeth at school, since he would be conspicuously different from his peers. Parents must remind their child, throughout school age, to brush his teeth, even if toothbrushing is a well-established routine. The dentist or dental hygienist will instruct the child in proper care, but parents need to observe and supervise him periodically. When he becomes concerned about appearance and bad breath, he will take increasing responsibility for dental hygiene.

School

School influences every aspect of the child's development: achievement in academics and motor skills strengthens his sense of industry, he can learn to work and play with children of different races, socioeconomic classes, and ethnic groups, and he observes and interacts with adults other than his parents. Because he is in the stage of concrete operations, he can look at concepts and relationships more objectively, and use them in different situations. He may adopt many new ideas due to this less egocentric point of view and question some family values and beliefs. He usually develops a more realistic self-concept as he compares himself with his peers and acquires social skills that ensure group acceptance. By the end of this period, he can apply much of what he has learned in school to the "outside" world and perform many adult-level tasks.

The child who is noticeably different in appearance, intellect, and behavior often does not have a positive school experience. He learns that he is a deviant. If he consistently excels in a subject or skill, he may attempt to hide the fact to avoid the disapproval of his less fortunate friends, become obnoxious about his ability, or become bored with the lack of challenge. If, on the other hand, he can seldom measure up to standards, he often stops trying to meet expectations and withdraws into his own world or develops undesirable behavior to gain attention.

Appearance is a very important aspect of acceptance among school-age peers. If the child's body is abnormal in any way, his peers and, too frequently, adults will initially react to the abnormality instead of to the total person he is. A highly visible defect, such as obesity or large facial birthmarks, brings more negative responses than a leg brace covered with long pants. The child with a good self-image usually feels able to be a contributing member of the group regardless of his problem, but this is not so when the child sees himself as undesirable. The impeccably dressed child or the shabby, dirty child may be ridiculed and rejected by the group. Throughout school age, the child develops an increasing need to conform to the standards of his peers.

Leta, aged eight, went to a middle-class neighborhood school where her academic achievement was above average. Her parents were alcoholics, so she was on her own much of the time. She had only one shirt, one sweater, and a pair of jeans to wear every day to school. Obviously, the shabbiest, dirtiest child in the class, she usually was left out of peer activities. She eventually gained a new friend, Sally, who was also not accepted by the other children because she had not been there very long. Leta and Sally played together on the swings, sang together in the hallways, and sat together in class. Such a happy time! Leta went to school every day, and her grades were excellent. Then Sally moved on to another place, and Leta felt outcast all over again.

The other children thought Maurice, aged ten, was a "nurd." His father required his son to project a "proper" image at all times; Maurice's hair was cut very short, with hardly enough to part down the middle. He wore pressed dress pants and shirts with a matching V-neck sweater. His leather shoes were always highly polished. When other children made fun of him, he had quick responses such as "At least I'm neat—not a mess like you," but Maurice was a bitter, lonely child. Fortunately, when the teacher and school psychologist advised his parents that he needed counseling, the whole family entered therapy and made slow but positive changes. Maurice's parents relaxed the rigid restrictions they had placed on him.

The child who is markedly below average intellectually is usually at a disadvantage in school. The intellectual deficiency is quickly recognized by other children, and the unfortunate child is called "dummy," "stupid," "retard." If the school program is not carefully designed to allow the child some success, he will soon stop trying. The very bright child, on the other hand, may succeed in school and study new and interesting things in his extra time, or he may disrupt the classroom when he becomes bored. Many schools have small classes for remedial instruction, and some schools have classes for advanced study (Figure 7–6). Teaching machines, teachers' aides, and volunteers can also provide individualized instruction for students of inferior or superior ability.

The average school-age child adapts to

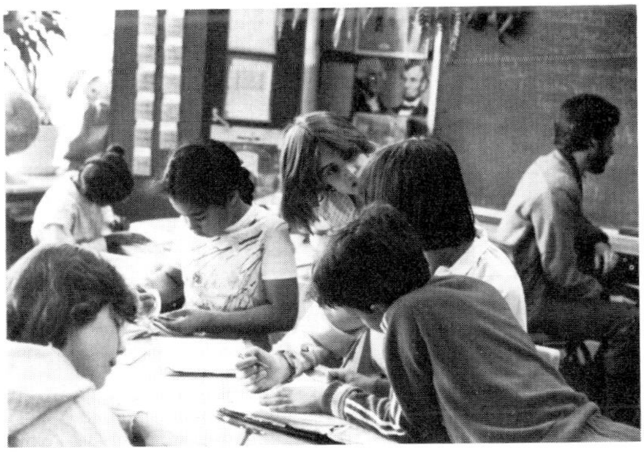

Figure 7–6. *A class of children with special learning needs.*

classroom routines and expectations quickly. Teachers impose greater limits and expectations as the child grows older, but they tolerate an occasional misdeed from the child. When his behavior is consistently disruptive to the class, however, his teacher may spend much of her time controlling him instead of teaching the other children. The child is likely to be punished frequently and this will reinforce his already lowered self-concept. Withdrawn behavior is less often recognized since the child causes no trouble in the classroom; his teacher may notice that he has a problem only if his work is deficient. The child whose behavior deviates noticeably from the norm usually needs evaluation by the school psychologist in order to identify problems and plan solutions with parents, teachers, school nurses, and community resources as needed.

In order to obtain federal funding, schools must now provide free education for every child, regardless of his physical, emotional, or intellectual ability. The child who has abnormalities is *mainstreamed* into regular classrooms during some part of his day. The rationale for mainstreaming is that the child should go to school with all types of children (not just those who have similar problems), since the outside world is comprised of mostly "normal" people. Some teachers protest that they have too many students to allow extra time for a special child and that they do not have preparation in special education. Parents of special children often are distressed because their child does not seem to learn as well in the regular classroom. The child will suffer if his learning experiences are geared to the average, if he has no peers with similar problems, and if he is treated with cruelty by classmates. With a greater number of specially trained teachers, mainstreaming could prove to be beneficial not only to the special child but to his classmates as well.

Jimmy, aged eleven, was much taller and heavier than the other fourth-graders. He was educably retarded and was able to learn at the lower level of his class. Unfortunately, when he was ridiculed, he would swing at the tormentors to shut them up. One day, someone gave Jimmy a large "chocolate candy bar" that was actually a potent laxative. Jimmy developed severe diarrhea and soiled his pants, socks, and shoes. His parents agonized over what to do. The principal was horrified that such cruelty had occurred, but he could not guarantee that it would not happen again. Jimmy's teacher explained to the class what had happened, and many of the children began to help him as necessary. They began to defend him when he was made the butt of jokes. His parents remain uneasy about public school attendance, but they feel safer as Jimmy copes with the situation week after week.

PLAY

Hobbies are popular pastimes during school age. The child may collect such items as insects, dolls and doll clothes, football cards, or the latest hit records. He may learn basic skills in needle work, painting, carving, or playing a musical instrument, and may advance rapidly as his motor coordination improves. Hobbies can provide pleasant, self-paced learning experiences in which the child can be productive and creative. He need not compare the product of his efforts to those of others, but he often does.

Games of all kinds are fun for the child, especially when he wins. Card games, spelling contests, sports, board games, and hopscotch all have built-in competition. Every child must win at least some games to feel that he compares favorably with his peers.

Many parents and teachers use the school-age child's competitiveness to manipulate his behavior. Parents and teachers can encourage the child to compete with his own past record, as with miniature golf and swimming, instead of constantly comparing himself with others. Opponents in games can be "equalized" by handicapping the better player until each player has a chance to win.

Lenny, aged eight, and Chris, aged eleven, were the only two children left in the convalescent home during the holiday season. Chris consistently won all games they tried, so Lenny refused to play anything. The nurse intervened by giving Chris fewer checkers, giving Lenny a free point at the beginning, and moving Chris a wheelchair-length further away from the dart board. Chris initially had difficulty losing to an eight-year-old, but he soon accepted it as "fair."

The school-age child can work with his peers toward a common goal, spending much time and energy building hideouts, forts, and tree houses, completing school projects and devising money-making schemes. One child often assumes a leadership role and directs the members of the "task force." In these cooperative endeavors, the child learns to share responsibility and rewards with others. These activities strengthen his developing sense of industry and make him feel that he is securely a part of a peer group.

Organized sports are available in many communities for children as young as five (Figure 7–7). Some teams are led by gentle coaches who spend most of their time teaching and encouraging the children to practice coordinating their movements. The guiding principle of this kind of coaching is that winning a game is not as important as making sure every child has some success before the game is over. Other teams are coached by adults who are so determined to win that only the most capable children compete. These coaches have loud

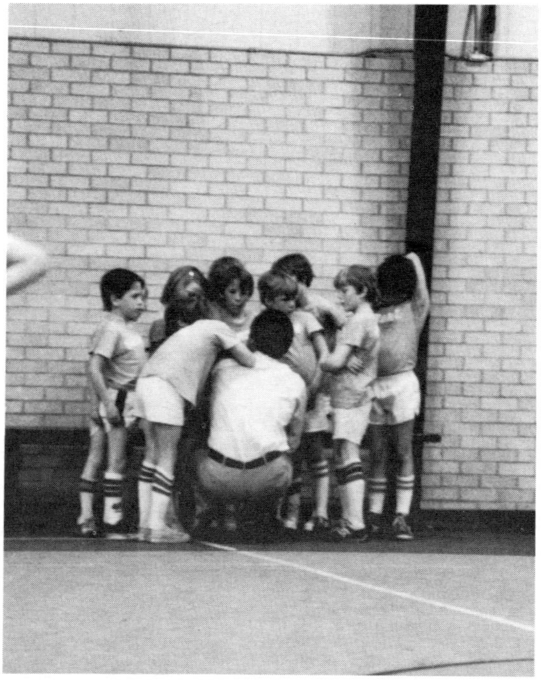

Figure 7–7. *A neighborhood basketball game. Note the coach who is stooping while he talks to his team and the child who is leaning on the coach.*

arguments with the referees, are openly critical of the players on the court or field, and punish the child's mistakes with instant removal from the game.

Participation in team sports can be a very positive experience when the child gradually relinquishes the strong drive to win as an individual and acquires a sense of team spirit. The experience can also be emotionally damaging to the child whose coach pressures him to win and whose parents want him to be the best player.

Girls do not usually have as many opportunities to participate in organized sports as do boys. Increasingly, girls are being allowed to join boys' teams, but, unless they excel, they are highly resented by their male counterparts. Frequently, a girl will go to one or two practice sessions and decide that she cannot tolerate insulting remarks, being left out unless the coach intervenes, and giving up certain feminine dress and habits. More girls' teams, however, are being formed to meet their athletic needs.

The child learns much about play from his parents. If they allot time to sports, indoor games, and hobbies, the child will learn to value these activities. If parents seek new and interesting activities for the family, the child will gain the self-confidence that will allow him to try new activities at school, camp, and community centers. Play continues to be the child's "work" throughout this period, teaching him much about himself and his world.

COMMON PROBLEMS

Bedwetting

The average child gains nighttime bladder control (with the exception of occasional accidents) before five years of age. After this age, regular bedwetting is called nocturnal enuresis and is considered abnormal. Because developmental, emotional, and physical factors can affect the child's ability to hold his urine throughout the night, each of these factors must be evaluated. Developmental factors include increasing bladder capacity, maturation of neurological pathways, and changing patterns and levels of sleep. Emotional aspects of bedwetting may be related to problems of the child, his parents, and the whole family, such as overdependence of the child on his parents, abuse of the child by his parents, or severe marital discord. Physical causes of bedwetting include anatomical deviations and infections of the urinary tract, anomalies of adjacent structures, such systemic diseases as juvenile diabetes mellitus and reactivity to bladder irritants such as cola. Although a child may be emotionally upset, or the family frankly chaotic, physical causes must be identified and treated before exploring other possibilities. Emotional problems may require referral to a behavioral specialist; developmental delays will improve with time and patience.

The average child plagued with nocturnal enuresis is greatly disturbed by this problem. There may be little he can do to keep his bed dry, since forcing him to decrease fluid intake and to get up to void during the night can make him feel punished and/or anxious.

Lea, aged eight, wet the bed almost every night. Her mother was terminally ill, and her father was an alcoholic. For years, Lea's life had been a series of chaotic and unpredictable events. She did enjoy some pleasant days with friends, but the nights were filled with anxiety and shame. She would lie in bed for hours, getting up frequently to empty her bladder in hopes of avoiding wetting the bed. Once she was placed in a children's home, which she disliked but tolerated; her bedwetting problem was never mentioned or even acknowledged there except that she was given instructions on how to get clean sheets for changes as needed. Her bed was soon dry in the mornings, much to her relief.

The child should not be ridiculed, punished, deprived of fluids, or awakened to empty his bladder; none of these techniques works. Increasing fluid intake during the day and helping the child to hold more urine for longer periods of time will increase bladder capacity, but this will not necessarily decrease the incidence of bedwetting. Giving the child more responsibility for his problem (e.g., having him change the sheets or teaching him to limit his own late afternoon and evening intake of fluids, especially colas and other caffeinated drinks) in accordance with his age, may help.

Almost nothing will save face for the child when he is at camp or at a friend's house. Some children will risk putting on a disposable diaper behind a locked bathroom door in hopes of keeping the sheets dry. The older child may benefit from a buzzer system that awakens him when the first drop of urine hits the pad on his bed; he may learn to wake up when his bladder feels full before he voids. This method keeps the bed dry, but the child wakes up to empty his bladder instead of sleeping through the night, but the benefits usually are well worth the inconvenience. Unless the reason for bedwetting is purely physical, the child usually gains nighttime bladder control by late pubescence regardless of the techniques used.

School Phobia

School phobia is a term used for varying degrees of fear related to school (See Ch. 12). Mild, transient fear is not generally considered a phobia, but it may account for many trips to the physician. The child develops a stomachache, headache, or earache that miraculously disappears as soon as the school bus is out of sight. Parents cannot decide whether or not their child is ill, so they consult their physician, or, increasingly, the nurse practitioner, who finds nothing on examination. Questioning the child may easily reveal that a bully threatens him, that he is afraid of a certain teacher, or that he has a report to read aloud to the class.

Richard, aged seven, refused to go to school one morning because his stomach hurt. He felt fine later in the morning but had another stomachache the next morning. In the physician's office, Richard explained that he had a loose bowel movement at school two days earlier, and the odor was so bad that the other children called him "stinky." He also had had to sit on a toilet seat wet from the urine of careless little boys. Richard was able to tell the understanding physician of his fears that he would have another loose bowel movement at school. Unfortunately, careful study of the situation revealed no way to provide better toileting facilities. Richard was told in a sympathetic manner that he would have to accept the situation and that he must attend school. He was reassured that he could handle the problem but that his mother would pick him up at school if he had more than one loose bowel movement. He was encouraged to carry a tissue in his pocket to wipe off the toilet seat if necessary.

Confronting the child with the cause of his fears, helping him to see methods for solving his own problem, intervening for him when necessary, and insisting that he go to school usually will resolve this type of problem. A severe and persistent dread of going to school requires the assistance of a behavioral specialist. Often, the child is overdependent on his mother, who often has her own difficulty in being separated from her child. This is a complex situation in which the child and mother may need individual psychotherapy, and therapy for the family as a whole may also be beneficial. Parents, teachers, school nurses, guidance counselors, and behavioral specialists must coordinate their services in order to provide consistency and continuity of care for the child. Regardless of the situation, the team must ensure that the child attend school to overcome his fear.

Constipation

Every school has its routines, which may interrupt the child's bowel habits. He may not have time or the urge for a bowel movement at home in the morning. There often is little opportunity to drink water regularly during a normal school day. If the child feels the need to have a bowel movement at school, he may be upset by the lack of privacy or the lack of cleanliness in the bathroom at school. Adjusting schedules to provide time on the toilet either before or after school, increasing bran and fluid intake to soften stools if necessary, and exercising regularly will help the child overcome this temporary problem.

Long-term, severe constipation is frequently overlooked by parents of the school-age child, since he is responsible for his personal hygiene, and the parents are simply unaware of his bowel habits. They may be surprised when he tells the physician of hard, painful stools and excessive flatus (gas).

Tobie K., aged nine, was deserted by his mother at age two. His grandmother, Mrs. K., moved in with him and his father to care for them, but she became bitter about her predicament. She controlled Tobie's every move. When they visited the nurse practitioner, Mrs. K. described Tobie's horrible constipation, which she treated with laxatives, suppositories, and enemas. She required him to leave his stools in the toilet until she could see them and "break them up with a coat hanger" when necessary. He simply had no bowel movements except when he could no longer hold it—about every 10 days. Mrs. K. seemed to want to help. Tobie's eyes sparked with defiance. The nurse practitioner recommended the following:

- Mrs. K. was not to mention, look at, or treat Tobie's stools in any way.
- Tobie was first to take laxatives, followed by stool softeners, until his stools were soft and passing painlessly. He was to keep his medicine in his room.
- Tobie was to call the nurse practitioner every other day for a week, then weekly.
- Tobie was to return in two weeks for another talk with his nurse.
- Mrs. K. was to set up an appointment with the family counselor to discuss alternatives to her present situation.

In two weeks, Tobie's situation had improved. Although many problems remained, he expressed great relief over his privacy in the bathroom and the assurance that he would not suffer further intrusions by his grandmother.

Orthodontic Braces

Braces on teeth during the later school-age period are no longer a problem for the average child, since orthodontic care is more common than it was some years ago, and many of the child's friends will have them; in fact, braces are often a status symbol. A child may, however, be extremely self-conscious about braces. He needs an opportunity to express his feelings. It does not help to say, "It will be worth it when it is over" because he either already knows that or doesn't believe it. Commenting on his positive features may redirect his attention somewhat, but he may resent such tactics. Regardless of whether he accepts the change in his looks or not, he still requires frequent reminders to keep his teeth very clean with brushing and flossing, tasks that are time-consuming and boring.

Obesity

Childhood obesity is a problem that profoundly affects every aspect of the child's life. He cannot hide his body with clothes or cosmetics, so he seldom has relief from acute embarrassment. There is always at least one classmate who torments him unmercilessly.

Fatty, fatty, two by four
Can't get through the bathroom door
So he does it does it on the floor
Cleans it up and does some more.

The obese child may strike back at cruel children, withdraw to a quiet and safe world of his own, or develop a self-deprecating sense of humor. He often avoids athletics, since he is usually clumsy and slow and his rolls of fat are painfully exposed in athletic uniforms. He selects, instead, quiet activities that burn few calories, compounding his weight problem.

The other members of the obese child's family often have poor eating habits, no exercise routines, and are often overweight themselves. The parents may be excessively critical of their child for some reason, increasing his desire for the sure pleasure of eating. If he is reprimanded for overeating, he frequently becomes a master at sneaking food from the refrigerator while feeding the cat or washing the dishes; he may hide candy under his mattress, put the wrappers in his pocket, and throw the incriminating evidence in the trash at school.

The treatment of childhood obesity that is not accompanied by underlying pathology usually requires the involvement of the parents. They need information about nutrition, exercise, emotional aspects of obesity, and ways to support their child during weight loss. The family cook should not make cakes, cookies, puddings, casseroles, breads, and so on, because the child simply cannot resist the temptation. If his parents reward or console him with sweets, he will console himself later the same way. Some families will need the help of a behavioral specialist or team to identify emotional problems. Occasionally, a child will diet and exercise in order to lose just enough weight to fit within the weight limit for an athletic team or to fit into a ballet costume. A physical education teacher or school nurse might influence the child to lose weight, and support him throughout his struggle with regular weight checks and encouraging talks, although the child himself must want to lose weight if any program is to succeed.

ACCIDENTS

As has been mentioned in earlier chapters, accidents are the most frequent causes of death throughout childhood. The school-age child has less and less supervision as he rides his bike to various places, travels for group activities, and explores new places and interesting phenomena. He still does not have enough awareness of his own motor skills and endurance to make consistently realistic decisions about how far to swim before turning back or when there is enough time to get across the street before the oncoming car arrives. This lack of judgement results in drownings and accidents involving motor vehicles. The child is also susceptible to accidents with fire because his curiosity about fires is not matched with an understanding of how fire and smoke spread and what precautions are necessary for safety. Trauma from burns or motor vehicles not only kills but, more frequently, results in extended hospitalizations and permanent disability. Other common accidents during the school-age period involve vision loss from flying or exploding objects, hearing loss from extremely high noise levels, and internal bleeding from injuries sustained during participation in contact sports. Parents can teach safety during school age by setting good examples and by explaining the logical consequences of unsafe behavior. When the child is not allowed to do "what everyone else is doing," parents can point out that he cannot be trusted to do what *seems to be* safe because his judgment is not yet fully mature.

Bud, aged eight, was riding with his mother when a friend on a bicycle swerved in front of their car. She slammed on the brakes and almost said, "See that idiot? I nearly killed him!" Instead, she struggled to regain her composure and said, "Children do not always stop and look when they are on their bikes. This is why you can ride only in our neighborhood where people usually drive slowly." Bud was visibly shaken by the incident.

When the child is in late infancy, parents begin to warn him of dangers simply by saying, "no," "hot," or "hurt," but of course they must provide protection at all times. Later, they become more explicit, saying, "If you touch the stove, you will get burned," "If you keep wading further out in the lake, water will get in your nose," or "If you run too fast, you will fall down and skin your knee." The child soon assumes that he is responsible for all his accidents whether or not he was careless. He believes in what Piaget calls *immanent justice,* the expectation that his wrongdoing (including disobeying a safety rule) will sooner or later inflict its own rightful punishment on him. When the child has suffered major trauma, he often feels that pain, disfigurement, and/or immobility are just punishments. Even the older child, who can verbalize that he had a faultless accident, will explain that it would not have happened if only he had stayed home that day, or if he had seen whatever caused the accident in time. Parents may compound his guilt by reminding him that he could or should have avoided the mishap, or that they are greatly inconvenienced by his hospitalization. They usually feel unrealistically responsible for his safety. Nursing care should include a frank discussion of these feelings with the parents and the child. The child needs reassurance that he is loved and forgiven (if necessary) throughout his recuperation.

SIGNS AND SYMPTOMS OF ILLNESS

The school-age child is usually free from illness other than common colds. Because many states require immunizations for admission to school, the child is often protected from most common childhood diseases. He also has acquired immunity to some diseases by contracting them earlier in his life. His body has grown bigger and his organs are farther apart, so infections spread less freely, swollen tissue is less likely to encroach on adjacent body parts, and mucous accumulation blocks vital passages less frequently. The child's skin, lungs, bowels, and urinary tract can conserve fluid more efficiently, so dehydration is a less frequent problem. His illnesses seldom have a very rapid onset now that his body systems can adapt somewhat to the stress of early illness.

Illness in the school-age child often causes him to look tired, pale, flushed, and generally unhappy. He usually refuses to eat regular meals but accepts his favorite juices and other drinks. His appetite may improve considerably when his body temperature is normal. He often prefers to lie on the sofa to watch television during a brief illness. Bowel and bladder habits may change somewhat as a result of dehydration, or elimination may cause a marked loss of fluid and electrolytes. Fever, respirations, and heart rate generally do not rise as rapidly or as high as with the younger child.

The school-age child is aware of body sensations and thus is able to locate and describe with some accuracy pain, nausea, itching, and so on. He may know that he is getting sick but hide signs of illness long enough to go to a long-awaited party. He may learn either consciously or unconsciously to "look" sick to avoid an unpleasant activity. *Functional disorders*, signs and symptoms of illness with no detectable physical cause, such as abdominal pain and headache, become more prevalent. Parents, child, and physician must work together to determine the cause of the functional disorders, which may usually be emotional stress.

HOSPITALIZATION

Most hospitals have routines that severely limit the well-established autonomy of the schoolager. There are rules that prescribe bed, bath, and meal times, types of diversions, and the minimum age of visitors. Hospital personnel intrude into his allotted space without even a knock on the door, depriving him of privacy and his own territory. Nursing care of the school-age child should be directed toward giving him reasonable control over and responsibility for his own behavior. Parents remain a very important source of support to the child, but he can draw strength from other caring individuals when he needs assistance if his parents are not available.

Admission

The school-age child enters the hospital with a mixture of fear, excitement, and curiosity. His parents, of course, are anxious because of his problem and the disruption of family security. To tell their story of the present problem is frequently the parents' most pressing need during admission. The child will want to give his version of the illness, but he often is more concerned about what will happen to him. The child may be quiet while his parents are talking but may have many questions in mind. Give him an overview of the admitting procedure; if he is not acutely ill, he will be interested in why you measure his blood pressure, height, weight, and vital signs. He will be relieved to know that you will try to keep his clothes on unless removal is absolutely necessary. If he asks how long he will be there or how many "shots" he will get, respond honestly that you do not know, unless you are absolutely certain of the answer. He may be delighted to find that his room has a television and a phone for him to use, that the unit has a playroom, and that he has a choice of food. He may appear quiet and shy while his parents talk, so you must give him time to ask questions. He may be angry if there is an early "lights out" time, or if his roommate is much younger than he. Provide an opportunity to discuss his feelings and try to individualize regulations whenever possible.

Preparation for Procedures

The school-age child is accustomed to following directions, listening to explanations, and solving problems. His thinking is logical although still somewhat egocentric. In preparing him for a procedure, first find out what he expects to happen. As with the preschooler, the school-age child and his parents should know what he will see, feel, and hear, whether he is going to the unit treatment room, the operating room, or the x-ray department. His expectations may be so accurate that you can concentrate on his feelings about the procedure; more often, his idea is incorrect or incomplete. Diagrams, slides, pictures, and movies are useful in teaching about equipment such as ventilators, traction or x-ray machines (Figure 7–8). However, the child needs more concrete experience, such as going through the motions of a procedure by participating in a "dress rehearsal."

The school-age child may be very reluctant to discuss his feelings about surgery or other procedures because he thinks "big" people are supposed to be fearless; parents may feel the same way. It is an important nursing function to identify and respond to the child's fears.

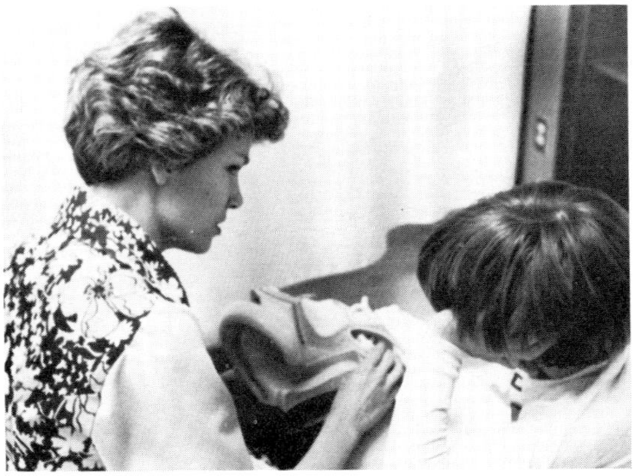

Figure 7–8. *A nurse uses a model of the ear to prepare a child for surgery.*

Larry S., aged eight, had been admitted to the hospital for a minor surgical procedure. The nurse was assessing Larry's previous experiences with surgery before preparing him for the next day's procedure. She learned from Mrs. S. that Larry's grandmother had died unexpectedly in the same hospital under anesthesia only six months earlier. Larry began to cry, "I'm going to die, too." His mother ran to him and began to sob almost hysterically, "No, no, not you!" After quietly listening to the whole story, the nurse called the physician, who cancelled the surgery. Larry and his mother were referred to a counselor for help in resolving their grief.

Jenny, aged nine, had had several operations to remove a large hemangioma (birthmark) from her face. The nurse who interviewed Jenny and her parents was impressed that they were well-informed and seemingly at ease. However, when Jenny used puppet play to demonstrate what she had been told about the latest operation she was to undergo, she had the little girl puppet say, "Over and over you say you're going to fix my face, but you never do and you probably never will." The nurse realized that she had said "fixed" when she described the surgery to Jenny, so she admitted that Jenny was correct but that the surgery would make the mark smaller. The parents and child described their disappointment with previous corrective attempts while the nurse listened. Later she noted their feelings on Jenny's nursing care plan and relayed them to the surgeon and to the pediatric nurse specialist for further evaluation and intervention.

Other Nursing Interventions

One of the greatest challenges to the nurse of a school-age child is to prevent boredom during an extended hospitalization (Figure

7–9). Soap operas and game shows on daytime television quickly become boring as do books, crossword puzzles, and solitary games. Established hobbies hold the child's interest if he feels energetic enough to work at them. He may enjoy learning new crafts, but he usually needs an instructor and materials. In some settings, tutors can keep the child abreast of schoolwork. Unfortunately, however, many hospitals have little other than a playroom. An adequate activities program takes time, space, equipment, and knowledgeable people. The child needs peers in order to enjoy his play fully because he enjoys competition and sharing; he also needs adults who listen to his ideas. Some large children's hospitals have outstanding activity programs; in smaller hospitals that have no organized programs, the child should be encouraged to call his friends and write them letters. If necessary, call his teacher and ask her to send letters from classmates. The school-age child listens to popular music, so a radio can help to pass the time. Limiting television will make a few selected shows seem better. Put at least two (and more if possible) children together for a talk or game, even if you have to move a whole bed to another room. Ask the child for ideas—he may surprise you.

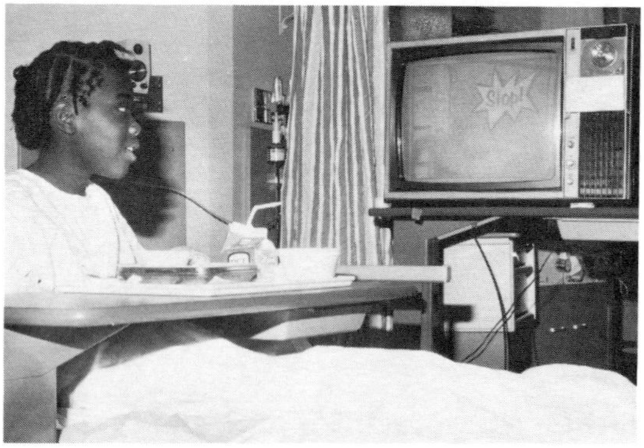

Figure 7–9. *Television can alleviate some of the hospitalized child's boredom, but it soon loses its appeal.*

Hospital staff members and even parents may mistakenly feel that the school-age child is old enough and secure enough to spend the night without parents, perhaps because he has spent the night at relatives' and friends' homes with little or no difficulty. They do not realize that a form of regression occurs when separation anxiety becomes very strong in a strange and frightening environment—the hospital.

Skipper, a "rough-and-tough" nine-year-old, was admitted to the hospital for a simple surgical procedure, which he tolerated well. He scoffed at the nurses' assurances that it is all right to express his fears or cry during injections. The next day he was to go home but he had to stay in his room alone for about 30 minutes while one parent settled the bill and the other parent kept his younger brother in the lobby. Suddenly, the usually self-confident Skipper was overcome with fear. He had his mother check his dressing, help him to the bathroom, plump his pillow, hand him the call bell, put his drawing pad on the bed, point out the car waiting for them, and so on. When big tears finally welled in his eyes, his mother realized that he could not tolerate being left alone at that moment for some reason and asked for a nursing assistant to sit with him for a few minutes.

Assess the child's separation anxiety if the parents must leave. Moving the child to the playroom, near the nurse's station, or into another child's room may help. Encourage him to call a friend on the phone, write a letter, or work on a hobby. Most important, spend a few minutes to explain that his feelings are normal, even for a school-age child. Parents also need the reassurance that their increased anxiety is to be expected when they leave their child in the hospital. If the child receives competent nursing care for an extended time, both he and his parents usually feel secure when the parents go home or to work, but the child does continue to need frequent contact with them.

The child learns to resist crying by observing adults stifle the urge to let their tears flow. The school-age child often has enough control to stifle cries, even during very painful experiences. Since it seems to be so important not to cry, he feels quite a failure if he does. Begin every procedure with an honest explanation, e.g., "You will feel a stick (burning sensation, pressure, and so forth), and it will hurt. I will be as quick as possible, and you may cry as loud as you want; it is always OK to cry when you hurt." Parents who were about to say "Don't cry" usually are visibly relieved and will agree with you. Your best efforts may convince neither the child nor parents that crying is acceptable during the "big" school-age period. Do not force the issue, because the child may become upset with the conflict between nurse and parent. Try to make your point with the parents later.

Discharge

The discharge procedure for the school-age child is different from that for the younger child because the former can learn to perform continuing procedures by himself or with a little help from his parents. Both the parents and the child, therefore, must develop competence in such skills as administering injections, cast care, "ostomy" care, and so on. It is important for the child to learn these techniques in the hospital if possible because parents may be either overprotective or negligent at home.

Johnny, aged nine, had had juvenile diabetes melliteus since he was nine months old. His mother could not bring herself to allow him to give himself his own injections. Intellectually, she knew she was meeting her own need to protect him, but she simply could not hand him the syringe and let him try. She refused to allow a home nurse to instruct him. He was admitted to the pediatric unit for three days where he was taught self-injection as his mother watched, tight-lipped, from the corner of the room. The pediatric nurse specialist persuaded Johnny's mother to allow him to go to summer camp alone. She slept very little as she struggled with her fierce need to go get him and bring him home.

There are fewer post-hospitalization behavioral changes in the child of school age, although he may have nightmares, cry over minor frustrations, wet the bed, or resist separation from his parents. Explain to the child and his parents that these changes are normal and temporary. As with earlier stages, a gradual resumption of routines and limits is helpful.

SUMMARY

The school-age child develops a sense of industry by successfully completing tasks, or a sense of inferiority, if he constantly fails. He progresses through the concrete operations stage of cognitive development, in which he is capable of logical, but not yet abstract, thinking. His vocabulary increases and his ability to use new grammatical patterns correctly improves. Growth is slow and steady until the pubescent growth spurt occurs. The school-age child's fine and gross motor coordination progresses remarkably, so he is able to complete many types of projects involving manual and motor skills. He becomes so involved with school and extracurricular activities that his daily routines are often disrupted. He begins to enjoy new foods, but he will eat large quantities of junk foods if permitted. School influences every aspect of the child's development. He learns to use concepts in problem-solving, and to expand his knowledge of the world around him. School-age play reveals the child's competitiveness and his strong desire to meet the standards of his peer group.

Common problems include bedwetting, school phobia, constipation, adjustment to orthodontic braces, and obesity. Accidents are responsible for more deaths among school-age children than any other cause; motor vehicle accidents account for the largest percentage of these accidental deaths. The child usually perceives an accident as justified punishment for his wrongdoing, real or imagined.

The school-age child is generally healthy. During an illness, he can describe his symptoms with some accuracy. Functional disorders such as headaches and abdominal pain become more prevalent. Hospitalization provokes fear in the school-age child, but his newly acquired logic enables him to learn about his problem and to participate in his own care. His parents are important sources of support, especially when he regresses to a more dependent state. Posthospitalization behavioral changes include nightmares, crying over minor frustrations, and anxiety caused by separation from parents.

CHAPTER **8**

The Adolescent

BEHAVIORAL OBJECTIVES

After studying this chapter you will be able to:

- Describe the adolescent's development of identity versus role diffusion.
- Discuss the formal operations stage of cognitive development.
- Describe the adolescent's language development.
- Discuss adolescent growth and physical changes; list, in typical order of appearance, the secondary sex characteristics.
- Describe the adolescent's motor development.
- Discuss normal nutrition and common nutritional problems of adolescents.
- Identify the activities that may comprise daily activities, including school functions.
- Discuss play in relation to the emotional and cognitive development of the adolescent.
- Identify common problems and accidents during adolescence.
- Describe signs and symptoms of illness in the adolescent.
- Discuss nursing care of the adolescent and his parents during hospitalization.

TERMS AND CONCEPTS

Identity
Role diffusion
Formal operations
Menarche
Acne vulgaris
Amenorrhea
Dysmenorrhea
Venereal disease

The adolescent is neither child nor adult. When he is hospitalized, treat him as an adult as much as possible, by encouraging him to assume maximum responsibility for his own care and behavior, although you will place him more in the child's role to the extent that you will include his parents in decision making. When parents provide strength and comfort to their adolescent, especially during major emotional or physical stress, support their efforts with comfortable facilities and willingness to listen. When parents arouse feelings of ambivalence and/or rebellion in their adolescent, avoid taking sides; try to understand both points of view, and offer a logical problem-solving approach in your counseling.

EMOTIONAL DEVELOPMENT

The adolescent faces the difficult task of developing a sense of who he actually is, i.e., a sense of *identity*, as Erikson calls it. The influences of his family, friends, society and, of course, his own personal attitudes and self-image, contribute to this sense of identity. The conflict and confusion that occur may hamper his efforts to determine life goals or may obscure logical ways to achieve his goals. This lack of direction, which Erikson calls *role diffusion*, is usually temporary and is resolved as the adolescent becomes better able to set priorities for himself.

The adolescent must detach himself somewhat from family ties, in order to decide which of their practices and values to make his own. Parents may be hurt, resentful, or angry when they see their offspring reject their way of life. He has a mixture of emotions resulting from not knowing the "right" thing to do. The adolescent has an almost adult body and demands adult privileges, but actually he is afraid of total responsibility for his life.

Jeff, an immature-looking sixteen-year-old, was receiving his college physical from a nurse practitioner. As he described his feelings about going far away to college, he made conflicting statements such as, "I'm going away to college no matter what my parents say," "My mother is really kicking me out of the house, but I guess it is time," and "I griped so much about moving to this town that I could not possibly go to the university here."

Katie, aged fifteen, demanded to go on an overnight skiing trip with a group of older teenagers. Her parents rejected the idea from the first, and Katie raved and ranted for two days. Suddenly she said no more and made arrangements to go to a local high school ball game instead. Later, when she was in a good mood, she told her parents that they "might" have been right about keeping her home, but she would not explain her change of heart.

Parents, too, are unsure about reasonable limits on their adolescent's behavior and are frequently too strict or too lenient. Parental ambivalence increases the conflict in the child.

Sherry, aged fourteen, was not allowed to date. When her friend, Pattie, began to date, Sherry demanded the right to double-date with her. Sherry's parents debated about her level of maturity and responsibility, boys she could date, how late she should be allowed out, and so on. Finally, they decided she was simply too young to date at all, and Sherry was infuriated. Her parents stuck to their decision but tried to cheer her up by offering to let her give a party for friends at home, go with a group to the movies, etc. Nothing suited Sherry. She felt sure that she could soon change her parents' minds since they had almost given in earlier.

When the adolescent lives in a family that has constantly allowed and encouraged making decisions and accepting the consequences, the adolescent will be less reluctant to make decisions and will have less need to rebel. He knows he must accept whatever happens as a result of his behavior, and his parents already have an idea of how he will react to many situations. Mutual trust and respect will assist the whole family, but even the most loving, stable, and democratic parents will have conflicts with their adolescent.

Friends are crucial to a developing sense of identity (Figure 8–1). The typical adolescent has a group of friends and a "special" friend. The group is usually tight-knit, with four to eight members who may be jealous of one another's achievements and possessions. They are usually of the same socioeconomic class, race, sex, and level of achievement in popularity, academics, and extracurricular activities. The "special" friend," who is more important to girls than to boys, acts as a sounding board for plans and dreams and shares the highs and

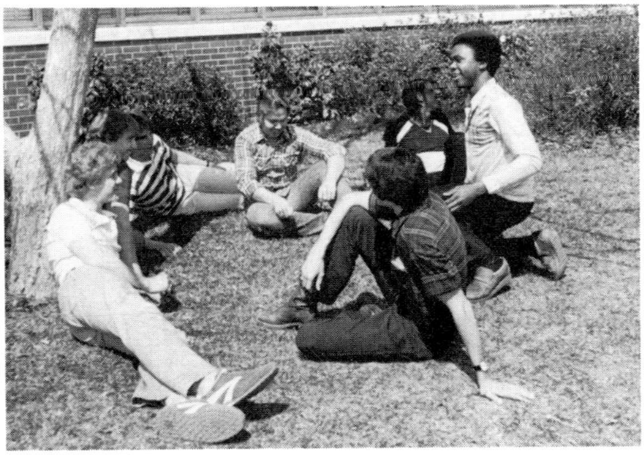

Figure 8–1. *Friendships are essential to the adolescent's developing sense of identity.*

lows of daily life. For a while, the adolescent may adopt almost all group values, including those regulating dress, activities, and relationships. This can be disastrous when the group indulges in alcohol, drugs, sexual promiscuity, theft, and so on. A more socially acceptable group, however, may actually improve a member's behavior. As he grows older, he can comfortably remain in the group but take a different position in some issues.

Society and its imperfections may overwhelm the adolescent. He feels that society should be "right"—that no one should be cold or hungry, but taxes should be lower; that there should be no wars, but some country should help struggling nations maintain their boundaries. Wavering between idealism and realism can be very disturbing; the adolescent may work to effect change within the system, fight the system, or give up on the system completely for a while. In young adulthood he usually becomes more realistic in his expectations of society.

The adolescent has his reputation at stake if he tries something new. In earlier periods of development, the child felt free to experiment with unexplored tasks because "try and try again" was acceptable to him and his friends. There were many things that he could not accomplish because of his age and size. Because the adolescent must maintain his image of being smart, athletic, or beautiful, he may hesitate to participate in the debating team or to attempt a new sport. The possibility of failure is a dilemma that prevents him from trying to learn to dance, asking a girl for a date, or wearing an outfit that is in "questionable" style among his peers.

Pat, aged seventeen, had always excelled in sports, but he had never skied on snow. His girlfriend, an accomplished skier, talked him into going to the slopes and taking lessons. The lessons were of little help, and he fell time and time again. When his girlfriend kidded him about his "skill," he threw his ski pole at her. He finally made it down the slope with one humiliating fall after another, stormed into the lodge, and refused to put on skis again for years.

Parents can set a good example by continuing to explore new places, people, and activities, and actively involving each family member regardless of his age.

Body image changes considerably during adolescence. The adolescent's body reaches adult size and proportion. Secondary sex characteristics become obvious. The adolescent becomes so acutely aware of every flaw that even a small pimple can seem as noticeable as a flashing red light. Clothes take on an increased importance as part of the external image, and members of the group dress very much alike to avoid being different. The adolescent whose body or clothes do not meet the standards of the group or of his school usually has marked feelings of inferiority. Reassurance from his parents that the teenager looks fine is worthless or worse. Adolescence also alters the internal body image with the appearance of menstruation and seminal emissions. This change may cause feelings of accomplishment, matter-of-fact acceptance, or dread. In time, the adolescent usually will begin to make the best of what he has and tolerate what he cannot change (Figure 8–2).

Megan, aged thirteen, visited the nurse practitioner only on her mother's insistence. One year earlier, she had had two periods a month apart and none since. She refused to wear pads and failed to insert a tampon after many attempts, so she sat on the toilet most of the time. She vowed not to have any more periods. She explained to the nurse that she was afraid she would "start" during a softball or tennis game, so she gave up these sports. The nurse listened to Megan's fears about menstruation and then instructed her on the proper method of inserting a tampon. Megan made an appointment to return in a month to discuss other ways to cope with the problems of menstruation. When she saw the nurse, Megan said, almost angrily, "I hope you are satisfied. I had another period!" She had, however, mastered the technique of inserting a tampon and had tolerated the experience well.

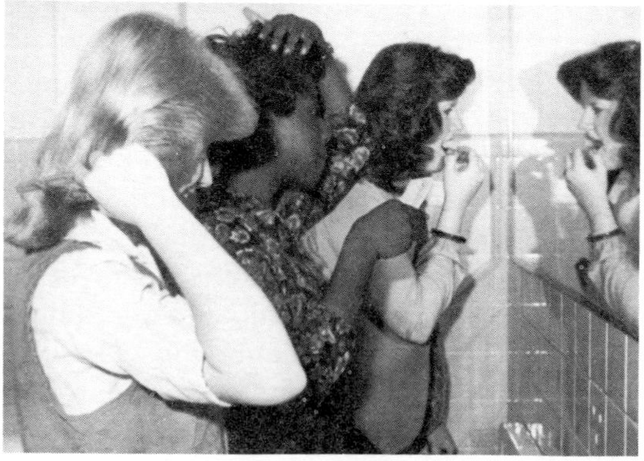

Figure 8–2. *Primping is a natural outgrowth of a positive body image.*

The child knows much about sex long before he enters adolescence, regardless of what his parents tell him. He learns from peers, school, television, movies, and books, as well as from parents. When secondary sex characteristics begin to emerge, he wonders increasingly how intercourse is accomplished and how it feels. He later fantasizes about sex as he knows it, which might be simply a loving embrace or a confused jumble of violent motions. He may brag to others that he actually enacted these dreams in real life. These fantasies may take up much of his time as he considers such questions as whether to try to touch his girlfriend's breasts on the next date. The adolescent girl, on the other hand, may have to decide how to entice her boyfriend to try touching her intimately, or whether she will let him if he does. Because there is often an almost physical ache or yearning to touch someone of the opposite sex, teenagers frequently hold hands, sit close together, walk with one arm around each other, in addition to engaging in more frankly sexual caresses. This desire to touch is probably related not only to a normal sex drive but also to the need for skin contact that is present in all people in a nonsexual context (Figure 8–3).

Sexual activity in the unmarried adolescent is now commonplace. Boys have intense sexual urges that they usually relieve with masturbation and intercourse, frequently with almost any willing partner. Girls, too, have sexual tensions that they may relieve in the same ways, but they seem to want more affection and caring along with sexual involvement. These male-female patterns may change as women continue to assume more assertive positions in all aspects of life, including sex. Ambivalence toward sex on the part of some parents is summed up in a teenager's

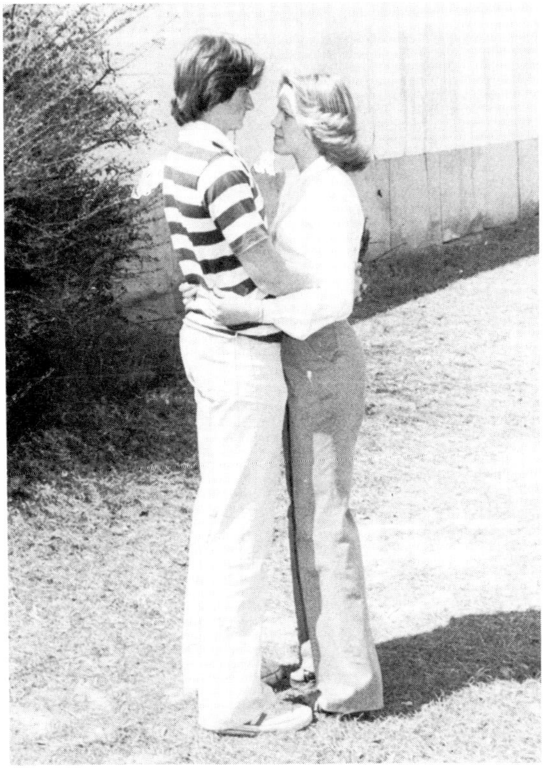

Figure 8–3. *Touch plays a part in most adolescent heterosexual relationships.*

comment to her mother, "You say 'Don't have sex, but if you do, be sure to use protection' ". Other parents forbid any sexual activity before marriage, citing religious and cultural values. Decision-making about sex is similar to solving any other problem. If parents have maintained open communications with their adolescent, they can discuss the advantages and disadvantages of an active sex life. They can state their own beliefs about human sexuality and offer insight about potential problems. Parents can set rules and guidelines for teenage behavior, but realistically, they cannot prevent sexual activity. Because of intense peer pressure, the adolescent may need support from parents and nurse when he decides not to have intercourse.

School age is a time for same-sex peer closeness, which continues during adolescence. When sexual urges arise, the teenager, especially the boy, may turn to his best friend or friends for relief. They may manipulate each other's genitals to the point of ejaculation, or a group may masturbate together. These sex acts are not truly homosexual, but common practices that may cause guilt and the fears that one is homosexual.

Jim, aged sixteen, had had diabetes mellitus for two years. He tried to deny his disease by drinking beer, taking his insulin late or not at all, and checking his urine only occasionally. He was sitting in the nurse practitioner's office with his head down, miserable as usual. He kept hinting that he had something unspeakably horrible but could not get the words out. Finally, he blurted out, "I'm not natural. God will not love me now." The nurse guessed his problem, and he described a sexual experience with another boy. After evaluating his emotional status further and reassuring him that he was not a homosexual, she referred him to an adolescent psychiatric agency.

Selecting a career is a difficult task that faces the adolescent (Figure 8–4). High school guidance counselors can provide assistance by giving the adolescent information, arranging for aptitude testing and developing a program of study which will meet his probable future career needs. The adolescent may be able to postpone the decision by working at odd jobs or taking general courses in college, but usually he has begun training for a career or working in a permanent position by the end of his teens. Once a career is definitely chosen, the adolescent feels more secure about who he is and what his life goals are.

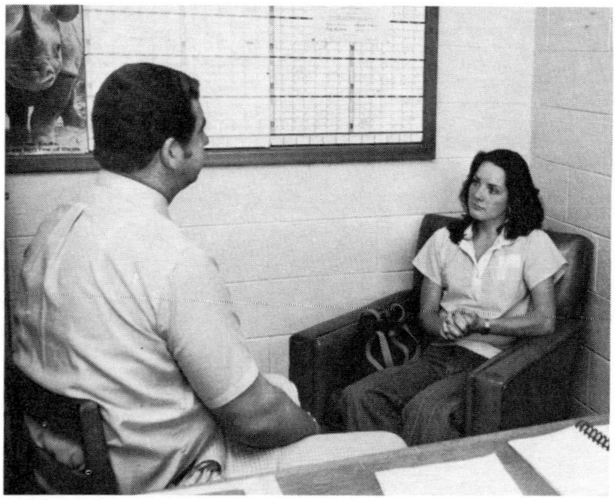

Figure 8–4. *The high school counselor assists in making a decision about a career.*

Lee, aged eighteen, never enjoyed studying, but he maintained above-average grades throughout high school. He was so depressed during the first half of his senior year that he hardly spoke to his family members and gave up dating altogether. Finally, he sat down with both his parents to tell them that he would not go to college after high school, although he was well aware that he was the first grandchild on both sides of a very large family to make such a decision. His parents discussed the disadvantages of lacking a college degree, but they accepted his decision. When Lee began to search for what he decided he wanted—the best-paying outdoors job available—he soon became more interested in his friends and family.

The ambivalence of the adolescent toward himself is evidenced by his extremely critical attitude toward his parents. His mother is too fat or her hairstyle is old-fashioned; his father should exercise and stay in shape; the family should do more for unfortunate members of society; his parents should hide any indication of sexual interest in one another. As the adolescent develops a stronger, more acceptable personal identity, he becomes more tolerant of others.

COGNITIVE DEVELOPMENT

The adolescent may remain in the concrete operations stage of cognitive development for the rest of his life and manage to live a productive adult life. The more intelligent and stimulated teenager, however, progresses to the stage of *formal operations* in which his thinking is much more abstract. He can see clearly from many points of view and can more objectively scrutinize his own viewpoint. He can use many hypotheses to construct his theories and state conclusions, tentatively, realizing that another theory can negate his own. His thinking becomes increasingly logical, and further cognitive growth in adolescence seems to be the result of individual interest in learning and opportunity.

LANGUAGE DEVELOPMENT

Language development is inevitably interrelated with cognitive development. The adolescent who remains in the stage of concrete operations increases his vocabulary and broadens his understanding of concepts to a degree. The adolescent who progresses to formal operations greatly increases his vocabulary, acquires a much fuller understanding of abstract concepts and relationships, and employs more complex sentence structures.

The adolescent develops a collection of slang terms and phrases that have a special meaning to his group. Members of other age groups usually sound foolish if they dare to use these words. Drug- and crime-oriented gangs have elaborate jargon that changes frequently to maintain some secrecy about their operations.

GROWTH AND PHYSICAL CHANGES

The change in physical appearance caused by growth is only one of many significant changes to which the adolescent must adjust. The growth changes occur in the same sequence; however, onset, speed, and the amount of the changes are extremely variable. The variability in the growth patterns is contributed to by race, sex, heredity, nutrition, and environment. The increases in physical stature are accompanied by development of the reproductive organs and secondary sex characteristics.

Body Proportion

The adolescent experiences significant changes in bones, muscles, and adipose tissue. Young men begin adolescence with an increase in adipose tissue, followed by a decrease during accelerated skeletal growth. The changes in proportions are no less significant in young women, but they may seem less dramatic because the female's earlier growth spurt during school age makes the physiological transition to adulthood appear less abrupt.

Skeletal growth in the male and female involves increases in leg length, hip width, chest breadth, shoulder width, length of the trunk, and depth of the chest. The hormonal changes in men bring about greater increases in shoulder breadth, leg length, and arm length, especially in the forearm. The female hormonal changes affect the skeletal system by increasing the width of the hips and changing the size and proportions of the bony pelvis. Girls also have less increase in bone diameter than boys. The development of the facial skeleton, especially the mandible and maxilla, changes the facial appearance significantly. The rounded "baby face" is replaced by the more angular adult face. Many times this change will occur over a period of three to four months.

Rita C. had been away from her family for several months. She got a call that her mother was ill and made an emergency trip home. She was to be met at the airport by her favorite sixteen-year-old nephew, Jackie. After landing, she spent 15 minutes looking around the waiting room before a tall, thin, nice-looking young man, grinning facetiously, walked over and identified himself as Jackie. She was amazed that a person could change so radically in a few months.

Changes in muscle tissue development and distribution are significantly different in boys and girls. Girls have their maximum number of muscle cells by the time they reach the first menstrual period. Boys, however, increase the number of muscle cells until eighteen months after they have reached their maximum height. Boys also have a greater distribution of muscle tissue in the shoulder and back.

Height and Weight

The height gain in boys during adolescence is 10 to 30 centimeters (4 to 12 inches); girls' average increase is 5 to 20 centimeters (2 to 10 inches). The weight changes during the same period are 7 to 30 kilograms (15 to 65 pounds) for boys and 7 to 25 kilograms (15 to 55 pounds) for girls. Ninety-nine percent of the adult size is reached by age eighteen.

Hearing and Vision

It cannot be assumed that a child will not develop hearing or vision problems just because the problems have not developed during the first twelve years of life. The health practitioner must continue screening for these difficulties throughout adolescence. There is great potential for hearing loss among an adolescent population exposing itself to the high noise levels of rock music. Inner ear damage is almost a certainty with frequent, prolonged exposure, especially with the use of headphones.

The adolescent may feign hearing or visual loss, adding difficulty to screening. It is important that the screener be aware of this possibility. Reasons for feigning loss are as varied as individual personalities; however, the adolescent is always aware that he is deceiving the examiner. The examiner should attempt to rule out actual vision or hearing loss and recognize that the deception is a symptom of an underlying problem. Often it is an attempt to gain peer group attention.

Other Health Measurements

The adolescent's body temperature lowers to the adult average. Pulse continues to slow to an average of 60 to 65 beats per minute. Respirations also continue decreasing until age 18 when the average is 16 to 17 respirations per minute. Blood pressure generally rises to the average adult levels, and hemoglobin rises slightly, with a greater increase for boys (14 to 18 g/100ml) than for girls (12 to 16 g/100 ml). The hematocrit increases for both also, but again the increase is greater for males. The average range for men is 42 to 52 and 37 to 47 for women. These levels remain standard throughout adult life.

Teeth

The school-age child gains most of his permanent teeth. The second molars erupt in early adolescence (ages twelve to thirteen), and third molars (wisdom teeth) erupt five to eight years later, and they may be extracted because of lack of room in the jaw. The adolescent is particularly prone to dental cavities; a diet very high in carbohydrates is the norm for this age group, and frequent snacks are also common. These two factors increase the likelihood of bacterial growth. The carbohydrates provide good growth media for bacteria, and the frequent snacks prevent saliva from cleansing the teeth completely. The adolescent should be advised of the need to incorporate regular brushing, flossing, and twice-yearly visits to the dentist into his routines.

Secondary Sexual Development.

The onset of puberty and the appearance of secondary sex characteristics arouses very ambivalent feelings in boys and girls.

> Laura and her mother were discussing when Laura should start wearing a bra. Laura's breasts had begun to develop and were obvious beneath her shirts. All of a sudden Laura burst into tears and wailed, "Oh, Mommy, I don't want to grow up. Everything gets so complicated."

It is very important for the parents to recognize this ambivalence as a normal reaction to changes in the body. Also, they need to reassure the adolescent that it's OK to talk about these feelings.

The physical changes in both sexes follow an orderly pattern. The first indication of puberty in boys is a general enlargement of the penis and testes with textural changes in the scrotum. There may also be a small amount of long, fair pubic hair apparent. As the general increase in size of the penis and testes continues, spermatogenesis begins. These primary changes usually occur during the first year of puberty. During the second year, further growth of the penis, testes, and scrotum occurs, and pubic hair darkens and curls. The completion of these physical changes can take from 1.8 to 4.7 years in males.

Pubertal change in females occurs in breast tissue and in the genitals. The onset of puberty is evidenced by the fine growth of hair on the external genitals and the slight elevation and enlargement of the breasts. This is followed by increasing amounts of darker pubic hair and further enlargement of the breasts. The final stage is the adult amount and distribution of pubic hair. Girls may take 1.5 to 3 years to complete breast and genital development. *Menarche,* the first menstrual period, usually occurs between age twelve and fourteen years, when pubic hair spreads from the labia over the pubic region, and the nipples begin to take their adult shape. Menarche may occur as early as age nine or as late as age seventeen and still be within the normal range. Menstruation may be irregular and sparse initially, causing the adolescent either concern that her body is malfunctioning or great relief to be spared this monthly inconvenience.

The extended family gathered at the beach house for their usual summer reunion. Sara, aged twelve, had saved babysitting money, and Dean, aged eleven, had saved lawnmowing money for the trip. All year long the cousins had made plans to swim, body surf, fish, and so on. When she was changing to her swimsuit on the first afternoon, Sara found a spot of blood on her panties and more on the toilet tissue. She was well-prepared for menstruation, but she called her mother and began to cry. Her mother offered to help her insert a regular-sized tampon, but Sara ordered her out of the bathroom so she could try in privacy. After several unsuccessful attempts, she resorted to a pad and put her shorts back on. Sara took out her frustrations on her frantic mother and angrily rejected all suggestions. Dean could not understand why Sara suddenly decided to watch television instead of going to the beach. After everyone left, Sara's aunt, a nurse, convinced her to try again with small tampons and explained how to use them. The next day Sara was swimming with Dean, but she still seemed a little strange and aloof to him.

It is important to remember that this sequence of developmental changes is generalized, and not all adolescents will follow the same pattern. Girls especially may show deviations from the norm, for example, enlarged breasts but sparse pubic hair. Be aware of individual differences.

MOTOR DEVELOPMENT

The adolescent achieves all the gross and fine motor skills of adulthood and works to refine them. He strives to perfect his abilities in sports, hobbies, and occupational endeavors. During the peak period of the growth spurt, a period of clumsiness may ensue; reassure the teenager and his parents that this is a temporary problem, but encourage them to express any concerns. If parents are concerned that this clumsiness is prolonged, a thorough physical exam may calm them.

Adolescence is the optimal time to start physical fitness programs. Since variations in the rate of development is so broad, it is important to provide programs that can be adapted to individuals.

NUTRITION

The increased body awareness of the adolescent results in the desire to have the "perfect" body. The boy often exercises to increase chest measurements, and the girl diets to ward off unwanted pounds. Teaching nutrition to this age group can provide a great deal of satisfaction or frustration, since the adolescent wants to be trim but cannot resist eating junk food with friends after school. Use a positive approach, such as "These are things you can do to improve your body" instead of "You're too heavy because you eat all the wrong foods." Parents should be included in discussions about nutrition, but they should be advised to avoid taking responsibility for their teenager's diet. If they monitor his intake and criticize him for overeating, he may very well eat twice as much in rebellion. Parents can help by buying nutritious foods and snacks, and by preparing well-balanced meals. Setting a good example for their adolescent is advantageous.

The adolescent growth spurt demands a greatly increased calorie intake, 2800 to 3000 calories for the boy and 2300 to 2500 for the girl. The girl's calorie needs drop quickly after the period of rapid growth, but the boy's requirements remain high throughout adolescence, because his basal metabolism is higher and his growth takes longer. The boy eats so much food to meet his calorie requirements that he usually acquires enough other nutrients to have a well-balanced diet. The girl's caloric requirements, however, decrease earlier in adolescence, so she frequently gains weight or tries fad diets that do not provide a balance of nutrients. Of course, activity level is another determinant of calorie needs in both sexes. Increased protein is essential during growth peaks to achieve maximal height. Vitamins and minerals are an important part of the adolescent's diet. Calcium and iron are especially important for growth, but the adolescent diet, especially that of the girl, is often low in these nutrients.

DAILY ROUTINES

The adolescent fills his days with school and homework, athletics, hobbies, household chores, being with friends and family, and perhaps a part-time job. He may be so overwhelmed by ambivalence and indecision that he establishes no priorities and accomplishes little. Whether or not this is true, the adolescent is unlikely to maintain a set routine every day.

Sleeping

Sleep is highly valued by the adolescent, especially when he can sleep late in the morning after a night out with friends. He needs extra sleep during this period of increased activity and rapid growth, but he rejects his parents' suggestions that he go to bed earlier. The teenager may complain to the physician or nurse practitioner that he is "tired all the time." An assessment of his activities, sleeping patterns, nutrition, and sources of stress may reveal a probable cause for fatigue. He may be too active or bored and depressed. He may sleep very little one night and long hours the next in an attempt to "catch up." A hemoglobin or hematocrit check will indicate whether anemia, which can cause fatigue, is present. Another possibility is that the teenager is facing a problem he cannot handle, and sleeping to avoid the problem. If there is no identifiable reason for a noticeable increase in sleeping, further medical evaluation is indicated.

Eating

The adolescent often eats "on the run," picking up fast foods and eating in the car. The average teenage boy has such a big appetite that he will eat large amounts of almost any food served when he has time to sit down for a meal. The teenage girl (and, less frequently, the boy) who is overweight alternates between a diet that is heavy in empty calories and various fad diets that are deficient in some nutrients. She may try to reduce her calorie intake by skipping breakfast and lunch, but she often is so hungry by mid-afternoon that she eats continually until bedtime. A typical complaint of the teenager on such a diet is: "I just don't understand why I keep gaining weight, because I never eat breakfast or lunch." Some high school cafeterias provide salad bars that serve fresh vegetables, cheese, and eggs to support students' and teachers' efforts to eat a nutritious lunch while avoiding unnecessary calories. Eating three well-balanced meals and a protein or fruit snack in the afternoon is best for maintaining stamina throughout the day while controlling weight.

Personal Hygiene

The average adolescent is so concerned with peer approval that the use of soap, shampoo, toothpaste, mouthwash, underarm deodorant, and even genital deodorant is part of the average teenager's daily personal hygiene routine. Occasionally, a teenager who has offensive breath or body odor is mercilessly ridiculed or ostracized by his peers. Halitosis (bad breath) is usually caused by bacterial action on food particles in the mouth, and body odor results from bacterial action on material secreted by sweat and oil glands at the base of the axillary and pubic hair follicles. Health and physical education classes are ideal for teaching the cause of odors and the reactions of others who must tolerate them. If the teenager does not have the benefit of such classes, a teacher, school nurse, or counselor should point out the problem as nicely as possible and offer to assist him in obtaining the necessary supplies if possible.

Melvin, aged fifteen, had the worst body odor imaginable. His classmates tormented him until one day he ran from class before Mrs. D., the new teacher, arrived. She looked for Melvin until she found him, and confronted him about his problem. She explained that he must eliminate his body odor and that she would help him in any way possible. Melvin decided that he would shower after the daily physical education class and, if Mrs. D. would lend him a dollar to buy the first can, he would use deodorant. He arranged to help her after school to repay her. A further investigation revealed a deplorable lack of facilities in his home.

Douches destroy the vagina's natural defenses against infection and should not be used routinely. Perfumed douching solutions may cause severe vaginal irritation, and perfumed deodorizing sprays for the external genitals may also cause inflammation of the contact areas. Uncircumcised boys should retract the foreskin of the penis when bathing in order to remove accumulations of smegna (sebaceous secretions).

School

Most high schools offer a variety of academic courses, counseling services, some vocational training, limited health screening, and extracurricular activities, including academic and honor clubs, athletics, literary competitions, and orchestra and band. Some high schools have better specialty programs than others, but the average adolescent has the opportunity to prepare for immediate employment in semi-skilled jobs, or for entrance into college or vocational schools.

Almost every adolescent who is aware of

the importance of education wishes to do well in school. He is most likely to succeed when he comes from a middle-class family, when he believes he can control his own fate, and when he associates with friends who appreciate education. Position in the family among siblings (that is, birth order, or ordinal position) affects achievement, the eldest child often being the most ambitious. The child of a minority group and/or a lower socioeconomic class who is below average in intellectual ability, or who has a physical or cosmetic abnormality usually does not achieve well in high school pursuits, whatever they are. The adolescent, struggling with his ambivalence toward authority, society, and himself, may feel lost in a large school and be unable to take advantage of its many offerings.

A high school athletic program can draw a community together and give its members a sense of belonging (Figure 8–5). Aside from the obvious physical benefits of an athletic program, sports provides an emotional outlet for the players and spectators, including students, teachers, parents, and interested others. In addition, important social functions often accompany the highlights of the school athletic seasons.

High schools are faced with the problems of increases in assaults on teachers, drug use, and vandalism. Occasionally, schools must be patrolled to protect lives and property. The threat of violence is disturbing to everyone but especially to the timid, insecure student who feels unable to defend himself.

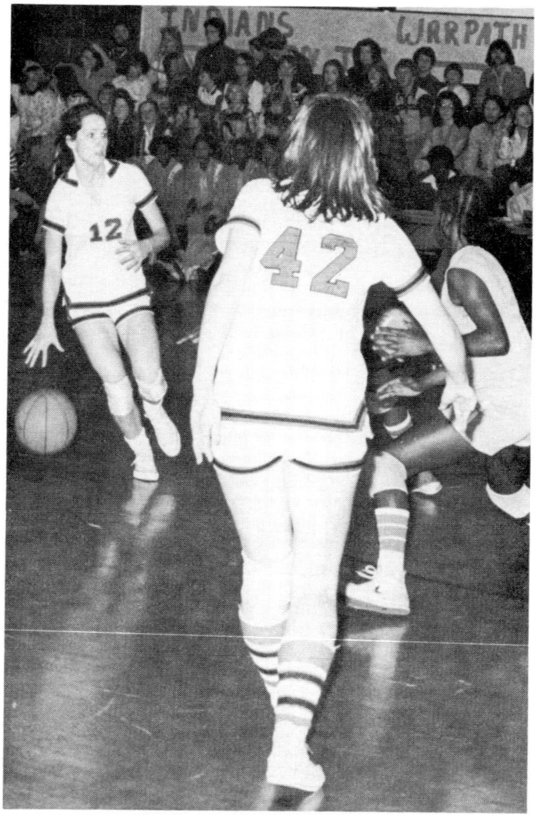

Figure 8–5. *Girls gain valuable team skills by playing basketball.*

Marti, a tiny fifteen-year-old, had only enough intellectual ability to hold her own in lower level classes in her new high school. Her parents had never shown much interest in Marti, and she had learned not to bother them. First she carried her lunch money in her purse, but it was stolen when she was in the gym. Then she put her lunch money in her sweater pocket, but Jane, a tough-looking girl, took it out, daring Marti to complain. Next Marti simply brought no money to school, but Jane threatened to "knock her head against the wall" if she showed up with no money. Marti brought the same amount of money daily until the physical education teacher observed the money change hands and instantly recognized what was happening. Jane was suspended for a week, and Marti was transferred to another gym class. Marti never again took money, gum, food, or extra supplies to school, because she feared someone would take them.

Officials have unsuccessfully attempted to control drug traffic. Marijuana is easily obtained from students, some of whom attend school only to sell drugs.

David, a sixteen-year-old tenth-grader described his marijuana habits to a school counselor. He smoked three "joints" on the school bus in the morning, another during the five-minute break, one at lunch, and two more on the way home on the bus. He never sold "the stuff" except as necessary to buy his personal supply. Psychometric testing indicated that he was of average intelligence, but that he was on the sixth-grade level of achievement. He was so shocked to learn this that he left the counselor's office and went straight to his regular "smoking spot" for relief.

The problems of pregnancy and venereal diseases are a concern of the high school faculty, administrators, counselors, and nurses. Sex education, including information on how to obtain birth control measures, is offered in health, family life, home economics, biology, and physical education courses, but the sexual problems of the adolescent persist and multiply. Parents in many communities block efforts to provide frank discussion and instruction about sex in schools because they fear that their children will be enticed to experiment with sex. With or without a formal sex education program, high school staff members often find that they are asked for information or assistance regarding a pregnancy, suspected venereal disease, and so on.

Mrs. C., the eleventh grade guidance counselor, cultivated a good working relationship with a nurse practitioner in a nearby family practice center. She had a great need for "emergency" services, usually pregnancy or venereal disease testing, for her students. Mrs. C. would bring them to the office and wait with them for the results so that she could provide continuing support. Mrs. C. and the nurse would then co-counsel the students.

Some schools respond to the problem of teenage pregnancy by offering special classes on childbirth and child rearing, the opportunity to talk with homebound teachers, and/or group sessions designed to meet the emotional needs of the pregnant adolescent. Many community agencies now coordinate the programs available to the high school student, relieving the schools of much responsibility after referral.

Play

The adolescent spends much of his free time with his peer group or with a best friend, talking about themselves and their world (Figure 8–6). The average teenager can talk

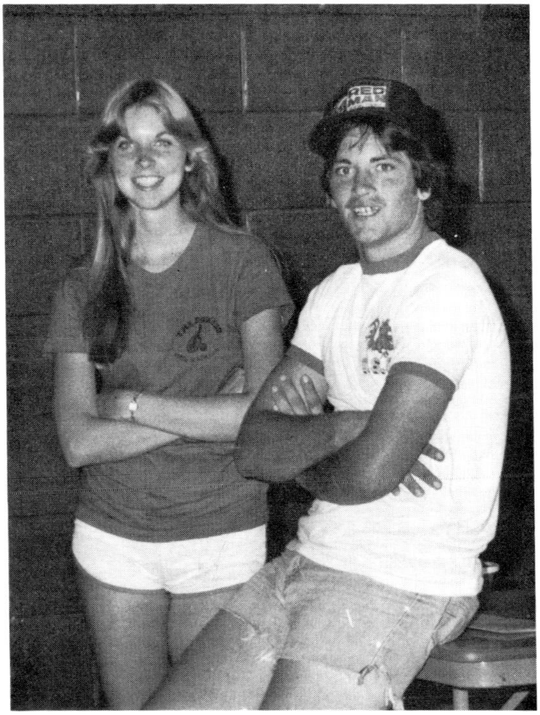

Figure 8–6. *The adolescent can enjoy the company of the opposite sex without romantic involvements.*

to a friend for hours on the telephone, and then meet the friend at a pizza house to continue the conversation. He may experiment with different roles, such as that of the parent, through babysitting, the teacher, by instructing younger children, and spouse, by developing an intense and interdependent heterosexual relationship. He learns or refines such skills as sewing, carpentry, and auto mechanics, which will prove to be valuable throughout life. He continues to enjoy competitive sports, academics, and complex games such as bridge and chess. The adolescent may seem to waste a lot of time in his room daydreaming and listening to popular music, but he needs thinking time to find out who he is and where he is going (Figure 8–7).

COMMON PROBLEMS

Some problems that occur frequently during adolescence are, unfortunately, not minor disturbances that are resolved with a little time and effort. These problems can have a profound emotional and/or physical effect on the teenager for the rest of his life; treatment may be long and expensive, requiring the expertise of a vast health care team, as in the case of drug-related problems. Of course, other problems can be resolved more easily.

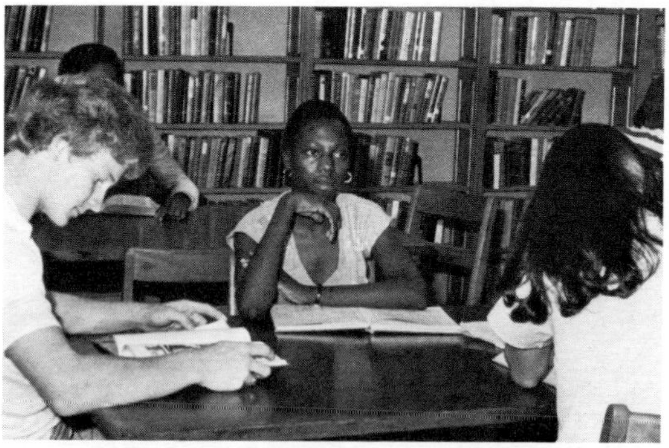

Figure 8–7. *The indecision and ambivalence that are usually a part of adolescence usually lead to daydreaming.*

Acne Vulgaris

Acne vulgaris is a chronic inflammatory skin condition caused by the excessive production of sebum (oil) at the base of the hair follicles, resulting in comedones (blackheads), papules (pimples), pustules (whiteheads), and, in severe cases, cysts deep within the skin layers. Androgen, a hormone that is secreted in increased amounts during puberty and is responsible for the appearance of male secondary sex characteristics, causes the increased oil production in both males and females. Emotional stress seems to exacerbate acne, as do hormonal changes that occur before menstruation. Diet does not usually directly affect oil production in the skin, but occasionally a specific food causes acne in an individual.

Success in the control of acne depends on the adolescent's willingness to follow a prescribed regimen that may be quite involved. Some teenagers begin a program zealously but soon become annoyed with the inconvenience or with side effects, such as peeling of the skin. Parents then blame the adolescent for his acne and often badger him to wash his face and to use the expensive medicine they bought. The teenager often reacts by neglecting his skin even more, frustrating both parents and health professionals.

A good approach to the problem of acne is to place the responsibility squarely on the adolescent. Explain the treatment and its rationale to him, and suggest that the parents not mention acne treatment at all. Only small amounts of medication should be bought for a trial period. If the teenager does not feel that his acne is troublesome enough to warrant treatment, his parents should ignore the fact that his skin looks worse. Many adolescents, however, are so delighted with clearer, healthier skin that they develop a twice-daily routine on their own. A deficient diet may lead to further skin problems, so a well-balanced diet may help the adolescent's appearance.

Acne causes more anguish than any other problem during adolescence. Since most acne responds well to treatment, even the teenager whose problem seems minor should receive the benefit of a prescribed regimen of cleansing and medication. Mild cases of acne can be treated with regular washing of the area with a mild soap and the application of a drying agent. Worse cases may require additional peeling/drying agents and systemic antibiotics to combat infected lesions, topical antibiotics for further protection from bacteria, and corticosteroid preparations to decrease inflammation. Management of severe cases of acne may include all of the treatments mentioned plus the application of dry ice (frozen CO_2) to the area, prescribing oral contraceptives to inhibit androgens, and surgical procedures to correct existing cysts or to smooth pitted skin. (See Table 13–1).

Menstrual Disorders

Common menstrual disorders include irregularity, pain, and excessive or lengthy flow. Irregularity, especially just after menarche, is caused by hormonal interactions that are not yet stabilized. A strenuous exercise regimen can cause extended *amenorrhea* (absence of menstrual periods) as can severe emotional stress and malnutrition. *Dysmenorrhea* (painful menstruation) can result from infection, anatomical anomalies, or physiological disorders, or for no obvious reason. Excessive or lengthy menstrual flow may also be a sign of pathology or of a functional problem. The adolescent girl with menstrual problems (except for irregularity following menache) should receive medical attention to identify pathological conditions; a doctor's care will also provide relief and reassurance that the problem is only a nuisance.

Preparation for a pelvic examination should include a step-by-step explanation of the whole process, using pictures, vaginal speculum, and a hand mirror. Identify the parts of the genitals as the client looks with the mirror. Encourage her to take regular, deep, slow breaths, inhaling through the nose and exhaling through the mouth, to relax her pelvic muscles. During the pelvic exam, remind her frequently to continue her breathing pattern. Holding the teenager's hand is an excellent support technique, but if you are assisting the examiner, this may not be feasible. Although you may feel awkward, talk to the patient, not the examiner, during the examination. The person undergoing a pelvic exam feels very alone if the examiner and assistant converse between themselves at the foot of the examining table.

Pregnancy

Pregnancy carried to delivery creates a physical and emotional crisis for the adolescent girl. Her body is frequently not mature enough to provide an optimal uterine environment or to allow a safe vaginal delivery. The pregnancy may be complicated by eclampsia (a toxemia of pregnancy) and delivery by cesarean section (abdominal incision) may be necessary. Such complications occur more frequently in adolescent pregnancies. The typical adolescent girl's poor nutrition habits and insufficient or erratic sleep pattern compound the health problems of the pregnant teenager, and her emotional status is affected by the fact that the normal need to develop a sense of identity is compounded by the need to cope with the pregnancy, by even greater changes in body image, and by the reactions of peers and family members.

The number of unwed adolescent mothers is increasing as the number of adolescent marriages decreases. The grandparents, especially the grandmother of the new baby, usually share parenting responsibilities with the mother until (or if) she can manage a household alone, or until she marries. This extended family arrangement is much more prevalent in lower-class families in which the unmarried mother frequently opts to keep her child rather than resort to abortion or adoption. She often returns to school to pursue a high school diploma. She is faced with conflicting roles—that of daughter/student and that of mother—that affect her identity development. Pregnancy of the unmarried adolescent still carries the stigma of immorality in much of society, but few barriers hamper educational and employment endeavors. The adolescent father suffers far fewer consequences of the conception, but he may feel guilt or may have to contend with family pressure to marry his partner.

Abortion

Early pregnancies (up to twelve weeks) can be terminated by suction removal of the conceptus, while later pregnancies require induced labor and delivery. Abortion, a highly controversial religious and political issue, is presently available only to people who can afford to pay for the service except in cases of rape or threat to life. No federal funds are available for elective abortions.

The adolescent girl whose pregnancy is aborted often feels guilt, shame, and disappointment. She may have subconsciously allowed herself to become pregnant in hopes of having a baby, who would give her unconditional love. She often wonders what would have happened if she had had the baby, how it would have looked, and so on. An image of an infant may haunt her for years, and she may feel that any misfortune that befalls her later is just punishment for her wrongdoing. The father may also have guilt feelings.

Fred and Fran were inseparable since their early teens. When Fran was sixteen she discovered she was pregnant, and she had an abortion in a clinic. She began to take birth control pills, and they enjoyed frequent sexual intercourse without further fear of pregnancy. They married after college and soon decided to have a baby. They made elaborate plans and arrangements for the baby's arrival. When the baby was born with severe deformities and it was obvious that he would not survive, Fred sobbed as he sat in the "Father's Room." When all the relatives left to get something to eat, he confided in the nurse: "I know this was because we had the abortion. I knew better, but we did it anyway."

Never advise a person or couple to have an abortion. Always discuss the full range of alternatives, giving the pros and cons of each, and let those involved make the decision. If you are strongly biased for or against abortions, you should avoid counseling the pregnant adolescent.

Venereal Disease

Venereal disease (VD) is any disease transmitted through sexual intercourse. Some diseases can be transmitted sexually and otherwise; an example is trichomoniasis, which can be traced to intercourse or to clothes-swapping. A venereal disease can be passed from the genitals to the rectum or mouth, depending on the contact site. Syphilis, gonorrhea, genital herpes, chancroid, granuloma inguinale, and genital warts are transmitted sexually. The incidence of venereal diseases, especially gonorrhea, has risen sharply due to the adolescents' frequently unstable sexual relationships and his fear of seeking professional help. Lack of treatment may result in severe illness requiring hospitalization. Supporting both parents and child may be difficult when they harbor such emotions as fear, anger, hurt, and disgust. Maintaining a nonjudgmental attitude is essential. Venereal disease in the adolescent or younger child may sometimes be traced to incest as a form of child abuse.

Teaching the adolescent about venereal diseases is an important part of health education. The adolescent frequently relates easily to a caring nurse who brings up the topic and gives him permission to talk about his sexual concerns and interests. Take advantage of opportunities to explain how the diseases are transmitted, prevented, recognized (by himself), diagnosed, and treated. Include possible complications in your discussion. Because many states allow adolescents to be treated without their parents' knowledge or permission, you should be aware of laws governing your area.

Drug Abuse

The incidence of adolescent drug use is rising at an alarming rate. The teenager often begins by smoking cigarettes (Figure 8–8). then tries beer, wine, and liquor, progresses to marijuana, and then to other drugs. He may stop at any point on the ladder, but

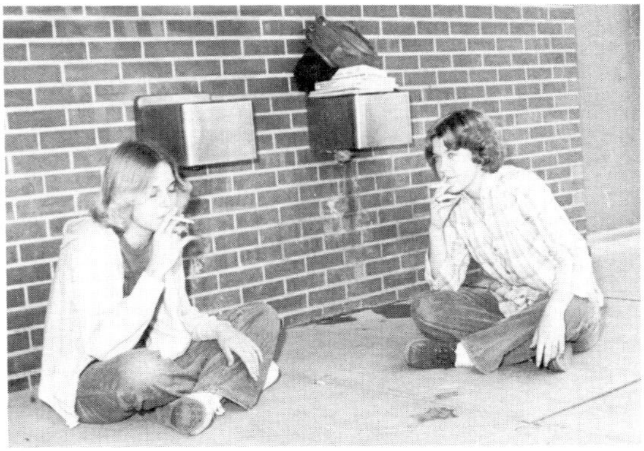

Figure 8–8. *Cigarette smoking is increasingly common among adolescent girls.*

usually tries drugs in this order; almost every teenager tries alcohol and cigarettes before he tries smoking marijuana, and he has usually smoked marijuana before using other drugs. Many factors influence drug use. The adolescent often adopts his parents' habits of consumption, and since the majority of adults in this country drink on occasion, it is no wonder that their offspring do, too. He may consume drugs as a way to rebel against his parents' wishes or to conform to peer expectations. If he cannot form a sense of identity and set life goals, he may use drugs to block out reality. Drug education programs have not decreased the rate of smoking, alcoholism, or other drug abuse; statistics do not usually impress the adolescent who receives satisfaction from drugs.

The treatment of drug addiction may require admission to a residential program or frequent contacts with an outpatient unit for withdrawal, followed by intensive psychotherapy. Parents are usually ineffective in dealing with their child's drug problem, so they, too, will need support and counseling. Sometimes the adolescent is a patient on an acute care unit for another problem when he begins to have withdrawal symptoms.

Louis, aged fifteen, had a compound fracture of the tibia. On the third day after his surgery, he began to pick at imaginary objects on his overhead trapeze. He began to shake a little at first and later shook the whole bed. Although the surgeon knew Louis was under the effects of alcohol when he broke his leg, he had no idea that Louis was experiencing delirium tremens (DT's) from severe, long-term alcoholism. The team of nurses and physicians in the intensive care unit were barely able to save his life. When the crisis had past, he was moved to the adolescent psychiatric unit for treatment of his addiction.

An overdose of drugs may be accidental or suicidal, but it is always an indication that the adolescent needs help (See Ch. 12).

Suicide

Suicide and attempted suicide is an increasing problem in adolescence and it is known to be a leading cause of death among teenagers. The teenager may try to kill himself by running his car into a telephone pole, hanging himself, shooting himself, or overdosing himself with drugs. Attempts, however far from successful, should be viewed seriously as a cry for help, and psychotherapy should be provided (See Ch. 12).

When an adolescent attempts suicide, he frequently experiences shame and guilt. He must face people who "know." Health professionals may have little sympathy for his plight.

Jimmy, aged fifteen was under the influence of several drugs when he showed up at the family practice center. He wanted to change his lifestyle and live without drugs. As the nurse practitioner was trying to locate an agency that would admit him that afternoon to help him withdraw from the drugs immediately, he went outside and cut his wrists just deep enough to bleed a little. The nurse practitioner, who had been on the phone for hours, did not feel sorry for him as she cleaned up the blood on his fingers and wrists. She was exasperated as she thought about how far behind she was and how needless such an act seemed.

You may need help from another nurse or a behavioral specialist to cope with your feelings of frustration and, occasionally, anger. Be sure to allow the adolescent and his parents to discuss their feelings about the attempt. Prepare them for the questions—or total lack of questions—from friends who do not know what to say or do when the adolescent goes home and back to school.

ACCIDENTS

Accidental deaths increase sharply during adolescence, and motor vehicle accidents are responsible for most of the increase. The teenager, especially the boy, is often a reckless driver. Many accidents occur while the driver is under the influence of alcohol and/or drugs; others occur when a teenager attempts to impress his friends with his skill at maneuvering a car or motorcycle at top speed. It seems that the adolescent is actually trying to "outsmart" death as he endangers his life time and time again; in fact, reckless driving may be a form of attempted suicide. Parents can manage the adolescent's driving as they would any other responsibility: if he obeys safety rules, he can continue to drive; if he breaks the rules, he loses his driving privileges. The consequences of unsafe driving can be discussed, but as with drugs, teenagers are not usually impressed with statistics. Driving lessons, which ensure that the adolescent has the necessary skills, and which often entitle the driver to reduced insurance premiums, are recommended for the beginning driver.

Other accidents occur during various athletic endeavors. Contact sports can result in musculeoskeletal and neurological trauma. Such activities as water and snow skiing, swimming, running, or even dancing can cause sprained muscles and broken bones. Occasionally, parents must decide for their adolescent whether or not to continue participation in a sport, or to take time out for recuperation, and this may result in considerable conflict.

SIGNS AND SYMPTOMS OF ILLNESS

The adolescent's reaction to illness is very similar to that of the adult. He has a tired look on his face, and his skin hangs loose when he is dehydrated. He usually will not eat solid foods but may take plenty of fluids if his gastrointestinal tract is not severely disturbed. The very busy teenager may convince himself that he is not ill and continue his activities until he is obviously sick. He may, however, suddenly require more sleep than usual or choose not to participate in a favorite activity. He is, of course, responsible for his own elimination, so he will recognize changes in these habits. His vital signs, approaching adult measurements, respond to many illnesses with increases in temperature, respirations, and pulse.

Body awareness, both internal and external, peaks during adolescence. Minor variations of functioning, such as in bowel movements, or appearance, e.g., acne, can cause undue concern; the teenager may be too embarrassed to discuss the problem with anyone, especially if the problem concerns the genitals. Unfortunately, some health professionals are equally ill at ease when such concerns are voiced, making the teenager's embarrassment seem justified.

Jake, aged fifteen, had had no sex education from his parents or his school teachers. His understanding of intercourse was so jumbled in his mind that he wasn't sure if he'd experienced "it" or not after a petting session with his girlfriend. He noted that some physical activities, such as running and swimming, caused erections and even ejaculations, so he gave up these sports. On a routine visit to his long-time family physician, he summoned enough nerve to ask if these ejaculations were normal. His physician looked away, said "I don't know," and changed the subject. Jake was too embarrassed to pursue the matter any further.

Connie, aged thirteen, developed vulvar itching and irritation during the swimming season. Although her mother was easy to talk to, Connie was afraid she would have to be examined by their male physician if she revealed her problem. When the itching became unbearable, she finally told her mother, who called the physician's office for an appointment. Connie was humiliated when she had to undress for an exam. She later recounted the experience to her best friend, who vowed she would never submit to such an indignity.

Overconcern with the body may lead the adolescent to seek the advice of a health professional when he feels the slightest ache or pain. He may fear cancer if he feels a swollen lymph node in his neck or if he feels tired several days in a row. A simple diagnosis and an explanation of why the sign or symptom occurs usually satisfies the adolescent, but he may return several times before he is convinced he is well.

HOSPITALIZATION

Nursing care of the adolescent should allow him maximum control of his environment and treatments, while maintaining medical and unit requirements. Parents continue to be essential health team members, but they usually expect their child to assume much responsibility for his own decision making, even during hospitalization.

Admission

The adolescent enters the hospital with doubts about how he should act and fears about what will happen to him. If he is admitted to a pediatric unit filled mostly with infants and young children, he probably will feel totally out of place; he may worry that he will be treated as a child. He may come to the hospital with a reputation for being "super cool," mature, and responsible, and he may try to maintain this image even when he is under severe physical or emotional stress. Tell the adolescent that you understand his need to be himself during his hospitalization. Describe such provisions as game rooms, planned activities, telephone and visiting privileges, and freedom to wear his own clothes to reassure him that you are willing to help him continue his activities and relationships as far as possible. Discuss his perception of the reason for his hospitalization, bearing in mind his increased concern for his body. He may have a distorted picture of his problem, but you usually will be able to correct any misunderstandings. If you do not have enough information upon admission to describe what will happen to him, be sure to give him additional information as you receive it.

Parents, also, do not know what is expected of them when their adolescent is hospitalized. They may have an intense need to stay with their child continuously, although he may need to show himself and others that he can do without them. In general, unless the child is seriously ill, his parents should visit daily and stay only a portion of the day. This allows the adolescent patient to establish new friendships with staff members and other patients, to have his friends visit without his parents' presence, and to develop proficiency in his own care. If he is seriously ill, the adolescent may want his parents nearby at all times and then provisions for rooming-in should be made. If the seriously ill adolescent feels hostility because he is totally dependent on his parents, the nurse should take responsibility for most of his care. The decision of whether to have parents room-in must be made on an individual basis and it must be kept in mind that the situation may change during the hospitalization. In any event, continue to keep parents informed of their child's progress.

The adolescent needs to know what he will see, feel, and hear during a procedure, as a person of any age. He can learn what he will experience through discussions, movies, pictures, etc. He can prepare for certain procedures with such exercises as deep breathing, but he probably will be embarrassed or insulted if you offer a dress rehearsal or puppet show. If a procedure will be painful, explain to the adolescent that you will help him be as comfortable as possible. Discuss the fact that teenagers may need to cry when they are in pain, and that you think crying is "OK," but do not overdo the subject; the teenager may think he will be faced with unbearable pain. Assess his need for his parents' presence (or his parents' need to be present) during a procedure before deciding whether they should attend. Parents can be very supportive to their child, but they may also overprotect him.

Jerry, aged eighteen, was scheduled to receive chemotherapy every other Monday morning. First he would undergo a series of blood tests and then wait for the results before the drug would be administered. He became very tense while he waited. He wanted his mother to be near him during the wait and also during the injection of the drugs. This need caused great conflict in Jerry, since he was ashamed to admit that he, a normally self-confident and independent college freshman, required the security and comfort of having his mother nearby. Fortunately, he was able to discuss these feelings with a nurse specialist, who explained that this increased dependency was normal.

Jan, aged fifteen, developed a vaginal discharge while she was in a body cast. Her physician asked her mother, Mrs. S., to step outside while he examined Jan. Mrs. S. seemed very upset, but she finally left the room, apparently to Jan's relief. The nurse talked with Mrs. S. about being sent out of the room and learned that Mrs. S. supervised many of Jan's daily routines at home. She monitored Jan's menstrual periods to make sure "they weren't too long or too heavy," and kept up with the number of pads used each month. The nurse noted on the nursing care plan Jan's need for independence and Mrs. S's need for Jan to remain dependent. Jan went home a few days later without having made any progress toward self-sufficiency.

Illness interrupts the usually busy life of the adolescent. A brief episode in the hospital usually has mild and transient effects on his emotional status, while a long-term or serious illness forces him to reorganize his life. If, as is typical with adolescents, his life lacked direction in the first place, he may have difficulty in setting goals that are compatible with his illness. He may concentrate on going home in time for a special event, such as a tournament game; gently bring him back to reality if you are certain he will not be able to go. Express your sympathy and say that you can imagine how hard it must be to stay in the hospital while life goes on in the outside world.

Dot had had a good first semester in the tenth grade. She began to tire so easily after exams that her mother took her to the family physician. The day before the new semester began, he diagnosed Dot's illness as infectious mononucleosis, but he expressed hope that she could return to school soon. Dot seemed better but her spleen suddenly began to enlarge remarkably; her physician decided that her spleen must be removed, and Dot was hospitalized for surgery. Dot was depressed; the alternate cheerleader took her place on the squad. Her friends talked about the new semester's courses and soon she was too far behind to catch up with them. After her nurse had spent much time talking with and listening to her, Dot one day said, "I can go to summer school and earn two credits. That will allow me to be in the same grade as my friends next year." Her parents agreed to the idea. Dot called her guidance counselor to make the necessary arrangements; from that point on, her convalescence was more interesting.

The adolescent often resists authority, including that of a nurse. Bargain with him and offer compromises whenever possible. If you find yourself telling him what to do, stop for a few minutes to search for a better way to accomplish your goal. If there is a choice, let the teenager decide for himself what he will eat, wear, watch on television, and who may visit him. Give him maximum control over his activities and treatments. Keep schedules flexible so that he will not feel bound to rebel against a rigid routine, and so that he can plan some diversions for himself. If the teenager breaks several rules or manipulates the staff by telling conflicting stories to different staff members or to parents, look for his basic problem. Are the necessary regulations strictly enforced or are staff members inconsistent? Is a specific limit particularly offensive to several patients, and, if so, why? Does the adolescent have any outlets for the frustrations that multiply during hospitalization? Is he bored? Is this usual behavior for him at home and at school? Has anyone asked him what his problem is? Answers to these questions may help to identify the reason for his behavior and guide you in planning more effective care; on the other hand, your efforts may elicit a negative response from the adolescent that will leave you feeling angry and hurt.

Alice, aged sixteen, confided in her nurse that she had been having sexual intercourse with her boyfriend for a year. She had been taking birth control pills since her sixteenth birthday, the legal age for receiving pills without parental permission. Alice complained that her boyfriend wanted to have intercourse several times in one night in the back seat of his car, but that it hurt and she wanted sex only once a night. In the course of a lengthy discussion of sexuality, the nurse suggested that masturbation might relieve the boyfriend's intense sexual urges. Alice asked if masturbation could meet her own needs and the nurse answered, "Possibly." The next day Alice's mother called the physician angrily, complaining that some nurse had told her "daughter to start masturbating." Alice's nurse, only somewhat comforted when the physician explained that Alice pitted her parents against each other in the same manner, vowed that adolescent patients would arrive at their own conclusions about their sex lives in the future.

Seek the advice and support of the health team when you find you are angry with the adolescent; someone else may be more effective in providing care and setting limits on his behavior.

Regression is as much a problem with the hospitalized adolescent as it is with children at other developmental stages. As already mentioned, the teenager may suddenly want his parents with him during a painful procedure or throughout the night. He may begin to question decisions he made earlier. He may rely more on others to direct his activities and treatments. He may cry and/or daydream increasingly. He may be unable to tolerate other patients' mannerisms and habits. Regressive behavior in the adolescent can be confusing to parents and distressing to him. Explain that regression during hospitalization is normal.

When the adolescent is hospitalized, his previous standards for peers and activities usually change, at least temporarily. He is so glad to have compansionship his own age that he hardly cares if his new friend has stylish clothes or participates in organized sports. Almost all teenagers enjoy the same music and television shows, and they all have the same concerns about their identities and futures; just putting two or more in the same room usually results in satisfying interactions. Offer some leadership to groups of adolescents by listening to them and reflecting on what you hear being said. Avoid offering unsolicited advice and opinions; instead, support the group members' own logical conclusions and accurate observations. Plan some activities to allow creativity and productivity when possible. Darts, bumper pool, and pinball games can be played alone or with a partner. Arrange for excursions to the "outside world" to shop or watch a movie when extended hospitalization is required of a teenager who is ambulatory or confined to a wheelchair. The nursing staff must value activities as being therapeutic in order to maintain an effective program.

One half of the pediatric unit was reserved for adolescents. The game room in the corner was stark except for a ping-pong table. The ping-pong ball—the only one—remained in the nurse's station, *locked* in a cabinet because many had been lost in the past. No one ever bothered to ask for the ball; perhaps the patients did not know there was one.

Discharge Planning

As has been said, the adolescent should be encouraged to take maximum responsibility for his problem and its treatments throughout hospitalization, although allowances must be made for periods of increased dependency. The adolescent may be very dependent at first, so that his participation in his own care must be encouraged gradually. If he will require assistance or total care after discharge, his parents must be involved in the procedures early enough for them to perform them confidently. If you feel that the adolescent is struggling for a level of independence that is not possible because of his disorder, refer the family to community counseling services.

Once he returns home, the adolescent must assume his previous role as a family member. Since he was not quite sure of his role before hospitalization, he may have difficulty in meeting family expectations now. He may have enjoyed having had no household chores, watching television late on week nights, and receiving his parents' undivided attention on visits. Parents need to re-establish rules *gradually* during convalescence. The adolescent may require gentle reminders or a frank discussion about the family's need to return to normal.

SUMMARY

The great physical and emotional changes that characterize adolescence give rise to a sense of ambivalence and confusion; fittingly, the adolescent may have no fixed daily routines except for those that pertain to personal hygiene, which takes on a new importance as peer group approval and an interest in the opposite sex become prime concerns. As with the other stages of development, the emotional task of adolescence can be summed up in a pair of opposites, namely, the development of a sense of identity versus one of role diffusion.

Physical growth is marked by the attainment of near-adult size by age eighteen and the appearance of the secondary sex characteristics. Motor development is essentially complete by early adolescence, and the teenager works to refine his motor skills for the rest of the period. The adolescent's eating habits, especially the girl's, tend to be poor.

Common problems of adolescence include acne, menstrual disorders, pregnancy, drug abuse, and suicide. Accidental deaths are even more common than during childhood; motor vehicle accidents account for most of the increase.

The hospitalized adolescent is placed in a dependent role, which he may resist. Nursing care of the adolescent should take the parents into account, but should focus primarily on the adolescent and on encouraging him to assume maximum responsibility for his own care.

Bibliography

Alexander, M.M. and Brown, M.S. *Pediatric Physical Diagnosis for Nurses.* New York, McGraw-Hill, 1974.

Bellack, J.P. Helping a Child Cope with the Stress of Injury. *American Journal of Nursing* 74:1491, 1974.

Bishop, B. A Guide to Assessing Parenting Capabilities, *American Journal of Nursing* 76: 178, 1976.

Blust, L.C. School Nurse Practitioner in a High School. *American Journal of Nursing* 78:1532, 1978.

Brodic, B. Views of Healthy Children Toward Illness. *American Journal of Public Health* 64:1156, 1974.

Brown, J.B. Infant Temperature: A Clue to Child-rearing for Parents and Nurses. *American Journal Maternal-Child Nursing* 2:228, 1977.

Chinn, P.L. *Child Health Maintenance, Concepts in Family-Centered Care,* St. Louis, C.V. Mosby, Co., 1979.

Dansky, K. Assessing Children's Nutrition. *American Journal of Nursing* 77:1610, 1977.

Dowd, E.L., Novak, J.C., Ray, E.J. Releasing the Hospitalized Child from Restraints. *American Journal Maternal-Child Nursing* 2:37, 1977.

Elkin, F. and Handel G. *The Child and Society.* New York, Random House, 1978.

Erickson, M.L. *Assessment and Management of Developmental Changes in Children.* Saint Louis, C.V. Mosby Co., 1976.

Erikson, E.H. *Childhood and Society.* New York, W.W. Norton and Co., 1963.

Farrell, E. and Kierman, B.S. A Positive Approach to Nutrition for Hospitalized Children. *American Journal Maternal-Child Nursing* 2:113, 1977.

Galligan, A.C. Books for the Hospitalized Child. *American Journal of Nursing* 75:2164, 1975.

Grinder, R.E. *Adolescence.* New York, John Wiley & Sons, Inc. 1973.

Haggerty, R.J., Maroney, M.W., Nades, A.S.: Essential Hypertension in Infancy and Childhood, *American Journal of Disabled Child* 92:535, 1956. (Copyright, American Medical Association)

Hardgrove, C. and Rutledge, A. Parenting during Hospitalization, *American Journal of Nursing* 75:836, 1975.

Heagarty, M., Glass, G., King, H. Sex and the Preschool Child. *American Journal of Nursing* 74:1479, 1974.

Iliff, A. and Lee, V.A. Pulse Rate, Respiratory Rate, and Body Temperature of Children between 2 Months and 18 Years. *Child Development* 23:237, 1952.

Inglis, S. The Nocturnal Frustration of Sleep Disturbances. *American Journal Maternal-Child Nursing* 1:280, 1976.

Jelnek, L.J. The Special Needs of the Adolescent with Chronic Illness. *American Journal of Maternal-Child Nursing* 2:57, 1977.

Johnson, J., Kirchoff, K., Endress, P. Easing Children's Fright During Health Care Procedures, *American Journal Maternal-Child Nursing* 1:206, 1976.

Johnson, T.R., Moore, W.M., Jeffries, J.E. (eds). *Children Are Different: Developmental Physiology.* Columbus, Ross Laboratories, 1978.

Johnston, M. et al: Putting More Pep in Parenting. *American Journal of Nursing* 77:994, 1977.

Kempe, C.H., Silver, H.K., O'Brien, D. *Current Pediatric Diagnosis and Treatment.* Los Altos, California, Lange Medical Publications, 1974.

Krause, M.V. and Hunscher, M.A. *Food, Nutrition and Diet Therapy.* Philadelphia, W.B. Saunders Co., 1972.

Lawson, B.A. Chronic Illness in the School-Aged Child: Effects on the Total Family. *The American Journal Maternal-Child Nursing* 2:49, 1977.

Lopez, R.I. *Adolescent Medicine.* New York, Spectrum Publications, 1976.

Lynn, D.B. *The Father: His Role in Child Development.* Belmont, Ca., Wadsworth, 1974.

McCary, J.L. *Human Sexuality.* New York, Van Nostrand Co., 1978.

Mennear, J.H. The Poisoning Emergency. *American Journal of Nursing* 77:842, 1977.

Mills, G.C. Books to Help Children Understand Death. *American Journal of Nursing* 79:129, 1979.

Milne, A.A. The Friend, in *Now We Are Six.* New York, E.P. Dutton, 1926.

Mussen, P.H., Conger, J.J., Kagan, J. *Child Development and Personality.* New York, Harper and Row, 1974.

Muus, R.E. *Adolescent Behavior and Society.* New York, Random House, 1975.

Norbeta, M. Caring for Children with the Help of

Puppets. *American Journal Maternal-Child Nursing* 1:17 1976.

Pearson, G.A. Nutrition in the Middle Years of Childhood. *American Journal Maternal-Child Nursing* 2:376, 1977.

Penlaver, M. Helping the Child Handle his Aggression. *American Journal of Nursing* 73:1554, 1973.

Petrillo, M. and Sanger, S. *Emotional Care of Hospitalized Children.* Philadelphia, J.B. Lippincott Co., 1972.

Piaget, J. and Inhelder, B. *The Psychology of the Child.* New York, Basic Books, Inc., 1969.

Picke, J.C. Tell Me a Story. *American Journal of Nursing* 78:1188, 1978.

Robertson, J. *Young Children in Hospitals.* London, Tanistack Institute of Human Relations, 1958.

Robinson, C.H. and Lawlen, M.R. *Normal and Therapeutic Nutrition.* New York, Macmillan Co., 1977.

Schell, R.E. and Hall, E. *Developmental Psychology Today.* New York, Random House, 1979.

Slattery, J. Dental Health in Children. *American Journal of Nursing* 76: 1159, 1976.

Slattery, J.S. Nutrition for the Normal Healthy Infant. *American Journal Maternal-Child Nursing* 2:105, 1977.

Smart, M.S. and Smart, R.C. *Children.* New York, Macmillan Co., 1977.

Snell, B. and McLellan, C.L. Whetting Hospitalized Preschoolers' Appetities. *American Journal of Nursing* 76:413, 1976.

Southall, C. Family Life and Sex Education. *American Journal of Nursing* 77: 1473, 1977.

Stokan, R.E. The Right Formula for the Right Infant: Making Sense of Infant Nutrition. *American Journal Maternal-Child Nursing* 2:104, 1977.

Stone, L.J. and Church, J. *Childhood and Adolescence.* New York, Random House, 1979.

Torre, C.T. Nutritional Needs of Adolescents. *American Journal Maternal-Child Nursing* 2:118, 1977.

White, B.L. *The First Three Years of Life.* Englewood Cliffs, N.J., Prentice-Hall, 1975.

Zueig, I. A New Way to Get Acquainted with the Hospital: Pediatric Open House for Well Children. *American Journal of Maternal-Child Nursing* 1:217, 1976.

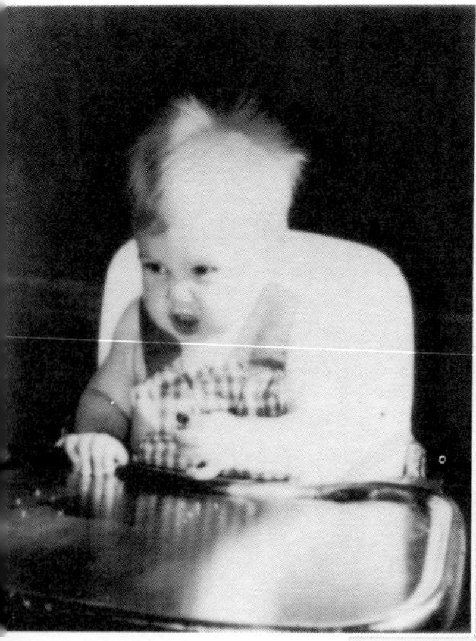

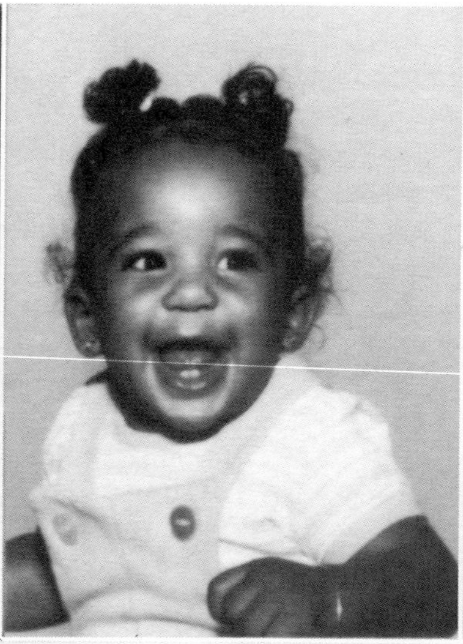

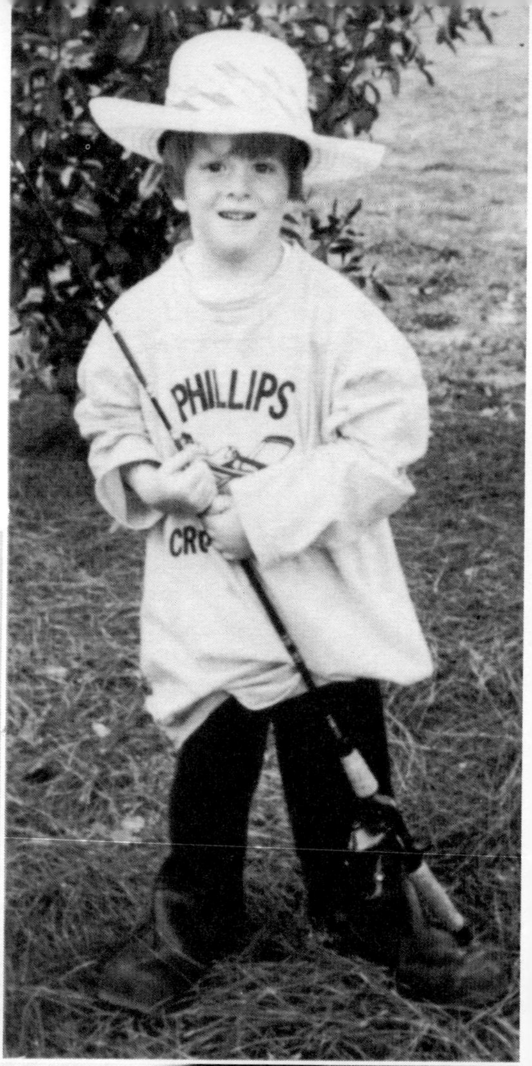
PHILLIPS

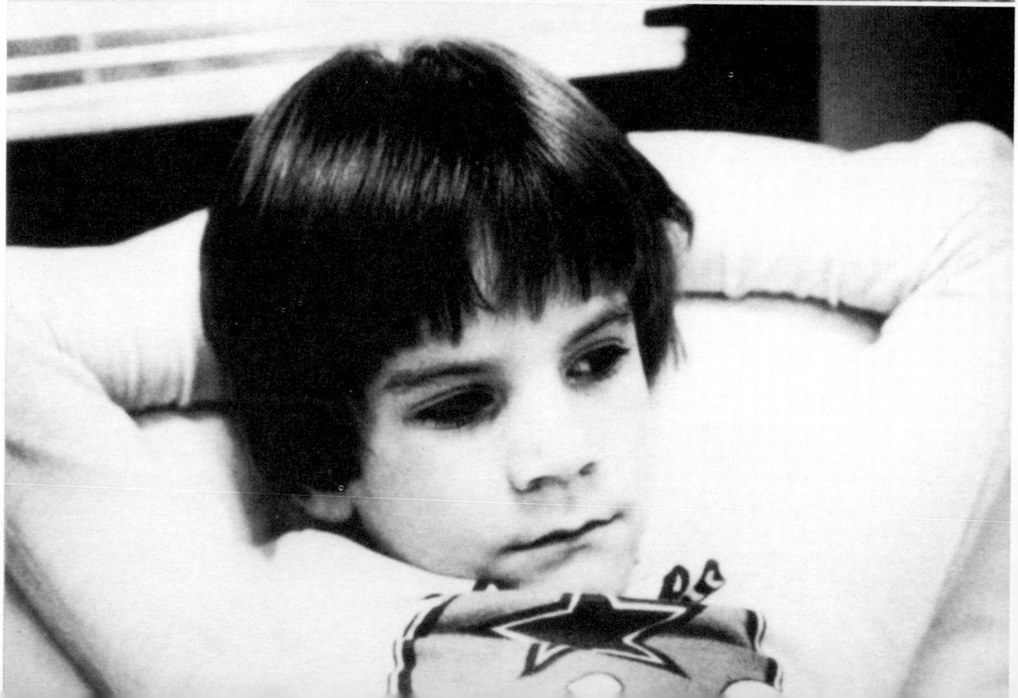

PART III

Child Health Needs

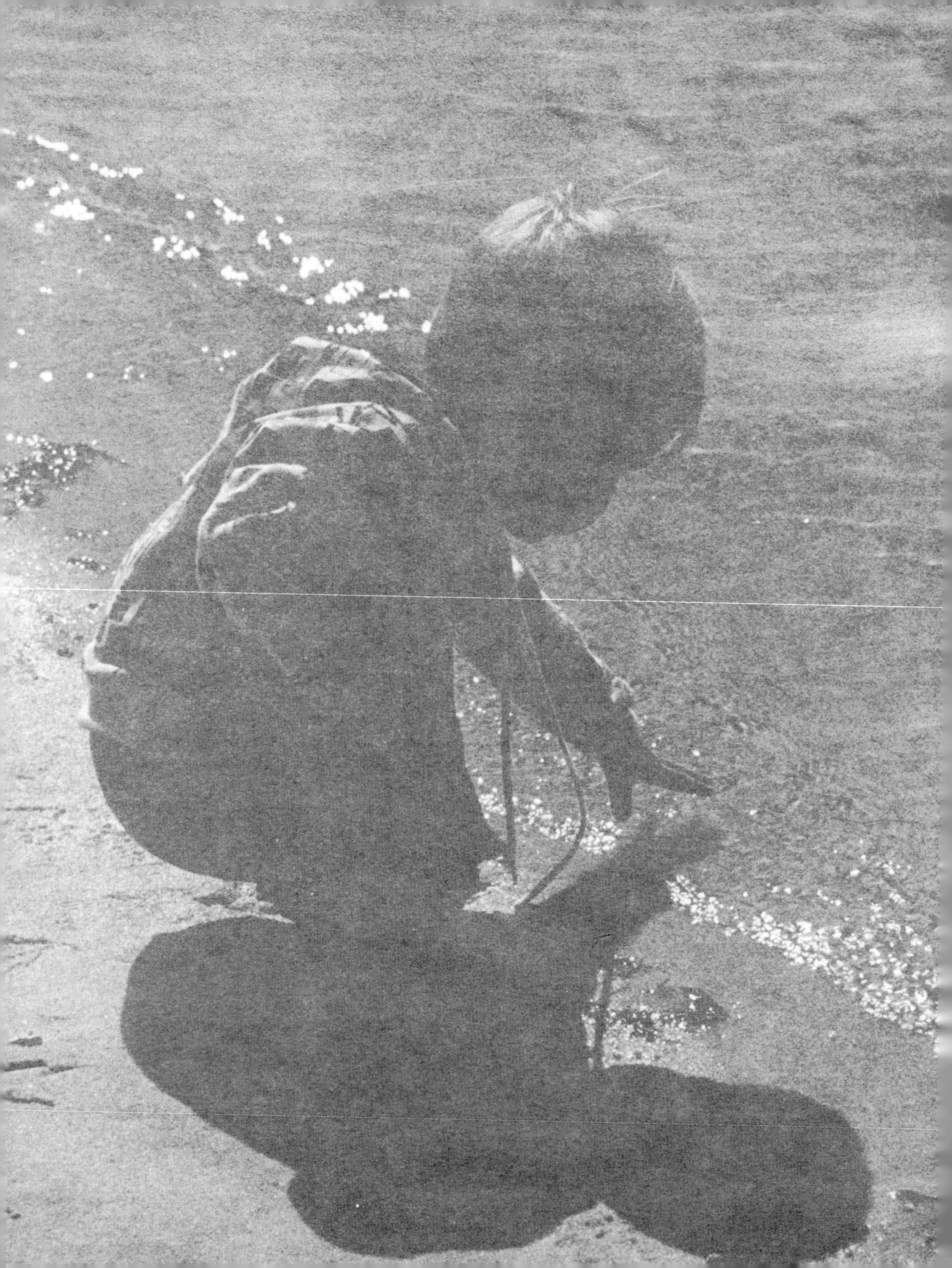

SECTION ONE:

Emotional Integrity

CHAPTER 9

The Child's Self-Concept

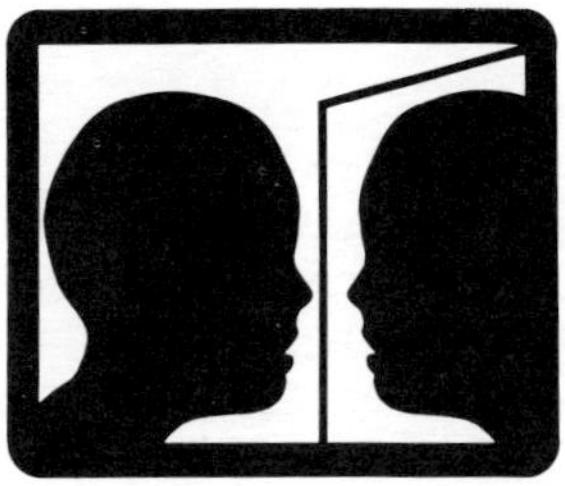

BEHAVIORAL OBJECTIVES

After studying this chapter you will be able to:

- Explain and discuss the meaning of self, self-concept, self-esteem, and body image.
- Identify and discuss the factors that affect a child's self-concept during a hospitalization.
- Assess the emotional integrity of the hospitalized child and construct nursing interventions that will promote coping.

TERMS AND CONCEPTS

Self-concept
Self-esteem
Body image
Self
Emotional integrity

Never static, ever-changing, the developing, maturing child forms a mental picture of himself; the perception a child has of himself constitutes his *self-concept,* or *self-image.* One's self-concept includes *self-esteem,* an evaluation of oneself, and *body image,* an abstract visualization of one's physical functions, characteristics, and limits. Body image is an inner sense of identity that includes one's abilities and limitations. Experiences that influence the body image occur at three levels: *physiological, behavioral,* and *topological.* Physiological responses that affect body functions and, subsequently, body image, include muscle sensations and activity, hormonal secretions, and chemical interactions. Behavioral responses that affect the body image include motor, intellectual, and emotional expressions. The developing motor ability of the infant versus the sophisticated, independent abilities of the school-age child radically affects body image. The intellectually impaired child, unable to understand abstract words, has a different body image from the articulate, conceptualizing child. Topological experiences are those that emanate from the characteristics of the child's body surface. The infant discovers and manipulates the openings and protuberances of his body as part of the process of distinguishing himself from others. As the child develops, he continues to explore such surface aspects as the genitals and skin color, incorporating his perceptions of these characteristics into his self-image. Naturally, any temporary or permanent impairment of the child's ability to perceive his body surface affects his body image.

THE SELF-CONCEPT

The *self* is an integrated whole that consists of body image, self-esteem, and nonphysical or spiritual factors. These elements make up the child's individual, unique concept of himself. The child's self-concept is fluid and continually changing to accommodate additional experiences. The child needs to have a strong, definite perception of himself in order to view others accurately and to test the reality of situations. The strength and resilience of the self hinges on the child's degree of success in mastering the various developmental stages and the accompanying relationships with significant others, especially his parents. If the child develops a healthy sense of identity from an initial trusting relationship with his parents that promotes autonomy and self-assertiveness, the years of learning and accomplishment will culminate in an integrated, adaptive self-concept that can accommodate emotional or physical illness. However, if the child experiences alterations in development (for example, impaired intellectual ability, or motor or sensory deficits) that hinder the experiences that are necessary for mastery of the various developmental stages, he will have difficulty interacting with the environment and will thus develop a weak, vulnerable self-concept. The child's *emotional integrity* depends on the ability, arising from his self-concept, to react adaptively to positive, growth-promoting stimuli or to negative stimuli that inhibit growth (See Table 9–1).

Each hospitalized child is exposed to stimuli that may adversely affect his self-concept. The effect of any illness or dysfunction depends on:

- Developmental age
- Physical appearance and visibility of the dysfunction
- Functional significance of the dysfunction
- Degree and rate of bodily change that accompany the dysfunction
- Previous experience of the child and his family with a dysfunction.
- The parents' and child's perceptions of and responses to the situation.
- Availability of rehabilitation resources

All these factors are interrelated and cannot be considered separately. In order to formulate a nursing plan, the nurse must appraise each factor.

Developmental Age

The assessment of developmental age includes taking a history from the parents of the child's growth and development, ascertaining which developmental skills the child has mastered, and determining his strengths, weaknesses, abilities, and disabilities (refer to Ch. 2). These data should be compared with the normal developmental expectations for the child's age, and a list should be made of the positive and

Table 9–1. **The Changing Self-Concept**

Infant	*Toddler (1–3 years)*	*Preschooler (3–6 years)*	*School Age (6–12 years)*	*Adolescent (12–18 years)*
Does not differentiate self from other persons or objects. Discovers body parts. Develops a trusting relationship with parents and/or other care giver.	Differentiates self from others. Learns motor, language, and social skills for exploration and mastery of environment. Controls body functions (e.g., elimination. Aware of approval or disapproval of significant others.	Identifies and learns sex-role behavior and difference between sexes. Egocentric. The child focuses on himself. Further growth of language, social, motor, and intellectual skills.	Refinement of sex-role behaviors. Enhanced intellectual abilities that are measured against peers. Same-sex peer interactions become more important (e.g., competitive games, secret clubs and codes). Concerned with peer acceptance.	Changes in self-image because of rapid physical growth and sexual maturation. Needs approval of changed physical appearance from peers. Heightened interest in physical appearance (e.g., clothes, hair styles, complexion). Increased interest in opposite-sex interactions. Body is perceived in terms of its physical features (i.e., size, contour, secondary sexual characteristics).

Growth-promoting Interventions	Immediate satisfaction of basic needs (e.g., hunger, sleep, and warmth). Stimulate the senses.	Encourage mastery of body and environment, including opportunities for self-feeding, self-dressing, and self-bathing. Promote development of motor, language, and social skills (e.g., play and peer interactions). Positive approval from significant others.	Provide a positive sex-role model. Permit sexual curiosity. Foster motor, social, language, and intellectual skills. Positive approval from significant others.	Provide opportunities for peer interaction (e.g., games, crafts). Approval from peers.	Positive approval from significant others.
Growth-inhibiting Situations	Lack of consistent care. Basic needs not met. Minimal or no stimulation.	A health problem that prevents body control (e.g., paralysis, blindness, mental retardation). Disapproval of assertive behavior from significant others.	No parental model for sex-role identification. An illness or dysfunction that inhibits or prevents the promotion of motor, language, social, and intellectual skills.	A health problem that decreases peer interaction (e.g., lengthy hospitalization, chronic illness). Disapproval by peers of motor, intellectual, social, or language abilities).	A health problem that alters normal growth and sexual maturation (e.g., a hormonal imbalance). Disapproval of significant others of physical appearance.

negative factors that could affect the child's self-concept. After the child's prehospitalization self-concept has been appraised, it should be used to direct appropriate nursing interventions.

Physical Appearance

The visibility and appearance of a dysfunction depend on which levels of bodily experience are affected. Physiological dysfunctions due to chemical imbalance can cause profound, frequently chronic, physiological changes, but these alterations are not necessarily visible; the child may not look different. Similarly, behavioral changes and intellectual alterations cannot readily be seen, although they become apparent as the child interacts with other persons. On the other hand, topological changes (for example, burns or deformities) are vividly apparent; the child receives many responses from everyone he encounters. At any age, a visible, physical dysfunction or deviation will affect one's interrelationships; a physical deviation may evoke strong responses from others. Children perceive their bodies as others perceive them, and body changes frequently produce uncertainty about the future, impose restrictions on ability, and may lead to rejection. The child who is pitied, secluded, and overprotected will feel humiliated, inhibited, and depressed; his self-image will not be able to integrate experiences normally. When caring for the child, anticipate anger, hostility or regression; remember that each child expresses his feelings differently. Acknowledge his feelings and provide appropriate opportunities for their release. (Chapters 10 to 13 discuss situations that foster appropriate emotional expression.) If the dysfunction of deformity is correctable, give the parents and child accurate, realistic information, and suggest how the child can do things for himself in order to preserve a measure of independence until the disorder is corrected. Thoroughly assess your own reaction to the child's physical appearance. Are you repulsed by it? Do you avoid the child except when treatment is required? If so, look closely at your own experiences and any situations that may explain your feelings. Acknowledge your feelings and identify your reactions, trying to understand their origin; total acceptance of the child and his family is required for a helping relationship.

Functional Significance

A dysfunction acquires functional significance to the extent that the dysfunction interferes with the child's ability to experience and process stimuli and interact with the environment. Temporary or permanent loss of hearing or vision, for example, reduces the child's ability to perceive his environment, to learn, and to integrate experiences into his self-concept. The inability to speak, to feed oneself, or to move affects independence and initiative; the child regresses in his ability to function. With parental assistance, identify the abilities the child still has and encourage their use. For example, if the chilc cannot see, make use of the child's senses of hearing and touch to acquaint him with his environment and with whatever procedures he is to undergo.

Degree of Change

The degree of change in body appearance and the rate at which the change occurs affect the adaptive capacity of the self-concept. Body image deviations that arise from conditions present at birth require the parents and concerned others to adjust. The infant, unaware of his physical deviations, seeks the same basic gratification as any infant. If his physical difference is accepted by his parents and his development is fostered, his body image will develop normally.

Trauma (e.g., burns, lacerations, or fractures), on the other hand, causes sudden, unanticipated changes in body appearance. The toddler and pre-school-age child are egocentric, judging the environment by their own physical appearance. Since the child of this age cannot mentally retrace the steps of an occurrence back to the beginning, he has difficulty imagining a return to his former physical state. Select nursing interventions that will offer tangible proof to the child that he is returning to his former state. For example, use a mirror to show the child his healing skin, x-ray pictures to show new tissue connecting a previously severed bone. Since the young child judges experiences almost exclusively by his perceptions, offer simple, direct explanations about any body image change, and about the equipment and procedures that surround the child. Encourage the child to verbalize and act out his perceptions so that any misconceptions or fears can be identified and corrected with appropriate information. The school-age child or adolescent, who is experiencing *normal* (and rapid) body image change, needs extra reassurance that his burns and fractures will heal and that he will be able to resume his previous activities, if this is true. Peer interactions and opinions decisively affect an older child's self-concept; self-acceptance hinges on peer acceptance. Try to arrange activities that will promote positive peer interactions for the older child.

Prior Experience

The family and child's previous experience with a health problem will determine how anxious they are and the type of stress response. If the child and his family have had several hospitalizations, they will be familiar with the equipment, procedures, and staff. If the child has developed appropriate stress responses to his hospitalization, his self-concept will be affected only minimally. However, if the child is hospitalized unexpectedly he has no repertoire of behaviors to manage his feelings of fright, uncertainty, and pain, his self-concept will be placed under considerable stress as he tries to understand new situations. To initiate a nursing plan, assess the child's and his parents' previous exposure to illness, their feelings, and reactions. How was stress managed in the past? Has the child experienced a recent change in body image? If so, what were his responses? What did he do and say? The child who can use a variety of means to express stress (e.g., crying, talking, playing) will put to use more appropriate and adaptive behaviors than the hospitalized child who has only a few means of expression. Encourage each child and family member to share their fears, anxieties, perceptions, and feelings about the child's alterations in body function. Encourage the parents and staff to focus on the child and not on the dysfunction. (Chapters 10 to 13 discuss this approach and the accompanying nursing interventions.) A child's self-concept and emotional integrity can be strengthened during a stressful event if his adaptive abilities have been assessed and encouraged.

Responses

Each child depends on his parents for safety and security. The young hospitalized child does not comprehend why his parents cannot remove his pain, stop the procedures, and take him home. Parental responses to the child's dysfunction will be echoed by the child: parents who remain calm, composed, and confident in the need for the hospital procedures will convey assurance to the child. With parental help, establish a nursing plan to acknowledge the child's responses (for example, crying, verbal protest, or physical resistance). Inform the child about hospital procedures and arrange acceptable outlets for his expression of pain and fear. Security and trust can be fostered by offering your hand to the child and permitting him to squeeze it as hard as he wants or by giving verbal assurance that crying is permitted. Tell the child in advance exactly what will happen and how the procedure will make him feel. Don't use false analogies when explaining the procedures; an injection does not feel like a pinch or a mosquito bite—it hurts. Be honest in informing the child and his parents of the side effects and desired outcome of medications and procedures. Show confidence in the child by letting him help, either by holding equipment or remaining still. Some children respond well to simple diversions like counting backward from ten or listening to a riddle or rhyme during a procedure. Reassure the child and inform him of the progress being made: "The needle is in and the medicine is entering your body" or "Two stitches are out, so there are three more to remove." These measures will promote an adaptive response to stress.

Rehabilitation

The availability of rehabilitation treatment services determines how much additional stress will be placed on the child and his family. The child who lives far from treatment and rehabilitation services will have to be away from his home, family and community. The separation may be lengthy, perhaps during a critical period of development. Long separations from parents that occur in infancy may permanently stifle personality development. The child whose hospitalization requires that he be separated from his family will experience a greater change in his self-concept than will the child who is hospitalized close to home.

With each hospitalized child, determine whether the dysfunction affects the physiological, behavioral, or topological level of self-image. More than one level may be affected, and then it is important to determine which level is affected most. Ascertain the child's developmental age and the image he has of himself. Evaluate the physical, functional, and rehabilitative significance of the dysfunction. Ask about the child's previous exposure to illness and the family's and child's earlier and present reaction patterns. (Table 9–2). This information will help to identify situations related to the dysfunction that are causing stress and what behaviors the child is using to cope. Select nursing interventions that will support and promote positive coping methods.

SUMMARY

For optimal health, the child must be emotionally integrated. Congenital, environmental, physiological, and behavioral alterations that interfere with or disrupt this integrity will affect the child's self-concept. How the child and his family perceive and integrate a dysfunction will determine whether the occurrence will inhibit or promote growth.

Bibliography

Anthony, J. The Child's Discovery of His Body. *Physical Therapy* 48:1103, 1968.

Table 9–2. Assessing Emotional Integrity During Hospitalization

Child's Name:
Age:
Developmental Age. (Refer to chapter 2 for assessment methods.)
Considering the dysfunction, which level of self-image is primarily affected?
Topologic _____ Behavioral _____ Physiological _____

Functional Significance
What functions previously performed by the child are presently altered or not possible due to the dysfunction?

	Not Altered	Altered (limitations)
Self-feeding	_____	_____
Self-toileting	_____	_____
Self-bathing	_____	_____
Self-dressing	_____	_____
Movement	_____	_____
Speech	_____	_____
Sight	_____	_____
Touch	_____	_____
Smell	_____	_____

Degree and Rate of Dysfunctional Change
Developmental age when change occurred (for example, birth, toddler) _____
How long will change persist? days_____ weeks_____ months_____ years_____
Prognosis for recovery.

Visual Significance
Is dystunction visible? Yes_____ No_____
Is body disfigured? Yes_____ No_____
Comments of child regarding physical appearance.
Comments of family regarding child's physical appearance.
Comments of staff regarding child's physical appearance.

(Continued)

Table 9–2. (Continued)

Child's Responses to Dysfunction and Related Care

Behavioral Responses	*Check Observed Behavior*	*When Does Behavior Occur*—meals, procedures, absence of parents?
Tries to escape		
Turns or pulls away		
Kicks, bites, spits		
Holds body rigid		
Clings to parent		
Looks for parent		
Looks for staff		
Turns away, closes eyes		
Lies quietly, maintains control		
Verbal Responses		
Cries, screams, moans, whimpers		
Protests, pleads, begs		
Bargains		
Expresses anger, pain, fear		
Tries to postpone activities		

Rehabilitation Resources

Will rehabilitation be necessary for restoration of normal function? ____________

Where are rehabilitation resources available? ____________

How far from the child's home are resources? ____________

Bellack, J.P. Helping a Child Cope with the Stress of Injury. *American Journal of Nursing* 74:1491, 1974.

Blaesing, S. and Brockhaus, J. The Development of Body Image in the Child. *Nursing Clinics of North America* 7:597, 1972.

Brown, M.S. Development of Body Image from Preschool through School Age, in Bower, F. (ed). *Normal Development of Body Image.* New York, John Wiley & Sons. Inc., 1977.

Clemmens, R. and Kenny, T. Prevention of Emotional Problems in Childhood: A Philosophy for Child Rearing. *Clinical Pediatrics* 16:122, 1977.

Fagin, C.M. Introductory Comments. in Fagin, C.M. (ed). *Nursing in Child Psychiatry,* ed. 1. St. Louis, C.V. Mosby Co., 1972.

Gelbert, E. Children's Concepts of the Content and Functions of the Human Body. *Genetic Psychology Monograph* 65:293, 1962.

King, C.N. Distortions in Body Image from Infancy to School Age, in Bower, F. (ed). *Distortions in Body Image in Illness and Disability.* New York, John Wiley & Sons, Inc., 1977.

———. Distortions in Body Image from School Age to Adolescence, op. cit.

McCloskey, J. How to Make the Most of Body Image Integrity in Children. *Nursing Clinics of North America* 7:651, 1972.

Roberts, S. *Behavioral Concepts and Nursing Throughout the Life Span.* Englewood Cliffs, N.J. Prentice-Hall, 1978.

Rubin, R. Body Image and Self Esteem. *Nursing Outlook* 16:20, 1968.

Stone, S. Emotional Reactions to Alterations in Body Image. *Journal of Practical Nursing* 26:24, 1976.

Wilson, M. and Cameron, J. Elements of a Psychological Assessment. *American Journal of Nursing* 77:235, 1977.

Zager, R. The Pediatrician and Preventive Child Psychiatry. *Clinical Pediatrics* 14:1161, 1975.

CHAPTER **10**

The Child with a Perceptual Deviation

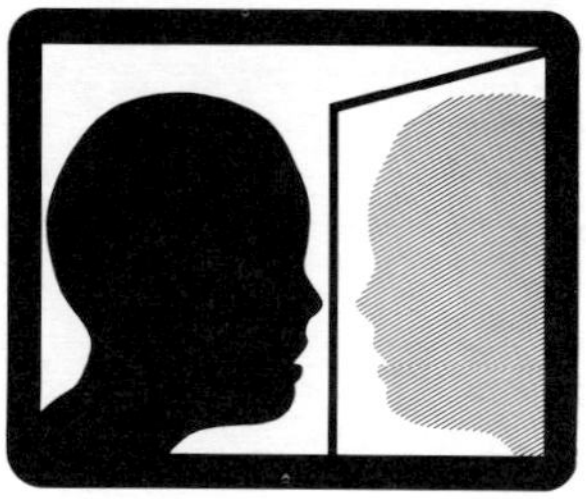

BEHAVIORAL OBJECTIVES

After studying this chapter you will be able to:

- Describe the major parts of the eye and discuss the process of seeing.
- Describe the major parts of the ear and discuss the process of hearing.
- Identify the signs of inadequate stimulus processing.
- Identify and explain two communication methods for the infant, toddler, preschooler, school-age child, and adolescent with an auditory deviation.
- Identify and explain two stimulation methods for the infant, toddler, preschooler, school-age child, and adolescent with a visual deviation.
- List three visual and three auditory assessment methods.
- Discuss the rationale and procedure for use of ophthalmic antimicrobial drugs, eye patches, and hot or cold compresses.

TERMS AND CONCEPTS

Sight
Hearing
Perceptual deviation
Sclera
Cornea
Lacrimal gland
Lacrimal fluid
Iris
Lens
Refraction
Hypometropia
Hypermetropia
Accommodation
Anterior chamber
Posterior chamber
Vitreous body
Retina
Rods and cones
Conjunctiva
Pinna
External auditory canal
Tympanic membrance
Eustachian tube

Malleus, Incus, Stapes
Cochlea
Organ of Corti
Conductive deafness
Sensorineural deafness
Central deafness
Stimulatory deprivation
Stimulatory communication
Ophthalmoscope
Tonometer
Otoscope
Tympanometer

A child learns, discovers, and assimilates information about himself, others, and the environment with his senses, especially *sight* and *hearing*. A change in the child's ability to see or hear, whether a temporary problem during a short period of infection or a lifetime permanent disability, alters his perception of the world. This chapter reviews the basic anatomy and physiology of the eye and ear, common problems of the child with visual or auditory impairment, problems of the family, usual diagnostic procedures, and treatment. Specific auditory and visual conditions are listed in Tables 10–1 and 10–2, together with definitions, means of treatment, and nursing considerations.

THE EYE AND VISION

One inch in diameter, the human eye (Figures 10–1 and 10–2) is formed by several layers of tissue enclosing a fluid-filled center. The outer layer consists of the *sclera,* the white of the eye, and the *cornea.* The sclera and cornea are strong and resistant to stretching and tearing, yet are flexible and resilient. The transparent cornea transmits light to the interior of the eye. The cornea is kept continually moist by the production of tears by the *lacrimal gland.* If allowed to dry, the cornea would lose its transparency and could scar.

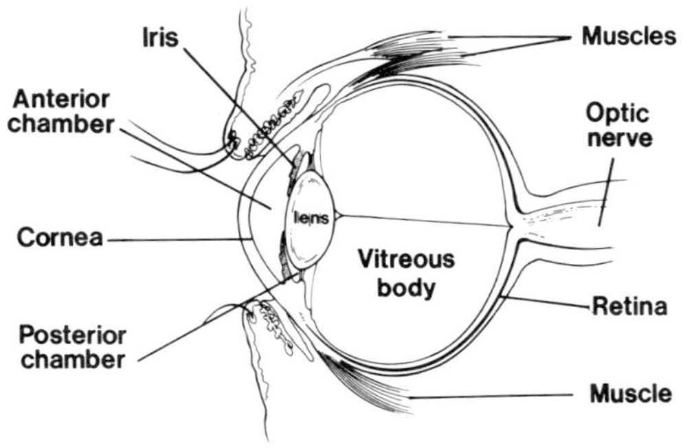

Figure 10–1. *The Eye:Lateral View.*

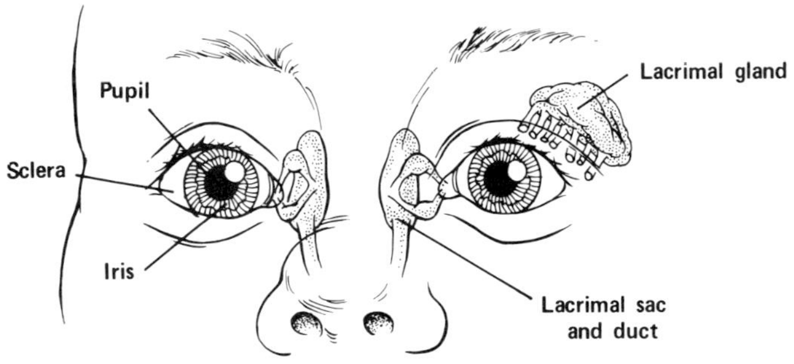

Figure 10–2. *The Eye:Anterior View.*

The middle eye layer is composed of the *iris, lens, muscles,* and *ligaments.* The iris is the contractible, circular diaphragm that one refers to in describing the color of a person's eye. It contains a circular opening, the *pupil,* in its center. Two muscles in the iris change the size of the pupil to control the amount of light that enters the eye. The pupil dilates in the dark and constricts in bright light. Behind the iris is the lens, a transparent structure that is encased in an elastic capsule. Ligaments suspend the lens behind the pupil. The lens focuses light on the retina by refraction. *Refraction* is the bending of light, which is necessary for focusing images on the *retina,* the seeing portion of the eye. The refractory ability of the lens depends on its curvature and the density of the structures within the eye that the light rays must pass through before striking the lens. If the eyeball is too long for the focusing power of the lens, vision is blurred, a condition called *hypometropia* (nearsightedness). The opposite condition, in which the eyeball is too short for the focusing power of the lens, is called *hypermetropia* (farsightedness). Images are focused through the combined effort of the lens, eyeball movement, and constriction of the pupil. The process of focusing is termed *accommodation*.

The components of the eye form three chambers. The *anterior chamber* (which lies between the iris and cornea) and the *posterior chamber* (which lies between the iris and lens) are filled with a watery nutrient solution. The space behind the lens is filled with a gelatinous fluid called the *vitreous* body. The innermost layer of the eye is the *retina*; it contains light-sensitive visual receptors, the *rods* and *cones*. The rods, which are receptors of low-intensity light, enable one to see at night. The cones, which are receptors of high-intensity light, enable one to see in daylight and to see colors. Visual perception occurs when an image is formed on the retina, stimulating the rods and cones. This formation of an image is accomplished by the combined processes of refraction, accommodation, and constriction of the pupil. The visual messages of the retina leaves the eyeball via the optic nerve and are processed in the visual areas of the cerebral cortex.

The eye is suspended in its bony cavity, the orbit, by muscles, ligaments, vessels, nerves, and cushion of fat. Six muscles act to aim both eyes at exactly the same point. A muscular imbalance can cause *strabismus,* which results in a deviation of the eye, such as "cross-eye."

The eyelids are flexible, protective coverings that spread tears over the eye when the lids are blinked. Secretions from small sebaceous glands along the margins of the lid prevent tears from overflowing onto the skin. An infection of one of these glands is called a *hordeolum* (sty).

The *conjunctiva* is a delicate membrane that lines the back surface of the eyelid and the front surface of the eyeball (except for the cornea). An infection of the conjunctiva is termed *conjunctivitis* (pinkeye).

Lacrimation (tearing), discharge, and pain are common responses to an eye insult. Tearing, usually due to an obstruction of the nasolacrimal duct (which extends from the lacrimal sac into the nose), may also be associated with inflammation, allergy, viral disease, and glaucoma. Purulent optic discharge is usually the result of a bacterial infection; mucoid discharge usually indicates a viral, allergic, or chemical irritation. Pain may be due to eye injury, infection, or disease. Refractive errors may produce headaches.

THE EAR AND HEARING

The ear (Figure 10–3) is divided into three parts: the *outer, middle,* and *inner* ear. The *pinna* and *external auditory canal* comprise the outer ear. The external auditory canal is lubricated and protected by cerumen, a brown secretion that is commonly called "ear wax." If cerumen accumulates, sound can be blocked from entering the ear. The outer ear gathers and transmits sound to the middle ear, which consists of the *tympanic cavity* and *eustachian tube.* The eustachian tube connects the middle ear to the throat, permitting secretions to drain from the middle ear to the throat. This is fre-

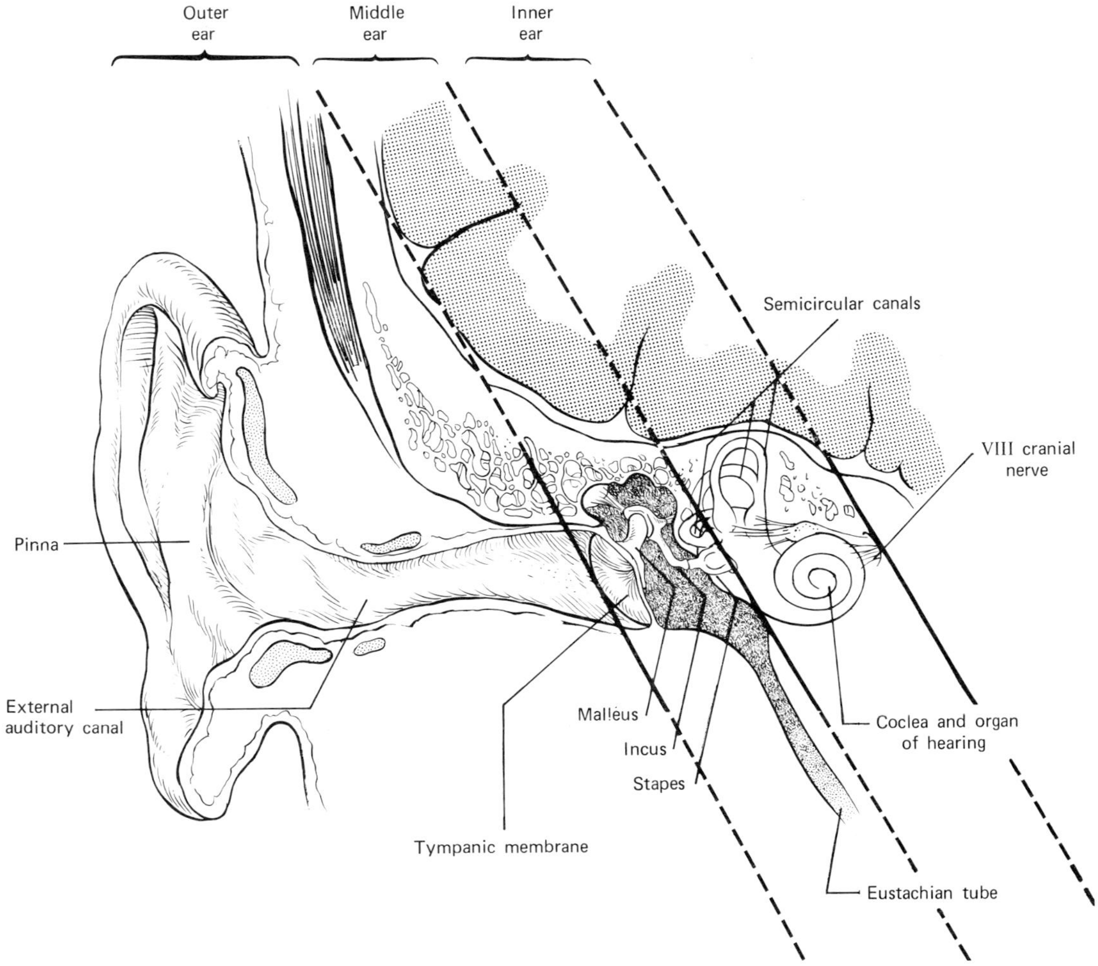

Figure 10–3. *The Ear:Lateral View.*

quently the route by which throat infections reach the middle ear. The function of the eustachian tube is to equalize air pressure on both sides of the eardrum, thereby preventing rupture. Three small bones, the *malleus, incus,* and *stapes,* which lie in the tympanic cavity, transmit vibrations of the eardrum to the *cochlea* and increase the force of eardrum movements; this increase in force is necessary because the organ of hearing, the *organ of Corti,* floats in the fluid of the cochlea and it takes more force to cause a structure to vibrate in fluid than in air.

The inner ear contains the cochlea, the organ of Corti, and *semicircular canals* that assist in maintaining balance. The organ of Corti lies inside the cochlea, a coiled, snail-shell-shaped structure that wraps around a central core bone. The organ of Corti contains hair cells that can convert movement into electrical impulses. These electrical impulses are conducted from the cochlea by the eighth cranial nerve to the auditory center in the temporal lobe of the cerebrum.

Hearing Deficits

Hearing deficits are classified as *conductive, sensorineural,* or *central.* If the sound does not reach the hair cells of the cochlea, because of problems in the external and/or middle ear, the child has a conductive hearing loss. Conductive hearing defects may be acquired or congenital. Examples include the absence of a malleus, incus, stapes, or tympanic membrane, or closure of the external canal. Most acquired conductive hearing defects result from the accumulation of fluid in the middle ear. The fluid which results from an infection, can be removed surgically or medically. In conductive deficits, the loudness is reduced but the clarity of sound remains the same; mild conductive losses often remain undetected.

Sensorineural hearing loss can be hereditary, congenital, or acquired. Half of all cases of congenital hearing loss are genetic, considered to be a recessive trait. Premature birth, hypoxia at birth, birth trauma, and maternal rubella may cause congenital sensorineural hearing loss. Acquired problems include trauma, the use of ototoxic drugs (drugs that cause damage to the eighth cranial nerve), noise exposure, and acute infections. Certain diseases (for example, mumps and meningitis) can cause an almost total and permanent hearing loss. Sensorineural hearing defects generally cause a greater handicap than do conducive losses because they can be corrected only rarely.

A third type of deficit, which is attributed to cerebral impairment, is termed a central hearing loss; like conductive and sensorineural deficits, central loss may be either congenital or acquired. Deafness, the inability to hear, occurs in 1 of every 1,000 births in the U.S. Twenty-five of every 1,000 children are born with a moderate to severe hearing loss. Detection, diagnosis, and rehabilitation measures should be undertaken early because hearing loss is directly related to delayed speech development.

COMMON PROBLEMS AND NURSING INTERVENTIONS

The following discussion applies to children with a severe, usually permanent, visual or auditory deficit.

Stimulatory Deprivation

A child's growth and development will lag if his means of communicating are impaired. The cooing, laughter, smiling, and eye movement that parents and siblings depend on for reinforcement and reward of verbal interactions are altered or nonexistent if a child has severe visual or hearing impairment. Without vocal and facial responses from the child, parents, siblings, and staff may become frustrated, turn away, and decrease their interactive efforts. Deprived of essential stimulation and communication, the child may seek bodily stimulation by rolling, rocking, head banging, swaying, and thrusting his fingers into his eyes and ears.

Stimulatory Communication

Using parental suggestions and guidance, develop a plan for communicating with the child while providing stimulation. Hold the child close to your body, talk, and place the child's hands on your face. The child will identify you as a source of communication.

Give the child tactile and motor signs for activities. If the child cannot rely on sight or hearing in order to understand daily care activities, offer consistent cues. For example, lay your hand gently on the child's back for a few seconds before picking him up. Put the child's hand in water before beginning the bath. Pull on the diaper two or three times before each change. Tap his hand several times before holding it for safety, a walk, or procedures. Patting the child's back several times can signal that you are departing. Offering consistent cues will enable the child to become familiar with the hospital environment, know what to expect, and to reduce his anxiety and fear. If cues have been used at home, incorporate them into your nursing care, if not, develop a plan and post it on a card file, door, or bedboard.

Observe the child's visual ability and capitalize on it. Does the child consistently turn his head in one direction, indicating that he sees better in that direction? Place the crib or bed next to the window for maximum light exposure. Hang shiny, light-reflective mobiles made from pie plates and foil-covered objects. Provide the child with large, colorful, moving, noisy toys such as music balls, drums, trucks, and dolls. When placing the visually impaired child on a pallet or in the playpen, scatter the toys so that the child will touch them as he rolls, creeps, and stretches. When communicating with the child who has a hearing deficit, draw attention to your face by raising an arm or hand. Do not touch the child first because this may startle him and does not encourage him to develop the habit of watching someone with whom he is attempting to communicate. Stand with the light on your face, look directly at the child, and speak normally and distinctly, avoiding mannerisms or gestures that could make lip reading more difficult. Avoid one word answers (except "yes" or "no"). Try not to show annoyance or frustration in your facial expressions because the child with a hearing deficit depends on visual cues for acceptance. Smile and speak each time the child looks at you. A simple "hello" will convey to the child that language is worth "watching" for.

Movement and locomotion are also frequently delayed in the perceptually impaired child. Frequent holding, cuddling, and stroking should be associated with activities that the child will view positively rather than in connection with the discomfort of procedures. Hold the child in your lap, play pat-a-cake, touch, stroke, and handle him in different positions in order to minimize his reluctance to be touched and to develop motor balance and coordination. Use an infant seat, swing, high chair, playpen, and floor pallet in order to change the child's position and facilitate interactions. Using parental opinions and help,formulate a stimulation plan with definite times and activities. Inform the staff about the plan and post it on the door, at the nursing station, or at the bedside or other appropriate place accessible to all personnel. If the child is beginning to walk, hold his hand and support him from behind. The child with a perceptual deviation cannot hear a reassuring, encouraging voice or see an enticing smile, so it is important to offer security and reassurance with a firm supportive hold using strokes and pats for encouragement.

Additional signs resulting from inadequate processing of stimuli are disturbed sleep-wake schedules and decreased nutritional intake. The child with a dysfunction may resist going to sleep at bedtime, wake up for extended periods during the night, and have difficulty establishing a sleep pattern in the hospital. Incorporating previously established home routines, devise a consistent wake-sleep schedule by setting a time for naps and bedtime. Provide sufficient physical activity so that the child will become tired, limit social interaction once the child is in bed, and require the child to stay in bed even if not asleep during the prescribed sleep period.

Frequently, the child with a permanent hearing or sight impediment is below normal height and weight for his age. Strive for a positive feeding experience by being patient, persistent, and consistent at meal time. Show the parents how to touch food to the child's mouth, allowing him to smell and touch the food. Put the cup of milk or juice to his mouth with some of it on the rim. Try to avoid procedures or any kind of stress for 30 minutes before and after meals. Eating with others and social interaction can provide an additional incentive to eat more. Emphasize this point to the parents, offering your participation and support during the child's hospitalization.

Another problem the child with a perceptual deviation has is a distorted body image and self-concept. (Review Ch. 9 on the effect of perceptual deviation on self-concept.)

The perceptually impaired child is also likely to experience an altered parent-child bond. The parents of a child whose vision or hearing is impaired do not receive the familiar response cues from the child. The child may not speak, may remain emotionally immature, and may not attain certain achievements at the usual age. The child may be infantile in his impulse control and ability to understand. His behavior may be erratic, with sudden, unpredicted outbursts of unintelligible sounds or inappropriate behavior. Parents wonder if it is fair to punish the child, not knowing what of if he understands; help the parents to make a distinction between punishment and discipline. The purpose of discipline is to teach the child socially accepted behavior, and this is essential for his development. Be gentle but firm and consistent with discipline; behavior that is not appropriate for a hearing or seeing child is not appropriate for a handicapped child. The lack of stimuli produces many frustrations, which lead to anxiety that finally culminates in anger. Frustration and anger are normal; on the unit as well as in the home, there should be appropriate channels for the child's anger, such as pounding-boards, blocks, and finger paints. Encourage the child to verbalize his anger if possible. Punishment is appropriate but must not be a positive reinforcer. For example, if the child tends to isolate himself, then isolation should not be used as punishment.

COMMON DIAGNOSTIC PROCEDURES

The Eye Examination

Eye inspection includes external and internal observation. In an external examination, the size and position, as well as any growths, discharges or inflammation of the eyeballs and lids are noted. Muscle balance and alignment can also be observed. An *ophthalmoscope* is used for internal inspection of the fluid chambers, retina, cornea, and lens. The *tonometer* is used to measure intraocular pressure. The device, which is hand-held, is equipped with a plate that is placed on the anesthetized cornea. The procedure (tonometry) is simple and painless.

Visual acuity is measured with either the Snellen test or the E chart. Both tests evaluate the ability to see at a given distance; the Snellen test is given to children who recognize the letters of the alphabet, and the E chart is used with younger children. The chart shows a capital "E" in different positions; the child is asked to point in the direction of the normally horizontal lines of the letter.

The test for color blindness is simple and should be done before the child enters school. The child is shown a series of multicolored designs; a person with color vision will be able to see numerals hidden within the designs, but the numerals are invisible to a person with red-green or yellow-blue color blindness. The test is especially important for boys because color blindness is a sex-linked recessive disorder that occurs more frequently in males.

The Ear Examination

The external ear and tympanic membrane are examined with an *otoscope*, a speculum that is inserted one-quarter to one-half inch into the ear canal. The Rinne and Weber tests use a tuning fork to determine how effectively the bones conduct sound. For the Rinne test, the stem of a vibrating tuning fork is placed against the child's mastoid bone; when the child says he can no longer hear the sound, the examiner moves the fork, without striking it again, closer to the ear canal, and asks if the sound can be heard and for how long. Normally, the child will still be able to hear the sound when the tuning fork is held in front of the ear canal, since air conduction is more efficient than bone conduction. For the Weber test, the tuning fork is placed against the center of the child's forehead and the child is asked where he hears the sound; it should be heard with equal acuity in both ears.

Close observation of the child's behavior enables one to distinguish a conductive from a sensorineural hearing loss. The child with a conductive deficit fails to respond to soft voices. His speech and language development are delayed, although his articulation is normal. The child with a sensorineural hearing loss fails to respond to any kind of sound.

The *audiometer*, which produces sounds that are heard through earphones, tests the child's ability to respond to sounds of different intensity (loudness, which is measured in decibels) and frequency (pitch, which is measured in hertz units); the results of the test are recorded on an audiogram. For a screening test, the audiometer is set at 25 decibels (dB) and from 500 to 6,000 hertz (Hz).

Tympanometry is an objective assessment of middle ear function. It is a quick, efficient, and easily tolerated procedure for assessing both the presence of fluid in the middle ear and eustachian tube function. The *tympanometer* is a hand-held automatic probe fitted with a soft rubber cuff that is pressed into the external auditory canal. Middle ear pressure, mobility, and any perforation of the tympanic membrane can all be assessed in less than 30 seconds for each ear. The typanometer also evaluates the improvement of *otitis media* (inflammation of the middle ear) and the patency of tubes placed in the middle ear for drainage.

Careful restraining of the child may be necessary for parts of the eye or ear exam. A sheet wrapped snugly around the child encasing all his extremities is called a mummy restraint. Another restraint method is to lay the child on an examining table, raise his arms above his head, and hold them firmly against the side of his head. A second person may be needed to secure the child's body and legs.

COMMON TREATMENTS AND NURSING IMPLICATIONS

Numerous surgical interventions exist for children with visual or auditory impairments. (The student is referred to chapter 2 for general information on preparing the child for a surgical procedure and postoperative care.)

Eye Surgery

Special nursing considerations before eye surgery include preparing the child for decreased vision, the use of patches and restraints, and comfort measures. Show eye patches to the child, placing a patch on a doll. Have the child apply a patch to a doll, yourself, or a parent, and then allow him to patch his eye. Discuss the pressure that patches produce. Promote security by having a favorite toy at the bedside when the child awakes from surgery, place the call bell within easy reach, and reassure the child that the patches are temporary.

Eye pads are used to absorb secretions of blood, provide comfort by preventing excessive eye motion, and decrease swelling; they are usually worn after eye surgery. To apply an eye pad, have the child close both eyes (it is difficult to close only one eye), gently place a pad on his eye without touching the eyeball, and place two pieces of paper or plastic tape across the pad diagonally from center forehead to center cheek.

Restraints may have to be used with a young child after surgery to keep the eye pads in place. Introduce the restraints to the child as one way of helping him to remember not to pull at his bandages. Talk about his eyes as being fixed, made better, or helped. Never use words like *cut* or *slice* to explain surgery. Show the child a picture of an eye and explain that the doctor uses tiny tools to fix the eye. Emphasize that the eye stays in its place; children commonly hold the misconception that the eye is taken out of the socket for an operation. Children are frequently burdened with guilt, feeling that eye surgery is punishment for watching television or for not eating their carrots. The use of illustrated material, audiovisuals, and play involving simulated procedures can correct misconceptions that may be worrying the child. Evaluate your teaching session by asking the child afterward to explain what he has learned.

An artificial eye is necessary if the eye must be extracted for certain ocular conditions. For example, a sudden trauma may require extraction. In this case, the family will be in a state of shock, needing support and understanding. Ocular prostheses are made of plastic or glass. Specific instructions for care vary according to the institution and physician. Cleansing the prosthesis includes washing it with soap and warm water. Alcohol and very hot or cold water should not be used. The plastic prosthesis should be stored in a container of tap water, while the glass prosthesis should be dried and stored in its case. Normal saline irrigations are done before the prosthesis is inserted. Sterile disposable tissue should be kept handy for wiping the accumulated watery discharge from the eye socket.

Ear Surgery

Common surgical interventions for hearing deficits include the tympanoplasty, myringotomy, mastoidectomy, and insertion of tympanostomy tubes. The *tympanoplasty* is not a single operation but a group of operations that are designed to improve the hearing of a child with a middle ear or conductive hearing loss. This procedure may be required because of perforation of the tympanic membrane, necrosis of the middle ear bones, congenital absence of middle ear bones, or trauma and dislocation of auditory bones.

Myringotomy is an incision into the tympanic membrane in order to remove pus due to middle ear infection. If pus remains in the middle ear, bone necrosis and eardrum rupture are possible. The child is given a local or general anesthetic for the procedure. Fortunately, this operation is seldom necessary if antimicrobial drugs are initiated and maintained for the prescribed period.

Tympanostomy tubes, commonly called polyethylene (PE) tubes, are inserted to allow drainage of middle ear fluid and to provide a source of air. The tubes are inserted into a myringotomy site.

Mastoidectomy is an incision behind the ear to remove diseased bone that results from acute mastoiditis.

Adenoidectomy is the removal of enlarged adenoid tissue that obstructs the eustachian tube opening and thus interferes with adequate ventilation of the middle ear and drainage of secretions.

Medications and Comfort Measures for the Eye

Medications for the eyes usually include antimicrobial drugs and/or ointments. *Steroids* are used for their anti-inflammatory effect. To ease examining the eye and during eye surgery, *mydriatics* (drugs that dilate the pupil) and *cycloplegics* (drugs that paralyze the muscles used for close vision) are used. The home use of eye patches and/or eye exercises may be prescribed, especially for strabismus. When exercises are ordered, written instructions with a suggested schedule that fits in with the family's life is helpful to both the child and family. Eye exercises can become boring and a chore for both child and parent. The use of a card that notes the date and depicts a star or smiling face for each exercise completed helps to motivate the child. Siblings and neighbors can learn the exercise regime in order to assist parents.

To hasten the formation of a head on a sty, or to soften crusted matter, hot compresses may be ordered. Use a washcloth wrung out in hot water and allow the cloth to remain over the eye until cool; repeat for 15 minutes. After the matter has softened, gently wipe the exudate away. Although cold compresses are not used in treating infections, they help to relieve itching, irritation, swelling, fatigue, or pain. Prepare cold compresses in the same manner as hot compresses, substituting ice water for hot water. The use of an ice bag, or ice wrapped in a washcloth, is helpful for reducing edema following strabismus surgery or for lid bruises; however, ice should not be applied directly to the lid. Remember that the eye does not need washing or irrigation except after a chemical burn.

Medications and Comfort Measures for the Ear

Common regimens for ear disorders include the use of systemic antimicrobial drugs for 10 to 14 days to eliminate ear infection and restore eustachian tube function. Decongestants may be used to improve tubal drainage and ventilation. Analgesics are administered for pain and general discomfort. Prophylactic antimicrobial drugs may be used for children with recurrent otitis media.

If secretions of ear wax are plugging the ear canal, cerumen removal may be ordered. The standard syringe flushing of ear wax is being replaced by irrigations with a dental irrigator (such as a Water Pik) in some institutions. The irrigator emits a fine stream, allowing space for the return of water and cerumen; it is especially well-suited for the tiny ear canal of a child. Children are often familiar with a dental irrigator; if an irrigator is ordered for removal of cerumen, prepare the child by allowing him to see, touch, and operate the machine. Use a towel to drape the child and hold a kidney-shaped basin below the ear to collect water and cerumen. It is important to use warm water because cold water can cause vertigo (dizziness). The pressure of the water jet should be set at its lowest point and increased as needed. Stop when the canal is clear. Insert cotton to dry the canal and remove it promptly. If a syringe is used, the principles of explanation, draping, and procedure remain the same.

Hearing aids are frequently prescribed and are available in a variety of styles and strengths. The hearing aid helps the child to use his residual hearing, to discriminate among different sounds, and to acquire language; it does not restore normal hearing. Parents need instruction on replacement of batteries, cords, and receivers. The child must be encouraged to care for the equipment as soon as he is able. Hearing aids are expensive and need to be kept dry at all times, however, they should not be stored on or near a heat source. For daily use, be sure the hearing aid is turned on and the volume control is set correctly. It is important to keep the child's ear clean by removing visible dirt in the outer ear with an applicator and alcohol. A light film of petroleum jelly may be used to grease the exterior of the ear, thereby making insertion of the ear mound of the hearing aid easier. The ear mold, which delivers sound directly into the ear, should be kept clean and dry. It may be washed with soap and water, dried thoroughly (a pipe cleaner is suitable for this purpose), and snaped back onto the receiver. Do not use alcohol to clean the ear mold. Whistling, the most common malfunction of the hearing device, is heard when the hearing aid is turned on but the ear mound is not making a tight seal in the ear. Hair tucked under the ear mold will prevent a tight fit. Is the ear or ear mold dirty? Check for proper fit because ear molds can be outgrown like clothes. Take the ear mold out of the ear and reinsert it. If the hearing aid will not operate, check the batteries. If the batteries are dead, insert new ones with the plus and minus signs matching. Finally, check the microphone of a malfunctioning hearing aid. Has spilled food clogged the tiny openings? If so, wipe the food off with a cloth. Dampness from spilled fluid can ruin a hearing aid. Do not poke the hearing aid with a pin because the delicate machinery may be hurt. It is preferable to consult the manufacturer.

Lastly, educational rehabilitation is recommended for the child with a visual and/or hearing deficit. Special textbooks and sight-saving classes are available to the visually impaired child. Auditory training enhances the deaf child's ability to discriminate among similar speech sounds. Speech training, lip reading, and sign language form part of a total communication program designed to maximize the child's potential. Information about special camps, parent groups, and educational programs can be of great help to the child with a *perceptual deviation* and his family.

There are many misconceptions about the care and treatment of the eyes. Factual information can help to eliminate fear and reduce anxiety. Some common misconceptions are depicted in Figures 10–4 through 10–8.

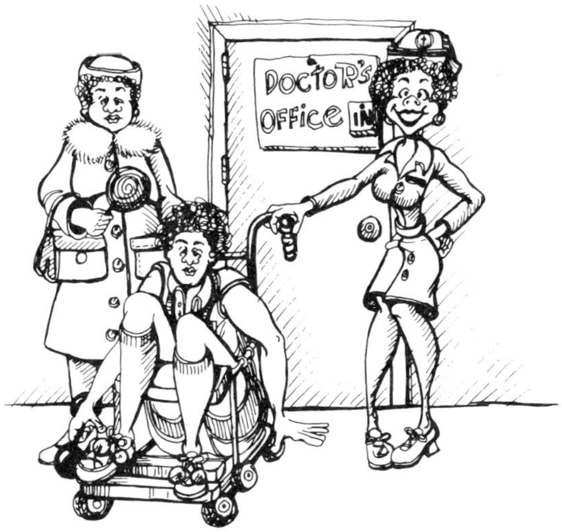

Figure 10–4. *Myth: The preschool child is too young to take to the eye doctor. Fact: Eye examinations can be performed on infants, and the acuity of the eye can be measured without the child reading from an eye chart.*

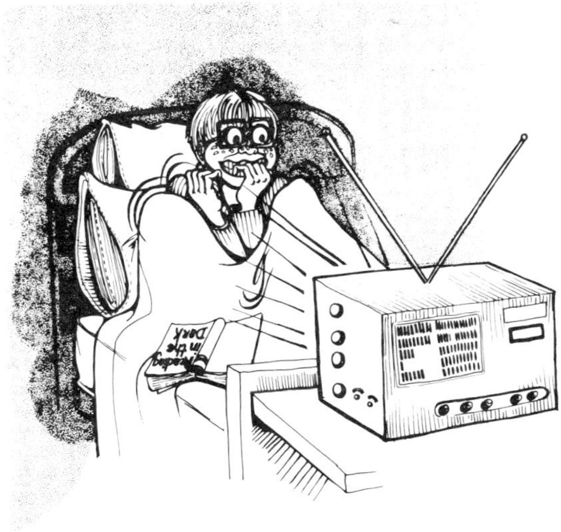

Figure 10–5. *Myth: Too much TV will hurt the child's eyes. Don't read in bed, in a car, or under a dim light.*
Fact: No structural damage to the eyes results from watching TV, or reading in bed, in the car, or in dim light.

SUMMARY

The child with a hearing or visual dysfunction cannot adequately process communication stimuli; therefore he lags behind in language, motor, and cognitive development. Mobility, sleep, and feeding patterns are also affected. A plan of stimulation, communication cues, and varied modes of interaction serves to decrease the child's fear and maximize his development. The parent-child bond is altered in these children; familiar child behaviors are replaced

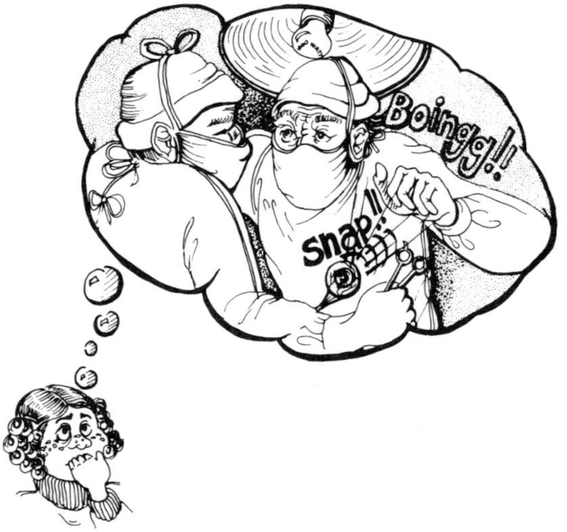

Figure 10–6. *Myth: The surgeon takes the eye out to operate on it. Fact: Eye removal and replacement is impossible. Delicate eye surgery is done with the eye in the orbit.*

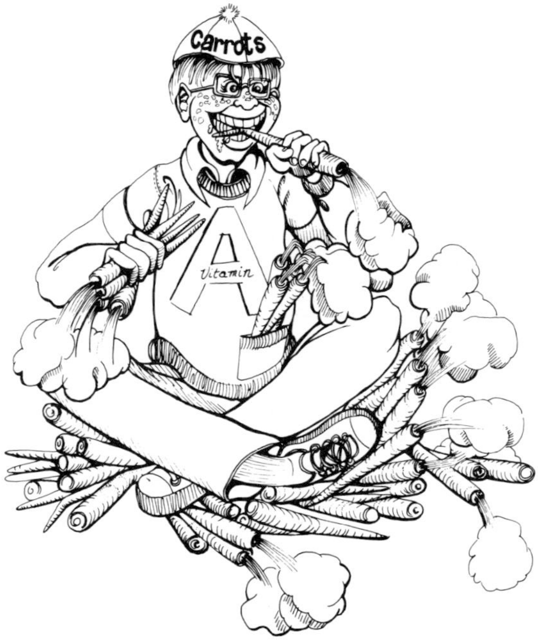

Figure 10–8. *Myth: Vitamins are good for your eyes. Eat a lot of carrots. Fact: There is no evidence that more than the required amount of vitamins will enhance vision.*

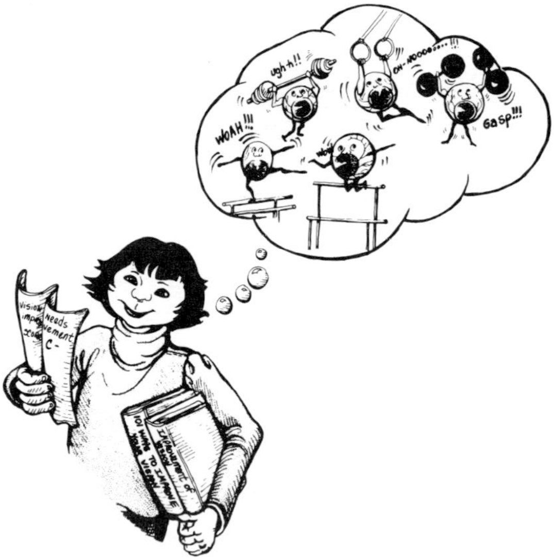

Figure 10–7. *Myth: Exercises will correct weak eyes. Fact: Errors in refraction are determined by the length and curvature of the eye; these are genetically controlled characteristics. Refractive errors cannot be altered by exercises.*

with erratic, immature, and unpredictable actions. The child must have discipline and appropriate outlets for his anger and frustration.

The eye is a fluid-filled structure composed of a cornea that transmits light, a lens that focuses and bends the light, and a retina that receives visual images and transmits them to the brain. The eye is protected by a bony orbit and eyelashes, and moistened by lacrimal duct secretions. Six muscles move each eye. Common reactions to eye disorders are tearing, purulent or mucoid discharge, and pain.

Common diagnostic tests for visual disorders include use of the ophthalmoscope, tonometer, and visual acuity charts. The following specific treatments are used for eye conditions: surgical procedures, eye patches and exercises, antimicrobial ophthalmic medicines, and hot or cold compresses.

The ear is composed of three parts. The outer ear and the external auditory canal gather and transmit sound into the middle ear. The middle ear, the site of most infections, consists of the tympanic cavity and the eustachian tube. The eustachian tube equalizes air pressure and connects the middle ear to the throat. Three small bones—the incus, malleus, and stapes—force sound into the organ of Corti, where hair cells conduct the sound impulses to the brain. Hearing deficits are due to dysfunctions in sound conduction or nerve function. Hearing losses may be genetic, congenital, or acquired.

Diagnostic measures for hearing disorders include the use of the otoscope, tympanometer, and audiometer. The most common operative procedure for correcting conductive hearing loss is the insertion of tympanoplasty tubes. Education programs include training in speech, speech reading, sign language, and auditory discrimination, as well as occupational training and guidance. Various types of hearing aids are used to amplify sound.

Tables 10−1 and 10−2 list specific conditions of the ear and eye and the nursing considerations for each condition.

CLINICAL REVIEW SITUATIONS

- Blindness and deafness affect self-concept (see chapter 9). What are the functional and visible effects of an auditory or visual disorder that influence a child's ability to adapt?
- How can the nursing process (ch. 2) be used to assess perceptual ability and to promote a positive self-concept (ch. 9) for the child with a visual impairment? With a hearing impairment?
- Select a developmental period and review normal tasks for that age. Choosing one task of that period, state how you would foster its performance during the hospitalization of a child with a hearing or visual dysfunction.

Tables 10−1 and 10−2 follow.

Table 10–1. **Specific Ear Conditions**

Condition	*Definition*	*Treatment*	*Special Nursing Considerations*
Otitis externa	Inflammation of the skin lining the ear canal, commonly due to accumulated water (e.g., after swimming). The water erodes the skin and leads to infection. Trauma to the ear with cotton-tipped applicators, insertion of a paper-clip or eraser can also lead to otitis externa. The child has pain and itching in the ear.	Analgesics for pain. Cleansing of the ear canal. Antimicrobial ear drops. Oral antibiotics for signs of a systemic infection (e.g., fever, tender lymph nodes).	Instill ear drops (See Skills Manual). Inform parents of importance of follow-up visit to make sure tympanic membrane is intact.
Acute Otitis Media	Inflammation of the middle ear that leads to swelling and closing of the eustachian tube. The inflammed middle ear discharges fluid into the tympanic cavity, where it collects. The child has sharp pain in the ear, high fever (40°C) and inflammation of nasopharynx. Small child is restless and fretful; the infant may pull at his ear or shake his head back and forth. The ear infection is frequently preceded by an upper respiratory infection. Impaired hearing and deafness are possible complications.	Antibiotics Analgesics (e.g., aspirin or acetominophen) for pain. Antihistamines to reduce inflammation in respiratory mucosa. Decongestants to dry up mucosal membranes and relieve stuffiness.	Dry heat (e.g., a hot water bottle wrapped in a blanket or a heating pad) applied next to the affected ear offers comfort. Instill ear drops. Inform parents that during illness and for six months afterward the child may have a conductive hearing loss.

Chronic Otitis Media	A constant or recurrent inflammation of the middle ear. Decreased hearing and a painless discharge from the ear.	Cleansing of the ear. Antibiotic ointment or drops. Systemic antibiotics Myringotomy Tympanoplasty	Instill ear drops. If a myringotomy is necessary, an incision is made on the tympanic membrane so pus and/or blood can drain from the middle ear; the procedure is painful and general anesthesia is necessary. Observe the bandage closely for amount and color of drainage.
Mastoiditis	Inflammation of the mastoid bone with necrosis. The child has pain, fever, and acute otitis media. Although not common, mastoiditis can occur if acute otitis media is not adequately treated with antibiotics.	Myrinotomy before treatment to reduce pus in the middle ear and to collect material for a culture. Antibiotics Mastoidectomy	Because the facial nerve is close to the middle ear, observe for signs of facial paralysis (e.g., drooping mouth or difficulty in drinking).
Serous Otitis Media	The accumulation of sterile fluid in the middle ear, commonly due to eustachian tube obstruction. The eustachian tubes may be closed due to an allergic inflammation, enlarged adenoids or insufficient treatment of a previous acute otitis media. The child complains of hearing loss but has no pain or fever.	To supply air to the middle ear. Use of oral decongestants to shrink mucosa of the eustachian tubes Have child "pop" his ears (see nursing considerations) Myringotomy and insertion of ventilation tubes (tympanostomy tubes). Adenoidectomy when eustachian tube blocked by enlarged adenoids	To "pop" ones ears, sufficient pressure must be built-up in the nasopharynx to open the closed eustachian tube. Have the young child (aged three to six) blow up a balloon while holding his nose closed. Another approach is to have the child hold his nose closed, and at the same time, blow his nose and then swallow. The child will hear his ears "pop." If ventilating tubes are in place, the child cannot participate in water sports (e.g., swimming, diving) that might allow water to enter the ear. Ear plugs are necessary for hair washing or a shower.

Table 10–2. **Specific Eye Conditions**

Condition	*Definition*	*Treatment*	*Special Nursing Considerations*
Blepharitis	An infection or allergy of the eyelid margin. The lids may be red, burning, itchy, and crusted. Sometimes the eyelashes are matted with exudate and may cease to grow and fall out. Commonly caused by seborrheic dermatitis (cradle cap).	Lid margin cleansed of crust and scales. Antimicrobial medicine applied to lid conjunctiva. If allergy caused, use of steroids.	Apply warm compresses for 10 to 15 minutes to soften and remove crust and scales. To treat cradle cap, oil the scalp with mineral oil or petroleum jelly to soften the crust, then shampoo to remove the crusted material. Repeat this process daily until crusting is gone. Shampoo daily thereafter to prevent cradle cap.
Cataract	Opacity of the lens caused by congenital factors, trauma, or infection. Opacity may involve one or both eyes. The child's pupil appears white, not black. Vision may be slightly or severely reduced.	Lens removed if both eyes are involved and vision cannot develop. Surgery is postponed until age two if cataracts are result of maternal rubella; the rubella virus may be activated if the operation is done sooner. Children with corrected vision of 20/50 are not operated on.	Prepare for surgery and postoperative care (see ch. 2). The child will probably have an eye patch following surgery. The patch will be removed after three or four days and eye drops instilled several times a day. Observe for signs of increased intraocular pressure (e.g., excessive restlessness, crying, general irritability).
Conjunctivitis	Infection of the conjunctiva due to bacterial, viral, or fungal organisms. Vision is not affected. Common types and symptoms include:		
	Gonococcal neonatorum: red conjunctiva, thick pus, and edematous eyelid. If not treated may lead to corneal ul-	Antibiotics (systemic and as eye drops). Eye irrigations to remove purulent material.	Instill eye drops. When irrigating the eye to remove purulent discharge, direct the stream of sterile saline

	cers and blindness. Prophylactic instillation of 1 percent silver nitrate solution or an antibiotic is required in most states to prevent gonococcal neonatorum in newborns.		solution toward the outer edge of the eyelid, away from the other eye. Apply cold compresses to relieve swelling of the eyelids.
	Acute purulent (pinkeye): red conjunctiva, watery discharge, adhesion of eyelids upon awakening.	Antimicrobial ophthalmic drops into the affected eye four to five times daily.	Instill eye drops. Teach parents treatment procedure and importance of continuing medication for prescribed period because infection may recur. Apply wet, warm compresses to soften and remove exudate; assure the child that his eyes will reopen. An epidemic may occur; nurse, child, and parents must maintain careful hand-washing. Isolate the affected child.
	Viral (usually adenoviral): red conjunctiva, thin watery discharge.	Because the infection is caused by a virus, antibiotics are of no value, but they are instilled into the affected eye to prevent a secondary infection.	Same as acute purulent.
	Allergic (noninfectious): red conjunctiva, lacrimation, stringy discharge, and itching.	Steroid eye drops.	Use of cold compresses.
Dacryostenosis (Lacrimal duct obstruction)	Congenital occulusion of the nasolacrimal duct by a membrane or epithelial debris. When the lacrimal gland cannot drain, tears overflow into eyes. If untreated, static tears in the lacrimal sac become infected and pus drains from the eye.	Digital pressure over lacrimal sac to express secretions. If no spontaneous correction in three to six months, surgery is necessary.	Teach parents procedures of hand-washing, restraint methods for infant (See Skills Manual), and application of pressure on lacrimal duct to express secretions. Suggest a routine time for the procedure, such as before each feeding or diaper change.

Continued

Table 10–2 *(Continued)*

Condition	*Definition*	*Treatment*	*Special Nursing Considerations*
Dacryocystitis	Inflammation of the lacrimal duct, frequently secondary to dacryostenosis. May occur during sinusitis if infected matter is forced back into the nasolacrimal duct.	Digital pressure to evacuate secretions from the duct. Local and systemic antibiotics. Probing to free duct of obstructing debris.	A frightening condition for parents who fear the child's sight might be affected; assure parents that the infection lies inside a gland near the eye and that vision is not altered.
Eye trauma/ injury	Foreign bodies, burns, lacerations, or abrasions that cause trauma or injury.	Embedded foreign bodies require removal by an ophthalmologist. Foreign bodies not embedded may be removed by gently touching the object with a moistened, cotton-tipped applicator.	Embedded foreign matter should not be removed manually. Use cold compresses and analgesics for relief of discomfort.
Glaucoma	Increased intraocular pressure due to inadequate drainage of fluid in the posterior and anterior chambers (Fig. 10–1). Increased pressure causes stretching of corneal and scleral tissue. Without treatment blindness occurs. Glaucoma may be caused by infection, trauma, or congenital factors. In congenital glaucoma, the angle of the anterior chamber is altered in fetal development; consequently, fluid from the chamber cannot drain properly and increased pressure results.	Medications to decrease production of fluid in the anterior chamber and increase drainage. Immediate surgical intervention. Several operations are frequently necessary.	General surgical preparation and postoperative care (see ch. 2).

Hordeolum (sty)	Inflammation of the sebaceous glands of the lids usually caused by staphylococcus organisms. The lid may be swollen, with pain and redness localized at one point.	Use of warm, moist compresses three to four times daily. Antimicrobial drugs.	When sty develops a head it may be incised and drained. Eye is painful and child is reluctant to allow anyone to touch the area. Never squeeze a sty.
Keratitis	Inflammation and infection of the superficial layers of the cornea. Causative organism may be bacterial, fungal, or viral.	Topical or systemic medication, depending on causative organism. Corneal transplant may be necessary.	General surgical preparation and postoperative care (see ch. 2).
Retrolental fibroplasia (RLF)	Acquired partial or total blindness in premature infants; caused by administration of oxygen concentrations exceeding 40 percent, which cause mild to severe scarring of the retina, distortion, and detachment.	Retinal surgery in cases of extensive damage.	Ensure that oxygen concentration does not exceed 40 percent unless specifically ordered. Advise parents to arrange for follow-up examinations.
Strabismus (cast, squint, crosseye, walleye)	Muscular imbalance of the eye causing an inward (esotropic), outward (exotropic), upward (hypertropic), or downward (hypotropic) cast. Occurs in 1 to 2 percent of all children; half of all affected children have a family history of strabismus.	Surgical alignment of eyes; use of corrective lenses, eye exercises, or patch occlusion of good eye to develop muscles of the deviant eye.	Surgical preparation and postoperative care (see ch. 2). Children may be admitted on morning of surgery. Find out whether fasting (no food or fluids since midnight or prescribed time) has been observed.
Trachoma	Bacterial infection of the conjunctiva, usually associated with deprivation and poor hygiene. Trachoma is the major cause of blindness in the world.	Antimicrobial medicines locally and systemically.	Instruct parents in eye drop administration and need for long-term follow-up care to identify any visual impairment.

Bibliography

Albert, D. and Scheie, H. *Textbook of Ophthalmology,* ed. 9. Philadelphia, W. B. Saunders Co., 1977.

Bumbalo, J. and Seidel, M. Identifying and Serving a Multiply Handicapped Population. *Nursing Clinics of North America* 10:341, 1975.

Crouch, J. and McClintic, R. *Human Anatomy and Physiology,* ed. 2. New York, John Wiley & Sons. Inc., 1976.

Dupont, J. What to Do for Common Eye Emergencies. *Nursing '76* 7:17, 1976.

Fisch, L. Causes of Deafness in Children. *Nursing Mirror* 143:48, 1976.

Freeman, F.D. Psychosocial Problems of Deaf Children and Their Families: A Comparative Study. *American Annals of the Deaf* 120:391, 1975.

Freeman, G. Middle Ear Diseases. *Nursing Times* 73:56, 1977.

Havener, W., Saunders, W., Keith, C. *Nursing Care in Eye, Ear, Nose and Throat Disorders.* St. Louis, C. V. Mosby Co., 1974.

Klein, J. Middle Ear Disease in Children. *Hospital Practice* 11:45, 1976.

Larsen, S. Removing Cerumen with a Water Pik. *American Journal of Nursing* 76:264, 1976.

Lesser, S. and Easser, R. Psychiatric Management of the Deaf Child. *Canadian Nurse* 71:23, 1975.

Levenson, L. and Levenson, J. Corneal Transplantations. *American Journal of Nursing* 77:1160, 1977.

Machol, L. Total communication: A New Hope for Deaf Children. *Family Health* 8:44, 1976.

Moor, P. Foster Family Care for Visually Impaired Children. *Children Today* 5:11, 1976.

Northern, J., Rock, E., Frye, D. Tympanometry: A Technique for Identifying Ear Disease in Children. *Pediatric Nursing* 1:32, 1975.

Petrillo, M. and Sanger, S. *Emotional Care of Hospitalized Children: An Environmental Approach.* Philadelphia, J.B. Lippincott Co., 1972.

Scharf, J. and Zonis, S. Perforating Injuries of the Eye in Childhood. *Journal Pediatric Ophthalmology* 13:326, 1976.

Tsappis, A. Audiological Aspects of the Identification of Hearing Impairments in Early Childhood. *Pediatric Nursing* 3:40, 1977.

Wright, J. Deaf But Not Mute. *American Journal of Nursing* 76:795, 1976.

CHAPTER 11

The Child with a Cerebral Dysfunction

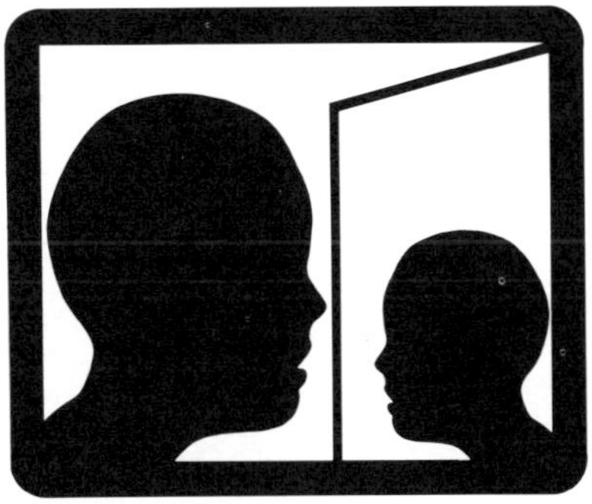

BEHAVIORAL OBJECTIVES

After studying this chapter you will be able to:

- Discuss the common behavioral alterations of a child with a cerebral dysfunction.
- Compare and contrast the causes, signs and symptoms, course, and nursing interventions for the child with an intellectual impairment versus the child with minimal brain dysfunction.
- List self-care behaviors and the principles of teaching the behaviors to children with an intellectual impairment.
- Describe the cyclic behaviors of parent and child in a stressed parent-child bond.
- List the components and discuss the principles of behavior modification.

TERMS AND CONCEPTS

Mental retardation
Minimal brain dysfunction
Cerebral dysfunction
Self-care behaviors
Behavior modification
Positive reinforcers
Negative reinforcers
Punishers
Target behaviors

The *mentally retarded* child has an intellectual impairment that is usually permanent. The child with *minimal brain dysfunction* has an alteration in cerebral function that hinders his learning ability, although the child's IQ is almost always normal. Cause and prognosis differ radically in these two disorders, but the nursing care problems are similar. Both conditions alter behavioral patterns and place stress on parent-child interactions (Figure 11–1). The specific causes, prognosis, common diagnostic, methods, and treatment plans are discussed for both disorders.

COMMON PROBLEMS, SYMPTOMS, AND NURSING INTERVENTIONS

Altered Behaviors

Ten to 30 percent of school-age children in the United States have difficulty adapting

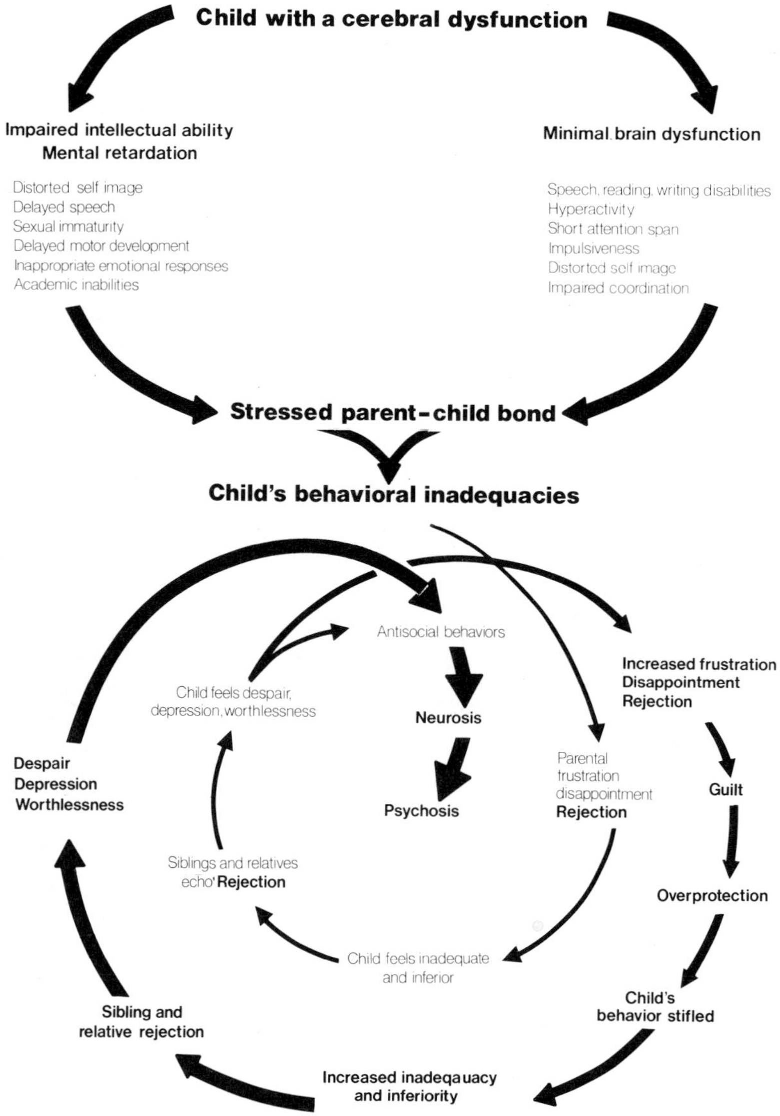

Figure 11–1. *Stressed parent-child bond.*

to their grade placement. The difficulty may be due to specific academic disabilities, inappropriate peer relationships, or hyperactivity. These children have a *cerebral dysfunction.* Common signs of cerebral dysfunction are delayed motor and language development, hyperactivity, emotional immaturity, and difficulties in reading, writing, spelling, or arithmetic.

Approximately 13 percent of the U. S. population are characterized as suffering from borderline mental retardation, or as being subaverage in intellectual functioning. An additional 3 percent are mildly to severely retarded. Many of these people are children; all have a cerebral dysfunction. When children with cerebral dysfunctions enter the hospital for medical or surgical attention, an awareness of their behavioral alterations, and an assessment of their current abilities can promote nursing care approaches specific to their needs.

The Mentally Retarded Child

Mental retardation is an impairment of intellectual function. Maturation in the retarded child is slow and incomplete, learning ability is impaired, and social adjustment is poor. Any child may be classified as mentally retarded if his performance on a standardized psychological test is two or more standard deviations below the mean. Mental retardation is classified by degree of severity, as mild, moderate, or severe. Seventy-five percent of children with mental retardation are classified as mildly retarded, having IQs of 50 to 70. These children are termed *educable,* and can be expected to learn basic academic and social skills within a specially designed program. Twenty percent of mentally retarded children are termed *trainable,* having IQs of 30 to 50. Five percent of mentally retarded children have IQs below 30, are severely retarded, and need custodial care. Children with IQs of 70 to 89 are classified as slow learners (90 to 120 is generally considered normal).

The child's potential for future development is as important as his IQ. The mildly retarded child can be expected to attain a sixth grade academic level and to perform at the mental age of twelve by adulthood. With training the adult can do semiskilled work. The moderately retarded youngster should attain a fourth grade academic level and be semi-independent by childhood, although frequent guidance and supervision will always be needed. The severely retarded person does not usually benefit from academic education, but can learn to complete self-care functions (e.g., bathing, eating, elimination) and carry out routine tasks (e.g., bed-making and cleaning). Most severely retarded children will need a sheltered environment such as an institution all of their lives.

Causes of Mental Retardation

Although more than 100 different factors have been identified as causes of mental retardation, they apply to fewer than 25 percent of retarded children. There are no known biological or organic causes for 75 percent of the cases of retardation; the cause in these cases may be environmental or sociocultural deprivation. These children have not received adequate and appropriate stimuli for normal intellectual development.

The primary known causes of mental retardation are infection, intoxication, and injury. Infections can occur prenatally (e.g., as a result of maternal rubella or syphilis) or during childhood (e.g., as a result of bacterial meningitis, influenza, or encephalopathy). The antepartal ingestion of certain medicines, toxemia of pregnancy, or childhood lead poisoning are examples of intoxicating causes of mental retardation. Injury or trauma may occur prenatally (e.g., irradiation, uterine hemorrhage) or at birth (e.g., anoxia, injury during delivery, or prolonged use of anesthesia). Disorders of metabolism or chromosomal alteration, e.g., Tay-Sachs disease, phenylketonuria, or Down's syndrome, (Figure 11–2) are clinical disease states of syndromes that cause mental retardation (see Table 11–1). Cerebral trauma or new growths such as an intracranial neoplasm or hydrocephalus may predispose the child to mental retardation. Despite this elaborate list of possible causes, the cause of retardation is unidentified in most cases. An unknown origin generates uncertainty, and possibly, guilt, as parents ponder the cause of their child's retardation.

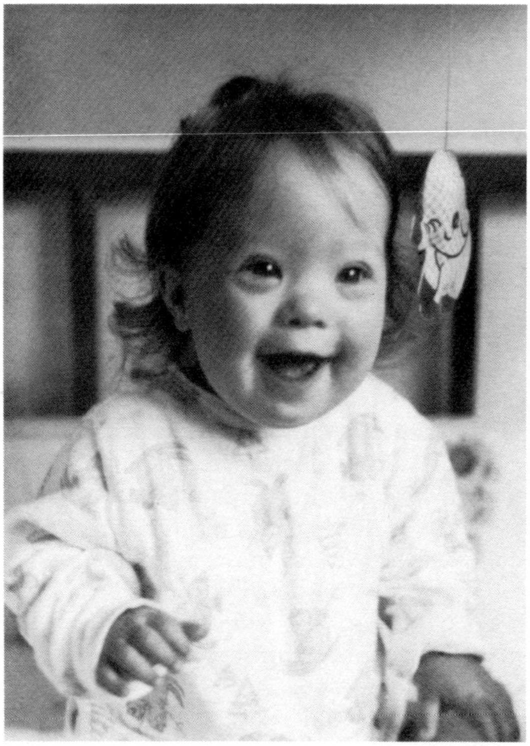

Figure 11–2. *A child with Down's syndrome enjoying the visual stimulation of a mobile* (From Smith, D.W. and Wilson, A. *The Child With Down's Syndrome* (Mongolism) Philadelphia, W.B. Saunders Co, 1973).

Assessment of the Child With Altered Development

Although one encounters children in the hospital who have been diagnosed as mentally retarded, far more undiagnosed children, who seem "slow" and delayed in motor, language, or social development, will be seen. The majority of children with delayed development are not diagnosed until four or five years of age. Another large percentage are not assessed until later, when the use of language expressing abstract concepts is required. If indicators of delayed development are assessed and diagnosed early, with appropriate educational treatment begun, the child's chances of maximizing his potential and making a healthy emotional adjustment to life are optimal.

The developmental status of each hospitalized child should be measured against the standard for the child's age (See ch. 2 and chs. 4–8). Children should sit by eight months, walk by fifteen to eighteen months, and respond to verbal commands and use expressive language by age two. If gross delays exist, discuss them with staff and parents. If a child is "slow" or diagnosed as mentally retarded, ascertain what concerns the parents have regarding the child's development. What *self-care behaviors* (e.g., feeding, bathing, dressing, toileting) can the child perform? What self-care or other behaviors do parents want to foster? What does the child want to achieve? Self-care is essential for independent functioning and a positive self-concept. Many preschool programs require independent care for entrance. Self-care behaviors are important to parents and crucial for peer and societal acceptance. They give the child a feeling of accomplishment and self-sufficiency, promoting emotional integrity. Awareness of the importance of these daily self-care behaviors can foster their consistent continuation in the hospital even though it may be faster and easier for others to dress, feed, or toilet the child.

After listing the self-care tasks the child can perform, assess how well they are performed, and whether the child is developmentally ready for the behaviors his parents expect. Do parents realize the child's progress will be slow? (The child of average intelligence requires six or seven years before complete self-dressing is possible!) Does the child have limitations other than intellectual ones that may affect his learning? If the child is not capable of independent locomotion, for example, then total independence in toileting is unrealistic. Have realistic goals been set for each skill? Self-care skills can be broken down into a series of small tasks; the completion of each small task is a step toward the accomplishment of the larger goal.

A Plan For Self-Feeding

Feeding oneself is the first major self-care behavior mastered by the child. Signs of readiness for self-feeding include the ability to sit without support, balance the head, control the arms, bring hands to mouth, grasp and hold a cup and spoon, bite, chew, and swallow.

Children need not master all these skills before they can feed themselves; however, if the child has difficulty with several of the above skills, he is not developmentally ready to feed himself, and if he is forced to perfect self-feeding, both parent and child will become frustrated and feel the child will never learn. Determine what the child can do and set realistic short-term goals.

Review ch. 5 and the steps of self-feeding for the normal child; extra time and patience must be allowed for the intellectually impaired child. If the child has normal motor control, regular utensils can be used, but if he has associated motor problems such as those associated with cerebral palsy (ch. 28), modified equipment such as spoons with curved handles, suction cups on the bottom of plates, and weighted bottoms or a wet wash cloth on the bottom of the tray or plate to stabilize the food container will be needed. The use of a small plastic cup or glass and flexible straws makes drinking easier. Serve mashed potatoes, squash, bananas, or other foods with a thick consistency. Retarded children must be helped with each motion: a parent's guiding hand moves the child's hand through the process of moving a spoon from bowl to mouth and back to bowl. As the child acquires skill and confidence, the guide is gradually removed. Training sessions should be held at the beginning of the meal, lasting 15 to 20 minutes. Give praise lavishly during the entire session.

Self-feeding is best taught as a series of small tasks. For example: 1) child can hold spoon; 2) child can take spoon to mouth; 3) child can hold spoon with food and take to mouth; 4) child can remove food from spoon with lips; 5) child can return spoon to bowl. If each task is seen as a goal in itself, then a feeling of accomplishment is felt by child and parent at each step. Patience is crucial, and if your tolerance or that of the

Table 11–1. **Conditions of Mental Retardation**

Condition	*Definition*	*Treatment*	*Special Nursing Considerations*
Down's Syndrome (Mongolism, Trisomy 21)	The presence of three chromosomes in the 21 group, occurring 1:600 births. A protruding tongue, almond-shaped eyes and short, broad hands and feet are characteristic features. The child has poor muscle tone. Intelligence quotients vary greatly.	Special education.	Increased susceptibility to infection (e.g., pneumonia, gastroenteritis). Congenital heart malformations in 40 percent of children.
Klinefelter's Syndrome	The presence of an extra sex chromosome, (XXY) occurring 1:500 males.	Special education. Testosterone replacement therapy (to promote development of male secondary sexual characteristics, although the boy will remain sterile).	Children with the syndrome have small testes and are sterile; the syndrome may not be detected until puberty.
Phenylketonuria (PKU)	A defect of protein (phenylalanine) metabolism transmitted by an autosomal recessive gene. Excessive amounts of phenylalanine accumulate in body serum, cerebrospinal fluid, tissue, and urine, causing severe mental retardation. Occurring 1:10,000 births, most often in children with blond hair and blue eyes. To be diag-	To keep blood level of phenylalanine between 3 and 8 mg/100 ml (normal range is 1 to 4 mg/100 ml), phenylaline in the diet is restricted. This is difficult because *no* natural protein exists that is low in phenylalanine and contains others essential amino acids. Lofenalac, a synthetic milk substitute, or Product 3229 (syn-	Monitoring of special diet. Help parents locate recipes that use Lofenalac to make ice cream, puddings, and milk shakes. Regular monitoring of blood and urine for phenylalanine levels. Most states require screening of all newborns for phenylketonuria before discharge from hospital. Emotional support to minimize

	nosed as having **PKU**, the infant's blood plasma level of phenylalanine must be 20 mg/100 ml or higher.	thetic amino acids) is given. Solid foods are added gradually, avoiding high-phenylalanine foods (e.g., meats, eggs, green vegetables, cheese, milk). Controversy exists as to how long the low-phenylalane diet must continue. Some experts recommend five years, others feel dietary restrictions are needed throughout adolescence.	behavioral problems due to dietary restrictions. Assure parents that if **PKU** was diagnosed shortly after birth and blood levels of phenylalanine are controlled, the child's intelligence should be that of a nonaffected child.
Tay-Sachs Disease	A condition characterized by abnormal deposits of lipids (fats) in the cells of the cerebral cortex, spleen, liver, and lymph nodes, transmitted by an autosomal recessive gene. Carrier rate 1:30 for Ashkenazic Jewish population.	Symptomatic and supportive care.	Blindness, muscular degeneration, seizures, and death by age three to four. Identification of carriers possible by means of simple blood test.
Trisomy 13 (Patau Syndrome)	Presence of an extra chromosome in group 13, occurring 1:5,000 births. The child is severely retarded.	Symptomatic and supportive care.	Cleft lip and palate, deafness, extra digits, death in early childhood.
Trisomy 18	Presence of an extra chromosome in group 18, occurring 1:4,000 births.	Symptomatic and supportive care.	Renal and cardiac abnormalities. Death in infancy.

parents wanes, it is best to stop and begin again at the next meal. Allow the child to play with eating utensils, such as a plastic spoon, cup, and bowl, between meals. After learning spoon-feeding, the child can progress to using a fork and knife. Sitting positions, napkin use, and other manners can be taught later. Guard against teaching and expecting too much at one time.

Toileting and Dressing

After the child can feed himself, he is ready to be toilet trained. Readiness indicators are the ability to stand and walk alone, to remain dry for two or more hours, to have regular bowel movements, and to be aware when elimination has occurred. The principle of dividing the end goal into a series of small tasks, the use of appropriate equipment, and consistent, daily practice sessions are helpful. Dressing, grooming, and hygiene are other habits important for independent functioning. Self-dressing requires the ability to stand, walk, balance on one foot, extend the arms and legs, and the development of a thumb-forefinger grasp and finger dexterity. Clothing conducive to self-dressing includes slip on, polo-type or turtleneck shirts, elastic-waisted pants, slip-on or zippered shoes, and front-buttoned or zipped pants or dresses. Age-appropriate clothing and hair styles are important for peer acceptance and the promotion of a positive self-concept.

Play

Play provides stimulation and a context for peer interaction, which is essential for emotional growth and integrity. The child with impaired intellectual ability may be excluded from peer interactions or, when included, criticized for his ineptness. Hospitalized children who form play groups are quick to single out the "slow" child, labeling him "retard" or "dummy." In the hospital and at home, advise the parents of the retarded child to choose toys and group activities that involve the use of large muscles, repetitive motions, and no fantasy play. For example, paints, clay, blocks, ball games, and cooking are suitable group activities. Avoid paper-and-pencil and abstract activities that frequently go beyond the mentally retarded child's intellectual ability.

Sexuality

The development of a sexual identity and the appropriate expression of sexual feelings are part of normal sexual maturation. The child who is mentally retarded may show delayed or incomplete sexual development. Because of limited expressive abilities, the child may be unable to express feelings adequately, or may make inappropriate use of emotionally potent words like *love* and *hate*. The mentally retarded adolescent needs instruction on menstrual grooming and reproduction. Pictures and films give clarity to sexual instruction. Identification of feelings is the first step in learning how to handle them. If the family and others accept the child's sexual needs, the child also will be able to incorporate physical and emotional changes into a positive self-concept.

The Child With Minimal Brain Dysfunction Syndrome

Minimal brain dysfunction refers to a cluster of altered behavioral and intellectual patterns. The behaviors characteristic of affected children are not different from those of normal children; however, the intensity, duration, and frequency of certain behaviors is very different. The child with minimal brain dysfunction has a cerebral dysfunction but not necessarily an intellectual impairment; the child may have near-average, average, or above-average intelligence. Any combination of the following characteristics is typical of the child with minimal brain dysfunction: a short attention span, susceptibility to distraction, hyperactivity, hypoactivity, impulsiveness, emotional lability, impaired coordination, perceptual difficulty with time, space, form, sound, or sequencing, and impaired language skills, particularly in speech and reading. The cause of minimal brain dysfunction varies; it may be genetic or organic. *Minimal brain dysfunction* is defined as an immaturity of cerebral functioning; specifically, it is a defect in neurotransmissions that results in difficulties in cognitive-perceptual skills or behavioral control. Symptoms may change; a child may have only a behavioral alteration, such as hyperactivity (excessive and disorganized activity), at one age, and may have certain academic difficulties and no behavioral alterations at a later age. A diagnosis of minimal brain dysfunction is made in 5 to 20 percent of all children between the ages of 4 and 14; boys are affected three times as frequently as girls. Most of the affected children are referred for behavioral or learning problems in the early primary grades, frequently years after the first symptoms of minimal brain dysfunction have gone undiagnosed. Learning disorders are the major single cause of children dropping out of school and constitute one of the major problems of children and adolescents who have been referred to clinics and juvenile courts for behavioral disorders. Sometimes, symptoms of minimal brain dysfunction, especially hyperactivity, are present at birth (although hyperactivity, for one, is not necessarily a symptom of minimal brain dysfunction). Particularly suspicious is the newborn who is exceedingly restless, has colic for an extended period, and has head-banging and rocking episodes.

The child with minimal brain dysfunction may be so diagnosed when he is hospitalized for an infection, surgery, or a childhood disease. If the diagnosis is made, assess the parents' and child's understanding of the child's problem. What routines have they established at home for daily activities? What type of environment is most conducive to increasing the child's self-control and decreasing hyperactivity?

With the family, devise a daily plan of consistent, predictable times for eating, bathing, rest, play, and sleep. Select a location that offers a minimum of distractions and extraneous stimuli. Decide on firm but reasonable limits; discipline must be consistent. Hyperactive behavior is increased when the child is fatigued or overstimulated. During rest and sleep periods, turn the television and radio off and restrict social interaction. Provide for small-group play periods with two or three other children. Provide a positive, accepting environment. Spending time with the child, listening attentively, and using touch are simple ways to convey interest and concern. The child needs to experience success in personal achievement and interpersonal relationships. Use doll play to simulate experiences the child will have. When informing the child of procedures, guard against misunderstandings by avoiding ambiguous words and by using illustrations. Children with minimal brain dysfunction experience frustrations and anxiety because of their behavioral or learning disabilities. Providing safe means for them to express their frustration through creative art, water or sand play, and large-muscle activities can ease their tension while helping them to maintain self-control.

A Stressed Parent-Child Bond

When normal development is replaced by alterations in performance, stress is placed on the child and his family. Parents notice the child's inadequacies and inabilities, a different pace of activity, varying emotional responses, or an inability to understand; they will normally become anxious as they become aware of the child's persistent difficulty in basic motor function, learning, or behavioral reactions. They may feel anger and disappointment as their child fails to develop elementary skills. Even when given extra time and patience, the child does not equal the performance level of his siblings and peers. The child experiences emotional pain as he becomes acutely aware of his failure to meet parental and sibling expectations and demands; love and acceptance are linked to performance, and the child cannot perform. Feelings of inadequacy and inferiority smother him as he desperately tries to meet unrealistic demands. Despair and depression threaten to take control of the developing self. Emotional integrity is assaulted by a distorted self-concept in which the child sees himself as worthless.

Antisocial behavior, an adaptation to the stress of the dysfunction but not otherwise related to it, may emerge. The child may begin to display such behavior as lying, cheating, stealing, being disobedient and defiant to parents or other authority figures, or bullying other children. Habit disorders, such as enuresis (bedwetting), excessive masturbation, or regression to an earlier developmental stage, may also occur. All these behaviors are reactions to the emotional trauma that the child encounters as he tries to perform. If a negative self-concept continues to exist, neurotic or psychotic behaviors may result (See ch. 13). During this progression of stressed parent-child interactions, the parents may experience guilt arising from their unconscious and conscious rejection of the child. These feelings may be displayed by overprotection of the child. Overprotected, the child does not attempt as much, and the parents are not reminded of the child's limitations. As a result, the child falls below his already limited level and is burdened with increased feelings of inadequacy, difference, and depression.

The stressed parent-child bond (Figure 11–1) warrants early attention and active intervention. Families should be told that feelings of frustration, disappointment, rejection, and guilt are normal and understandable, as are the child's expressions of depression and worthlessness. The nurse can alleviate the stressed parent-child bond by coordinating special resource persons the child may need during his hospitalization, explaining procedures, and offering instruction and readiness assessments in self-care skills. Acknowledging accomplishments, no matter how small, increases the child's sense of self-worth and motivates parents and child to improved interactions with one another.

COMMON DIAGNOSTIC STUDIES AND NURSING IMPLICATIONS

At admission to the hospital, a physical examination and a perinatal and developmental history will be completed. The physical examination gives special attention to congenital stigmata, head size, and a systems review. An allergy history should be taken because a significant number of children with minimal brain dysfunction display at least minor allergic symptoms. Information on the ages at which developmental tasks were completed will be elicited and appraised. A behavioral history, assessing activity, attention span, speech, muscular coordination, and emotional maturity is also recorded. A profile of the family, including data on sociocultural and economic status, environment, educational backgrounds, and recreational habits, is constructed. A neurological examination and an electroencephalogram (EEG) may be performed, and cytogenic studies may be ordered if a chromosomal disorder is suspected.

Psychological testing evaluates intellectual capabilities and potential, personality traits, and special interests and abilities. Intellect is classically measured by a structured system of questions that requires specific responses from the child; among the most commonly used intelligence tests are the Stanford-Binet and Wechsler. Personality traits are typically measured by unstructured, or projective, means such as the Rorschach test, in which the subject is asked to interpret a series of ambiguous ink-blot designs.

The results of psychological testing are frequently recorded as *mental age* (MA), expressed in years and months. If a child receives an MA score of 10 years, 2 months on a given test, the child did as well as an average child of 10 years, 2 months. Explaining the rationale for a developmental history, socioeconomic assessment, and the battery of psychological tests is an important supportive measure.

The diagnostic period can be long and stressful for child and family. The parents will be requested to recall developmental milestones that may have occurred five or ten years earlier. It is difficult for any parent to recall the exact age at which the child sat, said "dada," or pedaled a tricycle. Be patient and try to aid the parent's memory by linking developmental questions to holidays, birthdays, or seasons of the year. If the child was born in the summer, was he sitting by Christmas and walking by his first birthday? Grandparents and baby books can be excellent sources of information.

In many cases, even following the long battery of tests, no cause can be offered to explain the child's impairments, and the child's future potential is difficult to predict. When and to what degree basic learning skills and social and developmental abilities will be attained are unknown. Unlike most families, who plan for the purchase of a tricycle and bicycle, entry into school, and music and swimming lessons, these families cannot plan. How parents and siblings adjust to the indefinite and unpredictable nature of the child's future greatly influences the child's perceptions of his self-worth and ability.

During the diagnostic period, parents are usually receptive to suggestions and recommendations that will facilitate the child's development, and because the hospital affords the opportunity to observe family interaction patterns, the nurse can assess how parents and child relate to one another. Is the child touched, held closely, and cared for in a way that shows tenderness and love? Does the child reciprocate? Is the child allowed to play, roughhouse, tease, and be teased by parents and siblings? Is the child permitted some control over choice of food, clothing, and play? (A choice between ordering a hamburger or a hot dog teaches discrimination between two foods, but equally important, the child can influence his environment and observe what happens to him after making a decision.) Do the parents help the child relate actions, results, and feelings? (Although the child is not responsible for feelings elicited by a situation, the way the feelings are expressed is subject to social sanction.) Do the parents help the child identify feelings of sadness, disappointment, and guilt, discussing the feelings and providing means for their resolution? Or do parents flounder when the child is frustrated, appeasing the child with food or toys in an attempt to stop unattractive behavior? How accepting are parents and siblings of the child's inabilities? Is the child encouraged and praised for attempting new skills, or do parents seem to consistently prefer to act on the child's behalf? Do the parents express pride in the child's abilities or is a subtle or obvious negative-rejective attitude apparent when new skills are attempted?

When evaluating the family of a child with a cerebral dysfunction, bear in mind the pattern depicted in Figure 11−1, and identify any family interactions that suggest guilt, rejection, or overprotection. Early identification of stress behaviors and appropriate interventions by trained personnel can usually prevent the development of the more serious problems of neurosis or psychosis.

COMMON TREATMENTS AND NURSING IMPLICATIONS

Education

Educational programs for the child with a cerebral dysfunction are most effective if they provide an environment of minimal distraction and competition, practical education, and a teacher who is trained in various strategies that encourage the child's abilities. No unnecessary pressure should be placed on the child; realistic goals must be established. Depending on the child's needs, he may be able to participate in a regular classroom. *Mainstreaming* is the practice of placing the child with a cerebral dysfunction in a regular classroom where he, like other classmates, follows curricula tailored to his ability level. The use of a tutor or special educational setting are other alternatives.

Behavior Modification

Behavior is reciprocal. Parents affect their children's behavior and children affect their parent's behavior. *Behavior modification* is a method of changing behavior by the use of reinforcers. Reinforcers encourage a given behavior. *Positive reinforcers* add something desirable to the child's environment—a smile, a hug, money, toys, or praise. *Negative reinforcers* remove an unpleasant stimulus from one's environment. For example, assume that a whining child is smiled at and given a cookie, and that the child stops whining and eats the cookie. The person who gave the child the cookie has been negatively reinforced, since an unpleasant stimulus (whining) has been temporarily removed. The child has received a positive reinforcer. Positive and negative reinforcers reinforce the behavior that follows.

Punishers decrease the behavior they follow. A punishment is the application of an adverse consequence, such as a frown, a reprimand, isolation, or the removal of a positive reinforcer. Reinforcers and punishers can be used to modify or change behavior when they are given immediately after the behavior. For example, when the child is learning self-feeding, each time the desired behavior occurs, positive reinforcement should be given. To use behavior modification, first assess the child's developmental level, (for example, by observing that a child can sit unaided and hold a spoon), identify behavioral areas of concern, (such as no attempt to put spoon in mouth), and note the situations that elicit the behavior—mealtimes. Next decide on a *target behavior,* the action that the behavior modification program is designed to encourage or discourage. (Target behaviors may be desirable acts to which positive reinforcers are applied, or undesirable acts to which measures are applied to decrease the behavior.) The target behavior must be observable, measurable, and controllable by the child. In the above example, the target behavior is the child taking food from a spoon with his lips. Reinforcers are selected; for example, each time the child removes food from the spoon with his lips, a pat and verbal praise are given. If the food is spilled, no reinforcement is given. The plan is implemented, and behavioral changes are recorded.

Behavior modification is one way to increase adaptive behavior. The principles of behavior modification can be used in the home, at school, and in the hospital. Parents can be instructed in the basic principles and referred for further education, support, and supervised practice. In applying principles of behavior modification, follow the steps as in the nursing process: assess the child's behavior, identify target actions, establish a plan and implement and evaluate the plan.

Medication

Drugs called psychostimulants are commonly prescribed for the child with minimal brain dysfunction, although medication does not replace an individually adapted educational experience and parental involvement. Such drugs as Dexedrine and Ritalin promote learning by reducing distractibility and hyperactivity. The risk of addiction is minimal; be certain to assure parents of this. The side effects of anorexia and insomnia do not persist if dosage and schedule of administration are adjusted for individual needs.

Diet

If allergic symptoms are present, the child may be placed on a hypoallergenic diet for one month and then reassessed to determine if changes in behavior and physical well-being have occurred (e.g., less irritability, decreased fatigue, increased attention span). Considerable information exists in the lay literature on certain food additives and their possible effects on behavior. Parents may ask the advisability of children eating certain foods. A knowledge of basic nutrition and an awareness of the ingredients in foods are essential to nutritional guidance.

SUMMARY

The child with a cerebral dysfunction may have permanent intellectual impairment and be classified as mentally retarded, or he may have an alteration in behavioral or intellectual patterns classified as minimal brain dysfunction. In either case, the child's behavior is altered. The behavioral changes may consist of delays in motor development, impaired academic achievement, or immature emotional responses. The behavioral changes place stress on the parent-child bond, causing a negative self-image, which in turn affects emotional integrity adversely. Diagnosis and an appropriate environment must be promptly established for the child. Behavior modification and certain drugs are used to control symptoms and maximize the child's potential.

CLINICAL APPLICATIONS

John, an eight-year-old, sits before the television in his hospital room, engrossed in daily game shows. He was diagnosed as having minimal brain dysfunction and hyperactivity at the community clinic and placed on Ritalin twice a day. He has always done poorly in school and is repeating the second grade this year. He was admitted with arm burns caused by a fire he started. He screams, fights, and spits with each dressing change. John uses the call cord every five or ten minutes and has rung the emergency bell twice in three days. John is in a four-child ward and threatens to beat up the younger children if they do not obey him. He intentionally broke several of the younger children's toys this morning. John lives with his mother, who works at a factory during the evening, leaving John to care for himself. His mother states that he has always been "mean" and she does not know what to do with him.

1. Considering the environmental needs of the hyperactive child, suggest appropriate room placement, games, and an activity and rest schedule for John.
2. Review the cyclic behavior indicative of a stressed parent-child bond. At what stage are John and his mother? What support measures can you offer them? Explain minimal brain dysfunction, the accompanying behavioral changes, medication, and emotional and academic needs to John's mother.
3. Review behavior modification principles; select one of John's inappropriate behaviors as a target behavior and write a plan to decrease it. What type of reinforcers are you going to use? What behaviors are you going to record? Why?

Joan, a two-year-old with mild mental retardation, sits quietly by the window, licking a popsicle while clutching her teddy bear. She has been hospitalized for a week, choosing to remain in her room and not to play with other children. Her mother maintains a constant vigil, anticipating all her needs, and states that Joan has always been a "slow" child who needs her constant attention. Joan watched with interest at noon as the toddler across the hall fed himself. However, when she reached for her own spoon, her mother quickly reminded her she would spill the food. Joan can put on her dress but is unable to button it, a further indication, according to her mother, that she is unable "to do for herself."

1. What are the readiness indicators for self-feeding? What self-feeding readiness indicators does Joan exhibit? What questions should you ask in order to assess the mother's understanding of how children learn to feed themselves and her willingness to allow Joan to handle utensils and food?
2. The mother is doubtful but willing for Joan to learn self-feeding. Identifying small tasks and positive reinforcers, plan a 3-day self-feeding experience, allowing for increased participation at each meal. What behaviors will indicate Joan is ready for additional tasks? What behaviors will indicate a need to revise your plan, allowing extra time for task mastery?
3. Reviewing the cyclic behavior indicative

of a stressed parent-child bond, identify the stage at which Joan and her mother are. What anticipatory guidance can you offer?

Bibliography

Amundson, M. Nurses as Group Leaders of Behavior Management Classes for Parents. *Nursing Clinics of North America* 10:319, 1975.

Barnard, K. and Erikson, M. *Teaching Children with Developmental Problems,* ed.2. St. Louis, C.V. Mosby Co., 1976.

Bean, M. and Bell, B. Nursing Interventions in the Care of the Physically Handicapped, Severely Retarded Child. *Nursing Clinics of North America* 10:353, 1975.

Boder, E. School Failure—Evaluation and Treatment. *Journal of Pediatrics* 58:392, 1976.

Conway, B. Adaptive Problems in School and Learning, in *Pediatric Neurologic Nursing.* St. Louis, C.V. Mosby Co., 1977.

Dodge, P. Neurologic Disorders of School-Age Children. *Journal of School Health* 46:338, 1976.

Frazier, S. Minimal Brain Dysfunction. *Medical Times* 103:68, 1975.

Gross, M. and Wilson, W. *Minimal Brain Dysfunction,* ed.1. New York, Brunner/Mazel, 1974.

Hegarty, J. Psychological Assessment of Mentally Handicapped. *Nursing Mirror* 143:59, 1976.

Holmberg, N. Serving the Child with MBD and His Family. *Nursing Clinics of North America,* 10:381, 1975.

Hunt, M. and Gibby, R. *The Mentally Retarded Child: Development, Education, and Treatment,* ed.3. Boston, Allyn and Bacon, 1976.

Jobe, P. Therapy of Childhood Hyperkinesis. *Current Concepts in Psychiatry* 3:2, 1977.

Kinsbourne, M. MBD—A Fuzzy Concept Misdirects Therapeutic Effort. *Postgraduate Medicine* 58:211, 1975.

Kluss, K. Training the Mentally Retarded Child in Self Help Skills, in Brandt, P., Chinn, P., Smitt, M. (eds). *Current Practices in Pediatric Nursing.* St. Louis, C.V. Mosby Co., 1976, p. 157.

McCormick, D. Pediatric Evaluation of Children with School Problems. *American Journal Disabled Child* 131:318, 1977.

Niemeier, D. and Allison, T. Nurses Can Be Effective Behavior Modifiers. *Journal Psychiatric Nursing and Mental Health Services* 14:18, 1976.

O'Neil, S. Behavior Modification. *Nursing Clinics of North America* 10:373, 1975.

O'Neil , S., McLoughlin, B., Knapp, M. *Behavioral Approaches to Children with Developmental Delays,* ed. 1. St. Louis, C.V. Mosby Co., 1977.

Patullo, A. The Socio-Sexual Development of the Handicapped Child. *Nursing Clinics of North America* 10:361, 1975.

Phenylketonuria—Low Phenylalanine Dietary Management with Lofenalac. Evansville, Indiana, Mead Johnson Laboratories.

Reyzer, N. Diagnosis: PKU. *American Journal of Nursing* 78:1895, 1978.

Rogers, M. Early Identification and Intervention of Children with Learning Problems. *Pediatric Nursing* 2:21, 1976.

Walker, J. and Shea, T. *Behavior Modification* St. Louis, C.V. Mosby Co., 1976.

Wyatt, D. Phenylketonuria: The Problems Vary during Different Developmental Stages. *Journal of Maternal-Child Nursing* 3:296, 1978.

CHAPTER 12

The Child with a Behavioral Deviation

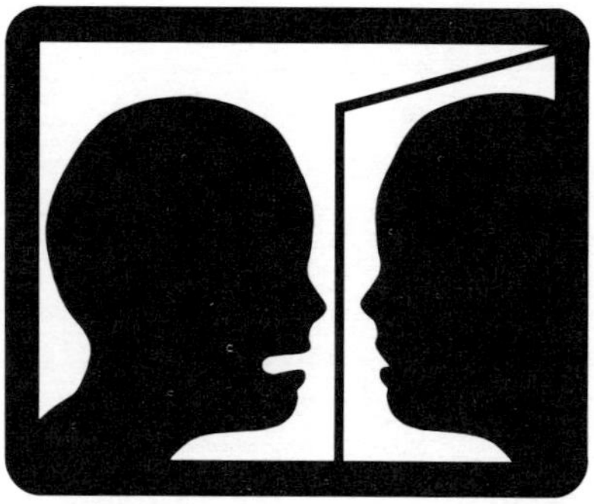

BEHAVIORAL OBJECTIVES

After studying this chapter you will be able to:

- Explain and discuss common causes, signs and symptoms, and nursing interventions for anxiety.
- Differentiate between neurotic and psychotic behaviors, giving examples and nursing interventions.
- Define psychotherapy and discuss individual, group, directive, and nondirective therapy.
- Name common misconceptions about drug abuse and suicide, listing behaviors of presuicidal and drug-abusing youth.
- Compare and contrast group versus individual delinquent behavior.
- Differentiate between normal, adaptive behavior and deviant, maladaptive behavior.

TERMS AND CONCEPTS

Anxiety
Neuroses
Phobia
Conversion hysteria
Obsession
Compulsion
Antisocial behavior
Juvenile delinquency
Drug abuse
Drug addiction
Habituation
Drug withdrawal
Suicide
Psychoses
Delirium
Illusions
Hallucinations
Childhood schizophrenia
Infantile autism
Psychotherapy
Individual therapy
Group therapy

Milieu therapy
Family therapy

Unexpressed anxiety can produce behavioral deviations of varying duration, frequency, and intensity. In this chapter, assessment factors for the child at risk for maladaptive, growth-inhibiting behaviors, and the appropriate nursing interventions and anticipatory actions are discussed. Terms used to designate behavioral deviations are discussed and related to specific examples. Diagnostic and treatment methods of supportive and curative value are listed and a table of specific behavioral deviations is presented (Table 12–1).

COMMON PROBLEMS AND NURSING INTERVENTIONS

Anxiety

To be loved and accepted is a basic human need. Love provides the child with physical and emotional security. A feeling of security comes from having one's needs met and knowing they will continue to be met. With love and security, the child completes developmental tasks while receiving the recognition needed to motivate the child toward other achievements. The mastery of developmental tasks leads to independence and self-confidence. The child feels adequate and worthwhile, and he is able to reinvest his love, affection, and trust into relationships with others. When emotional integrity is thwarted because basic needs are unmet or interrupted because of parental illness, absence, or rejection, the child experiences anxiety. *Anxiety* is the feeling of tension or dread that results when part of the child's self-concept is threatened. Anxiety is learned; a parent who was absent yesterday may leave again today. The possibility produces anxiety. Anxiety can inhibit development, cause physiological changes, distort perceptions, and render the child incapable of coping with daily situations.

Anxiety in its elementary form can produce excitement, motivation, and self-expression. It can promote and sustain growth and emotional maturity. However, anxiety that is unresolved, repressed, or not expressed may surface in the form of fear, anger, resentment, and frustration that stifle growth and batter the self-concept. When the child is unable to cope, he seeks to relieve his anxiety. If acceptable ways of relieving anxiety have not been learned or are not available to the child, fear and panic, aggression, withdrawal and depressive sullenness, or physical complaints emerge. Anxiety also consumes the energy needed for development.

Children experiencing anxiety are in special need of a positive, accepting environment in which their basic needs of love and security are met. As a nurse, you should not panic, pass judgment on, or become distraught with the child whose anxiety produces undesirable behavior. Act as the child's advocate by acknowledging his fears and complaints, protecting his feelings and allowing their expression without ridicule; bear in mind that although his expressions of anxiety may be inappropriate, he presently has no other means of expression. Do not try to remove the child's fears by forcing him into the situations that provoke the fear. Instead, discuss the child's fears with him, acknowledging them, and help the child to verbalize them. Acknowledging one's anxiety is the first step in learning to deal with it appropriately. Use touch to de-

Table 12–1. **Behavioral Deviations**

Behavior	*Definition*	*Treatment*	*Special Nursing Considerations*
Anaclitic Depression (Maternal Deprivation)	Failure of infants to thrive following prolonged separation from parents. Characterized by crying, followed by withdrawal, depression, and developmental retardation.	Presence of parents during hospitalization.	Promote parent-infant emotional and physical interactions during hospitalization (see ch. 4).
Encopresis	Involuntary defacation after the second year, not due to neuromuscular disease, and usually occurring during the day several years after bowel control is established. Causes include lack of parental affection, separation from parents, domination, or nagging.	Tranquilizers, psychotherapy.	Parental counseling and education to correct child-rearing misconceptions (e.g., as regards age of toilet training and expected independence). Halt punitive measures (e.g., shaming, scolding, spanking, threats, limiting fluids). Improve parent-child interactions that will decrease anxiety and increase bladder and/or bowel control. Provide positive, confidence-building experiences for the child and assure him that his problem can be helped.
Enuresis	Involuntary bladder emptying during the day or night beyond age four, not associated with loss of bladder control (i.e., incontinence). Causes include hereditary, emotional, organic, or socioeconomic factors.	Imipramine hydrochloride (Tofranil), psychotherapy.	

Pica	An appetite for and ingestion of unsuitable substances (e.g., sand, earth, grass, soot, paint from furniture or walls). Causes are obscure; lead poisoning is the primary hazard in homes with lead-based paint.	Parental education.	Offer parent education on oral needs and suitable articles for chewing, supervision during play, and dangers of lead intoxication.
Rumination	Purposeful and pleasurable regurgitation of ingested food, usually in infancy, with subsequent malnutrition and electrolyte imbalance. Causes include a detached, indifferent parental attitude.	Appropriate parenting.	Encourage fondling and stimulation of the infant and diversional activities after feeding.
Tics	Frequent, abrupt, purposeless, involuntary, habitual movements of a muscle group, usually involving the face and/or neck. Children eight to twelve most commonly affected, due to anxiety and tension.	Tranquilizers, psychotherapy.	Counsel parents against shaming or calling attention to the tic. Provide ample rest and appropriate physical activities for the child.

crease anxiety; calm the frightened child with long, smooth strokes or rocking motions. Holding the shoulders, arms, or a hand firmly while saying "slow down" or "take it easy" can calm the aggressive, "acting-out" child and aid him in regaining control. Patting the head, shoulders, or hands when the child regains composure indicates your approval, which reinforces his self-image. Be slow and unobtrusive when approaching the withdrawn, sullen, or depressed child. Place your hands on the child's shoulders briefly and stand nearby, allowing the child to sense your presence. Be careful not to overpower or startle the child. Act as a role model, explaining to the child's parents various methods to use in approaching their anxious or distraught child. Parents frequently become incapacitated during their child's outbursts of anxiety-related behavior and don't know what to do; they will usually welcome support and assistance.

Suggest a consistent daily routine for the child, specifying periods of activity and rest. Avoid needless restraint, confinement, or overly strict requirements. Provide activities that are appropriate for the child's age and level of development, and explain to parents the importance of not doing for the child what he can do for himself. The child who is experiencing increased anxiety needs independence and autonomy. Be clear and precise when speaking to the child, avoiding vague or indirect language: "Stop throwing the ball" is clearer than "Wouldn't it be nice if you were to stop throwing the ball?" Discourage temper tantrums, showing off, and teasing by ignoring the behavior, provided that the behavior poses no threat to safety; these behaviors increase when acknowledged. Remain calm and nonjudgmental; reasoning with a child during an outburst of temper is useless. Discuss teasing, showing off, or temper tantrums alone with the child, after the episode. Place emphasis on the child, not on the behavior. Encourage self-expression; talking and play decrease anxiety, and satisfying interactions can replace fears, complaints, and aggression.

Neurosis

Behaviors caused by repressed or unresolved conflicts are *neuroses*. Anxiety is the source of the neurosis; the neurotic behaviors reflect unrelieved anxiety. When anxiety is unrelieved, it may cause such physical symptoms as diarrhea, abdominal pain, headaches, insomnia, and constipation to surface. Phobias, conversion hysterias, and obsessive-compulsive acts are abnormal behaviors that reflect anxiety. A *phobia* is a fear of a particular object or situation (e.g., dogs, darkness, school). The child experiences uncontrollable apprehension when confronted with the phobic object. School phobia is common among chronically ill and overprotected children. The illness or hospitalization of a parent, or discord between parents, can also precipitate school phobia; the child wants to be at home to make sure nothing bad happens. Previous academic failure, embarrassment at physical or intellectual deficits, or a difficult home situation may also cause intense fear and provoke a school phobia. The child needs the reassurance that others understand his fears. Positive interactions and improved family communication patterns are needed to bolster the child's self-concept. An assessment of previous school attendance and achievement, coupled with an awareness of the possibility of school phobia after a lengthy hospitalization, can help the family recognize early signs of a problem and seek help. Statements such as "It is difficult to return to school after a long absence" or "It is hard to make up schoolwork" acknowledge to the child that you are aware of his concerns. Discussing ways to catch up on assignments (e.g., a visiting teacher, tutoring, or extra parental assistance in the evenings) can help relieve anxiety.

Conversion hysteria is the temporary loss or alteration of a sensory or motor function unaccompanied by detectable physical damage. The loss, such as blindness or paralysis, which is voluntary, serves to express unrelieved anxiety.

Obsessions are persistent and disturbing ideas. When a child feels compelled to act out obsessive thoughts in repetitive, ritualistic acts, *compulsions* result. The child may wash his hands abnormally often or walk in an unusual way. Many obsessive-compulsive behaviors begin in normal children; the behaviors are considered abnormal only when they interfere with school performance, general functioning, and the child's overall adjustment.

All children experience anxiety and handle it with varying degrees of appropriateness; normal, adaptive behavior becomes abnormal and maladaptive when the degree, frequency, and duration of the behavior interfere with functioning and exceed the bounds of social acceptance. It is important for parents to understand this difference between normal and abnormal behavior, or they will experience unnecessary alarm during normal developmental stages. It is advantageous to review with the family the normal growth and development patterns for their child's age, emphasizing that each child is an individual and will have unique ways of expressing his developmental problems (See chs. 4–8).

Antisocial Behavior

The extreme and impulsive behavioral expression of anxiety caused by unconscious, unresolved conflicts arising from hostility or love characterizes *antisocial behavior*. The antisocial youth frequently has poor judgment and lacks insight. Juvenile delinquent acts are an example of antisocial behavior.

Juvenile Delinquency

Juvenile delinquency is youthful behavior that violates the law. Much of the behavior is illegal only because of the child's age (as in the case of school truancy or "running away" from home). Three percent of American children appear in juvenile court every year for reasons other than traffic offenses. Twelve percent of all children between ten and seventeen, or one in every nine youths, will make one court appearance. Twenty percent of all boys will appear in court. These national figures are minimal because most youths who commit illegal acts are not apprehended, and of those who are apprehended, only a fraction appear in juvenile court; thus the actual incidence of delinquent behavior is higher than the figures indicate. Between 1973 and 1974 the number of fifteen- to seventeen-year-olds in the general population declined, but the incidence of violent crimes (homicide, rape, and assault) attributed to this group increased by more than 100 percent. This trend continues to accelerate. Since children with a history of delinquent behavior will be among those hospitalized, it is desirable for the nurse to have an awareness of their behavioral problems in order to understand these children and to be able to offer meaningful emotional care.

Most juvenile delinquent behavior occurs in the context of a gang. *Group delinquency* occurs in all socioeconomic strata; it is motivated and goal-directed, the goals being achievement, peer acceptance, and recognition. The gang delinquent feels secure, satisfied, and accepted in the gang. These youths possess a capacity for interpersonal relationships that can be exploited in their treatment, which should direct them toward social action programs that provide jobs and athletic activities, and neighborhood-based programs that provide legal recreational and income-producing activities that satisfy the need for recognition, acceptance and security.

A second form of delinquency is individual delinquency. The acts of the individual offender represent expressions of frustration and the need for recognition; the youth always manages to be caught in the act or shortly afterward. These youths are in need of effective rehabilitative programs, such as individual and family counseling, crisis intervention, jobs, and alternate educational programs.

In a third type of delinquent behavior, the individual has little concern for the impact of his behavior on others. The youth is a loner, extending trust and loyalty to no one. He has no regard for others or their feelings; he seeks to satisfy his needs by the most direct route. The youth is amoral, aggressive, impulsive, and narcissistic. His delinquent acts tend to be chronic, and frequently one of the child's parents showed similar behavior patterns. Intensive individual therapy is the treatment of choice. It is important to consider the type of delinquency in order to provide an atmosphere of acceptance and security and age-appropriate group activities (e.g., crafts, board games, table tennis, pool) that allow for individual and group achievement.

Drug Abuse

Excessive or compulsive use of a drug that damages the user's health, social, or vocational functioning, or is harmful to society, as in the case of driving while intoxicated, is called *drug abuse*. Among youth the most commonly used drugs are alcohol, nicotine, and marijuana. *Drug addiction* is characterized by a physical dependence on a drug, including a tolerance to the drug, and withdrawal illness if the drug is removed. Addiction occurs only with depressants (e.g., alcohol, sedatives, narcotics). *Habituation* is a psychological dependence and can occur with any drug or, for that matter, with reading, watching television, or listening to music.

The two abused drugs that cause most deaths, disabilities, and addiction are alcohol and tobacco; these drugs affect more youths than all other drugs combined. Although the sale of these substances to persons under 18 is illegal in most states, casual observation reveals their easy accessibility to young consumers.

Myths and misunderstandings surround drugs and drug use; educating youths and parents is crucial. Drugs do not affect all people the same way, or affect the same person the same way each time the drug is taken. No ingested drug, by itself, can cause a sexual experience, produce a genius, cause a burglary or killing, produce a solution to a school problem, or produce new friendships. Any drug experience is a product of the individual character, personality, mood, attitude, previous experience, and expectations of the user; the drug experience is first what the person is and second what the drug does.

Affluence, the mass media, peer pressure, parental influence, and twentieth-century technology have all been accused of causing and perpetuating the use of drugs by the young. It has been said that Americans are immersed in a drug culture; it is certainly true that youths have ready access to drugs, especially alcohol and tobacco. National statistics compiled in 1976 indicated that 50 to 70 percent of teenagers drink regularly, yet less than 30 percent find drinking enjoyable. Six out of ten traffic fatalities among youth involve alcohol. The effect of alcohol and other drugs is determined by the amount, purity, frequency of use, combination with other chemicals, interval since ingestion, and, most important, the personality of the user as he interacts with his environment. All drug overdoses are treated as emergencies. The medical concerns are to ensure an adequate airway (with the administration of oxygen if necessary), to assess cardiovascular integrity, and to begin intravenous fluids as a first step toward drug detoxification.

Drug Withdrawal

Discontinuance of a drug on which one is physically dependent may result in *drug withdrawal,* characterized by such symptoms as insomnia, vomiting, diarrhea, tremors, muscular aches, confusion and, in the case of withdrawal from depressant drugs, seizures. The symptoms occur 4 to 12 hours after the drug is withheld. Drugs can be withdrawn without any medication ("going cold turkey"), or with a medication that substitutes for the addicted drug (e.g., methadone for heroin) or with an agent that produces unpleasant effects when the addicted drug is taken (e.g., Antabuse given before alcohol ingestion). Drug withdrawal is a lengthy process requiring extensive emotional support of the patient and understanding of the patient's particular problems (see Table 12–2 for specific drugs used in a withdrawal program).

Numerous health problems are associated with continued drug abuse. The youth may be malnourished and have vitamin deficiencies. Record what the person's usual dietary intake is, discussing acceptable foods of high nutrient value that are affordable and available. Vitamin supplements are frequently necessary. Look for dental cavities and loss of teeth, making dental referrals as needed. Since drugs are frequently injected under septic conditions, assess the general condition of skin and check for abscesses and infected lesions. Because some drugs cause constipation, menstrual irregularities, and impotence, inquire if the youth has experienced any of these effects.

Identification of the drug-abusing adolescent (Figure 12–1), education to dispel myths and stereotypes, and referral to community help programs are the responsibilities of the nurse. Commonly abused drugs, their primary and long-term effects, and respective nursing interventions are listed in Table 12–2.

Suicide

Suicide is the fourth leading cause of death among American adolescents, preceded by accidents, malignant neoplasms, and homicides. Most suicide attempts and deaths are reported as "accidents," making the true number of cases much higher than statistics indicate. The ratio of suicidal gestures or attempts to actual deaths is 100:1.

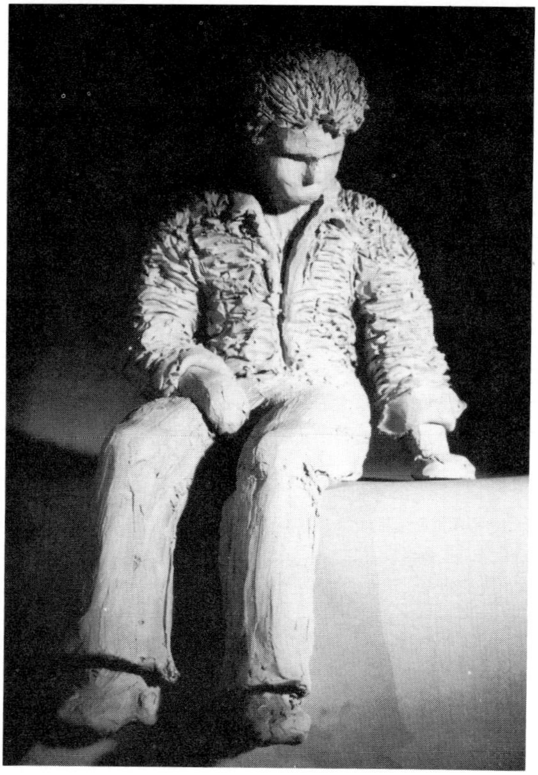

Figure 12–1. *The drug-abusing adolescent may have red, watery eyes and red, raw nostrils from glue-sniffing; a running nose from taking heroin, morphine, or codeine; raw lips, chapped by constant licking to relieve the dryness caused by amphetamines; profuse perspiration and body odor from taking amphetamines; long-sleeved garments worn constantly to hide needle marks; drastic weight loss from taking heroin or opium; staggering, disoriented appearance from taking barbiturates.*

Suicidal gestures frequently involve the ingestion of drugs or poison, although gunshot wounds are the most frequent cause of death in suicides of young people. Suicidal gestures are more common among girls. Suicide by youths is usually the expression of hostility toward a parent that has been transferred to the self. Feelings of rage, helplessness, and worthlessness dominate; the youth may perceive a real or threatened loss of a relationship with a parent or other loved person. The youth feels isolated, rejected, and guilty. He is depressed and may complain of constipation, loss of appetite or sleep, fatigue, or restlessness.

The only intervention in cases of suicidal youths is prevention. Suicide is a form of communication; when, how, where, and to whom the suicide is directed is the message. In assessing the depressed youth, be alert for suicidal warnings. The child who says "I'm going to shoot myself" or "People will be sorry when I'm dead" should be taken seriously. Never ignore statements of suicidal intentions. Explore the statement with the child as well as with parents and staff; the child who says "I'm no good" or "Everything I do is bad" is asking for help. The suicidal messages may be nonverbal; a drastic personality change or the giving away of personal possessions is an indicator of contemplated suicide (see Figure 12–2). The adolescent who attempts or completes a suicide often has a history of trying to communicate his inner distress by nonsuicidal means. A history of failing school grades, drug abuse, or delinquent behavior is a request for help. The child who talks about suicide, has a deflated self-image, is depressed, or makes suicidal gestures is at great risk.

Suicide attempts require immediate medical intervention. Respiratory maintenance, detoxification from an offending chemical agent, fluid and electrolyte management, and circulatory stabilization are first concerns. Next, psychological care is begun, with the goal of the resolution of the precipitating crisis and the restoration of behavioral function. Long-term goals include the elevation of behavioral function-

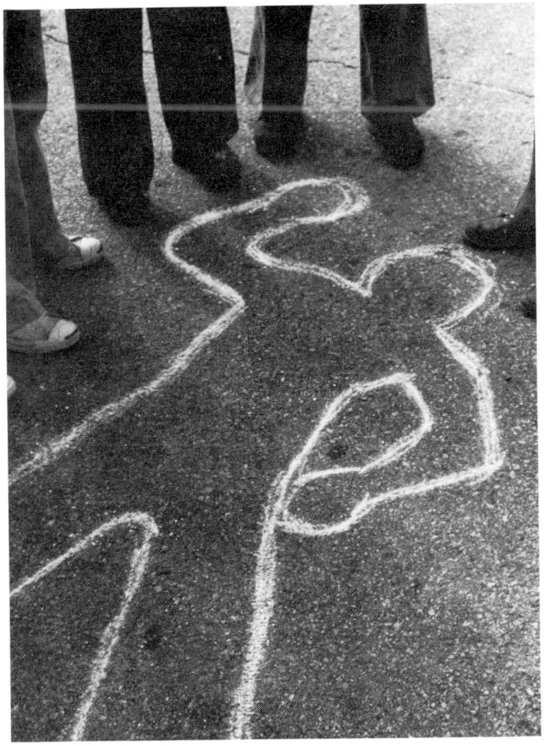

Figure 12–2. *Myth: People who talk about suicide never commit suicide. Fact: Eight out of ten people who kill themselves have given prior warning. Suicide threats and/or attempts are real and serious. Myth: Suicide happens without warning. Fact: Suicide persons give many verbal and nonverbal cues. Suicide attempts are a cry for help. Awareness and assessment can prevent suicide. Myth: Suicide is inherited; it runs in families. Fact: Suicide does not discriminate. It occurs in all socioeconomic, racial, and ethnic groups. It is an individual occurrence. It can be prevented. Myth: All suicidal children are "mentally disturbed," or insane. Fact: The suicidal child is extremely unhappy; he is not necessarily mentally ill or disturbed. The unhappiness may be from a temporary emotional crisis, a long and painful illness, or a loss of hope.*

ing to a state above the precrisis level. The hospitalized youth contemplating or having attempted suicide needs concern, care, and acceptance with attention given to basic needs and the promotion of feelings of security and worth. Traditional nursing safeguards, such as 24-hour vigils and the removal of all harmful objects including utensils, have been curtailed in many hospitals, with responsibility for behavior being placed on the youth, and a caring, trusting, and hopeful relationship with the nurse being offered instead.

A suicide increases anxiety in others. Repressed self-destructive urges are aroused. Suicide and suicidal attempts of others bring into focus our own mortality and its implications. The nurse is responsible for being aware of her anxiety, managing it, and not communicating it to the suicidal youth.

Suicide stigmatizes the victim's family, friends, and other concerned persons. Frequently, significant others do not know what to do or say to the family, so they remain silent and do nothing. The family is left isolated and senses rejection, which adds to existing guilt. The family feels inadequate, pondering what cues and signs they missed. They are compelled to relive over and over the events of the days immediately preceding the suicide. Many families will not accept a therapy program and the hours of grief-work needed to lessen the effects of loss. Although there is little information on ways for nurses to help families after a suicide, some general nursing interventions include being available to the family, being nonjudgmental, and *listening*. Although you are not a therapist, your accepting, noncritical attitude can pave the way for the family's willing compliance with a referral for therapy. This is a time to make no demands on the family and to assist them in simple, practical ways. Your concern, conveyed in such seemingly

Table 12–2. Commonly Abused Drugs

Drug (Slang Names)	*Immediate Action*	*Chronic Abuse Effects*	*Special Nursing Considerations*
Alcohol (booze, suds)	Central nervous system (CNS) depressant; decreased alertness, drowsiness, reduced inhibitions, impaired perception.	Impaired coordination and judgment, permanent liver and brain damage, addiction.	Antabuse, a medication, causes nausea when followed by alcohol and is used for withdrawal. Recommend self-help groups (e.g., Alcoholics Anonymous).
Hallucinogens/LSD (acid, cubes)	Intensely distorted sensory experiences (especially visual); rapid flow of ideas; mood changes; pupil dilation; increased pulse and heart rate; chills and shivering; anxiety.	Hallucinations, confusion, impaired judgment. Some studies document chromosomal breaks that last up to six months. Children of women who took LSD in early pregnancy have chromosomal changes.	An overdose intensifies distorted sensations. The person is afraid and anxious. Provide a quiet, destimulating place with soft lights and minimal noise. Reassure that the drug intensifies feelings and the drug will wear off. Establish verbal and physical contact; touch or hold, listen, and reassure the person that you will remain with him.
Marijuana (pot, grass, weed, joint)	Mixed CNS effects; increased appetite, decreased alertness and inhibitions. Euphoria, hilarity, changed time perception, glazed eyes, dry mouth, increased pulse.	Acute panic or hallucinations, bronchitis.	

Narcotics/Opiates (e.g., heroin, morphine, codeine) (junk, smack, horse)	CNS depressant: sedation, drowsiness, analgesia, decreased alertness and inhibitions, slurred speech, coma.	Constipation, decreased appetite, weight loss, addiction, accidental death from overdose.	Naloxone hydrochloride is given IV for opiate overdose. For withdrawal, methadone is substituted for the opiate and gradually reduced.
Nicotine (cigarettes, cigars)	CNS stimulant: increased wakefulness, decreased appetite.	Heart attacks, strokes, lung cancer, bronchitis, emphysema.	Health education.
Sedatives/ Barbiturates (sleepers, barbs, reds, yellow-jackets, goofballs)	CNS depressant: drowsiness, sedation, decreased alertness, reduced inhibitions.	Impaired coordination and judgment, drowsiness, stupor, confusion, addiction.	For overdose, gastric lavage (see ch. 18) and induction of alkaline diuresis to increase elimination of barbiturates. For withdrawal, a long-acting barbiturate (e.g., phenobarbital) is given with daily dosage reduction of 10 percent.
Stimulants/ Amphetamines (pep pills, bennies, dexies, speed)	CNS stimulant: increased alertness, restlessness, decreased fatigue, reduced appetite, talkativeness, dilated pupils, dry mouth.	Sleeplessness; weight loss and malnutrition; irritability, delusions, and hallucinations.	An overdose may produce hyperactivity and combativeness. Do not approach the person from behind. Approach slowly, speaking in a calm, soft tone. Avoid touching.
Tranquilizers (e.g., Valium, Librium)	Decreased tension and anxiety. Suppression of neurotic or psychotic symptoms.	Destruction of blood cells, jaundice, hypotension, muscular stiffness, blurred vision.	

small gestures as providing a cup of coffee or a comfortable chair, will also be of great help.

Juvenile delinquency, drug abuse, and suicide attempts are all antisocial behaviors that require long-term management. The hospital experience after a suicide attempt or a drug overdose may bring about the family's earliest awareness of the child's problem. Requests for referral information are common; being knowledgeable about community resources can help ensure meaningful referral.

It is difficult for parents and family to admit that a member of the family has a serious behavior problem. Children are extensions of their parent's hopes and desires. To acknowledge that one's child has an emotional or psychological problem is to cast doubt on one's parenting and child rearing abilities, a difficult process for any parent. In talking with the family, acknowledge society's negative attitude toward behavior disorders and discuss coping mechanisms that the family can use during this difficult period. (Review Chs. 2 and 3.)

Psychoses

Psychoses are extreme, bizarre disorders in behavior. Psychotic disorders are classified as functional or organic. *Functional psychoses* are behavioral deviations unaccompanied by an identifiable structural or metabolic alteration. *Organic psychoses* have an identifiable structural or metabolic cause. Organic psychoses can be caused by infection (e.g., pneumonia, septicemia, or viral pathogens), chemical intoxication (e.g., drug abuse), trauma, growth anomalies (e.g., tumors), vascular insufficiencies (e.g., stroke), or febrile convulsions.

In children, psychotic behavior stemming from an organic cause usually persists until the infection or intoxication has abated; treatment therefore is directed at the illness. Delirium often accompanies febrile convulsions (see Table 27–1). Approximately 10 percent of hospitalized children will have some degree of delirium. *Delirium* is a dreamlike state of consciousness. The delirious child is unable to distinguish between mental images and perceptions. Illusions and hallucinations may occur. *Illusions* are false perceptions of real stimuli; for example, the child who hears a vacuum cleaner but perceives it as a wild bear growling at him. *Hallucinations* are sensory experiences occurring in the absence of external stimuli. Although hallucinations may involve any of the senses, auditory hallucinations (for example, hearing the voices of persons not present) are the most common. Both hallucinations and illusions can cause severe anxiety and restlessness, especially at night. The child is disoriented to time and place; he is confused. Disorders of memory may occur.

Strive to decrease the hospitalized child's anxiety by reducing stimuli and providing a restful atmosphere. Use night-lights and avoid repositioning of furniture and equipment to reduce confusion. Approach the child slowly and speak softly. Assure parents that the irrational state usually subsides as the child improves and that the medicine and treatments are directed to restoring health. Promote closeness of parent and child by having parents talk to the child, telling him they are present. Encourage parents to visit and remain with the child as much as possible.

Before age two, the child with a functional psychosis usually resists physical contact and prefers to be alone. The child appears aloof and seclusive, seeking minimal physical contact with other people. A distinct lack of interest in surroundings is displayed. Age-appropriate developmental and academic abilities, including self-care skills, are deficient; regression is the rule. The child is occupied with self-stimulating activities and repetition of motions and words. Speech is impaired or delayed. The sense of identity is vague and disorganized, and the child frequently refers to himself in the third person. Functional psychoses occur in 3 of 10,000 children; the cause is not understood.

Childhood schizophrenia and *infantile autism* are examples of psychotic behavior states. The former term is applied to children between 8 and 12 years of age; the latter to children who are 3 years old or younger. Both disorders are characterized by extremely distorted personality. Children with these disorders pay little attention to environmental stimuli and are engrossed in self-stimulating behaviors. Normal development and task mastery are severely impaired and delayed, and no improvement can be expected until the child's attention span is increased. It is important to assess the psychotic child's developmental level. With the parents' help, determine what communication means are available to the child. What vocabulary does the child possess? What emotions are expressed(e.g., fear, joy, hate)? Is the child aware of his body? Does he know the names of body parts? Can he distinguish himself from others? Does the child refer to himself in the first person (e.g., *I, mine, me*) or third person (*John, boy*)? Is the child withdrawn or aggressive? Does he sit close to others or maintain a distance? What are the child's general behavior patterns? When, how and what does he eat? How well does he sleep? What are his elimination patterns and self-help abilities? Using the assessed information, establish a communication plan. Touch can communicate your concern and acceptance as effectively as verbalizing. If some form of communication is established with the child, then a relationship can begin. The relationship is the foundation for nursing interventions that help the child maintain and promote his developmental abilities while hospitalized. When the psychotic child is hospitalized, the first nursing intervention is to meet the physical needs for nourishment, comfort, rest, and activity. Second, safety precautions must be taken so that the child will not hurt himself or others. Third, communication should be established. Finally, developmental abilities must be maintained and, if possible, advanced. The psychotic child will need long-term referral care, the ultimate goal being the reestablishment of the child's sense of identity and mastery of developmental tasks.

COMMON DIAGNOSTIC STUDIES AND NURSING IMPLICATIONS

The diagnostic methods discussed in chapter 11 also apply to the child with a behavioral deviation.

COMMON TREATMENTS AND NURSING IMPLICATIONS

Psychotherapy

Psychotherapy refers to any treatment for an emotional disorder that seeks to change thought, mood, and behavior. The treatment may be nondirective or directive, involve an individual or group, occur in a formal setting or an informal one, such as in schools, community mental health centers, or hospitals.

Nondirective and Directive Therapy

Nondirective psychotherapy places responsibility on the child. The principle of therapy is that the child has the resources for change and growth within himself. The therapist provides opportunities for the child to become aware of his strengths and resources. The relationship between therapist and child is characterized by warmth and concern, usually on a one-to-one basis. The focus is on the present, and activities are adjusted to individual needs. The therapist guides the sessions, but the child sets the pace.

In *directive psychotherapy* the therapist guides the youth into experiences that develop awareness. Behavioral therapy is a form of directive psychotherapy in which the therapist divides task behaviors into a series of smaller task behaviors, using reinforcers to increase target behaviors (see ch. 11). In directive therapy, the therapist assumes an active, intrusive role. The goal is to help the child with specific problems. Games, role playing, and psychodrama are among the techniques used in directive psychotherapy.

Play Therapy

Play is the usual context of psychotherapy for children. The play may be directed or nondirected. Play provides a means of communication as well as a way to express internal conflicts and anxiety. Different types of play have different therapeutic uses. For example, punching bags, toy guns, pounding boards, and ball games can provide an appropriate release for aggression, while doll houses, puppets, and blocks allow fantasy play and provide a stage for the portrayal of internal conflict. Board games (e.g., checkers, chess, Monopoly) can stimulate interpersonal contact and communications. Manual dexterity and developmental mastery are promoted with crafts, cooking, or sewing. Lastly, sensory stimulation is achieved with sand or water play. The trained play therapist carefully chooses the type of play according to the therapeutic goals.

Group Therapy

Group psychotherapy has bloomed since the 1960's. Among the types of groups are sensitivity, activity, "rap," marathon, encounter, and transaction groups. Group activities range from lecture and discussion formats to in-depth analyses of individual and group behavior. Various activities are used to stimulate the group interaction process, on which emphasis is placed.

Groups may or may not offer qualified, professional direction. Consumers should be advised to carefully evaluate any group program. Many self-help groups (e.g., Narcotics Anonymous and Alcoholics Anonymous) deal with specific problems in a group setting.

Milieu Therapy

The use of the social environment to treat behavior deviations is called *milieu therapy*. The physical atmosphere, the personal attitudes and interactions, and the social context of the living arrangement are examined in an attempt to alleviate behavioral disorders by providing relationships that satisfy emotional needs, reduce psychological conflicts and strengthen personality development. The child is an active participant in his care, making decisions about matters that affect him. Therapy is frequently education-oriented, using the teacher-pupil model to rehabilitate the child. The goal of milieu therapy is environmental manipulation for the purpose of facilitating adaptation to appropriate social interactions.

Family Therapy

Nuclear families or extended families participating as a unit in psychotherapy constitute the client in *family therapy*. The underlying assumption in family therapy is that disorders of the family are primarily responsible for the child's behavioral deviations. The goal is to change family interaction patterns, promoting individual growth and emotional integrity.

Behavior Modification

Behavior modification refers to the systematic application of reinforcement principles to change deviant, maladaptive behavior to adaptive behavior (see ch. 11).

Medication

Major tranquilizers such as Thorazine and Stelazine are used to reduce anxiety and psychotic symptoms (e.g., hallucinations, agitation, and withdrawal); minor tranquilizers such as Librium and Miltown reduce the mild-to-moderate anxiety associated with neuroses. Both types of tranquilizers act directly on the central nervous system to produce changes in thought, mood, and behavior. Stimulants or antidepressants are prescribed for the hyperactive child to decrease activity and lengthen the child's attention span (see ch. 11).

SUMMARY

Anxiety is the result of forces that thwart emotional integrity and interrupt basic need fulfillment. Repressed or unresolved anxiety, manifested in phobias, conversion hysteria, or obsessive compulsive acts, constitutes a neurosis. Nursing interventions for anxiety include the use of verbal and nonverbal communication to calm and reassure the child and to promote a feeling of security and acceptance.

Intense behavioral expressions of anxiety include such antisocial acts as juvenile delinquency, suicide, and drug abuse. Delinquency may involve a group or an individual. Gang delinquency is cohesive and goal-directed; individual delinquency communicates the anxieties and needs of the individual.

Drug abuse and suicide are still widely misunderstood; education and prevention are nursing responsibilities. Providing for basic needs and a communicating, trusting relationship with the nurse are basic to reestablishing the emotional integrity of the suicidal or drug-abusing child.

Perceptual distortions typify the psychotic child. Delirium, hallucinations, and illusions are alterations in sensory perception that require the maintenance of a safe environment where basic needs are met and some form of communication is established.

Psychotherapy is treatment directed at resolving emotional problems. The forms of treatment include individual, group, and milieu therapy.

CLINICAL APPLICATION

"Damn you, go to hell!" Rick turns the radio louder and buries his head in the pillow as his parents leave the room. At sixteen, Rick has been in juvenile court twice for stealing and has attempted to commit suicide with drugs. He has been hospitalized after an accident the previous night due to reckless driving. Although he has broken several bones, he did not injure any major organs. Rick will be on the adolescent unit for several weeks. He complains of pain hourly, stating that the medicine for pain is "no good." He refuses meals, indulging in the candy bars, crackers, and Coke his friends bring. You have requested a 30-minute interview with his parents this afternoon to assess their son's physical and emotional needs. In preparing for the interview, list questions that will assess:

- family communication patterns;
- family strengths and weaknesses;
- family awareness and perception of Rick's previous and present behavior;
- family concerns, worries, and needs.

Bearing in mind that anxiety is caused by a frustration of basic needs, list questions the answers to which will determine whether Rick's need for love, security, and acceptance is being met. If so, how? If not, what factors are interfering?

What questions about Rick's behavior at home, school, and with friends will aid your care plan?

After the interview you set the following goals:

1. Provided with appropriate inpatient activities, Rick will experience peer acceptance, accomplishment, and increased self-esteem.

   Considering the adolescent's needs and developmental abilities, list appropriate activities and a rationale for each.
2. You will talk with Rick twice daily for 15 minutes at each session.

   For two days you and Rick discuss sports and music. You find out he plays the guitar and has always wanted to take lessons. However, his parents dislike music, find it a waste of time, and have refused to pay for lessons. Rick smiles, uses appropriate language, and seems to enjoy each visit. He has not requested pain medication since the daily planned interactions began. After explaining the importance of regular meals and allowing Rick to make menu selections, snacking ceases. As you begin to leave today, Rick says, "No one really cares about me; I'm just no good." Discuss your possible responses and your rationale for them.
3. After a staff meeting, family psychotherapy is recommended to Rick's parents. Rick's parents angrily tell you "We are not a crazy family, only Rick. By the way, what is family psychotherapy anyway?"

   Briefly define psychotherapy, explain principles of family therapy, and guide Rick's parents in selecting a referral resource.

Bibliography

Anthony, E. The Behavior Disorders of Childhood, in Mussen, P. (ed). *Carmichael's Manual of Child Psychology,* vol. 2, ed 3. New York, John Wiley & Sons, Inc., 1970, p. 667.

Bakwin, H., and Bakwin, R. *Behavior Disorders In Children.* Philadelphia, W. B. Saunders Co., 1972.

Bourne, G. and Lindley, P. Suicide. *Nursing Mirror* 143:49, 1976.

Bragg, T. Teen-age Alcohol Abuse. *Journal of Psychiatric Nursing and Mental Health Science* 14:10, 1976.

Carter, M. *Psychosocial Nursing Theory and Practice, in Hospital and Community Mental*

Health, ed. 2. New York, MacMillan Co., 1976, p. 391.

Duffy, J. *Child Psychiatry: Medical Outline Series.* New York, Medical Examination Publishing Co., 1974.

Farberow, N., MacKinnon, D., Franklyn, L. Suicide: Who's Counting? *Public Health Reports* 92:223, 1977.

Fort, J. Youth: Drugs, Sex and Life. *Current Problems in Pediatrics* 6:40, 1976.

Haber, J., Leach, A. M., Schudy, S. M., Sideleau, B. F. *Comprehensive Psychiatric Nursing.* New York, McGraw-Hill, 1978.

Hofmann, A. D. Adolescents in Distress, Suicide and Out of Control Behaviors. *Medical Clinics of North America* 59:1429, 1975.

Hughes, J. G. Psychologic Aspects of Childhood, in *Synopsis of Pediatrics,* ed. 4, St. Louis, C. V. Mosby Co., 1975, p. 49.

Johnson, R. and Magrab, P. *Developmental Disorders: Assessment, Treatment, Education.* Baltimore, University Park Press, 1976.

McAnarney, E. Suicidal Behavior of Children and Youth. *Pediatric Clinics of North America* 22:595, 1975.

McDonagh, M. Behavior Modification Principles and the Use of Nursing Approaches as a Means of Reducing Enuresis and Encopresis, in Fagin, C. (ed). *Nursing In Child Psychiatry.* St. Louis, C. V. Mosby Co., 1972.

Nader, P., Bullock, D., Caldwell, B. School Phobias. *Pediatric Clinics of North America* 22:605, 1975.

Payne, D. *Psychiatric Mental Health Nursing: Nursing Outline Series.* New York, Medical Examination Publishing Co:, 1974.

Pinkerton, P. Pediatric Psychiatry. *Nursing Mirror* 143:60, 1976.

Pothier, P. *Mental Health Counseling With Children.* Boston, Little Brown and Co., 1976.

Schnoll, S. Guidelines for the Care of the Drug Abusing Patient. *Hospital Medicine,* 12:85, 1976.

Segal, J. (ed). *Research In The Science Of Mental Health: Report of the Task Force of National Institute of Mental Health.* Department of Health, Education, and Welfare, No. (ADM) 75–237, 1975, p. 1.

Trail, I. Symposium on Alcoholism and Drug Addiction. *Nursing Clinics of North America* 11:481, 1976.

Weiner, J. Juvenile Delinquency. *Pediatric Clinics of North America* 22:673, 1975.

Weinz, F. Effects of Seasons and Sociological Variables on Suicidal Behavior. *Public Health Reports* 92:233, 1977.

Weissman, M. Self Destructive Youth: A Problem in Primary Prevention. *Current Concepts in Psychiatry* 2:24, 1976.

CHAPTER **13**

The Child with a Psychosomatic Disorder

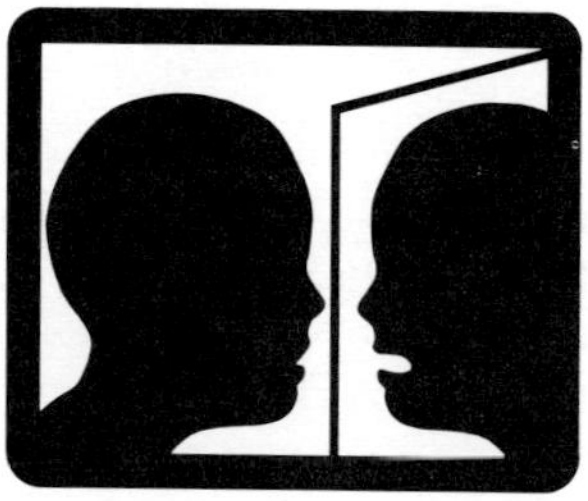

BEHAVIORAL OBJECTIVES

After studying this chapter you will be able to:

- Discuss the phenomenon of psychosomatic illness.
- Identify and describe the factors that contribute to a psychosomatic disorder.
- Differentiate between constructive psychosomatic reactions and destructive psychosomatic reactions, offering examples.
- Construct nursing care goals that minimize anxiety and convey concern and acceptance of the child with a psychosomatic illness.

TERMS AND CONCEPTS

Psychosomatic disorder
Psyche
Soma
Constructive psychosomatic reaction
Destructive psychosomatic reaction
Genetic predisposition

Disorders that are described as *psychosomatic* (from the Greek words *psyche,* meaning "soul," and *soma,* "body") are physiological dysfunctions and structural changes that result primarily from psychological factors rather than from physical ones, such as mechanical trauma, drug intoxication, or infection.

The concept of psychosomatic illness presupposes an integration of physical and emotional factors in health and illness. To this extent, psychosomatic medicine opposes the mechanistic and impersonal aspects of earlier, strictly physiological schools of medical diagnosis and treatment. The concepts of psychosomatic medicine have by now been scientifically tested and documented, and occupy a recognized role in health care.

This chapter will discuss the origins, manifestations, diagnosis, and treatment of psychosomatic disorders. Nursing interventions in prevention, support, and education will be presented with reference to the specific psychosomatic illnesses summarized in Table 13–1.

COMMON PROBLEMS AND NURSING INTERVENTIONS

Constructive and Destructive Psychosomatic Reactions

As was discussed in chapter 12, anxiety can cause behavioral responses that are adaptive and health-promoting as well as responses that are maladaptive and detrimental to normal growth and development. Anxiety can create a wide variety of physiological changes, including modification of the diameter of blood vessels with resultant changes in heart rate and blood pressure; alterations in the rate, depth, and regularity of breathing; changes in the formation and chemical composition of urine; and alterations in body secretions. If these physiological responses promote functioning, they are *constructive psychosomatic reactions*. For example, the internal mobilization of energy and strength for defense or protection are essential for individual survival.

Physiological changes that result from emotional stimuli and impede optimal functioning are *destructive psychosomatic reactions*. For example, the increased secretion of gastric juices that leads to a peptic ulcer, or changes in cellular production or destruction that are sustained, repeated, or intensive can result in psychosomatic disease.

Table 13–1 lists common psychosomatic disorders, their treatment, and nursing interventions. These disorders are psychosomatic in that they are physiological dysfunctions and frequently result in part from repression of frustration, conflict, or anxiety, that is, from psychological causes. However, each of the disorders may also result from organic causes or complications of an organic disorder.

Psychosomatic Illnesses Versus Behavioral Deviations

Psychosomatic illnesses differ from conversion hysteria neurosis (discussed in ch. 12). The child with a conversion hysteria resulting in blindness or paralysis experiences a temporary behavioral deviation; there is no detectable tissue and/or structural change. The behavior relieves anxiety and thus solves a problem for the child.

The child with a psychosomatic illness is also seeking relief from anxiety (Figure 13–1). A difficult home situation (arising from tension within the family, role confusion, lack of communication, overconcerned or abusive parents, etc.), peer pressures and demands, or prolonged illness can cause a behavioral deviation or a psychosomatic disorder. These two kinds of illness differ in that the child with a psychosomatic condition exhibits definite tissue and /or structural change. The condition is frequently lengthy and may be chronic; in some cases, such as in anorexia nervosa, the child may even die.

Predisposing Factors And The Needs Of The Psychosomatically Ill Child

All children experience emotional trauma, yet only a few develop a psychosomatic illness. Why? Each child is born with characteristics inherited from each parent. *Genetic predisposition* is a primary factor in psychosomatic disorders. In addition to obvious physical traits, the child inherits internal structural characteristics. These include the degree of strength and durability of muscles, vessels, and tissues. Each structure in the individual has its level of resistance to stress. Some muscles, vessels, and tissues will alter their function in response to stress far more rapidly than other tissues in the same person, or than the same

Table 13–1. Specific Psychosomatic Disorders

Disorder	*Definition*	*Treatment*	*Special Nursing Considerations*
Acne	Dermatitis of sebaceous (oil-secreting) glands and hair follicles of face, back, and shoulders causing *papules* (small, solid elevations) and *vesicles* (small, fluid-filled elevations), affecting 80 percent of adolescents. The acne lesions are an inflammatory reaction caused by exposure to oil. Tension and anxiety can increase the secretion of skin oils and the severity of acne.	Medications: Skin cleansing with sulfur and salicylic acid preparation (e.g., Fostex bar, cream and liquid). Antiseborrheic lotion containing sulfur that inhibits microbial growth and dries the skin (e.g., Fostril, Sulforcin). Additional preparations commonly used include benzoyl peroxide, resorcin, retinoic acid, sodium triosulfate. Systemic antibiotics (e.g., tetracycline) and/or estrogen in selected cases. Ultraviolet light weekly to increase peeling of the skin. Surgical removal of deep lesions. Cosmetic surgery for deep scarring.	Offer emotional support and acceptance. Body image is distorted at a crucial developmental period. Discourage squeezing, pinching, and picking at lesions; suggest the use of gloves while doing homework or watching television. Urge avoidance of greasy cosmetics. If ultraviolet light treatments are used at home, instruct in safety requirements; eyes should remain closed during treatment; advise parental supervision to guard against burns from overuse or accidents. Assess diet and advise the reduction of foods that aggravate acne (e.g., chocolate, nuts, carbonated beverages, fried or fatty foods).
Anorexia nervosa	Loss of appetite, severe weight loss, hyperactivity, and menstrual irregularities. Morbid fear of obesity. Excessive feelings of anxiety, fear, and guilt; distorted body image. Ninety percent of affected youth are females between sixteen and twenty-three years old.	Bedrest, immediate use of intravenous tube, or oral feedings to restore electrolyte and nutritional balance; 21 percent of affected youth die from malnutrition or intercurrent infection. Psychotherapy, behavior modification.	Avoid threats, pleas, and health advice. The youth is listless and depressed. Express concern and acceptance.

Bronchial asthma	Difficulty in breathing *(dyspnea)* caused by spasms of the bronchial muscles. Symptoms include shortness of breath, gasping for air; coughing, thoracic contraction, and a whistling noise on expiration *(wheezing)*. Bronchial spasms may be allergic responses (see ch. 16) or a reaction to emotional stimuli.	Psychotherapy. Hyposensitization, medications, physical therapy, avoidance of allergens. (Chapter 16 includes a detailed discussion of emergency and chronic care treatments for the child with altered sensitivity.)	Observe parent-child interactions during hospitalization, paying special attention to events preceding asthmatic attack. Provide a calm, concerned atmosphere, avoiding unnecessary tension and anxiety. Maintain consistent limits on behavior.
Constipation	Infrequent and difficult passage of hardened feces, frequently accompanied by pain and rectal bleeding. Child may begin retaining feces because of emotional reasons. The feces harden and are difficult to evacuate; anal fissures may develop, increasing stool retention and further constipation.	Medications: Mineral oil, 1–2 teaspoons, 1–2 times daily, mixed in orange juice. Stool softeners (e.g., Colace) Enemas (see Skills Manual). Dietary alterations.	Establish a consistent daily elimination schedule. Plan a diet of high-roughage foods (e.g., bran, whole wheat, fruits, and vegetables). Discourage use of laxatives, anal suppositories, or forced increased fluid intake because these procedures help only temporarily and produce additional frustration and hostility, usually worsening the constipation. Advise child and parents that stool retention is not dangerous; it only distends the colon. Focus attention on the child.
Dermatitis	Inflammation of the skin, accompanied by *erythema* (redness), papules, and vesicles. Oozing of the vesicles causes encrusting, scaling, and thickening of skin.	Avoid contact with or ingestion of irritants. Apply wet dressings (e.g., Burow's solution) for anti-inflammatory and antipruritic effect. Systemic antibiotics for infection; topical corticosteroid cream and ointments.	Tension, fear, and anxiety may cause the child to itch and scratch. The anxious child, who may be more aware of itching sensations, may inflict urticaria and excoriations on himself. Many allergic conditions are associated with emotional disturbances (see ch. 16).

(continued)

Table 13–1. *(Continued)*

Disorder	*Definition*	*Treatment*	*Special Nursing Considerations*
Gastric and Peptic Ulcer	An erosion of the mucous membrane of the stomach (gastric ulcer) or upper small intestine (peptic ulcer) caused by hypersecretion of acid gastric juices. Varying degrees of pain are experienced. Dangers include perforation and hemorrhage. Most ulcers in children heal rapidly and do not require treatment for more than three to four weeks.	Psychotherapy. Rest; bland diet, high in milk and dairy products: gradual resumption of normal diet thereafter. Medications: gastric antacids containing aluminum hydroxide (e.g., Maalox, Gelusil, or Mylanta) taken between meals; antispasmodic, anticholinergic drugs (e.g., propantheline bromide); multivitamins. Blood transfusions for hemorrhage. Surgical removal of ulcer *(gastrectomy)* if perforation or obstruction occurs.	Psychotherapy is very important because one-half of all children with chronic ulcers have recurrent ulcers as adults. Dietary restrictions can produce additional emotional stress and secondary behavioral deviations. Plan a palatable, easily digested and nonirritating diet, avoiding spicy and high-roughage foods. Evaluate for pallor and iron deficiency anemia (see ch. 24), which frequently develops because of bleeding and dietary alterations.
Headaches	Recurrent head pain, usually in late childhood and early adolescence. In headaches of psychosomatic origin, the pain is continuous, as opposed to intermittent organic head pain. The child may be depressed and is frequently anorectic and constipated. Anxiety is the primary predisposing factor.	Analgesics (e.g., aspirin, acetaminophen). Resolution of precipitating anxiety. Antianxiety drugs (e.g., Librium) may be prescribed in conjunction with psychotherapy.	Provide for ample rest and sleep in a quiet, darkened room. Seek to avoid or minimize experiences that provoke the pain.
Infantile Eczema	Dermatitis in young children, accompanied by redness, itching, and oozing of vesicular lesions that become scaly, encrusted, and hard. Exacerbated by certain foods or other allergens (see ch. 16).	Avoid allergens. Application of Burrow's solution soaks to relieve pruritus (itching). Medications: antibiotics for local infection; antihistamines (e.g., Benadryl, Periactin) for pruritus; tranquilizers to re-	Explain use of soaks, allowing child to handle gauze. Prewarm room to avoid chills when wet soaks evaporate and cool. Cut fingernails short and use gloves or sock mittens to discourage scratching. Provide

		duce anxiety and promote rest. Topical corticosteroids for improved appearance and comfort.	diversionary activities and assure parents and child that appearances are temporary and treatments will help.
Migraine	Recurrent headaches, usually on one side of the head, often preceded by a visual aura, and followed by nausea and vomiting. The pain is caused by expansion of cranial blood vessels following abnormal constriction of intracranial arteries (which produces the aura). Migraines usually run in families.	Psychotherapy. Medication: ergotamine preparations (e.g., Cafergot) taken orally or by suppository. Analgesics (e.g., aspirin, Tylenol) are used to reduce pain.	Medication must be taken during vasoconstriction (aura) period to prevent pain from vascular distension.
Obesity	Persistence of excessive fatty tissue beyond early childhood. Hereditary factors can contribute to obesity. Many obese children seem to satisfy an emotional hunger for love, security, or attention by eating. Although children are rarely hospitalized for obesity, it is a frequently encountered condition.	Psychotherapy. Reduction of food intake. Exercise. Anorexigenic drugs (e.g., amphetamines and related compounds) as an adjunct to above treatments. The drugs lose their effectiveness in 6 to 8 weeks.	Education on diet and exercise. Devise a plan with the family to increase energy expenditure, encouraging planned exercise and activities. Exercise does not increase appetite. Offer education on caloric values of various foods and an assessment of child's home diet. "What do you usually eat?" or "How often do you eat?" elicits little information; be specific. If yesterday was a typical day, ask exactly what the child ate and how it was prepared (e.g., fried or baked, fresh or cooked). Child is usually depressed and lacks self-esteem. Avoid judging attitude, teasing, or scare tactics. Provide concern and age-appropriate activities. Summer camps and obesity clubs help some youngsters.

(continued)

Table 13–1. *(Continued)*

Disorder	*Definition*	*Treatment*	*Special Nursing Considerations*
Ulcerative Colitis	Chronic inflammation and ulceration of the colon, causing abdominal pain and recurrent diarrhea and rectal bleeding, accompanied by loss of appetite and malnutrition. Hemorrhage and perforation are dangers. Diagnosed by sigmoidoscopy (see ch. 18).	Psychotherapy. Bed rest, liberal fluid intake, nonirritating diet. Blood transfusions if necessary. Colectomy (surgical resection of the colon) and ileostomy (the creation of an opening through the abdominal wall into the ileum). Medications: anti-inflammatory, immunosuppressive preparations (e.g., prednisone) to control symptoms; anticholinergic and antidiarrhea preparations (e.g., Lomotil, Donnagel-PG) to decrease bowel activity; tranquilizers for anxiety; analgesics for pain; supplemental vitamins and iron for malnutrition and anemia; sulfonamide preparation (e.g., Azulfidine) to control symptoms.	Encourage activity as tolerated. Provide appetizing diet and measures to decrease anorexia (see ch. 18). Establish a home routine for taking medications. Assess for pallor and iron deficiency anemia arising from bleeding and dietary alterations (see ch. 24). Surgical preparation and appliance education if an ileostomy is performed.

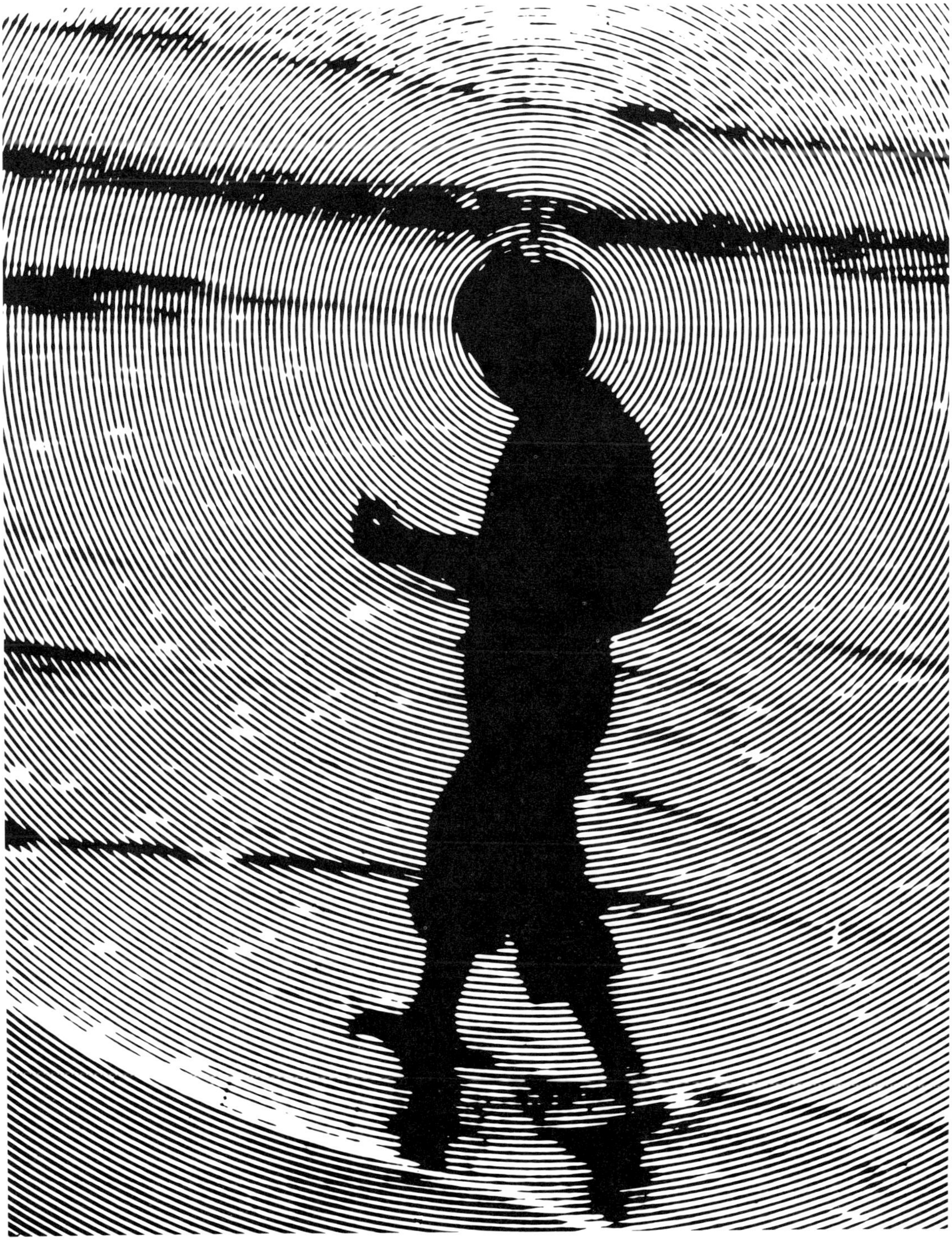

Figure 13–1. *I am angry, I am confused I do not understand me. I hurt but feel no pain. I cry but have no tears. PLEASE HELP ME.*

type of tissue in another person. Environmental insults can also predispose a structure to increased vulnerability. Air or water pollution and drug or chemical ingestion may alter resistance levels. Another determinant in the development of a psychosomatic illness is the intensity, duration, and frequency of the emotional stimuli; the more frequently the individual is affected by emotional reactions, the greater the likelihood of a psychosomatic disorder.

The child with a psychosomatic illness needs concern, acceptance, and basic need fulfillment. The nurse should seek to relieve feelings of shame and/or guilt in children suffering from psychosomatic conditions by reassuring them that their illness does not mean that they are "bad."

Avoid the common pitfall of lavishing attention when symptoms become most pronounced and ignoring the child as the symptoms diminish; be consistent, directing communication and activities toward the child, not toward the symptoms. "John, how do you feel?" fosters individual recognition and attention; but "How is the diarrhea today?" places emphasis on the symptom. Negative behavior will persist if reinforced. The child with a psychosomatic illness may use his symptoms to obtain sympathy, special attention, and such favors as exemption from school, chores, or other unpleasant activities. An awareness of the principles of behavior modification, and especially, of the principles of reinforcement, can be of great help to parents, siblings, and concerned others as they relate to the child.

Provide play and peer-interaction activities that ensure success and achievement and minimize frustration. Plan the child's daily routine with the parents, allowing for a balance of play, rest, sleep, and nourishment. Tell the child and family about diagnostic tests and procedures, allowing time for questions in order to alleviate unnecessary fear and anxiety.

Offer education and guidance about child-rearing practices to the parents. Find out when the parents feel the child should be eating, toileting, and dressing independently. What methods have they been using to teach these skills, and what have they been doing if the child does not succeed? Most emotional problems in children arise from surface conflicts between them and their parents, regarding such matters as developmental tasks, school, or family expectations. Psychosomatic illnesses, like perceptual deviations, cerebral dysfunctions, and behavioral deviations, place further stress on the parent-child bond. Special diets, medications, and procedures may hinder normal activities, resulting in anxiety and behavioral deviations that further complicate the disease state. For example, overly harsh, anti-allergy measures imposed on the child with asthma, such as forbidding pets, camp, or family or peer outings where environmental control is difficult, will produce resentment and anger portrayed in behavior that does not stem from the emotional stimuli that caused the psychosomatic illness.

Most parents would prefer not to believe that emotional problems can affect their child's physical state. The family with a psychosomatically ill child tends to "shop" for medical care, hearing what they wish, ignoring the rest. Be alert to the complexities of psychosomatic illness in children, and intervene with a plan of support, concern, and acceptance.

COMMON DIAGNOSTIC MEANS AND NURSING INTERVENTION

Physical Examination and Health History

The child with a psychosomatic illness will experience various procedures; support and education are primary nursing responsibilities.

A physical examination and health history can help determine if an organic disorder is partially or totally responsible for the symptoms. Give close attention to the family's medical history, noting other members with symptoms similar to the child's. Frequently, a family pedigree will be drawn, showing the sex, generation, and relationship to the child of each family member with similar symptoms. Assess developmental abilities by determining when self-care abilities were initiated and how they were taught. Explore parental goals, concerns, and frustrations as they relate to the affected child. The family health history will also assess family roles, parenting behaviors, communication patterns, and the child's relationship to each family member. Psychological testing may be performed.

COMMON TREATMENTS AND NURSING INTERVENTIONS

Psychotherapy

The goal of psychotherapy is to identify the emotions that are causing the child's symptoms and to enhance the child's coping ability and emotional stability. Therapy assists the child in recognizing the people, objects, events, ideas, attitudes, feelings, or situations that promote his symptoms. With awareness and identification, the child can learn how to cope more effectively with anxiety-provoking situations.

Medication

A variety of pain-relieving and function-promoting medications are used to temporarily decrease the symptoms until the underlying emotional problem is resolved. (See the specific psychosomatic conditions in Table 13–1).

Surgery

Structural changes due to a psychosomatic illness may require partial or total surgical removal of the affected organ. Fortunately, surgery is usually not necessary in psychosomatic disorders of children.

SUMMARY

Emotion shapes behavior. If emotional stimuli are positive, need-fulfilling, and rewarding, behavior is adaptive and growth-promoting; the child thrives. If emotional stimuli defer the fulfillment of the child's needs, produce conflicts, and cause frustration, destructive psychological reponses may produce symptoms of psychosomatic illness. Persistent negative emotional responses, genetic predisposition, or environmental insults can produce a psychosomatic dysfunction.

Nursing care procedures should place emphasis on the child, not on his illness. Offer the parents education and guidance in order to rid them of the misconceptions and to reduce their anxiety. Allow the child to express his emotional conflicts so that feelings can be dealt with more adaptively.

CLINICAL APPLICATION

"But I don't want to live with Grandma, I want you." Beth, an only child, was 10 last year when her parents separated and her mother accepted a demanding management job. Beth went to live with her grandmother, 100 miles away, until her mother would be able to support Beth and herself. Beth's mother tried to visit every weekend; however, her job demanded long hours and frequent weekend work, and lately she had begun to dread the visit because Beth cried and refused to eat for days after she left. Always a good student, Beth's grades had become progressively worse this year, and her only interest was watching television. Beth refused to play with girls her age in the neighborhood and last week decided to stop ballet and piano lessons. Beth asks daily when she can go live with her mother and although her grandmother was initially understanding and patient, she has become distraught with Beth's seemingly ungrateful attitude and her unwillingness to help around the house.

Two months ago, Beth told her grandmother she had begun her period for the first time; she had seen blood spots on her underpants that morning. Several days later Beth had a large, bloody bowel movement. Frightened, she told her grandmother, who told Beth that menstrual blood frequently drains into the toilet with a bowel movement.

During the past month Beth has had two episodes of bloody diarrhea with abdominal pain. Because she still refused to eat and was looking very pale, she was taken to the local family physician, who found that Beth was severely anemic; he recommended that Beth be admitted to the hospital for tests to determine the cause of the anemia and diarrhea. The studies indicated that Beth has ulcerative colitis, a disease of the large intestines. The bowel is inflamed and ulcerated, causing bleeding and abdominal pain. Although Beth can be given medication to make her more comfortable, the cause of the disease is almost always rooted in emotional problems that the family must work toward solving.

The next morning you enter the room to hear Beth expressing emphatically her desire to live with her mother. Beth's mother responds, "I just don't understand. Lots of children have parents that are separated or divorced and those children don't get sick. Why is Beth reacting like this? How can feelings cause stomach pain and diarrhea? I don't understand."

> Explain the nature of stress and the various responses of children to family disruption. Discuss what is meant by a psychosomatic disease.

Beth's grandmother is present and states that she had an ulcer as a young woman, and that Beth's mother had severe acne and constipation as a teenager. She asks if psychosomatic disorders run in families.

> Explain genetic predisposition.

Beth's mother tells you that she wants very much to care for her daughter but is fearful of Beth being alone in the apartment until she gets home from work after 9 P.M.. Beth quickly responds that she is 11 now and old enough to be alone. Beth promises to keep the door locked, do her homework, and follow her mother's instructions. Beth's mother sighs, "I just do not know what to do."

> This is a crisis period for Beth, her mother, and grandmother. To design a

care plan for Beth, list the developmental tasks of the school-age child. What intellectual, social, and motor skills does the child of this age have? List questions that will enable you to assess the mother's understanding of Beth's developmental level, her expectations of Beth, and her concerns. Also, list questions that will help you to assess Beth's concerns and expectations of living with her mother instead of with her grandmother. What is important to Beth? What information do you need to assess Beth's self-concept? Finally, the grandmother is an important family member; what questions will help evaluate her feelings about Beth's behavior, school performance, and emotional needs?

Beth tells you her grandmother will not allow her to wear a training bra, lipstick, or jeans. Beth feels different and embarrassed. You offer to talk to Beth's mother and grandmother.

Using information about the school-age child and the developing self-concept, what can you tell Beth's mother and grandmother about the importance of body image and its relationship to Beth's self-concept? Also, stress the importance of focusing attention on Beth, not on her symptoms of diarrhea and anorexia. Suggest ways the family can do this.

Following a medical conference, a referral for family therapy is offered to Beth's family. After two months of therapy, Beth begins staying with her mother on weekends with plans for a permanent move when school ends in two months. Beth has begun to choose and buy her clothes and lipstick from money earned at household tasks. Her grades are improving, and Beth has resumed ballet and piano lessons. Each family member is seeking to discuss feelings, not allowing emotions to fester.

Bibliography

Bakwin, H. and Bakwin, R.M. *Behavior Disorders in Children,* ed. 4. Philadelphia, W. B. Saunders Co., 1972, p. 557.

Carter, M. *Psychosocial Nursing Theory and Practice in Hospital and Community Mental Health,* ed. 2. New York, Macmillan Co., 1976.

DiKowitz, S. Anorexia Nervosa. *Journal Psychiatric Nursing and Mental Health* 14:28, 1976.

Finch, S.M. Psychophysiologic Disorders in Children and Adolescents. *International Journal Psychiatry in Medicine* 6:213, 1975.

Haber, J., Leach, A.M., Schudy, S.M., et al. *Comprehensive Psychiatric Nursing.* New York, McGraw-Hill, 1978.

Halmi, K. Anorexia Nervosa, Demographic and Clinical Features in 94 Cases. *Psychosomatic Medicine* 36:93, 1974.

Kempe, C., Silver, H., O'Brien, D. *Current Pediatric Diagnosis and Treatment,* ed. 5. Los Altos, California, Lange Publishers, 1975.

Lachman, S. *Psychosomatic Disorders: A Behavioristic Interpretation.* New York, John Wiley & Sons, Inc., 1972.

Miklich, D. and Tal, A. Emotionally Induced Decreases in Pulmonary Flow Rates in Asthmatic Children. *Psychosomatic Medicine* 38:190, 1976.

Rome, H. and Martin, M. Psychiatric Aspects of Gastrointestinal Function and Disease, in Bockus, H. (ed). *Gastroenterology,* vol. 4, ed. 3. Philadelphia, W.B. Saunders Co., 1976.

Stern, C. Dermatology in Adolescents, in *Adolescent Medicine Topics,* vol. 1. New York, Spectrum Publishers, 1976.

Stunkard, A. From Explanation to Action in Psychosomatic Medicine: The Case of Obesity. *Psychosomatic Medicine* 37:195, 1975.

Tolman, P. Acne and Acneiform Dermatoses, in Moschella, S., Pillsburg, D., Hurley, H. (eds). *Dermatology,* vol. 2, ed. 1. Philadelphia, W.B. Saunders Co., 1975, p. 1129.

Vaughan, V., McKay, R., (eds). *Nelson's Textbook of Pediatrics,* ed. 10. Philadelphia, W.B. Saunders Co., 1975.

SECTION TWO

Immunologic Homeostasis

CHAPTER **14**

The Immune System

BEHAVIORAL OBJECTIVES

After studying this chapter you will be able to:

- Describe the reactions of immunoglobulins, complement, leukocytes, and the lymph system to a pathogen.
- Explain the difference between innate immunoglobulins and antibodies.
- Explain how immunizations protect children from disease.
- List the steps of the inflammatory response.
- Describe the effects of local and systemic infection on the body.
- List and describe three types of altered immunity.

TERMS AND CONCEPTS

Pathogens
Antigens
Rejection reaction
Lymph network
Leukocytes
Immunoglobulins
Complement
Reticuloendothelial system
Phagocytosis
Chemotaxis
Ameboid locomotion
Antigen-antibody reaction
Antibodies
Opsonization
Lysis
Inflammatory response
Histamine
Pus
Immunity, active and passive
Immunization
Infection, local and systemic
Hyperimmunity (hypersensitivity)
Hypoimmunity (immunodeficiency)
Autoimmunity
Anaphylaxis
Atopy

The child's world is filled with disease-causing agents called *pathogens*. These agents can be found in his food, crib, air, clothes, pets, parents, friends, siblings—everywhere! Even the healthiest environment is teeming with germs. Although the child cannot escape exposure to pathogens without being totally isolated, his skin and mucous membranes keep the vast majority of pathogens outside the body. Once these barriers have been broken, however, the well child still receives a remarkable degree of protection from the immune system and inflammatory response. Most pathogens are stopped near the point of invasion, and many daily traumas are healed without notice. Every child will occasionally succumb to pathogens and develop disease, but he usually stays healthy without the help of medicine or treatment.

There are several types of pathogens. Chapters 14, 15, and 16 will focus on the pathogens that the body recognizes as foreign and on the trauma they produce. These pathogens, called *antigens,* can be infectious, chemical, allergic, malignant, or autoimmune. The infectious microorganisms are bacteria, viruses, fungi, and rickettsia, although larger parasitic organisms are also included in this group. Chemical agents include poisons, irritants, and the toxins produced by infection. Allergic pathogens (allergens) are particles that cause an abnormal, excessive reaction when they touch the skin or mucous membranes. Malignancies are growths that the body may attack as foreign invaders or that the body may allow to grow without resistance. Autoimmunity is a disease state in which, for some unknown reason, the body's own tissues are attacked as foreign matter by the body's defense mechanism. Grafted tissue and organs, such as transplanted heart and kidneys, are truly foreign tissue, and they initiate a *rejection reaction* by the immune system. The body reacts in essentially the same way to all trauma, whether caused by these antigens or by falls, cuts, burns, and so forth. The immune response and inflammatory response, therefore, will be discussed together.

The immune system is not easily identified or understood. Only recently have physiologists begun to recognize the relationship among several different body organs in protecting the body from all types of antigens. The immune system is made up of the *lymph network, leukocytes, immunoglobulins,* and serum *complement.* As a team, these components are highly efficient, attacking an antigen according to its specific properties. All other body systems, which depend on the immune system for protection, provide the chemical components of immunity and the transportation of the substances involved.

THE LYMPH NETWORK

The lymph network is composed of lymph, a system of vessels, and lymphoid tissue. Lymph is simply plasma, the fluid portion of the blood, that has passed from the blood through the body tissues into the lymphatic vessels, losing some protein along the way. These thin-walled vessels depend on muscle contraction to move the lymph forward and a series of valves to prevent backward flow. The entire system empties into the major veins for recirculation as plasma. Lymphoid tissue is found in the lymph nodes, the thymus gland, the spleen, the tonsils, and probably other areas of the body. All lymphoid tissue produces lymphocytes and plasma cells; it also filters lymph in order to trap and destroy unwanted particles (such as microorganisms and aged cells). The plasma cells and leukocytes that stay fixed in the lymph network make up another component, the *reticuloendothelial system* (RE system).

LEUKOCYTES

The leukocyte is a white blood cell. It differs from the erythrocyte (red blood cell) in color, structure, function, and number. The mature erythrocyte is round, smooth, biconcave, nonnucleated, and about 7 microns in diameter. It carries oxygen throughout the body. The white cell is round but somewhat irregular and nucleated; it ranges from 8 to 20 microns in diameter. It responds to foreign matter and trauma to the body. Depending on one's sex and age, the average well person has between 4.5 and 6 million erythrocytes per cubic millimeter of blood, but only 4.5 to 20 thousand leukocytes per cubic millimeter. Both leukocytes and erythrocytes originate in the bone marrow as stem cells. Of the different types of leukocytes, the smallest—the thrombocyte, or platelet—is a part of the body's clotting mechanism. The plasma cell produces immunoglobulins. The other five types of leukocytes—lymphocytes, monocytes, neutrophils, eosinophils, and basophils—all have varying capacities for *phagocytosis,* movement by *chemotaxis,* and *ameboid locomotion.* Phagocytosis is the process by which a cell engulfs an offending particle, destroys it, and then excretes the harmless remains. Cells capable of phagocytosis are called phagocytes: the large ones are called macrophages, and the small ones, microphages. Chemotaxis is the body's chemical mechanism for attracting the needed leukocytes to sites of trauma and invasion. Ameboid locomotion is accomplished by jelly-like extensions of the leukocytes' boundaries that "walk" the cells through capillary walls and body tissues to the problem areas (see Figure 14–1).

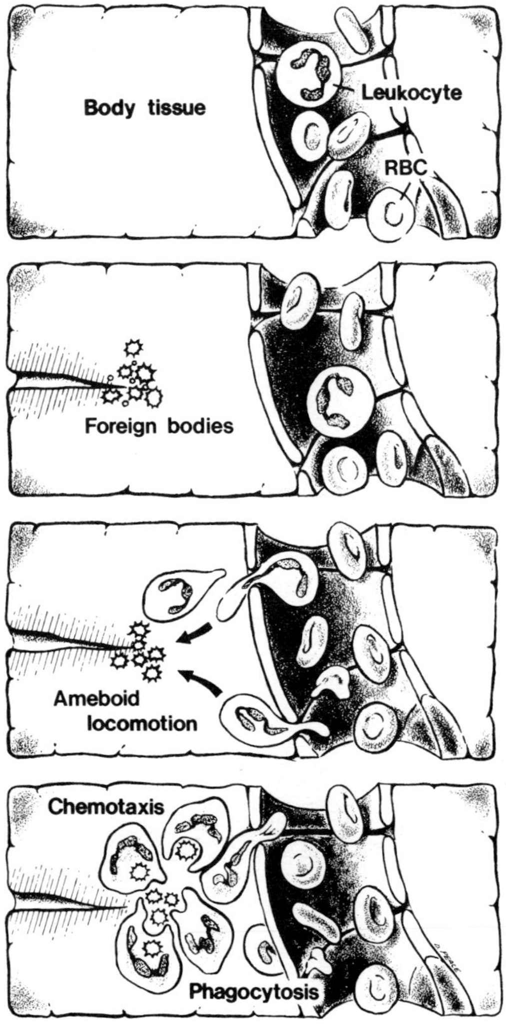

Figure 14–1. *Leukocytic response to foreign bodies.*

The lymphocyte is of great importance in protecting the body. It originates as a stem cell in the embryonic bone marrow. After being released from the bone marrow, the immature lymphocyte is influenced either by the thymus gland to become a T lymphocyte (thymus-derived) or by an area labeled "bursa-equivalent" to become a B lymphocyte. Both B and T lymphocytes migrate to lymphoid tissue and fill them by reproduction. When an antigen enters the body, some T cells begin to multiply and attack the offender, while others will circulate for the life of the individual, prepared to attack that one antigen in case it ever enters the body again. B lymphocytes can circulate in the blood or remain in the lymphoid tissue as plasma cells, producing immunoglobulins.

IMMUNOGLOBULINS

Immunoglobulins are complex proteins that are normally found in plasma, body secretions, and tissue fluid. Immunoglobulins bind antigens, inactivating them or marking them for phagocytosis or attack by complement. This process, the *antigen-antibody reaction,* may result in the clumping of reactive by-products in body tissues. There are two types of immunoglobulins: those produced innately in all normal humans, and those produced in response to individual invaders. The innate immunoglobulins are labeled with letters: A, D, G, E, and M (written IgA, IgD, IgG, IgE, IgM). These immunoglobulins protect the human being from many microorganisms that cause disease in other animals. IgG, the most abundant immunoglobulin, is responsible for most of our innate defense. Those immunoglobulins that develop in response to specific antigens are called *antibodies*. Once the body has been exposed to a specific antigen, the B lymphocyte enlarges and changes to a plasma cell that produces antigen-specific antibodies. With each successive invasion by that specific antigen, the already "sensitized" plasma cells respond by rapidly producing more antibodies (see Figure 14–2).

COMPLEMENT

Complement is a series of normally inactive proteins that are found in varying concentrations in serum; there are nine complement compounds. An antigen-antibody reaction activates the complement pathway, which results in the *opsonization* and *lysis* of foreign cells, mostly bacteria. In opsonization, complement coats the outside surface of the offending cell (see Figure 14–3). This coating makes the cell considerably more inviting to the phagocyte. Lysis is the destruction of a cell by means of a hole in the cell boundary that allows extracellular fluid to pour into the intracellular space until it bursts (see Figure 14–4). Complement components stack on top of each other until they all are working together to create the hole in the invader's cell wall. Once the hole has been made, the inward flow occurs naturally. The complement components also participate in chemotaxis and clotting.

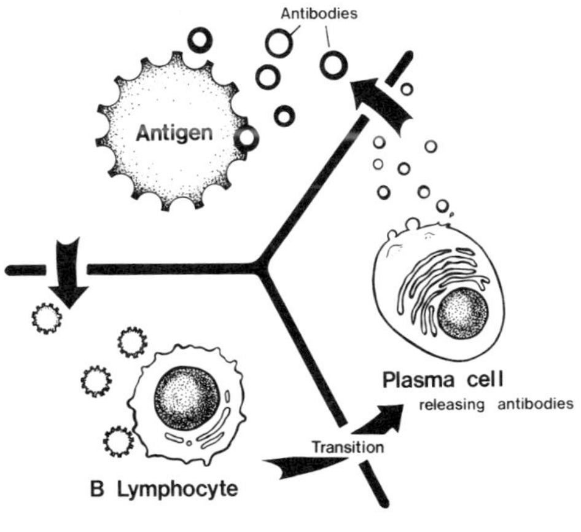

Figure 14–2. *Antigen-antibody reaction.*

THE INFLAMMATORY RESPONSE

The skin and mucous membranes provide the body with an excellent first line of defense. Immunoglobulins produced by the lymph glands in some of these surfaces

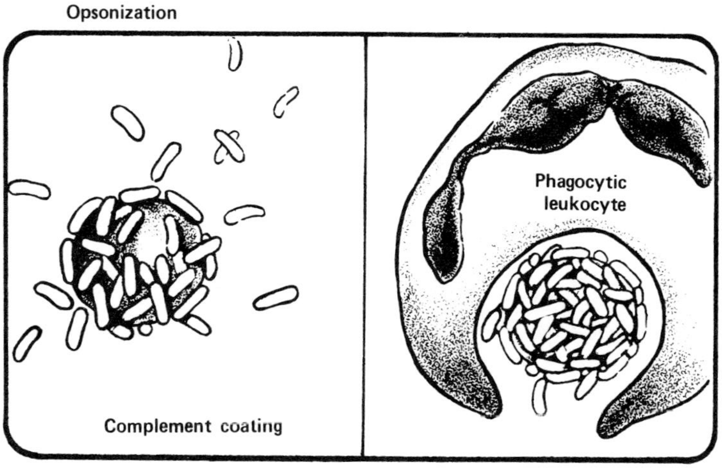

Figure 14–3. *Opsonization.*

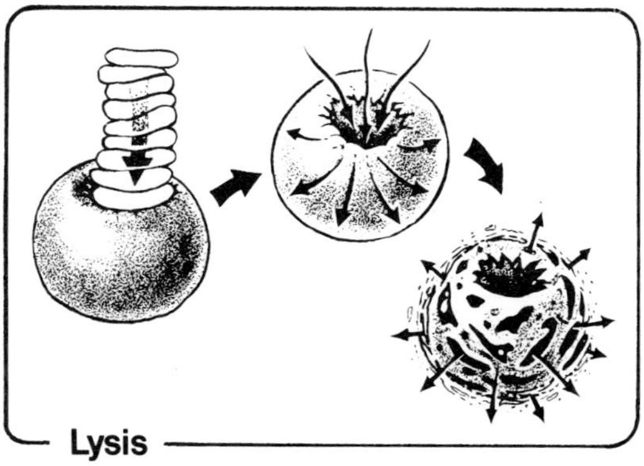

Figure 14–4. *Lysis and complement action.*

strengthen the barrier. When this defense fails and a pathogen invades the body, the immediate area becomes warm, reddened, swollen, and painful, a process called the *inflammatory response.* The function of inflammation is to destroy or neutralize the intruder and to help repair the damaged site.

When the tissues are invaded by pathogens, the damaged cells release chemicals that attract leukocytes to the area through chemotaxis. Some leukocytes line the blood vessels surrounding the insult and pass on through the vessel walls to help destroy the invaders chemically, or they completely fill the vessel, helping the thrombocytes in the clotting process. Other leukocytes engulf and remove the invaders and dead matter. The damaged cells also release *histamine,* which dilates the local vessels (vasodilation), increasing the amount of blood flow, and allows freer movement through the vessel walls (increased vascular permeability). Since the vessels are holding a substantial amount of leukocytes and fluid that can easily pass through to the tissues, the damaged area becomes edematous (swollen with fluid), warm, and red because of increased circulation, tissue fluid, and cellular activity. Local pain is caused by swelling of the tissues and, probably, by chemicals from damaged tissues.

Edema and leukocytes help contain the foreign substance near its point of entry. Leukocytes, dead material, and tissue fluid form a creamy discharge, *pus,* in the inflamed area. While the inflammatory response is in progress, the immune system is producing antibodies to the invader. The antibodies join with the antigen to form a unit that is easily removed by phagocytosis. If the invader moves through the tissue fluid, away from the site of invasion, it is filtered by a lymph node. The leukocytes in the lymph node multiply in order to attack, destroy, and remove the agent from the node. These actions may cause the node to enlarge and, occasionally, the node itself undergoes the inflammatory response. If the invader is released into the bloodstream, the protective mechanisms of the blood and the spleen usually destroy it before damage occurs in other parts of the body.

IMMUNITY

Immunity is the state of defensiveness against specific foreign substances, created by antibodies. In *active immunity,* the body produces its own antibodies, and in *passive immunity,* the body receives antibodies from other sources.

Active immunity is acquired either by contracting a given disease or by receiving an *immunization.* An immunization is a medication that contains weakened or killed organisms, organisms similar to the antigen, or modified toxins called toxoids. Both the disease *and* immunization stimulate the production of specific antibodies. The ability to produce more antibodies (antigenic memory) in response to a subsequent invasion by a given agent usually lasts a lifetime, although certain antibodies need the stimulus of a periodic booster immunization. Immunizations usually cause a subclinical inflammatory reaction, but in rare cases, they may produce a severe form of the disease.

Maternal antibodies received through the placenta and in breast milk provide the newborn with passive immunity. A child who has been exposed to a disease may be given an injection of antibodies from another person or animal who has already had the disease. These antibodies, which act as if they had been produced in the child, will weaken or kill the agent. Another type of passive immunity is afforded by injections of antibodies that have been pooled from many different people, and which attack a variety of pathogens. Passive immunity is never permanent, since the body cannot reproduce the antibodies acquired from other sources.

Immunization has drastically changed the entire world's health. At one time no one understood how infections came about, much less how to prevent them. Infectious diseases wiped out whole generations, towns, and armies. No one knew about germs. Physicians never washed their hands before surgery or before delivering babies. Many people died from infection soon after minor surgery or normal childbirth. The medical profession also had no knowledge about immunity from infectious diseases. Rural people, however, had long recognized that people who had had cowpox were somehow protected against smallpox. From that first piece of information emerged a whole range of immunizations that offer protection against such diseases as tetanus, diphtheria, pertussis, polio, and so forth (see Tables 14–1 and 14–2).

DEVELOPMENT OF BODY DEFENSE

The newborn leaves the protective environment of his mother's uterus relatively unprepared to defend himself against

Table 14-1. **Recommended Schedule for Active Immunization of Normal Infants and Children**

2 mo	DTP[1]	TOPV[2a]
4 mo	DTP	TOPV
6 mo	DTP	[2b]
1 yr		Tuberculin test[3]
15 mo	Measles,[4] Rubella[4]	Mumps[4]
1½ yr	DTP	TOPV
4–6 yr	DTP	TOPV
14–16 yr	Td[5]—repeat every 10 years	

[1]DTP—diphtheria and tetanus toxoids combined with pertussis vaccine.
[2a]TOPV—trivalent oral poliovirus vaccine. This recommendation is suitable for breast-fed as well as bottle-fed infants.
[2b]A third dose of TOPV is optional but may be given in areas of high endemicity of poliomyelitis.
[3]Frequency of repeated tuberculin tests depends on risk of exposure of the child and on the prevalence of tuberculosis in the population group. For the pediatrician's office or outpatient clinic, an annual or biennial tuberculin test, unless local circumstances clearly indicate otherwise, is appropriate. The initial test should be done at the time of, or preceding, the measles-rubella or
[4]May be given at 15 months as measles-rubella or measles-mumps-rubella combined vaccines (see Rubella, section 9, and Mumps, section 9, for further discussion of age of administration).
[5]Td—combined tetanus and diphtheria toxoids (adult type) for those more than 6 years of age, in contrast to diphtheria and tetanus (DT) toxoids which contain a larger amount of diphtheria antigen. *Tetanus toxoid at time of injury:* For clean, minor wounds, no booster dose is needed by a fully immunized child unless more than 10 years have elapsed since the last dose. For contaminated wounds, a booster dose should be given if more than 5 years have elapsed since the last dose.

Concentration and Storage of Vaccines

Because the concentration of antigen varies in different products, the manufacturer's package insert should be consulted regarding the volume of individual doses of immunizing agents.

Because biologics are of varying stability, the manufacturer's recommendations for optimal storage conditions (e.g., temperature, light) should be carefully followed. Failure to observe these precautions may significantly reduce the potency and effectiveness of the vaccines.

Table 14-2. **Primary Immunization for Children Not Immunized in Early Infancy** [a]

Under 6 Years of Age	
First visit	DTP, TOPV, Tuberculin Test
Interval after first visit	
1 mo	Measles[b], Mumps, Rubella
2 mo	DTP, TOPV
4 mo	DTP, TOPV[c]
10–16 month or preschool	DTP, TOPV
Age 14–16 yr	Td—repeat every 10 yr
6 Years of Age and Over	
First visit	Td, TOPV, Tuberculin test
Interval after first visit	
1 mo	Measles, Mumps, Rubella
2 mo	Td, TOPV
8 to 14 mo	Td, TOPV
Age 14–16 yr	Td—repeat every 10 years

[a]Physicians may choose to alter the sequence of these schedules if specific infections are prevalent at the time. For example, measles vaccine might be given on the first visit if an epidemic is underway in the community.
[b]Measles vaccine is not routinely given before 15 months of age (see Table 14-1).
[c]Optional.

pathogens. He has only a limited ability to manufacture innate immunoglobulins, antibodies, and complement, and his inflammatory response is immature. Because of these natural deficiencies, microorganisms can quickly spread throughout his small body. The human is born, however, with placental IgG, which usually contains specific antibodies for certain diseases such as rubeola (measles), rubella, and mumps. Also, the spleen acts as a filter for unwanted particles in the bloodstream. If the newborn is breast-fed, his gastrointestinal tract, part of the upper respiratory tract, and perhaps even the middle ear are protected from most infections by the immunoglobulins in breast milk. By six months of age, the infant is producing his own innate immunoglobulins and antibodies. With exposure to each new antigen, he develops a specific antibody that will prohibit further intrusions by that invader. Such activities as attending a day care center or kindergarten will cause him to be exposed to infections, which will result in the formation of new antibodies. As the child accumulates a variety of antibodies, he is able to withstand many different pathogens. By the time he reaches school age, the immune-inflammatory system is almost mature, and by adolescence it is complete.

INFECTION

Infection is a disease state in which microorganisms reproduce in the body, causing damage in the process. If the agent can move from one person's body to another and still multiply, the disease is contagious. Microorganisms can be transmitted through water, food, animals, direct contact, injections, infusions, human wastes, and airborne droplets from the nose and mouth. Infection is a biological accident, occurring only when there is a break in the body's defenses. The severity of an infection depends on the characteristics of the host, the invader, and the environment. The child's age will determine his susceptibility to many types of illnesses because of his developing immunity to specific microorganisms. Such health factors as other diseases and poor nutrition will lower his natural resistance. A person's previous exposures and immunizations can prevent some diseases thanks to antibody production in subclinical cases.

The characteristics of the invader that affect the severity of an infection are the number of microorganisms entering the body, their virulence, and their ability to produce damaging toxins. Some microorganisms require specific environmental conditions, such as tropical temperatures, humidity, or crowded living conditions, in order to thrive and spread.

Infections can be either localized or systemic. A *localized* infection produces the typical inflammatory response—redness, swelling, pain, warmth, and pus formation. There is a loss of function in the infected area. If the skin is affected, it can no longer protect the underlying tissues. If the brain is infected, the child exhibits neurological symptoms that may lead rapidly to death. If the infection is *systemic* (throughout the body), all tissues may function abnormally. The child usually has damaged cells, and this raises the overall body temperature. Whether an infection is localized or systemic depends on the magnitude of the inflammatory response.

Altered Immunity

The immunological mechanism is not always perfect. If a child tends to overreact to an antigen, he has *hyperimmunity*; if he does not react effectively to an antigen, he has *hypoimmunity*. If his body suddenly attacks its own tissue as if it were foreign matter, he has *autoimmunity*. In each of these conditions, the balance between beneficial and damaging inflammatory response is lost.

Hypoimmunity, also called *immunodeficiency* and *hyposensitivity*, is a rare disease caused by one or more missing, insufficient, or incompetent parts of the immune system. Primary immunodeficiency refers to a defect, usually congenital, in the system itself. The child may be born without a thymus, or he may have improperly functioning complement. His body may not produce innate immunoglobulins or antibodies. He may have too few leukocytes, or they may be abnormal. Children with various deficiencies develop serious infections as soon as the maternal antibodies no longer offer protection, i.e., around six months of age. If the defective part of the immune system can be replaced, the prognosis may be good. Immunoglobulin and antibody deficiencies can be successfully treated with gamma globulin. Other immunodeficiencies usually result in death. Diseases (cancer, infections), medication (steroids), and treatments (irradiation) may produce secondary immunodeficiencies, which are treated by replacing the depressed part of the immune system if possible.

Hyperimmunity, commonly known as *allergy* or *hypersensitivity*, occurs frequently in children today. The body responds abnormally to food, contact material (such as clothing and soap), and particles in the air with an excessive antibody response. The skin, mucous membranes, and surrounding tissues (such as respiratory and gastrointestinal tracts) may be affected. As with all inflammations, there will be edema, reddening, warmth, and increased mucous and leukocyte (mostly eosinophil) production. Normal functioning will be impaired. Unable to maintain a protective barrier, the skin and mucous membranes will permit pathogens to enter. The respiratory tract may be filled with mucus and the smooth muscles may constrict, hampering the supply of oxygen to the body. The gastrointestinal tract may respond with violent vomiting and diarrhea. A severe hyperimmune reaction that causes circulatory collapse, shock, and death is called *anaphylaxis*. The inherited tendency to develop abnormal antibodies to such antigens as pollen, dust, mold, and foods is called *atopy* (for example, atopic dermatitis).

Autoimmunity is an immunity to the presence of an antigen in the body's own tissue. The body reacts to this tissue as foreign and produces antibodies to it, causing tissue damage. Such a reaction is beneficial if the tissue happens to be a malignancy since it will stop the uncontrolled growth. Autoimmunity to the body's own malignant tissue is an adaptive process that probably takes place more often than anyone knows. Unfortunately, however, the autoimmunity may be to vital body parts. The symptoms will depend on which organ is attacked. For example, the body's autoimmune reaction to the kidney may result in a fluid and electrolyte imbalance. Researchers think that many unexplained diseases may prove to be caused by autoimmune reactions.

SUMMARY

The child's world is filled with pathogens. The well child's skin and mucous membranes usually prevent most of these from entering the body, and others are destroyed by the phagocytes in his immune system. If the pathogens do survive and multiply in his body, the various components of the immune system increase and the inflammatory response begins. The lymph system traps antigens and destroys them. Immunoglobulins (antibodies) fight pathogens by binding specific ones for easy destruction by phagocytosis. Once the body has produced antibodies to a specific disease, the child is actively immune to that disease. If someone else's antibodies are injected into the child, he is only passively immune; that is, protection will last only as long as these antibodies remain in the body. Infection occurs when pathogens manage to multiply, spread, and cause damage to the body. There are three types of altered immunity:

1. Hypoimmunity (immunodeficiency), i.e., not enough protection;
2. Hyperimmunity (hypersensitivity), i.e., an abnormal response that causes an excessive reaction;
3. Autoimmunity, i.e., destruction of the body's own tissues.

Bibliography

Crouch, J.E. and McClintic, J.R. *Human Anatomy and Physiology*, ed. 2. New York, John Wiley & Sons, Inc., 1976.

Dharan, M. Immunoglobulin Abnormalities. *American Journal of Nursing* 10:1626, 1976.

Glasser, R. Autoimmune Diseases. *Nursing '77* 8:38, 1977.

———. *The Body Is the Hero.* New York, Random House, 1976.

Guyton, A.C. *Basic Human Physiology*, ed. 2. Philadelphia, W.B. Saunders Co., 1977.

Hurley, J.V. *Acute Inflammation.* Baltimore, Williams and Wilkins Co., 1972.

Nysather, J.O., Katz, A.E., Lenth, J.L. The Immune System: Its Development and Functions. *American Journal of Nursing* 10:1614, 1976.

Sell, S. *Immunology, Immunopathology and Immunity.* Hagerstown, Md., Harper and Row, 1972.

CHAPTER 15

The Child with Infection

BEHAVIORAL OBJECTIVES

After studying this chapter, you will be able to:

- Name five types of infectious organisms.
- Describe common symptoms of children with infections.
- Discuss the complications of infections and methods of preventing and treating them.
- List principles of antibiotic administration.
- Describe nursing functions related to laboratory procedures for diagnosing and monitoring infectious diseases.
- Identify common infections in children and briefly discuss the symptoms, treatments, and nursing care of each.

TERMS AND CONCEPTS

Carrier
Virulence
Incubation period
Prodromal symptoms
Bacteria
Viruses
Fungi
Rickettsiae
Animal parasites
Mycoses
Fever
Febrile seizures
Hypothermia blanket
Antipyretics
Malaise
Exanthem, enanthem
Antipruritics
Abscess
Irrigation
Isolation
Aseptic technique
Infection, primary and secondary
Encephalitis
Culture
Sensitivity
White cell count and differential
Titer
Sedimentation rate
Antibiotics

By the beginning of the twentieth century, health care professionals accepted the fact that diseases are caused by germs that usually spread from person to person. There was no known way to kill the germs that managed to multiply in healthy bodies. Many children were stricken with infectious diseases, and too many died. Desperate to save children's lives, the health care team set about preventing the spread of disease by isolating all children admitted to the pediatric unit. Nurses stripped all children of their clothes and scrubbed them well from top to bottom.

The children's parents were sent home with the contaminated clothes. No one was permitted on the unit except the children and the team of workers. Parents' visits, limited in time and contact with the children, usually ranged from one hour a week to one hour a day, at most, and the parents were allowed only to look at the children through glass windows. Since all equipment was decontaminated regularly, there were no pretty, soft children's things about the place. All children were confined to their cribs, since it was thought that their playing with one another would spread germs. When it was time to go home, the children were upset with their parents for having deserted them, and either totally rejected them or clung to them for days to prevent being left again. The children did not eat and sleep as before. Parents swore they would never hospitalize their children again.

In the middle of the twentieth century, two major events occurred that radically changed the hospitalization of children. First, immunizations and antibiotics were used routinely to prevent and cure infectious diseases, decreasing admissions to hospitals and the need for long-term isolation precautions when admission was necessary. The other major event was the rising interest in child psychology. Health professionals began to look at how hospitalization and separation from parents adversely affected children.

By now, acute care units have fewer children with episodic infections and more with chronic diseases and secondary infections. Since many parents can care for moderately ill children at home, those who are admitted with infections are often quite ill. The use of isolation has decreased since antibiotics quickly render the child noncontagious. Parents are welcomed on most acute care units; favorite toys and blankets from home are encouraged. Children still experience emotional and behavioral changes because of the trauma of hospitalization, of course, but they often have positive experiences during their stays.

INFECTIONS

Children with infections are always present on pediatric acute care units. Since infections in children are very different from infections in adults, nursing care, too, is different. Some pathogens simply grow better in children. Immunity obviously plays a big role—maternal antibodies protect infants, and antibodies responding to previous invasions protect older children—but much age-related incidence is unexplained. Children become ill and recover faster, have higher fevers, lose proportionately more fluid, and develop greater electrolyte imbalances than do adults; children's anatomical structures are smaller and closer together allowing infections to spread more rapidly; only children have febrile seizures. Because of these factors, children must be watched more closely than adults so that the subtle changes that herald infection can be detected before the underlying condition worsens.

Infections begin with an invasion of mucous membranes or a break in the skin. Pathogens are "opportunists"; they depend on these breaks, or lowered body resistance, for continued survival. Some microorganisms are dormant until lowered resistance allows them to multiply. Occasionally, a person, called a *carrier,* will host a pathogen and spread it to others but will have no symptom of disease. The severity of an infection is determined by the number of invading pathogens, their *virulence* (strength), and the state of the body's defenses. If the *incubation period* (time from the initial invasion until the first symptom) is short, the illness is usually more severe, since the pathogens multiply rapidly. *Podromal symptoms* (symptoms that indicate the onset of a disease) often follow the incubation period, usually in the form of nonspecific complaints of fever, various aches, malaise, and irritability. Some infections are not considered contagious, since they are not passed from person to person, or from animal to person, except in bizarre circumstances. An example of noncontagious infection is otitis media at the stage when the pathogen remains trapped in the middle ear.

Infectious microorganisms are classified as *bacteria, viruses, fungi, rickettsiae,* or *animal parasites*. All are parasitic since they depend on living matter for survival, but each has different characteristics which generally produce different clinical pictures in children. The symptoms may be so similar that the actual organism must be identified before effective treatment is begun. The vast majority of these microorganisms either do not survive entry to the body, or they live without damage to the host. Occasionally, infection ensues because a child's resistance is low or the microorganism is especially numerous or virulent.

Bacteria, one-celled organisms, generally thrive on dead matter, but a few are able to exist on living matter. They multiply by simple fission, a process that can occur rapidly in the body (and laboratory) under favorable conditions. Some bacteria can live in almost any body tissue while others grow best in certain tissue. All bacteria appear microscopically as cocci, which are round, bacilli, which are rod-shaped, or spirilli, which are spiral. Bacteria are classified by shape, staining characteristics, and need for oxygen. While these microorganisms are responsible for most diseases of humans, they are also beneficial in numerous ways, especially by protecting the body from many pathogens, and in support of the environmental nitrogen cycle.

Viruses are the most primitive form of life; they are so tiny that only the largest can be seen through the conventional microscope, and the rest are visible only under the electron microscope. Viruses will not grow in regular culture media because they can multiply only within the living cell, which provides nutrients and energy. After killing the cell, the newly formed viruses enter healthy cells for further growth. This phenomenon prevented scientists from culturing them long after their existence was discovered. Viruses are now grown in laboratories in chick embryos and other living tissue. Since most viruses have an affinity for specific body tissue (e.g., the skin, liver, or the nervous system), and no simpler method of classification has been devised, they are usually classified according to the target organ.

Rickettsiae are microorganisms that have characteristics of both bacteria and viruses. They resemble bacteria in that they are about as large as small bacteria, they reproduce by simple fission, and respond similarly to broad-spectrum antibiotics. The life cycle of rickettsiae usually includes intracellular growth in the gastrointestinal tract of blood-sucking insects such as ticks and lice, which spread the disease to man.

Fungi occur in many forms—unicellular, multicellular, and branching. Since they cannot manufacture their own food, they live on living or dead tissue. They grow best in warm, moist, and oxygenated places.

Diseases caused by fungi are called *mycoses*. Fungi are present everywhere, waiting patiently for a weakness in resistance, but the body can usually control the growth of fungi with normal defenses, including beneficial bacteria. A troublesome cause of fungal infections that has arisen from modern medical advances is the use of antibiotics that destroy beneficial bacteria.

An animal parasite is any member of the animal kingdom that lives in the body of a host. Parasites usually spend part of their life cycles in the body of another host, so prevention is aimed at identifying the different habitats and avoiding transportation of the parasite or eggs. Not all parasites are pathogenic but live quietly in the body of a host. Parasites are classified as protozoa (one-celled organisms) or worms. Protozoa can cause severe bowel diseases such as amebic dysentery, blood diseases, for example, malaria, and acute vaginitis, such as trichomoniasis. Children with protozoan infections are rare on the typical acute care unit, but children with worms are frequently admitted with severe infestation or are found to have worms in addition to the original problem. Worms pose a major public health problem in warmer climates, rural areas, and poverty-stricken families. Most worms can be traced to unsanitary living conditions with the notable exception of pinworms (*Enterobius vermicularis*) (Figure 15–1), which affects members of all socioeconomic classes. External parasites grow in or on the skin and carry other disease organisms that infect the parasite's host. Even if the parasite carries no threat of infection, the body often recognizes it as foreign and develops an allergic reaction to it. Fortunately, the worms that are most common in children can be very effectively combated with medication.

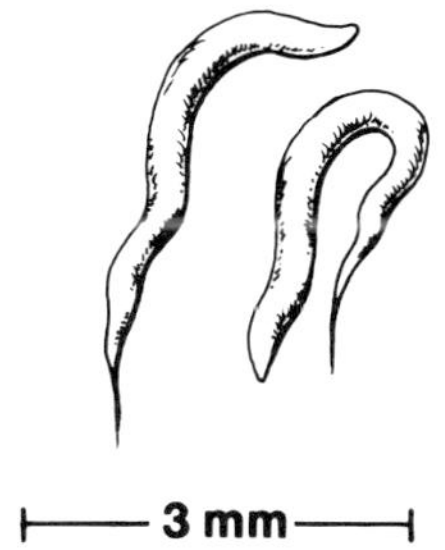

Figure 15–1. *Pinworm (Enterobius vermicularis).*

COMMON PROBLEMS, SYMPTOMS, AND NURSING INTERVENTIONS

Fever

Fever is an above-normal body temperature. Average normal temperature is 37.0°C (98.6°F) (oral), 36.5°C (97.7°F) (axillary), and 37.5°C (99.5°F) (rectal). Body temperature is usually lower than average in the morning, increasing as the day passes. Many factors in a normal child's life can cause an increase in body temperature; for example, overactivity, overexcitement, excessive clothing, playing in hot sunshine or in a hot room. The child's body can quickly compensate if the cause is removed.

Johnny's mother brought him to the nurse practitioner because of the events of the day before; Johnny, aged five, was outside playing with his friends in the sunshine. He came into the house with a headache, and since he looked flushed, his mother took his temperature. She was alarmed to find it was 38.3°C (101°F). She gave him aspirin, and he fell asleep. Two hours later he woke up with a normal temperature, felt fine, and was ready to play. His mother kept him inside until he could be "checked out" for illness. The nurse found a perfectly healthy little boy anxious to go home. She commended Johnny's mother for handling the problem correctly, explained the probability of overheating in this situation, and suggested that

Johnny's mother might be able to save herself a trip to the clinic by calling the nurse about similar occurrences in the future.

Fever is neither a disease nor a cause of illness; either it results from normal variations in environment and activity, or it is merely an indicator of an inflammatory process somewhere in the body. During the inflammatory process, damaged cells release chemicals that stimulate the hypothalamus to raise the body's temperature. The metabolic rate increases as do the heart and respiratory rates. These factors usually make the feverish child restless and irritable. Since a higher fluid intake is required to support the higher metabolic rate, but the child is in no mood to drink liquids, he often becomes dehydrated. Complicating the problem of fluid balance is the fact that the body cools itself with peripheral vasodilation, permitting fluid loss through the skin. The increased respiratory rate also results in fluid loss through the breath.

Fever in children rises and subsides more quickly than in adults. The child may be miserable when his temperature is up yet feels fine as soon as it is down a bit. Young children may have *febrile seizures* relatively frequently when their fever rises very rapidly because of common illnesses, but seizures related to body temperature in the adult usually occur only in cases of serious illness.

Many types of pathology involve the inflammatory process: infection, trauma (including surgery), and immunological deviations. Most children, therefore, will have a fever sometime during hospitalization. You will find yourself spending much time on any pediatric acute care unit assessing children's body temperatures, explaining the meaning of fever to parents, and using different measures to control fever.

Parents have the right and, usually, the desire to know their child's condition, which includes the degree of fever. Explain to the parents what causes fever, that body temperature fluctuates greatly in the child, and that it is normal to feel anxious. Tell them how they can help control the child's fever. If you can support the parents during this time, they usually can enhance your efforts at temperature control; not providing the parent with enough information often results in incorrect assumptions.

Karey J., aged four, was admitted with the diagnosis of "FUO" (fever of unknown origin). The nurse introduced herself to Mrs. J. when she began her afternoon shift. As she did with all parents, the nurse inquired about Mrs. J's recent amount of sleep and food intake, baby-sitting arrangements for the other children, and her use of facilities for a comfortable stay. Since Mrs. J. hardly answered, the nurse left with plans to spend extra time with Mrs. J. later in the evening. Karey's physician called the nurse ten minutes later. He angrily demanded to know why she implied to Mrs. J. that since Karey was indeed critically ill, she'd better resign herself to a long hospital stay. The nurse later learned that another parent had "diagnosed" Karey's problem as meningitis just before the afternoon shift began.

When you cannot adequately support the parents, the child senses their anxiety, and his temperature may rise as a result.

Assessment of body temperature is accomplished by placing a thermometer in the child's mouth, rectum, or axilla (see the Skills Manual). Since most young children resist rectal intrusions after infancy, you should try to take axillary readings whenever possible, although most alert four-year-olds can safely hold a thermometer in their mouths with continuous supervision. Hospital routines vary as to the frequency of temperature assessment. Most units will require checks morning and afternoon, immediately upon returning to the unit postoperatively, followed by a check in 2 hours and every 4 hours thereafter for 24 hours, every 4 hours for 24 hours after an elevation, and 30 minutes to 1 hour after antipyretic measures. Occasionally, the physician will leave several orders for temperature control requiring more frequent checks. You cannot limit yourself to these guidelines, however. The child who is hot to the touch, looks "dry," becomes restless or listless quickly, or has a sagging, loose scrotum or labia may have a fever. Other indications are sunken eyes and fontanelles, dried lips, and red cheeks.

A low-grade fever may not affect the child's behavior at all. However, if the child is uncomfortable or in danger of a further rise, you should begin conservative temperature control techniques. Undress the child except for one layer of light clothing; encourage him to drink as much as possible; keep the room slightly cool; remove blankets from the bed; and play quiet games with him to prevent restlessness which can easily cause some increase in temperature.

Moderate fever—38° or 39° C (101° to 103° F)—usually calls for more aggressive treatment. The child with a moderately high temperature is often cranky, restless, and anorectic. Water is effective in cooling the body, since it draws heat from surface blood vessels in the course of evaporation from the skin. Only tepid water should be used, because it is just below body temperature; cool water will make surface vessels constrict, routing the blood to the warm, inner parts of the body, or may even cause shivering, which produces heat, and warm water will impart its heat to the body.

The best method for cooling the child's body with water is probably the ordinary tub bath, which is fun for the average child. Be sure to get his own floating toy if it is available; if not, squeeze bottles, syringes without needles, small plastic basins, hoses attached to the faucet, and many other standard hospital supplies can provide much fun during this procedure. Parents are probably best for initiating the bath, but playing with the nurse can be a nice change for the child. Bubbles are entertaining, but they must be carefully rinsed from the child's body, especially from the girl's genitals. The water level should be at about mid-thigh when the child is sitting with the knees raised. Too much water will not allow for evaporation. Once in the tub, occasional sponging and splashing will keep enough water on the child's skin for cooling purposes. Add warm water periodically to maintain a constant temperature for approximately 20 to 30 minutes. When you take the child's temperature 30 minutes after completion of his bath, it should be about 1° C lower than before the bath. Unfortunately, many hospitalized children cannot get into a tub for various reasons. Sponging with tepid water accomplishes the task but it is restrictive and upsetting (see the Skills Manual). You may also put cool (not cold) cloths over the major blood vessels in the neck and groin areas; this measure will cool blood in the large vessels but will not cause shivering or constriction of surface vessels.

A high temperature is treated with medications and cooling techniques. If the fever is still high after medications and sponging, the child may be placed on a *hypothermia blanket*. This is a rubber blanket with coils of coolant that can be controlled manually by the nurse or automatically by the child's temperature as measured by a rectal probe or other type of monitor. The hypothermia blanket cools internal blood vessels, avoiding peripheral vessel constriction, chills, and subsequent temperature increase.

Nursing care of the child with a high fever, that is, 40° C (104° F) and above, includes not only attention to his body temperature but also to his usually distraught parents. When the hypothermia blanket automatically turns on and off, parents become aware of their child's rising temperature by totaling the number and length of times it cools the child. Some parents become visibly more anxious when the bedside console is running, and many health personnel use this reaction as an excuse for separating parents and child in the acute and critical care units. Listen to the parents' concerns, explain the value of the blanket, and answer their questions, repeatedly if necessary. Watch carefully for signs of chilling and discontinue antipyretic measures for a while if it does occur. The child is often uncomfortable on the hard blanket; it should therefore be covered with a thin cotton blanket. Explain each part of the procedure to the child; a child with a high temperature may perceive the cold as a punishment and you as the punisher, so he needs to hear frequently why he is receiving antipyretic measures.

Malaise

The problem of *malaise* (generalized restlessness, irritability, and discomfort usually increases with fever in a child with infection, although the reverse is not necessarily true. Infection, with its accompanying pain, loss of normal body function, boredom, fear of treatments, and so on takes up much of the child's energy; still more energy is needed to be pleasant, and the child usually lacks this extra energy. Parents often make the mistake of bribing, begging, or scolding to make the child eat, take medications, tolerate treatments and "be nice." Some parents bring bag after bag of toys from friends, family, nearby stores or the hospital gift shop. One toy after another is laid out on the bed until the child is nearly buried in them. This causes a sensory overload, and the child's irritability increases. A fine balance of limits, love, and sensory control, along with consistent parenting and nursing, is desirable but probably unattainable in many cases. Try limiting television to specific programs; "soap operas" are simply not an appropriate diversion for children in hospitals. Turn the television off when the play period begins, offer one toy at a time, and plan all recreational activities in accordance with age and stage of development.

Encourage parents to hold their child whenever possible; holding a child in pain, however, can increase his discomfort because of unexpected body movement and the body heat of the person holding him. Reassess the child's opportunity to rest and sleep and provide more if necessary. If he is in pain, try to time the administration of analgesics so that they will have their effect when relief is needed most, such as before procedures or play. Do not react to every spell of irritability, as a reaction may reinforce the behavior.

You may find that no tactic decreases the child's irritability; if so, accept the behavior as normal, and help the parents to do the same. Explain to the parents and to the child that this behavior is expected as a result of his condition, and that it will decrease as he improves.

Anorexia

The child with infection often has *anorexia*, a loss of appetite, but he has an increased metabolic rate to support. If the focus of infection is the gastrointestinal tract, intravenous feedings are appropriate. (See Chapter 18 for further discussion.)

Rashes

A rash is an eruption or "breaking out" of the skin or mucous membranes. An eruption of the skin is an *exanthem*; an eruption of a mucous membrane is termed an *enanthem*. Although rashes are frequently associated with systemic infections, such as rubella, or local infections, such as impetigo, they may be caused by overheating, rubbing together of skin (intertrigo), exposure to irritating substances, allergic reactions, or to congenital defects. A rash is usually temporary, spreading over the area of its normal distribution and fading, or healing, on removal of the offender. Rashes have very different characteristics and various symptoms. Most are erythematous (red) and pruritic (itchy). Some rashes appear as solid bumps (papules), some are filled with serum (vesicles) or pus (pustules), or they may be flat, colored spots on the skin (macules). The child has a weakened first line of defense since the skin is affected and since he often scratches to the point of breaking the tissues. Nursing care is directed at keeping the child as comfortable as possible and keeping the skin intact.

The child with a pruritic rash will certainly scratch himself. His nails must be cut short, but this is a difficult task with the infant and young child; they do not like to be held still, and their nails are tiny. Mittens may be sufficient to remind the older child not to scratch, and mittens that are held in place with rounds of tape at the wrist may stop the younger child. Restraints may be ordered to stop scratching, but this makes the child more upset, hot, sweaty, and chafed in the areas of restraint. If you absolutely must restrain the child, restrain all four limbs; one free limb can rip into itching tissue within a few seconds. Holding the child in a comfortable position and encouraging play with smooth, soft toys is the best method of restraint, but of course, this is not always possible.

Comfort for the itchy child is often a difficult objective to meet, but with careful planning he can be made less uncomfortable. Heat from body temperature, room temperature, or excessive clothing causes vasodilation, edema of the skin, and sweating. All of these reactions increase itching and should be guarded against by giving the child lightweight cotton clothing and linens, maintaining a cool environment, and using tepid baths and other controls of fever. Friction caused by clothing, bedding, braces, casts, or rubbing of two adjacent skin surfaces increases heat and sweating, causing more itching and possibly more eruptions. Cornstarch between the two surfaces will cut down on friction and keep the area dry for a while, but excessive moisture from sweating, urine, and so on will necessitate cleaning the surfaces and applying fresh cornstarch.

A wide variety of *antipruritics* (treatments and medications that relieve itching) may be prescribed. Generally, ointments and, occasionally, creams are used on dry lesions to prevent further drying, and wet treatments are used on oozing or crusty lesions. Ointments and creams are best applied in thin layers with firm, long strokes using at least three fingers or the flattened palm; strokes with too gentle a touch cause itching and tickling sensations. Thick layers of medications are no better than thin since only the actual contact is beneficial. (An exception to this rule is with antibiotic ointments for burns.) Baths and compresses should be cool to tepid to inhibit vasodilation and itching. Antipruritic baths may contain colloidal (gelatinous) additives, such as oatmeal or other chemicals, that are soothing. Wet compresses are applied when only certain areas of the body need treatment. Since baths and wet compresses usually last from 15 to 30 minutes, a child may become chilled if the temperature is not monitored carefully. Adding warm solution to maintain a tepid temperature will prevent this problem (see Skills Manual).

The physician often prescribes antihistamines, most frequently Benadryl, for the itchy child. Benadryl is a relatively safe medication that inactivates histamine, thereby decreasing vasodilation, edema, itching, and histamine-induced rashes. It also sedates the child somewhat, reducing his irritability and restlessness.

Abscess

An *abscess* is a collection of pus that occurs in response to infection in any part of the body. At first the infected area is hot, red, swollen, and painful. As the inflammatory process continues, a local area becomes "walled off" and the pus collects. The surrounding tissues do not have enough room for the pus, and pressure builds, causing pain and loss of function. Depending on the body part and amount of pressure, an abscess may be merely an annoyance or a severely disabling problem. If the abscess is in an area that does not allow expansion, such as the skull, severe pain and invasion of underlying tissues will occur. The pus may find a channel to the outside of the body through the skin or mucous membranes and drain spontaneously. Very often, the physician incises the lesion and may need to leave a drain made of gauze, or soft rubber with a gauze wick, to allow a continuous flow of old and newly formed pus.

An abscess in the child can be particularly dangerous if it is in or near a narrow passage such as the upper airway. Since the child is small, his organs are closer together, and an abscess is more likely to obstruct the original site or break into another area. An example of the latter process is the sinus abscess, which erodes the thin bone and tissues and infects the brain.

Nursing care of the child with an abscess is directed at providing physical comfort, facilitating the drainage of pus, preventing the further spread of infection, and helping the child cope with changes in body image. The child with an abscess is in pain and needs analgesics regularly, particularly before treatments or activities that require movement of the affected part; planning for analgesics 30 minutes beforehand will relieve the pain and, often, the child's anxiety. The child will usually immobilize the area on his own, but he needs to be up and about to stimulate circulation. Once the pus begins to drain through a spontaneous channel or an incision, immediate relief usually follows. Warm compresses applied to the drained area will increase circulation, which brings more white cells and serum to the affected area to combat the infection and increases drainage. The skin surrounding the drainage site must be kept as clean and dry as possible to prevent breakdown. Whenever feasible, showers and tub baths should be given for the generally clean feeling they provide; if they are not already prescribed by the physician, try to convince him of their benefit with an explanation of how a simple, removable plastic covering can protect the drainage site during a shower. Often all dressings can be removed for a soapy shower cleansing of the area. Exposing the site to air for a while will help prevent tissue breakdown. A 15 to 20 minute heat lamp treatment with a 20-watt bulb placed 12 to 18 inches away may be prescribed before dressing changes; remember that the danger of burns is ever-present, and careful supervision is required. After careful cleansing and airing, some protective covering of the skin, such as with an ointment, is usually applied before redressing. For continuous and heavy drainage, a stoma drainage bag of the type used for a colostomy (see Skills Manual) can keep the surrounding area (not the drainage site itself) clean and dry. Regardless of the apparatus used to collect pus, the child should be included in decision making and the procedure. For example, occasionally, he may be allowed to remove the adhesive tape holding the drainage apparatus in place himself, but he may prolong this step to avoid the next one. Indecision on the nurse's part will cause anxiety in the child, so offer only a few definite alternatives and proceed with the task if he cannot select one.

A dirty, smelly bandage saturated with pus from a hole in the child's body can be very upsetting to him. He may lose all desire to eat and even develop nausea and vomiting.

Phyllis, a prim and pretty fifteen-year-old, had been coping well with a moderate amount of continuous drainage from an abscessed appendix. One morning she woke to find her gown and linens soaked with pus. She began crying hysterically. Her nurse quickly removed all signs of the drainage, helped her bathe well, and took her to the dayroom until her room could be aired out. Phyllis became depressed and anxious about potential accidents, and cried frequently. She refused to eat a meal for the next two days.

Body boundaries can be partially restored with bandages and the child's own clothes; these should be used as necessary. Unfortunately, the child may require frequent changes of clothing, and parents would be greatly inconvenienced if they had to maintain a supply of clean clothes from home. Some other special object may help the child cope with the emotional trauma that may accompany an abscess.

Irrigation is frequently used in cases of abscess and other infections that are not on the surface of the body. Irrigation is accomplished simply by washing out the affected area to remove unwanted material, such as pus or blood, and/or by instilling medication. The injection of fluid loosens trapped debris and washes it out. The temperature of the liquid is routinely from 40° to 43° C (105°–110° F), depending on the reason for the instillation. Warm water or solutions stimulate further drainage. If the solution contains antibiotics, the temperature must be kept within the range indicated in the accompanying literature (usually room temperature or cooler, but well above freezing). If the irrigation is intended to soothe itching, the solution is usually cool. If the procedure is done to provide comfort and to stimulate drainage and decrease infection, maintaining the effectiveness of the antibiotics takes priority. The amount of solution, rate of flow, and length of time all may be prescribed, or you may need to irrigate until the solution returns clear, although each of the factors mentioned should be recorded with every irrigation. Sterile technique is required for irrigations of the bladder, eyes, and wounds. Common sites for irrigation are the eyes, ears, mouth, bladder, bowel, and wounds (surgical, infectious, traumatic). With all irrigations, outflow of the solution must be allowed to avoid undue pressure in the cavity. This may be accomplished through intermittent or continuous instillation and outflow. Outflow of solution (also called "return") is recorded as to amount, color, and sediment. Prepare the child carefully for this procedure, keeping in mind that he may have an irrational fear of popping wide open or of washing his insides out.

Isolation and Aseptic Technique

The child with an infection brings with him the threat of spreading disease to others when he enters a hospital. This problem is controlled with varying degrees of success by *isolation,* a process of separating a person from others, and *aseptic technique,* the modification of procedures to maintain freedom from infectious pathogens. Since the nurse spends more time with the child than any other care provider in the hospital setting (except parents), she shares a greater responsibility for protection. Numerous problems frustrate her best efforts. Many hospital workers (such as technicians, housekeeping staff, and therapists) who go into the child's room are not trained by and accountable to the nurse. Even if she has the right to report a person's error, she often may not be able to prevent his return. Another frequent offender is the physician who plans just to "peek in" but finds himself involved with the parent or child. You will find that each hospital has an elaborate set of rules for different types of isolation, applied to equipment in and out of the room and methods for the disposal of linen, food, excreta, and so on, facilitated by color coding, signs on doors, and so forth. In some hospitals, different units have different sets of rules. Regardless of the type of isolation, it is always contrary to the support of normal development in children who thrive on lots of human contact, freedom to move and explore their environment, and ability to control their lives as much as possible.

The five basic types of isolation are wound, enteric, respiratory, strict, and protective. The first four are designed to prevent the spread of a child's infection to others. The child, his excreta, discharges and drainages, and any articles that come in contact with the infected part are kept separate, in accordance with the type of microorganism and the method of transmission. Wound isolation entails protecting and/or separating anything that might contact the wound or its drainage, dressings, linens, clothing, and hands, as well as the clothing and body of anyone in contact with the patient. Enteric isolation usually applies to urine, feces, and anything contaminated by either, although, strictly speaking, it applies to feces only. Respiratory isolation is prescribed to prevent the spread of airborne diseases that enter the body through the respiratory tract. Strict isolation is achieved through total separation of the child, his clothing, linens, toys, food, and excreta from any exposure to other people.

Protective (or "reverse") isolation, the fifth type, is designed to protect an uninfected child from contracting an infection. It is strict isolation, but items and people are decontaminated by sterilization or covering before they enter the child's room, not after they leave. Optimally, air is filtered to remove airborne pathogens. Many hospitals have filtering mechanisms as part of the temperature control systems; others have equipment that maintains a flow of purified air in the child's immediate surroundings. Keeping the door closed may be the only way to decrease the influx of airborne particles. A child is placed in protective isolation when he is unable to withstand even minor threats of infection, such as the child with burns, leukemia, certain chronic diseases, and immunodeficiency.

The isolated child's care is very different from that of the isolated adult. The child does not stay still in a small area of a room unless he is confined to a crib. He may be too young to keep his hands away from dressings or excreta. Even if he is toilet trained, he may regress and contaminate chairs, floors, and toys with feces and urine. Observe carefully for unexpected sources of contamination, then extend precautions to eliminate them. The toddler who is on enteric isolation usually requires strict observation because his elimination is difficult to control. (See Chapter 30 for a discussion of the psychosocial implications of isolation.)

COMPLICATIONS

Lowered Resistance

The child with an infection has lowered resistance to other illnesses. As has been mentioned, he is often anorectic and thus may suffer from malnutrition and dehydration, which result in a less efficient immune system. The body is left vulnerable to microorganisms that usually are easily destroyed by the well child's immune system. Some infections render the body incapable of fighting other specific diseases; for example, measles temporarily depresses the body's ability to fight tubercle bacillus.

The location of infection affects the body's resistance to further infection. A local reaction (i.e., the inflammatory process) helps to resist the *primary* (first) infection, but the same reaction may leave the area open and edematous. Once the skin or mucous membrane is broken, the first line of defense is lost. When the underlying tissue is suffused with extra fluid, invading microorganisms have a warm, moist nourishing place to grow, and a *secondary* infection can develop.

Michelle, aged four, had been sick with viral bronchitis for a week. She had had low-grade fever, productive cough, and malaise. A leukocyte count ruled out bacterial infection. One afternoon, her fever went up, and she became noticeably worse. Lab studies indicated a bacterial infection. The chest x-ray revealed a lobar pneumonia. Michelle's mother was angry because the physician had not prevented the pneumonia with antibiotics earlier. The admitting nurse explained secondary infection to both parents and discussed briefly the disadvantages of administering antibiotics for viral infections.

Spread of Infection

The immune and inflammatory reactions usually prevent the spread of infection. If the reactions are not efficient, or if the pathogen is especially virulent or present in large numbers, the infection usually spreads through the blood. Normally, when bacteria or viruses enter the body, they will appear for a short period of time in the blood and then are removed by the immune system. This frequently happens with common colds, tooth extractions, and cuts. The microorganisms, however, can multiply and produce toxins within the circulatory system, causing septicemia (also called bacteremia or sepsis) or viremia. Septicemia can be mild and transient, or it can be an overwhelming disease, resulting in death in a few hours. Newborns and immunosuppressed children are particularly vulnerable to septicemia. Viremia is usually responsible for the chills and fever of viral illness.

Bacteria can enter the bloodstream via a break in the skin or mucous membrane, cause a mild bacteremia, and begin to multiply in body tissue already weakened for some other reason. For example, the child who has had rheumatic fever (see ch. 22) is left with heart tissues that are particularly susceptible to streptococcal infection. Streptococci entering the body through the pharynx or the site of a tooth extraction are transported throughout the body but may affect only the weakened heart valves. Prophylactic bood levels of penicillin are maintained in the child to prevent this complication.

Infection also can spread to adjacent tissue simply by multiplying, taking up available space, and eroding and invading adjacent tissues. This problem occurs frequently with local infections that are not controlled.

Freddie, aged two, uses his pacifier as a security object. Last week he developed a cold that caused a continuous, thick nasal discharge. The tissue below his nose became irritated and broken, and his frequent sucking on the pacifier irritated it more. A streptococcal infection developed and spread. By the time he arrived at the clinic, his nares, upper lip, and all surrounding tissue were covered with oozing, crusty lesions. He was still sucking his pacifier, spreading the secretions back and forth over the area each time he sucked.

Febrile Seizures

Febrile seizures are convulsions caused by a rapid rise in body temperature; they are usually brief; lasting no more than five minutes. Most febrile seizures occur at the beginning of an illness, when the temperature increase is so rapid that it goes unnoticed until the illness incapacitates the child. The seizure begins suddenly while the child is outside playing, or during or soon after a nap. Children from six months to three years of age are most vulnerable, but children from three months to six years old are susceptible. Fever is always present in moderate to high range. The seizure is labeled "febrile," however, only when the child has no other convulsive disorder, even when fever triggers a pre-existing tendency toward seizures. Once the child has a febrile seizure, he is likely to have subsequent seizures with progressively lower fevers. Only 3% of children affected by febrile seizures will later develop epilepsy.

The manifestations and nursing care of febrile seizures are the same as with other convulsions (see ch. 27). They usually are generalized but may be focal. Once the seizure is over, the child's fever should be brought down with routine antipyretic measures. If the child is at home, he should receive a medical evaluation. If the child has a seizure on the acute care unit or another health facility, the physician may order parenteral anticonvulsants. A lumbar puncture is performed to obtain cerebrospinal fluid if there is any suspicion of meningitis. Infants and young toddlers are frequently hospitalized for observation.

The prevention of recurring febrile seizures is the goal of the health team. With the first episode, the usual measures, plus a little extra caution, are used for temperature control. After the second episode, many physicians prescribe prophylactic phenobarbital which is continued until about five years of age. The practice of giving the child phenobarbital after he develops a fever is useless, since blood levels of the medication must be built up over a period of time to be effective. Since febrile seizures do tend to recur, watch for signs of a rapid increase in body temperature, and use antipyretic measures to control it. Parents must learn the same observational skills. Seizures are so fear-provoking, however, that you should encourage parents to avoid being too vigilant or overreacting to the child's temperature.

Immobility

After an infection process destroys healthy tissue, scar formation can tighten and bind underlying and adjacent tissue. The scarring may hold the joint in a flexed position, and the muscle will contract, forming *contractures*. Often a limb cannot be extended if the scar forms in the antecubital (anterior to the elbow) or popliteal (posterior to the knee) spaces; scarring around the mouth can hamper eating and even smiling. Infection alone does not usually cause severe immobility, but infection secondary to trauma, such as burns, results in further damage. Scar tissue that significantly reduces function is removed when possible and replaced with grafts (See chapters 26, 28, and 30).

The child with infection may be in such pain that he refuses to move. If the condition lasts for a brief time, immobility is brief. If, however, the child remains in a flexed position for several days or longer, the muscles begin to contract and hold the affected body part in the position of comfort. This is especially true with infections of bones, joints, and muscles, and prolonged illness may result.

Neurological Disability

Many childhood infections are complicated by *encephalitis*, inflammation of the brain. Edema of the cerebum can cause temporary brain dysfunction, resulting in a wide variety of problems from mildly blurred vision to hallucinations and seizures. As the edema subsides, the symptoms disappear. Unfortunately, a few children suffer residual damage. Motor damage resulting from damage to the brain is called cerebral palsy (see ch. 28). Intellectual loss ranges from mild dysfunction to severe mental retardation. Often the child with residual brain damage sustains both motor and intellectual impairment. It often takes weeks to months to determine the extent of permanent damage.

Eric, aged three and a half, had encephalitis following mumps. After three days of high fever and seizures, Eric lay in the bed with his left side limp. He was highly irritable and, as is to be expected, any bright light or loud noise brought loud, incoherent protests from him. His mother, a quiet, determined woman, kept stimuli to a minimum. She "worked" his limp limbs in a gentle, playful manner. Nurses cheered her on and relieved her periodically. Two months after discharge Eric and his mother revisited the unit. He was still a little weak on his left side but the improvement was remarkable.

Disfigurement

Scars, contractures, and other disfigurements can affect the child's self-concept. If the disfigurement lasts briefly, the child may be temporarily disturbed, but he usually tolerates the insult adequately. If the problem is prolonged or permanent, the child must incorporate the change into his self-image. Since the loss of the previous self-image will induce the grief process (see chs. 3 and 9), watch for the progression of stages and support the child accordingly throughout. Hopefully, the child will eventually accept the disfigurement as a part of himself with which he can live and cope. The older the child, the more difficult this adaptation will be. Very often, however, the child becomes self-conscious about the problem and may attempt to cover it in a way that draws attention to the site.

Lucy, aged eight, was in a car accident that broke her front teeth into jagged pieces. While undergoing various stages of dental procedures, she went to school at her parents' insistence. She tried to cover her broken teeth with her hand in school. Even now, as an adult, she covers her mouth when in an awkward social situation.

The child needs ample opportunity to talks about the change in his body image. Listen to him and encourage his parents to listen. Have the child suppose that his doll or a child in a picture has the same problem to encourage the child to talk about his feelings and thoughts. Have him imagine his first day back in school and role-play school childrens' possible questions or remarks about the problem. The child's teacher at school should be prepared to support the child without drawing undue attention to him. Parents often can talk with the teacher, but referral to a school nurse or public health nurse may be helpful.

COMMON DIAGNOSTIC PROCEDURES

Laboratory

When a child shows such indications of an infection as fever, anorexia, or pain, several questions must be answered before appropriate nursing and medical care can be provided. The first question—what category of microorganism is involved—is often answered by the physician by evaluating the child's overall health and any specific complaints. He then makes an educated guess and treats the child accordingly. Every pediatrician goes through this process daily, and as a result of their experience parents are spared the cost of expensive laboratory procedures, and the child is spared some pain. If the physician feels the need to confirm his diagnosis and wants to identify the specific microorganism involved and the medication that will combat it most effectively, he orders lab tests. The child with indications of infection on an acute care unit will almost always undergo laboratory procedures so that these questions can be answered.

A culture is a sample of microorganism taken from the site of infection and placed in a sterile environment that is favorable to the microorganism's growth. Different types of media and controlled temperature are used to nurture growth. After the microorganism has multiplied, it is identified, and its *sensitivity* to different medications is recorded; the microorganism is said to be sensitive to those medications that destroy it in culture.

Nurses are often responsible for obtaining a culture specimen. Never give the first dose of an antibiotic until the specimen is drawn or swabbed; question any order that seems to do so, since just one dose reduces the chance of an adequate culture. Use aseptic technique and sterile equipment. All cultures except cerebrospinal fluid can be kept in the refrigerator if they cannot be transported immediately to the lab. Since cerebrospinal fluid must be incubated soon after the lumbar puncture for best results, transporting the specimen to the lab as quickly as possible is a priority. Always label the specimen with the date, type of specimen, any medications given in the last 72 hours, and suspected microorganism if known. If more than one specimen is taken from the same site, number each one in order. Treat any specimen as contaminated material, taking the necessary precautions to protect yourself and others from infection.

Swabbing is a method of obtaining a specimen from skin lesions, abscesses, and mucous membranes of the eyes, mouth, throat, nose, rectum, and vagina. Good lighting is necessary, especially when swabbing a specific part of a body cavity, such as the tonsils. A sterile swab and aseptic technique are used to prevent contamination; the swab should be dry except when indicated otherwise. With viral cultures, the swab is dipped into the medium before swabbing. After clearing the infected area of debris, roll the swab so that contact is made completely around the cotton tip. Since many microorganisms need moisture to survive, moist culture containers are used to preserve the specimen until transportation to the lab is possible. If the specimen is to be placed in the culture medium immediately after swabbing, moisture is not required.

Children are not usually disturbed by swabbing the skin. Most mucous membranes, however, are inside the body, and swabbing these areas is an intrusive procedure. Infants and toddlers will require restraint, but many preschoolers can tolerate the procedure with proper preparation. To culture a child's throat, have him swallow first to clear the mouth of excess saliva, open his mouth, and stick out his tongue. If he seems to have good control of the gag reflex and you can see the throat well, place a depressor on his tongue lightly. If you cannot see the throat, depress the tongue in the area of the "hump" on the tongue; this usually elicits the gag reflex, which is very unpleasant, but it also clears the area briefly for swabbing. Swab the surface of both tonsils and the posterior pharynx (the back wall of the oral cavity behind the uvula). Nasal cultures are obtained by swabbing the inside of the nares. Nasopharyngeal cultures are similar to nasal cultures except that the swab is pushed gently into the back of the nose until it hits the posterior wall, causing pain to these sensitive tissues. Stool cultures are usually collected by swabbing the rectum one to two centimeters beyond the anal opening for the first specimen. A small amount of feces of each bowel movement thereafter is sent to the lab in a sterile container. Use a tongue depressor to remove the feces from the diaper or bedpan. If the stool is liquid, use a swab. A vaginal culture is obtained simply by swabbing the vagina; the real challenge is to prepare the child for this intrusive procedure.

Blood cultures are usually performed to diagnose bacterial disease but may also be used to determine the presence of other types of microorganisms. Venous blood is drawn into a special vacuum tube and transferred to a culture tube prepared with a blood culture medium. As with all cultures, *do not give* the first dose of an antibiotic until the blood is drawn. Laboratory technicians are usually responsible for venipunctures, but many nurses on pediatric units perform this procedure.

Urine is cultured from specimens obtained from voided urine, catheterization, or a suprapubic tap. The voided specimen is collected after washing the vulva or glans of the penis with an antiseptic solution (usually Zephiran) and rinsing well. The child is instructed to begin to void, stop, then void in a sterile container. The younger child is instructed to begin to void, and the container is quickly placed in the path of the stream of urine. Infants are cleansed and fitted with a sterile adhesive collection bag (see the Skills Manual). Catheterization carries with it the risk of infection, and urine specimens are rarely collected this way, although specimen is sometimes collected from an indwelling or suprapubic catheter. Aseptic technique is used throughout the procedure, and the urine is taken from the catheter tubing, *never* from the collection bag. The physician performs a suprapubic tap, puncturing the bladder through the abdomen just above the pubic bone with a needle. This procedure is usually done on newborns and infants whose voided urine is almost always badly contaminated before it reaches the lab. This method is less likely to cause a secondary infection. The nurse is responsible for preparing parents for this frightening experience and for restraining the infant. All urine specimens should be taken to the laboratory immediately after collection since contaminants inevitably overgrow the pathogens quickly.

Fluid for cerebrospinal cultures is obtained from a lumbar puncture. This can be a terrifying experience for the parents and the child, since the child is often acutely ill, and there is no time for adequate preparation. The child is restrained in a knee-chest, chin-on-chest position to expose the lumbar region of the spine and to increase intracranial pressure, facilitating specimen collection. Talking to the child throughout the procedure is crucial; all too often, the physician and nurse talk to each other, leaving the child to his thoughts and fears. When parent and child can be adequately prepared, the parent can support the child throughout the procedure (see the Skills Manual).

The cerebrospinal fluid specimen is cultured, sensitivity to medications is determined, and other studies, such as glucose and leukocyte cell counts, are done. Glucose usually decreases, and leukocytes increase, in cases of meningitis. The culturing of cerebrospinal fluid is usually an emergency, and the report from the laboratory is relayed to the physician immediately. Rarely, the puncture site will leak cerebrospinal fluid, decreasing pressure in the cerebrum and causing a severe headache; when this occurs, the child's head is kept low, fluid intake is increased to maximum tolerance, and stimuli are kept to a minimum. If the leaking continues, the physician may inject some of the child's blood into the intraspinal (intrathecal) space to encourage clot formation at the puncture site.

A sputum culture is obtained to identify microorganisms in the lower respiratory tract. Most children have difficulty with coughing up and spitting out secretions from their lungs and trachea because they usually swallow the material. Even after careful instructions and practice, children often produce saliva, which usually does not contain pathogens from the lower respiratory tract. Postural drainage (see ch. 23 and the Skills Manual) will frequently help the child to bring up a sputum specimen. Sputum may also be obtained through tracheal and bronchial suctioning. Again, sputum specimens are assumed to be infectious and must be handled with aseptic technique.

Hematologic Studies

When hematologic studies are indicated, it is the nurse's responsibility to supply information to the pathologist about the child's condition and previous medications, to prepare parents and child for the procedure, and, often, to interpret results for them. The nurse also may perform a venipuncture or a finger stick to obtain the sample, but this is usually done by the laboratory technician. Always indicate on the request form all medications the child has received in 72 hours, whether he has had recent surgery, whether he was receiving an intravenous infusion at the time of the venipuncture, and the actual or suspected diagnosis.

The *white cell count* is the number of leukocytes found in a cubic millimeter of blood. A white cell is usually indicative of a bacterial infection but may also arise from the administration of anesthesia, emotional stress, and blood disorders. The *white cell differential* is the identification of the type of white blood cells and the proportion of each. The differential helps to determine if the problem is bacterial, parasitic, allergic, or malignant, since the proportions change according to these factors. These two laboratory studies are frequently performed in the physician's office as well as in the acute care unit (see Table 15–1).

A *titer* is the amount of a specific antibody found in blood serum. Antistreptolisin O titer (ASO titer) indicates the formation of an antibody to a streptococcal enzyme. The ASO titer rises after a streptococcal infection. Rubella titer is important to women of childbearing age since rubella in pregnant women can cause severe damage to the fetus. Antibody titers are useful in diagnosing syphilis, mononucleosis, and many autoimmune diseases.

The *erythrocyte sedimentation rate* ("sed" rate) is a test that measures the rate at which red blood cells settle on the bottom of a test tube. The rate increases with any condition that destroys cells. This test is helpful in following the course of an inflammatory disease such as rheumatic fever; a decreasing sed rate indicates improvement.

Urinalysis

Urine tests can reveal infections of the urinary tract. The urine culture is the only reliable way to rule out a urinary tract infection. The microscopic exam is the next best method, since bacteria, and numerous leukocytes (white or pus cells), may be seen in the urine. Healthy children may have a few white cells in response to contamination of the urethra by the nearby rectum, vulva, and vagina in girls, and the foreskin in boys. Girls have a shorter urethra that is closer to the rectum, and they therefore have more white cells in the absence of illness. An increase above the normal number of white cells, therefore, is a sign of infection, although a lack of white cells does not rule out infection. Bacteria can be seen in the sediment of urine under the microscope, but they cannot be identified without cultures. The *specific gravity,* i.e., the measurement of the concentration of dissolved material in urine, increases because of two factors: an increase in dissolved particles such as erythrocytes, leukocytes, bacteria and debris, and/or degrees of hydration in which there is less water available to dilute the extra material. *Casts* are microscopic forms filled with erythrocytes, leukocytes, or albumin that have compacted in a kidney tubule and are passed out with the urine, retaining the shape of the tubule. Casts usually indicate a serious kidney disease since most normal kidneys wash solid particles from the tubules before they accumulate.

Table 15–1. Normal Leukocyte Differential Count in Peripheral Blood

	Segmented neutrophils		*Band neutrophils*[a]		*Eosinophils*		*Basophils*		*Lymphocytes*		*Monocytes*	
Age	%	*No./mm*^{3b}	%	*No./mm*^{3b}	%	*No./mm*^{3b}	%	*No./mm*^{3b}	%	*No./mm*^{3b}	%	*No./mm*^{3b}
At birth	47 ± 15	8,400	14.1 ± 4	2,540	2.2	400	0.6	100	31 ± 5	5,500	5.8	1,050
12 hours	53	12,100	15.2	3,460	2.0	450	0.4	100	24	5,500	5.3	1,200
24 hours	47	8,870	14.2	2,680	2.4	450	0.5	100	31	5,800	5.8	1,100
1 week	34	4,100	11.8	1,420	4.1	500	0.4	50	41	5,000	9.1	1,100
2 weeks	29	3,320	10.5	1,200	3.1	350	0.4	50	48	5,500	8.8	1,000
4 weeks	25 ± 10	2,750	9.5 ± 3	1,150	2.8	300	0.5	50	56 ± 15	6,000	6.5	700
2 months	25	2,750	8.4	1,100	2.7	300	0.5	50	57	6,300	5.9	650
4 months	24	2,730	8.9	1,000	2.6	300	0.4	50	59	6,800	5.2	600
6 months	23	2,710	8.8	1,000	2.5	300	0.4	50	61	7,300	4.8	580
8 months	22	2,680	8.3	1,000	2.5	300	0.4	50	62	7,600	4.7	580
10 months	22	2,600	8.3	1,000	2.5	300	0.4	50	63	7,500	4.6	550
12 months	23	2,680	8.1	990	2.6	300	0.4	50	61	7,000	4.8	550
2 years	25	2,660	8.0	850	2.6	280	0.5	50	59	6,300	5.0	530
4 years	34 ± 11	3,040	8.0 ± 3	710	2.8	250	0.6	50	50 ± 15	4,500	5.0	450
6 years	43	3,600	8.0	670	2.7	230	0.6	50	42	3,500	4.7	400
8 years	45	3,700	8.0	660	2.4	200	0.6	50	39	3,300	4.2	350
10 years	46 ± 15	3,700	8.0 ± 3	645	2.4	200	0.5	40	38 ± 10	3,100	4.3	350
12 years	47	3,700	8.0	640	2.5	200	0.5	40	38	3,000	4.4	350
14 years	48	3,700	8.0	640	2.5	200	0.5	40	37	2,900	4.7	380
16 years	49 ± 15	3,800	8.0 ± 3	620	2.6	200	0.5	40	35 ± 10	2,800	5.1	400
18 years	49	3,800	8.0	620	2.6	200	0.5	40	35	2,700	5.2	400
20 years	51	3,800	8.0	620	2.7	200	0.5	40	33	2,500	5.0	380
21 years	51 ± 15	3,800	8.0 ± 3	620	2.7	200	0.5	40	34 ± 10	2,500	4.0	300

[a] Note that these values are higher than those found in other references. They have been obtained by using strict criteria in differentiating segmented from band forms. We do not classify a neutrophil as a segmented form unless a typical threadlike filament is visible.

[b] To convert the number of cells in traditional units (cells/mm^3) to SI units (cells/l), the number in thousands is multiplied by 10^9; e.g., 8,400/mm^3 = 8.4 × 10^9/L.

Adapted from Miale, John B. *Laboratory Medicine: Hematology*, ed. 5. St. Louis, C.V. Mosby, 1977.

Always wash the vulva or glans (if the boy is uncircumcised) before collecting a specimen. Send the specimen to the lab within an hour of collection to prevent disintegration of the cells and overgrowth of contaminant bacteria. If there are signs of infection, another urinalysis for culture and sensitivity is in order.

Cytologic Studies

A *cytologic study* is the visualization of cells under the microscope. It is useful for diagnosing fungal infections, some bacterial infections (e.g., syphilis), parasitic infestations, some viral infections, and rickettsial infections. Discharges are swabbed onto a slide, a drop of solution specific for the suspected microorganism is added, and the specimen is studied microscopically for the pathogen. Other specimens are dried and stained for microscopic observation. Occasionally, a lesion is scraped and the scrapings are studied. Stool specimens are frequently observed for blood cells, ova from parasites, or the actual parasite ("stool for BOP"). Blood and urine may be studied cytologically, i.e., the cells themselves are assessed. All cytologic specimens must be preserved in the refrigerator or sent to the lab immediately, since cells disintegrate quickly and, once they do, the test will reveal little.

X-Rays

X-rays are often used to reveal changes in body structures caused by infection. The chest x-ray is a valuable tool for diagnosing lower respiratory infections when the physician is aware of a potential error in diagnosing because of indefinite clinical symptoms. The chest x-ray will reveal early changes in the lung fields, infiltrates, foreign bodies, tumors, pneumothorax, and pneumomidiastinum. The chest x-ray also is ordered to follow the course of a disease. Skeletal x-rays are taken to identify defects in bones; for example, bone infections (osteomyelitis) are easily detected after the initial stages of infection. X-rays of the sinus cavities in the bones of the nose, face, and forehead can show if these cavities are filled with fluid.

Prepare the child for x-rays, explaining how a picture will be taken. Emphasize that it does not hurt, nor does it require an intrusive procedure. Have the child practice taking a deep breath and holding it for five seconds for chest x-rays, and holding still for x-rays in general.

Mark, aged seven, is profoundly deaf. A chest x-ray was ordered because his breath sounds and symptoms suggested pneumonia. One look at the room brought terror to Mark. His mother was not allowed in the room. After listening to his muted screams for 10 minutes, his mother demanded to have her son. She asked for a film to take home where she acted out "camera and picture." Mark went back to the x-ray department later that night and maintained control easily.

COMMON TREATMENTS

Medications

Antipyretics are prescribed frequently on the acute care unit. You will find that a good understanding of these preparations will help you to control the child's temperature and, as important, to teach parents about their use at home. Acetylsalicylic acid (aspirin) and acetaminophen (Tylenol,

Tempra, Datril and many others), the two most commonly used antipyretic medications, are sold "OTC," i.e., over the counter, without a prescription, in huge quantities.

Children's aspirin is pleasantly flavored and parents sometimes tell their child it is candy in an attempt to encourage them to take it for fever; unfortunately, some children are apparently convinced that it *is* candy, with tragic results. A large bottle of children's aspirin can be lethal to a small child. Recent changes in packaging have drastically reduced deaths due to aspirin ingestion. "Childproof" tops are put on the bottles and, increasingly, only a limited number of tablets (usually 36) are dispensed in each bottle. Occasionally, parents may overdose their child accidentally, although they follow the recommended dosages because the child does not rid his body of the previous dose, and the drug has a cumulative effect. Acetaminophen can also be toxic in large doses and poisonings have increased with its widespread use.

If the child has ingested large amounts accidentally, first remove remaining aspirin from his stomach by gastric lavage (see the Skills Manual) and/or inducing vomiting. Intravenous infusions help to dilute and remove excess acidity through urine. Peritoneal dialysis may also be used for the same purpose. (See chapter 29 for a discussion of the fluid and electrolyte imbalance that results from aspirin overdose.)

Aspirin and acetaminophen are essentially equally effective in lowering fever. A major advantage of aspirin is its anti-inflammatory qualities, but disadvantages include gastric irritation and a relatively narrow zone between therapeutic and toxic doses. Signs of toxicity include increased respiratory rate in response to acidosis, tinnitus (ringing in the ears), and a tendency to bleeding evidenced by increased bruising and blood in stools.

Antibiotics are medications used to weaken and/or kill pathogenic microorganisms, including bacteria, some rickettsiae, a few large viruses, and fungi. Antibiotics interfere with the metabolism and/or normal reproduction of the pathogen. These medications may be very specialized and may control only a few microorganisms (narrow spectrum), or they may be effective against many different pathogens (broad spectrum).

Antibiotics come in many forms so that the highest possible concentration of the medication in the infected site can be afforded. Topical preparations (i.e., creams, ointments, and drops) are applied to an infected surface or instilled into an infected cavity or canal. These medications, absorbed in very small amounts by the body, are effective only for the actual contact area and not underlying structures. Oral preparations (liquids, pills, tablets, capsules, and powders) are absorbed by the gastrointestinal tract; anything delaying or decreasing general absorption will have the same effect on the medication. Parenteral preparations are liquids prepared for intramuscular (never subcutaneous) injection or intravenous infusion. Because intramuscular injections are painful, physicians now tend to prescribe that antibiotics be given intravenously through an existing infusion or intermittent needle therapy (INT). This change has resulted in an "IV orientation" to antibiotics on the acute care unit; even young preschoolers learn to protect their IVs to avoid an injection. Regular parenteral injections of antibiotics maintain blood levels of the drug more efficiently than oral preparations. Protect all liquid forms of antibiotics from heat and always check the expiration date.

Finding the drug to which the microorganism is most sensitive is becoming more difficult as resistant mutations are formed. Drug companies continue to produce new antibiotics to combat the mutants, which evolve very easily in hospitals. As an evolutionary/survival mechanism, resistant strains of microorganisms develop in the patient who has had extensive antibiotic therapy, and the resistant strains are spread to other patients by personnel, equipment, food, and so on. Antibiotics have greatly reduced the mortality and morbidity rates of children, but some pharmacologists fear that someday the resistant strains will develop more rapidly than new drugs to control them.

Many children on the acute care unit require antibiotics. These medications usually are prescribed for an acute infection but may also be used to prevent infection in the child before and after surgery, in children who have been exposed to a specific illness, and in the child at risk due to a chronic or acute disease. The nurse has a grave responsibility for the administration of antibiotics to a child. Always determine whether the child has had an allergic reaction to the prescribed drug or to any other member of that drug's class. Be sure to ask about rashes, swelling, trouble with breathing, and fainting; many people do not understand the question "are you allergic to anything?" Numerous drugs cause local irritation of the gastric mucosa, causing nausea and vomiting. If the child has had such a reaction to a drug, report the fact to the physician before administering it, although this is usually not an allergic reaction. As with all allergies, the child must have been exposed to a drug to have formed an antibody to it. The next course of the same medication, required by another illness, or the later doses of an initial course are recognized by the body as foreign, i.e., as an antigen, initiating an antigen-antibody reaction. The first reaction may be a mild rash, or it may be severe, resulting in anaphylaxis, shock, and death. The reaction may be immediate (as is more frequently the case with parenteral administration) or delayed. Frequent observation of the child on antibiotics is obviously an important nursing responsibility. Among the medications usually prescribed to alleviate adverse reactions are antihistamines (e.g., Benadryl) for mild symptoms and epinephrine (Adrenaline) for more severe symptoms. Check your hospital's procedure manual for policy concerning this emergency, which may require cardiopulmonary resuscitation (CPR). Discontinue the medication immediately if there is any sign of allergic reaction. Before discharging the child, write the name of the drug on a card for the parents to keep until the child is old enough to carry it in his own wallet. If the reaction is severe, the child should wear a tag identifying the allergy around his arm.

Drugs taken orally are usually best absorbed on an empty stomach. However, many are so irritating to the gastric mucosa that the child cannot tolerate them; in such cases, the physician may prescribe that the drug be taken after eating or that it be administered parenterally. Some oral antibiotics are rendered useless by other medications. (Increasingly, pharmacology texts list drug counteractions.) To maintain the antibiotic blood level, doses are usually given every six to eight hours but may be given three or four times during waking hours to allow for uninterrupted sleep. Although it is difficult or impossible to give every antibiotic on time (within 30 minutes before or after the prescribed time), maintaining blood levels of the drug is a priority for the child with an infection.

Another nursing responsibility is observation for adverse responses to the antibiotic. One very common problem is an overgrowth of fungi in the gastrointestinal tract; this occurs because the antibacterial medication destroys the beneficial bacteria that normally control fungi. The child may develop thrush (fungal infections of the mouth), a monilial rash (a fungal rash originating in the perianal area and spreading over the buttocks, genitals, lower abdomen, groin, and legs), or diarrhea. Report these reactions to the physician immediately; he usually will change the medication or prescribe another medication to alleviate the problem. Yogurt may be given to stimulate the production of normal gastrointestinal flora.

Occasionally, a child will be discharged while he is still receiving his antibiotics. Explain to the parents the importance of looking for allergic reactions, giving the medication on time and every time prescribed, and notifying the physician of changes in the child. Compliance can be encouraged by explaining the written regimen, having the parents repeat the explanation, and sending written instructions home for future reference.

In summary, the following steps can serve as guidelines for antibiotic administration: 1) obtain all cultures, 2) rule out any allergy to the drug or other members of its class, 3) explain to parents and child how antibiotics work, 4) administer the drug according to prescription, 5) observe for immediate and delayed allergic reactions, and 6) observe for problems secondary to the antibiotics.

SPECIFIC CONDITIONS

Roseola

Synonyms: Roseola infantum, exanthem subitum

Causative Organism: Virus

Vaccine: None

Incubation Period: Two weeks

Prodromal Symptoms: None known

Complications: Febrile seizures

Roseola is a mildly contagious disease most often occurring in children between six months and three years of age. The child suddenly registers a temperature of 39.5° to 40.5° C (103° to 105° F) and may have febrile seizures. The fever may be brought down by antipyretic measures, but it may rise again after their effect is gone. If the child has meningeal irritation, he is often hospitalized for a lumbar puncture and observation. If he has other concurrent bacterial infections, such as otitis media, his fever does not decrease with antibiotics, and 3 to 4 days after the fever begins, a light macular or maculopapular rash erupts on the trunk and spreads to the arms and neck. The child's fever drops shortly before or soon after the rash appears.

A child hospitalized with roseola is admitted with a diagnosis of "FUO" and undergoes many diagnostic procedures. Usually, he has a very high fever or an atypical form of the disease. About the time the physician decides he is dealing with roseola, the rash appears. Nursing care is directed toward preventing febrile seizures, and maintaining hydration.

Rubella

Synonyms: German measles, three-day measles

Causative Organism: Virus

Vaccine: Injectable in children fifteen months of age

Incubation Period: Two to three weeks

Prodromal Symptoms: Catarrhal symptoms, lymphadenopathy of head and neck

Complications: Congenital rubella syndrome in children of women affected while pregnant

Rubella is a highly contagious exanthem. After the mild prodomal phase, the maculopapular rash appears on the face and spreads over the trunk. The rash may disappear so quickly that it is not noticed, or it may last as long as three days. The child almost never feels sick, although he may have headache and malaise.

Rubella presents the greatest danger to the fetus of a pregnant woman. When the expectant mother contracts the disease, the virus crosses her placenta and infects and damages the fetus. Once the baby is born, he sheds the live virus for some time and demonstrates evidence of infection during the first months of life. If he was infected early in the pregnancy, the effects are usually devastating. The congenital rubella syndrome includes deafness, blindness, cataracts, cardiovascular defects, and mental retardation.

Most prenatal centers determine the pregnant woman's immunity status during the initial visit. If she is susceptible to rubella, exposure to the disease is a medical emergency. First, she may be offered the option of abortion. If this is unacceptable to her, large doses of gammaglobulin may be administered in hopes of preventing the disease. Spontaneous abortion occurs in 30 to 40 percent of the women who were infected during the first trimester. This tremendous waste of life could be a rarity if every child were immunized between 15 months and childbearing age, since it is during this period that the disease is usually contracted. The nationwide immunization program has resulted in a decrease in occurrence of rubella and congenital rubella syndrome.

Nursing care of children with rubella centers around the prevention of the spread of the organism. Because it spreads by airborne droplets, respiratory precautions are necessary from about a week after the child is exposed until the rash is gone. Children are seldom hospitalized with acquired rubella except with the rare complication of encephalitis.

Varicella

Synonym: Chicken pox

Causative Organism: Virus (Herpesvirus varicella)

Vaccine: None

Incubation Period: Two to three weeks

Prodromal Symptoms: Malaise, faint rash

Complications: Secondary bacterial infections, encephalitis, pneumonia

Varicella is a highly contagious disease; although a child of any age can contract the disease, it usually affects the school-age child. The rash first appears on the trunk in the form of several red papules (crops). The papules fill with clear fluid, which later becomes cloudy and either crusts over or dries up. For several days, new crops appear (the number and extent vary with the severity of the disease), over the whole body, including the mouth and nose; the gastrointestinal tract may also be affected (Color Plate 3).

Nursing care of the child with chickenpox focuses on the alleviation of itching and the prevention of the spread of the disease, which is spread by droplets or actual contact with the lesions. Strict isolation is required on the acute care unit. Once all lesions are crusted, the child is no longer contagious.

Varicella is caused by the same organism that causes herpes zoster, another viral exanthem that occurs in older children and adults. Children may develop varicella after exposure to herpes zoster. Most people who contract herpes zoster have had childhood chickenpox. The organism obviously lies dormant until the person is weakened in some way.

Rubeola

Synonym: Measles, red measles

Causative Organism: Virus

Vaccine: Injectable in children fifteen months of age

Incubation Period: Ten days to two weeks

Prodromal Symptoms: Koplik's spots, fever, cough, conjunctivitis white, on inside of mouth

Complications: Encephalitis, pneumonia, otitis media

Rubeola is a contagious viral disease. When the prodromal phase is over and the maculopapular rash develops, the child's fever peaks and all other symptoms worsen. The rash begins on the face and neck and spreads over the arms, chest, and the rest of the body. The lesions may be hemorrhagic (having blood evident in the center) or confluent (meeting each other's borders). Fortunately, antibiotics have now eliminated many complications, but deaths still occur occasionally.

Nursing care of children with rubeola is concerned with the control of fever, avoiding direct or harsh light in the room, providing relief from the itchy rash, and maintaining hydration.

Diphtheria

Synonym: None

Causative Organism: Bacteria (Corynebacterium diphtheriae)

Vaccine: Injectable series and boosters from infancy

Incubation Period: Two to six days

Prodromal Symptoms: Malaise, fever, headache

Complications: Secondary bacterial infections, toxic effects on body organs

Diphtheria is a contagious disease in which bacteria invades a mucous membrane, usually those of the nose and throat. The bacteria do not invade the underlying tissue but produce a toxin that destroys the cells of the membrane. The body responds to this insult with fibrin production, and tough white or gray pseudomembrane develops.

Symptoms are specific to the location of the membrane involved. The most serious location is the upper respiratory tract, which may be occluded. If the toxin from the membrane is absorbed into the bloodstream, the heart, kidneys, liver, and nerves are also attacked, producing symptoms for weeks. Both the bacteria and the toxin of diphtheria require prompt treatment. Antibiotics are effective against the bacteria, and an antitoxin neutralizes free toxins but does not affect toxins already in the cell. This deadly disease is now uncommon, thanks to immunizations. If there is some question about a child's status, the Schick test can be administered to determine immunity. dx DIPHTHERIA

Nursing care is specific to the membrane and organs affected. Strict isolation is required to prevent the spread of the organism. When the child is receiving the antitoxin, observe for allergic reaction. The antitoxin, which is extracted from the serum of horses, is composed of antibodies to the diphtheria toxin. Horse serum can cause a severe allergic response after the initial dose.

Pertussis

Synonym: Whooping cough

Causative Organism: Bacteria (Bordetella pertussis)

Vaccine: Injectable series up to age six years

Incubation Period: One to two weeks

Prodromal Symptoms: Catarrhal symptoms

Complications: Respiratory arrest, secondary infections

Pertussis is a highly contagious respiratory disease of young children, susceptible older children and adults, who may contract a mild form of the disease. The affected newborn and young infant have a high mortality rate. There is a two- to three-week prodromal stage that resembles a bad cold. The child's cough gets worse until he develops the characteristic "whooping cough." On inspiration, the "whoop" is heard as the child struggles to take in air; the expiration is a terrible cough marked by evident anxiety, red face, bulging tongue and eyes, and mucus bubbling from the mouth and nose. These spasmodic coughs occur in paroxysms a few or many times a day, ending with vomiting; the coughing stage lasts two to three weeks. Antibiotics do not seem to shorten the illness. Once the first immunization is received, the chances of getting a severe form of the disease are lessened, but a whole series is required for immunity.

Nursing care of infants and young children is specific to symptoms. The disease usually occurs in children from very poor families in rural or inner city areas. Once one child in a family develops the disease, other siblings can be expected to contract it, since it is highly contagious and children of same families are not likely to have been immunized. During the coughing spells, hold the child upright and wipe excess mucus from his mouth and nose. He usually will receive moisturized oxygen in a croup-tent, making the job of support more difficult. Be prepared for the child to vomit; allow for a rest period after the vomiting and feed him after the rest period. Maintaining hydration is important; the child may accept some fluid immediately after vomiting. Strict isolation is required for the younger child and respiratory isolation is required for older children. Antibiotics may be given to render the child noncontagious, or during the incubation period to weaken the organism.

Tetanus

Synonym: Lockjaw

Causative Organism: Bacteria (Clostridium tetani)

Vaccine: Injectable series and boosters

Incubation Period: One to two weeks

Complications: Respiratory distress, malnutrition, fluid and electrolyte imbalance

Tetanus is a severe infection that is rarely seen in this country today. In order to infect the child, the organism or its spore must get into the body tissues where no direct oxygen is available. This most frequently occurs after a puncture wound, delivery of an infant under unsanitary conditions, burns, or so on. The central nervous system is the focus of the infection, which causes spasms in the jaw ("lockjaw"), the back and neck (opisthotonos), abdomen, and, potentially, any other part of the body. The child remains mentally alert, so he is terrified. The mortality rate for tetanus is still high, but it has been reduced by the use of antitoxin, gammaglobulin specific for tetanus, antibiotics, and better techniques to maintain nutrition, hydration, and oxygenation until the disease subsides.

Nursing care of children with tetanus is provided on the critical care unit. All body processes must be supported. The nurse should determine the immunization status of each child admitted to her unit, inform the physician of deficiencies, and educate parents as to the value of protection for their children.

Conjunctivitis

Synonym: Pinkeye
Causative Organism: Bacteria, viruses
Vaccine: None
Incubation Period: Variable
Prodromal Symptoms: None
Complications: Rarely, corneal scarring

Conjunctivitis is an inflammation of the clear lining of the eyeball up to the cornea (bulbar conjunctiva) and of the underside of the eyelid (palpebral conjunctiva). Neonates develop conjunctivitis by passing through an infected birth canal, but the instillation of silver nitrate or other antibiotic drops in each eye at birth usually prevents infection. This instillation, required by law in most states to prevent gonococcal conjunctivitis, which causes blindness, causes transient irritation of and discharge from the membranes. Older children develop infectious conjunctivitis, usually viral, which causes mucopurulent discharge, swollen lids, and pain. They may wake up with their lids crusted together from the discharge and/or swollen shut by edema. This frightening condition can be relieved by gently irrigating the lids with a cool saline solution until the crusts loosen and the edema subsides. Some children have severe common cold symptoms along with conjunctivitis. Treatment is specific to symptoms except when the agent is identified as bacteria and area treated with antibiotics. Infectious conjunctivitis is transmitted by direct contact with secretions and often by droplets from the respiratory tract. This highly contagious disease spreads quickly through schools, dormitories, nursery schools, etc.

Acute Sinusitis

Synonym: None
Causative Organism: Variety of bacteria
Vaccine: None
Prodromal Symptoms: Fever, pain, sense of fullness in sinuses
Complications: Brain abscess, orbital cellulites, Osteomyelitis

Sinusitis literally means "an inflammation of a sinus," which is any cavity with a relatively narrow opening; The term *sinusitis,* however, generally refers to an inflammation of the boney sinuses that drain into the nose. The infant is born with some of these cavities in the surrounding bone, and others develop with age. Sinuses usually become infected with bacteria secondarily to a nasal allergy or a viral upper respiratory infection. The problem is much more prevalent in children with debilitating diseases. The sinuses fill with pus, causing foul-smelling discharge and breath, headache, anorexia, sore throat, and cough caused by drainage in the area. Antibiotics are given to combat the bacteria, and decongestants are prescribed to shrink the mucous membranes in hopes of promoting drainage from the sinuses. Occasionally, sinuses are drained surgically. Any underlying problems must be treated to prevent recurrent infection. Can be very serious

Otitis Media

Synonyms: Middle ear infection, tympanitis

Causative Organism: Bacteria (Diplococcus pneumoniae, Hemophilus influenzae)

Vaccine: None

Complications: Meningitis, hearing loss, mastoiditis

Otitis media, inflammation of the middle ear, is caused by many agents, including a wide variety of bacteria. Suppurative otitis media (bacterial) is a condition in which the infected membranes produce pus and fill the cavity, pushing the tympanic membrane out until it bulges or bursts. The bacteria get to the area through the eustachian tube, or perhaps through the blood stream. The affected child feels extreme pain until the pressure is removed either by rupture, myringotomy, or antibiotic therapy. Decongestants are used to shrink the eustachian tube in order to promote drainage. Children with severe otitis media are occasionally admitted to the acute care unit because of a high fever and the possibility or presence of complicating meningitis. Children with acute suppurative otitis media do not require isolation precautions unless there is a primary or secondary contagious infection. (For further discussion see Chapter 10.)

Osteomyelitis

Synonym: None

Causative Organism: Staphylococcus aureus and various other bacteria

Vaccine: None

Incubation Period: One to two weeks

Prodromal Symptoms: None

Complications: Destruction of bone

Osteomyelitis is an inflammation of bone usually caused by bacterial infection. The bacteria travel from an infected skin lesion or from the pharynx through the bloodstream to the periosteum (lining over the bone), where an abscess is formed. Once the periosteum is penetrated, the infection spreads just under it to other parts of the bone and to the marrow, destroying tissue along the way. The child usually complains of pain, swelling, and heat in the area of a bone, and is weak, irritable, and feverish. The organism is identfied by cultures of the blood or of aspirate from the affected area. The prompt administration of intravenous antibiotics specific to the causative organism is of utmost importance. The child may require antibiotic therapy for three weeks or more to prevent chronic infection and/or permanent destruction of bone. Nursing care is directed toward the administration of medications, maintenance of nutritional, fluid, and electrolyte balance, and the relief of pain. If there is an open wound, use wound isolation precautions to prevent the spread of infection.

Gonorrhea

Synonyms: GC, clap, drip, strain

Causative Organism: Neisseria gonorrhoeae

Vaccine: None

Incubation Period: Three to five days

Prodromal Symptoms: None

Complications: Blindness (newborns), arthritis, pelvic inflammatory disease and sterility (female), urethral strictures (male), gonococcal arthritis

Gonorrhea is a major health problem in contemporary society. This venereal disease is spread by direct contact with an infected mucous membrane or, rarely, with an object (fomes) that has absorbed the infected discharge and touches a healthy mucous membrane. Most cases of gonorrhea involve sexual contact with the genitals, rectum, or mouth. The conjunctiva of newborns may become infected as they pass through an infected birth canal. Children at increasingly younger ages are contracting the disease from sexual activity that includes sex play with other children, or from rape or other forms of molestation. Incest (sexual activity between close family members) as a form of child abuse also accounts for instances of the disease in children. The adolescent incidence rate has been rising rapidly with changes in sexual standards, and reinfection is to be expected. Adolescent parents are notorious for not seeking prenatal care, and the offspring of an affected teenager travels through an infected, untreated birth canal. The nurse in a hospital will see children with gonorrhea in the newborn nursery, children with gonococcal arthritis on the acute care unit, teenagers with inflammatory complications on the adolescent unit, and, on the maternity units, affected mothers. Children with other admitting diagnoses are sometimes found to have gonorrhea after routine testing.

Gonorrhea usually causes a painful urethritis with discharge in males and endocervicitis in females. Prepubescent girls often have vulvovaginitis. Unfortunately, since the disease may cause no symptoms at all, the male can spread the disease unknowingly, and females can develop pelvic diseases, and the resultant sterility is the first indication of infection. Penicillin is the treatment of choice except for penicillin-resistant strains which require other antibiotics. Surgery is often necessary to drain pelvic abscesses. The infected mucous membrane, or drainage from an abscess, requires wound isolation precautions to prevent spreading to others.

Syphilis

Synonyms: Pox, bad blood, syph, old dog

Causative Organism: Treponema pallidum

Vaccine: None

Incubation Period: Three weeks

Complications: Congenital: Deafness, keratitis, chorioretinitis, optic atrophy
Acquired: Cardiovascular changes, neurological degeneration

Syphilis is categorized as congenital or acquired. The incidence of both forms of the disease has risen with the increased number of sexually active adolescents, but many affected persons are cured unknowingly by having taken penicillin for other reasons. In the past, federally funded programs have been successful in decreasing the incidence of syphilis through prompt treatment and the location and notification of contacts. As with all venereal diseases, private physicians frequently do not report syphilis, allowing contacts to go untreated.

In congenital syphilis, the fetus contracts the disease through the placenta when the mother has either an active or a latent case. He may show signs of the disease soon after birth, or the first indications may appear after infancy. The infant may show such nonspecific signs as poor feeding, various skin problems, and bone involvement. If untreated, he may develop a flat nasal bridge, peg-shaped central incisors (Hutchinson's teeth), bowing of the tibia, and, later, deafness and blindness. Diagnosis is difficult because of the variety of symptoms. Once congenital syphilis is suspected, however, several lab tests, including direct visualization of the spiraled bacterium (spirochete) and serologic studies, usually confirm the diagnosis. Treatment consists of the administration of penicillin.

The incidence of syphilis is much lower than that of gonorrhea, but it is on the rise. Children acquire syphilis just as they do any type of venereal disease, i.e., through sexual activity with infected family members or other children, adolescents, or adults. There are three active stages (primary, secondary, and tertiary) and a latent stage. The primary stage begins with the eruption of a chancre, an ulcerated or crusted, painless lesion at the site of exposure, usually the genitals, mouth, or rectum. The chancre is highly infectious, but it disappears in six weeks or less even if untreated. The secondary stage is more generalized and is characterized by malaise, headache, weight loss, low-grade fever, and an infectious rash in the moist ano-genital area; this stage also resolves in six weeks or less with or without treatment. Some people do not experience the first two stages but develop the manifestations of tertiary syphilis, which include cardiovascular, neurological, and skin changes. This stage seldom occurs in children or adolescents. In latent syphilis there is no indication of disease except for positive serologic tests. All stages of the disease are treated with penicillin or other organism-specific antibiotics. The tertiary and latent stages, noninfectious except to the fetus, require no isolation precautions.

Mumps

Synonym: Epidemic parotitis
Causative Organism: Virus
Vaccine: Injectable, probably throughout life
Incubation Period: Two to three weeks
Prodromal Symptoms: Rarely, fever, malaisc, muscular pain
Complications: Meningoencephalitis, orchitis, epididymitis, deafness

Mumps is an inflammation of either or both parotid glands and, occasionally, other salivary glands. It most frequently affects children between five and twelve years of age. Swelling occurs just below the ears and spreads downward and forward. Any heavy salivation causes pain. The virus enters the bloodstream and may infect various organs, including the meninges, brain, testicles, epididymis, and ovaries.

Nursing care of the child with mumps is specific to symptoms. Since there is no treatment known to shorten the course, providing comfort and maintaining hydration are the nursing goals. Children on an acute care unit with mumps are most often afflicted with postmumps encephalitis or meningoencephalitis. These children may have fever, and central nervous system irritability, headaches, vomiting, and even convulsions. Orchitis (inflammation of the testes) occurs in about 25 percent of adolescent cases occasionally resulting in decreased fertility. Deafness arising from mumps is rare, but mumps is a major cause of sensorineural deafness in children. These complications are reason enough to encourage parents to have their children immunized against mumps.

Poliomyelitis

Synonyms: Polio, infantile paralysis
Causative Organism: Virus
Vaccine: Oral series and booster
Incubation Period: One to two weeks

Prodromal Symptoms: Coryza, central nervous system symptoms

Complications: Paralysis, gastrointestinal bleeding

Polio is transmitted by contact with the gastrointestinal tract. Before the development of the first (Salk) vaccine in the 1950's, polio left many children and adults with a flaccid paralysis that occasionally affected the respiratory muscles. Vaccines have decreased the incidence of the disease, but periodic outbreaks of polio occur in groups of people who are not immunized. The most important function of the nurse in relation to polio patients is to advise parents of the value of polio vaccines. The infant should receive the first immunization at about two months of age.

The child with acute polio receives care in a critical care unit. Extreme irritability of the central nervous system is evidenced by headache, nausea and vomiting, and convulsions; the child may also have muscle pain and spinal rigidity. Nursing care centers around maintaining comfort, hydration, respiratory function, nutrition, skin integrity, and mobility of the limbs.

Smallpox

Synonym: Variola

Causative Organism: Virus

Vaccine: Scratch, pressure techniques, usually cowpox lymph

Incubation Period: Two to three weeks

Prodromal Symptoms: Fever, headache, rashes

Complications: Secondary bacterial infections, respiratory involvement, bone destruction

Smallpox is a highly contagious viral diseases characterized by exanthems that erupt in a short period of time and progress from papular to vesicular to pustular form. The lesions crust over and are contagious until the last crust is gone. Smallpox has been eradicated in this country through vaccination and the control of immigration of nonimmunized persons. A few underdeveloped countries still have incidences of smallpox, but most countries have long been free of the disease. In rare cases, the smallpox vaccination, usually resulting in a single lesion, spreads over the body as generalized vaccinia, leaving scars and sometimes causing death. Since the threat of vaccinia is much greater than having the disease, smallpox vaccine is no longer routinely administered. Your major responsibility is to convince parents that their child is safe without the vaccine unless he goes to a country in which the disease is endemic.

Pharyngitis

Synonym: Sore throat

Causative Organism: Bacteria (Streptococcus) or virus

Vaccine: None

Prodromal Symptoms: Fever, malaise, coryza

Complications: Involvement of total respiratory tree and adjacent structures, rheumatic fever and acute glomerulonephritis following streptococcal infection

Pharyngitis in children is usually caused by viruses but may be caused by streptococcus (Figure 15–2) or, rarely, by other bacteria. (Also, allergies of the nasal membranes that cause mouth breathing and postnasal drip can make the throat very sore, especially in the morning). Streptococcal pharyngitis is a more severe illness, characterized by a more abrupt onset,

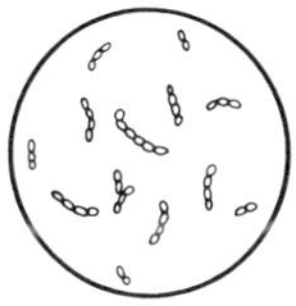

Figure 15–2. *Streptococci are responsible for a variety of illnesses in children, including pharyngitis, rheumatic fever, acute glomerulonephritis, and impetigo.*

more inflammation and pain, higher fever, and more exudate than in the viral forms. A throat culture is required for diagnosis since the clinical picture may be imprecise. Streptococcal pharyngitis is the more significant disease since rheumatic fever and acute glomerulonephritis may follow. If the child does not have antitoxin antibodies, he may develop a bright red rash, or scarlet fever. The streptococcal form is treated with antibiotics, while viral pharyngitis is treated only symptomatically.

Nursing care of children with pharyngitis on the acute care unit focuses on the control of fever and pain, maintaining hydration, and preventing the spread of infection. Cool drinks will soothe a sore throat and ensure fluid intake. Gargling with a warm normal saline solution and/or a topical anesthetic decreases pain and can help remove foul odor and taste from the mouth. Sucking on hard candy keeps saliva flowing which, in turn, soothes the sore throat. Earache may be caused by an infection of the middle ear or an inflammation of the eustachian tube.

Nasopharyngitis

Synonym: Common cold

Causative Organism: Rhinoviruses

Vaccine: None

Incubation Period: 12 to 72 hours

Prodromal Symptoms: Fever, malaise, and sneezing

Complications: Secondary bacterial infections of respiratory tract and adjacent structures, including middle ears, lymph nodes, and paranasal sinuses

The common cold occurs more frequently than any other disease in children. The average early school-age child will have three to six colds a year, but factors such as other illness, exposure to other children, and allergies will increase the incidence in some children. The virus invades the mucous membranes of the nose and throat, causing inflammation, a thin drainage, sneezing, fever, headache, and malaise. Later, the drainage becomes thicker and often purulent. The cold itself produces only minor annoyances for a few days, but complications can be extensive and severe, since anatomical structures in the infant and child are close to each other, and the respiratory tract has continuous mucous membranes. Once the mucous membrane is invaded by a microorganism, it is left vulnerable to bacteria. The body has various mechanisms to stop the progress of the infection, but they occasionally fail. Children on an acute care unit with pneumonia, laryngotracheobronchitis, and acute sinusitis usually had colds initially.

Nursing care of children with colds includes the provision of comfort, maintenance of hydration, and the control of fever. Since mucopurulent drainage from the nose can block airways, clearing the passages will allow the infant to breathe while sucking, and the older child to drink or eat more comfortably. You may have the responsibility of explaining to parents that their child should not have antibiotics with an uncomplicated cold. They may feel that the administration of antibiotics will prevent complications, but there are no indications that this is true; in fact, antibiotics affect the normal body balance, and infections secondary to antibiotic therapy may occur.

Croup

Synonyms: Acute spasmodic croup, laryngotracheobronchitis, epiglottitis

Causative Organism: Viruses, occasionally bacteria

Vaccine: None

Incubation Period: Variable; a few days to a week

Prodromal Symptoms: Coryza, malaise, fever

Complications: Respiratory arrest, secondary bacterial infections

Croup is a term used to describe acute infections of the larynx and/or adjacent structures that partially obstruct the larynx, causing a barking cough and inspiratory stridor ("crowing"). Infections of the larynx, epiglottis, trachea, and bronchi may produce these symptoms. Most are only mild infections, but they may be severe enough to obstruct the larynx totally, requiring artificial respiration. Epiglottitis is a medical emergency in which the child has a high fever, cherry-red epiglottis, extreme pharyngeal pain, drooling, and hyperextended neck. He should be examined only in the presence of emergency medical personnel and equipment because of the extreme danger of further epiglottal edema and obstruction. Laryngotracheobronchitis (LTB) may be mild, but it may progress to obstruct the larynx, trachea, and/or bronchi. Infectious laryngitis may also become rapidly obstructive. Children with these conditions are placed in a critical care unit for continuous observation and emergency intervention.

Acute spasmodic croup is a viral disease of young children; children whose admitting diagnosis is "croup" usually have this form of the disease. It tends to recur and seems to be familial. The child often has a mild cold and cough when he goes to bed, but he wakes up in the middle of the night with a croaking, barking cough accompanied by anxiety approaching panic. After struggling for breath for several minutes, he may vomit, quit coughing, and go to sleep, only to wake up later with another bout. Moist air, either warm or cold, decreases spasms. Children may be treated at home by having them sit in a closed bathroom with a hot shower running full force during the spasms. A calm parent can allay the child's anxiety considerably. Conversely, many health professionals relate the anxious parent to the anxious, croupy, child, but such a causal relationship has not been established.

Robbie, aged twenty-two months, woke up at 11 pm with a croaking, barking cough. His mother, Mrs. H., aged eighteen, rushed to the room, picked him up, and paced the floor until vomiting occurred and coughing ceases. At 12:45 P.M., another paroxysm occurred; Mrs. H. managed it adequately but with increasing fear. When Robbie began barking again at 2:45 P.M. Mrs. H., lying beside him and waiting for the next attack, lost control and started sobbing hysterically as she paced the floor with him. Mr. H. called the pediatrician, who instructed them to ride, with the window down, to the emergency room. He met the three of them and admitted Robbie, who was essentially asymptomatic, probably thanks to the moist night air. The nurse who admitted the family to the acute care unit found a helpless-looking father, an exhausted and anxious mother, and a sleeping baby. Robbie was placed in a croupette, Mrs. H. in a sleeper cot, and Mr. H. in a comfortable chair. When Robbie began barking just before daybreak, his nurse, encouraging Mrs. H. to sit him up in the croupette and talk quietly to him, stayed with the family until he was quiet again.

Spasmodic croup can result in complete obstruction of the larynx; careful observation is therefore required, either by the parent at home or the nurse in the hospital. Antibiotics are given only in the case of bacterial croup. Antihistamines, expectorants, and antitussives are ineffective. A brief course of steroids may be given to decrease inflammation of the larynx, but careful observation for masked infection is essential. The child with croup requires only routine precautions against the spread of infection except that he is not allowed contact with other children.

Pneumonia

Synonym: None

Causative Organisms/Matter: Bacteria, viruses, fungi, aspirates

Vaccine: Pneumococcal only

Incubation Period: Variable

Prodromal Symptoms: Fever, malaise, cough

Complications: Pneumothorax, lung abscess, atelectasis

The term pneumonia encompasses a variety of conditions including infiltration of interstitial tissue, lobules, or lobes of the lungs. Pneumonia can be an infectious disease caused by a variety of microorganisms, or it can be caused by aspirated matter. Generally, bacterial pneumonia is an acute systemic illness. The child exhibits a high fever, malaise, irritability, diminished breath sounds, and rapidly progressive respiratory distress. Bacterial pneumonias are treated with antibiotics and by the removal of accumulations of pus in the lungs and pleural space. Nursing care is directed toward the maintenance of respiratory function and fluid and electrolyte balance.

Viral pneumonias usually have a slower onset and less severe symptoms. Most children do not require hospitalization and receive care at home or in out-patient settings. Bronchiolitis is a form of viral pneumonia that causes enema of the bronchioles in infants. The swollen tubes allow some air into the alveole with each breath but trap it there. Both onset and recovery can be abrupt. Aspirated objects and chemicals can result in inflammation and infiltration of the lung. petroleum distillates, when swallowed, result in a chemical pneumonia either from inhalation or transportation by the circulatory system. Nursing care is of utmost importance with all pneumonias, but especially so with viral and aspirate pneumonias, which are not usually responsive to medications.

Gastritis, Gastroenteritis, Diarrhea

Synonyms: None

Causative Organisms: Viruses, bacteria, protozoa, fungi, rickettsiae and animal parasites

Vaccine: None

Incubation Period: Variable; a few hours to weeks, depending on organism

Prodromal Symptoms: Malaise, nausea, abdominal pain

Complications: Fluid and electrolyte imbalance, malnutrition

Inflammation of the gastrointestinal tract results from many disorders, including infections by each category of microorganism. Viral infections (usually caused by echoviruses) are usually self-limiting and milder than bacterial infections (cholera, salmonellosis, dysentery, and so on), which cause acute systemic illness in addition to gastrointestinal symptoms. Viral infections are treated symptomatically, while bacterial infections require antibiotic therapy. Protozoa can cause diarrhea severe enough to cause death in children. Fungal infections can produce mild to severe symptoms, especially when fungal food poisoning is involved. Each type of gastrointestinal infection requires a careful watch over the child's nutritional, fluid, and electrolyte balance. If the child is vomiting or has involuntary bowel movements, expect him to be upset by the loss of control of his body functions. Enteric isolation must be maintained in all cases of gastrointestinal disorders until they are proved noninfectious. A culture series of stool and, occasionally, vomitus is necessary in many types of infections.

Animal parasites also cause gastrointestinal disease. The pinworm (Enterobius vermicularis) is usually only an annoyance, causing anal itching, but this white, threadlike worm can migrate to the vagina or upper colon, irritating the mucosa of these organs. Some children complain of stomachaches, but more frequently the child is simply irritable. The "Scotch tape test" used to diagnose pinworms is performed by placing the sticky surface of cellophane tape over the anus for less than a minute in the early morning to obtain the ova for diagnosis. The ova of pinworms are almost light enough to be airborne and fly easily from person to person while changing clothes, linens, and so on. All members of a household, therefore, should receive anthelmintic medication to destroy the organism.

The roundworm (ascaris) looks like a large earthworm. Its life cycle includes ingestion by the child of soil contaminated with feces, migration to the liver, to the lungs where they are coughed up and swallowed, then back to the small intestine where they live and mate. They are passed out of the body through vomiting and/or diarrhea (see Figure 15–3).

Janie, aged three, had had a tracheostomy since birth. When her mother reported recent respiratory difficulty, the public health nurse suctioned a healthy-looking roundworm from the tracheostomy tube during her next visit. Janie was admitted to the acute care unit so that the infestation could be treated, and Janie's mother's knowledge and skill in caring for Janie could be reassessed.

Since the larvae migrate to the lungs, a pneumonia often develops. Some children develop sensitivity to the worms and display allergic symptoms. Roundworms can be destroyed with anthelmintics, but infection from this type of parasite is related to poor sanitary conditions, found most often in poverty-stricken families. Since aspects of lifestyle that arise from poverty are extremely difficult to change, reinfection can be expected.

The nurse may have difficulty in overcoming a feeling of repulsion when a child's diaper is full of worms, but these children need as much holding and affection as any other child—just be sure to use enteric precautions.

Impetigo

Synonyms: None

Causative Organism: Bacteria (Streptococcus [b-hemolytic; group A] or Staphylococcus auereus [hemolytic])

Vaccine: None

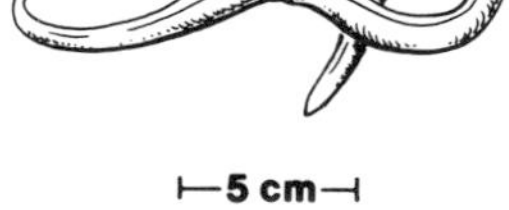

Figure 15–3. *Roundworm (Ascaris).*

Incubation period: Variable; four to ten days

Prodromal Symptoms: None

Complications: Acute glomerulonephritis following infection with nephritogenic strains of streptococci

Impetigo is an infectious disease of the skin. The causative microorganisms grow wherever there is a break in the skin. First, a vesicle forms, then it changes to a pustule, which then becomes crusted over. Itching is intense, and scratching spreads the infection to other parts of the body. The treatment of impetigo is simple; soften the crusts by soaking, remove them by rubbing with an antiseptic solution and terry cloth, and apply an antibiotic ointment three times a day. The lesions clear quickly with this routine, but since some strains of streptococci cause acute glomerulonephritis, oral antibiotics may be given to eliminate the organism from the body. Children of all socioeconomic classes develop impetigo, but poor children often have much worse infections due to a lack of cleanliness. Curing the illness may be difficult because parents hesitate to remove the crusts, and medications cannot reach microorganisms beneath them.

Impetigo is seldom an admitting diagnosis, but many children on acute care units have the disease. Parents of children with acute glomerulonephritis need to understand its relationship with impetigo and the importance of prevention.

Urinary Tract Infection

Synonym: UTI

Causative Organism: Bacteria (Escherichia coli and others)

Incubation Period: Variable, according to organism

Prodromal Symptoms: Urinary frequency

Complications: Chronic infection, permanent renal damage

Infections of the urinary tract are usually caused by bacteria normally inhabiting the large intestine. Usually, the whole tract is affected to some degree when one portion is infected; terms that describe an infection as being localized in the upper portion (pyelonephritis) or the lower portion (cystitis) of the intestine are incorrect to this extent. Girls have a significantly greater number of urinary tract infections than boys due to the proximity of the rectum and urethra. Many infections have no symptoms whatsoever, but they may lead to complications and permanent damage to the kidneys. Diagnosis and treatment of a urinary tract infection always includes a culture and sensitivity analysis. After a complete course of antibiotic therapy, urine cultures are obtained to rule out a continuing infection.

Most children with urinary tract infections are treated at home, but may require admission in cases of severe acute infection, chronic infection, or conditions requiring surgery. No specific isolation precautions are required since these infections are not contagious. Nursing care centers around the maintenance of fluid and electrolyte balance, providing comfort, and the administration of antibiotics.

Meningitis

Synonym: None

Causative Organism: Bacteria, virus, fungus

Vaccine: None

Incubation Period: Variable, depending on organism; one to ten days

Prodromal Symptoms: Fever, irritability, headache, gastrointestinal upsets

Complications: Cerebral edema, paralysis, mental retardation, hydrocephalus, sensory impairment

Meningitis is known to many people as "spinal meningitis," but since the meninges actually line the spinal cord and the brain, the word "spinal" is restrictive in that spinal meningitis involves only the meninges of the spinal cord. The disease causes extreme fear in parents who have heard stories of paralysis, mental retardation, and/or a swift death due to meningitis. The infection can indeed cause these complications, but meningitis also exists in a mild form that causes only discomfort, with no residual effects. In general, bacterial meningitis is more severe than viral (aseptic) meningitis. The bacteria that cause the infection in children are usually Hemophilus influenzae, pneumococci, and meningococci. The onset is often so sudden that diagnosing bacterial meningitis before it becomes well established in the child is very difficult. Diagnosis involves a study of cerebrospinal fluid obtained by a lumbar puncture. Other symptoms, such as increased protein and cell counts may be present.

Bacterial meningitis is treated with intravenous antibiotics specific for the organism, while viral meningitis is treated symptomatically. Nutritional, fluid, and electrolyte balance is maintained intravenously. Great care is taken to prevent or reduce any agents that might stimulate the already irritable central nervous system and cause spasms or convulsions. Since fever aggravates central nervous system irritation, close monitoring and control of body temperature is essential. Children with severe meningitis receive care in critical care units, but children with milder cases remain on acute care units.

Neonates born in circumstances in which the mother herself and/or the environment is unsanitary are especially susceptible to meningitis. Children who suffer from chronic illness or immunodeficiency are also at risk for the disease, as are children living in crowded, poverty-stricken areas. Outbreaks of meningitis occur among new recruits of the armed forces, who are housed in barracks and are under physical stress. Meningitis is spread by airborne respiratory droplets, but strict isolation (not just respiratory isolation) is usually necessary because of involuntary movement and vomiting. Isolation techniques are usually unnecessary after 24 hours of antibiotic therapy. Residual neurological damage requires a team approach in discharge planning. The services of a home health nurse, physical therapist, speech therapist, occupational therapist, psychologist, educational specialist, and many other professionals may be required. Whenever possible, make referrals to community agencies before the family leaves the hospital.

Encephalitis

Synonym: Sleeping sickness

Causative Organism: All types of infectious microorganisms

Vaccine: None

Incubation Period: Variable; 7 to 21 days according to organism

Prodromal Symptoms: Malaise, headache, upper respiratory symptoms

Complications: Cerebral edema, convulsions

Encephalitis means "inflammation of the brain,"; it is caused by infectious microorganisms, by allergic reactions to invaders when the infection has almost run its course, by reproduction of the microorganism in the brain after the initial illness, and by many other factors. Most cases of encephalitis, however, are of uncertain origin. A more precise term for the illness is *meningoencephalitis* since the meninges are inflamed, resulting in meningeal symptoms.

Most encephalitis known to be of infectious origin is caused by viruses that can be transmitted from person to person or from animal to person (e.g., a mosquito that bites an infected bird and then bites a child). Children with severe encephalitis require continuous critical care; convulsions, coma, cardiopulmonary arrest, and fluid and electrolyte imbalance are among the possible complications. The hypothermia blanket is frequently used to stabilize or maintain a below-normal body temperature. Anticonvulsants and antibiotics (when indicated) are administered intravenously.

Encephalitis frequently follows common childhood diseases (e.g., mumps and measles), most of which can be prevented through immunizations. Since many types of encephalitis are still of unknown origin, strict isolation techniques are used until noninfectious status is determined.

Influenza

Synonym: Flu

Causative Organism: Virus

Vaccine: Injectable for specific strains

Incubation Period: 36 to 48 hours

Prodromal Symptoms: Sudden onset

Complications: Pneumonia, severe croup, cardiac failure, secondary infections of entire respiratory tree and adjacent structures, Reye's syndrome

Influenza is a highly infectious respiratory disease that is responsible for acute illness in many children each winter. Symptoms include high fever, aching throughout the body, sore throat, and a dry, hacking cough. The affected child usually has no energy; he may even require help in going to the bathroom. Often, the disease seems to be waning when the fever rises once again before returning to normal. Treatment is specific to symptoms; complete bed rest is necessary. Influenza lasts three to four days, if no complications occur.

A significant complication of influenza is Reye's syndrome, which comprises encephalopathy accompanied by fatty degeneration of the viscera. This problem seems to be on the rise, but some of the increased statistical incidence may be the result of widespread recognition of the syndrome. Symptoms range from mild liver dysfunction to severe neurological involvement. The child appears to be recovering from influenza when he suddenly begins vomiting; convulsions and coma follow in one to two days. The child requires intensive nursing and medical care at all times to support body processes. Since a respirator may be required, close monitoring of respirations and blood gases is essential. Exchange transfusions and peritoneal dialysis are performed to alleviate the chemical imbalances resulting from liver dysfunction. Even with the best of care, the mortality rate remains high.

SUMMARY

Infections are no longer killers of well children, except in rare instances, thanks to the discovery and widespread use of immunizations and antibiotics. Even so, every nurse on a pediatric acute care unit will encounter many children with infections. An increasing number of children with chronic illnesses are hospitalized because of secondary infections. Sophisticated laboratory procedures closely monitor the infectious process and guide the health care team. Nursing care is directed toward maintaining comfort and physiological balance in the child, administering antibiotics, preventing the spread of infection to others, and supporting the child's parents.

Bibliography

Anthony, N. et al. Immunization: Public Health Programming Through Law Enforcement. *American Journal of Public Health,* 67:763, 1977.

Benjamin, J.T. Pharyngitis Due to Group C Hemolytic Streptococci in Children. *Journal of Pediatrics,* 89:254, 1976.

Brown, M.S. Syphillis and Gonorrhea: an Update for Nurses in Ambulatory Settings. *Nursing '76,* 6:71, 1976.

Castle, M. Help Stamp Out Infections: Be an Infection Control Coordinator. *Nursing '76,* 6:90, 1976.

Cohen, S. and Glass, G.K. Skin Rashes in Infants and Children (Programmed Instruction). *American Journal of Nursing,* 78:1041, 1978.

Derbes, V.J. Rashes: Recognition and Management. *American Journal of Nursing,* 78:54, 1978.

Furste, Ward and Aguirre, A. Preventing Tetanus. *American Journal of Nursing,* 78: 834, 1978.

Garrettson, L.K. The Child Resistant Container: A Success and A Model for Accident Prevention. *American Journal of Public Health,* 67:135, 1977.

Jenny, G. What You Should Be Doing about Infection Control. *Nursing '76,* 6:78, 1976.

Krugman, S., Ward, R., Katz, S.L. *Infectious Diseases of Children,* Saint Louis, C. V. Mosby Co., 1977.

Lake, A.M. Enterovirus Infections in Neonates. *Journal of Pediatrics,* 89:787, 1976.

Lindberg, J. Long Term Outcome of Hemophilus Influenzae Meningitis Related to Antibiotic Treatment. *Pediatrics,* 60:1, 1977.

Lopez, R.I. *Adolescent Medicine.* New York, Spectrum Publications, Inc., 1976.

O'Grady, R. Whooping Cough in Infancy. *American Journal of Nursing,* 76:114, 1976.

Pearce, J.L. Phenobarbital in the Acute Management of Febrile Convulsions. *Pediatrics,* 60:569, 1977.

Strangert, K. Respiratory Illness in Preschool Children with Different Forms of Day Care. *Pediatrics,* 57:191, 1976.

Treves, S. Osteomyelitis: Early Scintigraphic Detection in Children. *Pediatrics* 57: 173, 1976.

CHAPTER **16**

The Child with Altered Immunity

BEHAVIORAL OBJECTIVES

After studying this chapter, you will be able to:

- Define immunodeficiency, allergy, and autoimmunity.
- Describe similarities and differences in nursing care for the child with each type of altered immunity.
- Discuss diagnostic procedures designed to differentiate among immunological deviations.
- List major bronchodilators and common side effects.
- Discuss the use of corticosteroids in the treatment of the child with altered immunity.

TERMS AND CONCEPTS

Primary immunodeficiency
Secondary immunodeficiency
White blood cell count (WBC)
White blood cell differential
Immunoelectrophoresis
Transplant
Allergy
Inhaled allergen
Injected allergen
Contact allergen
Skin testing
Eosinophil smear
Radioallergosorbent test (RAST)
Hyposensitization (Immunotherapy)
Corticosteroids
Cushingoid appearance
Bronchodilators
Antihistamines
Decogestants
Eczema
Allergic rhinitis
Asthma
Status asthmaticus
Hives
Anaphylaxis
Autoimmunity
Lupus erythematosus (LE) cell

Today members of the health care team are focusing on the child with altered immunity. Researchers are pursuing new, exciting areas that promise a sure cure for cancer, prevention of all infectious diseases, and the successful transplantation of healthy organs to replace defective ones. These breakthroughs may seem to be only fantasy today, but hope for them is very real. In the meantime, the nurse's understanding of basic immune alterations and knowledge of the latest research will help the entire health team to provide the best possible care.

IMMUNODEFICIENCY

The immune system of the normal child is such an active and effective, yet interdependent system that any deficiency results in infections. These infections can be mild and transient or so severe that all types of microorganisms overwhelm the body. *Primary immunodeficiency,* a disorder of the immune system itself, is very rare. *Secondary immunodeficiency,* the suppression or alteration of the immune system, is much more common, and is increasing in incidence. Regardless of the type of deficiency, however, the clinical picture is essentially the same and requires similar nursing care.

Primary immunodeficiency usually is not evident at birth. A pattern of recurring, persistent illness develops as maternal immunoglobulins from the placenta and breast milk decrease. Virulent infections (often caused by normally nonpathogenic bacteria or fungi), severe reactions to live vaccines. and infections at unusual sites all suggest a defect in the child's immune system. Deficiencies can occur in the T cell, B cell, and a combination of the two. T-cell defects leave the body vulnerable to viruses, fungi, and protozoa. A common example of T-cell deficiency is fungal infections of the mouth (thrush), skin, and diaper area. B-cell deficiency, by far the most prevalent, results in severe bacterial infections. Affected children do not have normal immunoglobulin formation and/or do not produce antibodies to specific antigens. Combined immunodeficiency creates both T- and B-cell problems for the child. In rare instances inadequate or incompetent phagocytes or complement may cause the recurrence of bacterial infections and abscesses.

A secondary immunodeficiency is a malfunction of the immune system caused by outside factors. Most children in hospitals have some immunodeficiency, while others have marked immune incompetency. A variety of drugs, including some antibiotics, cortiocosteroids, and antineoplastic agents, suppress the immune system. Infections generally can suppress the system, and some specific infections can reduce the body's ability to fight other specific organisms. For example, measles temporarily leaves the body vulnerable to tuberculosis. Since malnutrition also causes immunodeficiency, all conditions resulting in malnutrition (such as cystic fibrosis, celiac disease, short-gut syndrome, and pylorospasms) may also result in immunodeficiency. Such acquired diseases of the system as leukemia are classified as secondary immunodeficiencies. Children with secondary immunosuppression not only have the danger of the deficiency but also a serious underlying cause.

COMMON PROBLEMS, SYMPTOMS AND NURSING CARE

Infections

The child with an immunodeficiency cannot fight infection properly, and since exposure to simple infections can be life-threatening, nursing care is directed toward the prevention of contact with pathogens. Unfortunately, this process, while decreasing the chances of infection, also deprives the child of many developmental opportunities.

Usually, the child with immunodeficiency is protected with such methods as protective isolation (see ch. 15). This technique is easily incorporated into hospital routines, but is a very difficult procedure for parents to implement in the home. All visitors and family members with any indication of infection must not be allowed in the child's room. All the doors and windows must be kept closed; every article used by the child must be disinfected and the air purified.

The strictness of protective isolation is determined by the child's vulnerability. Many families cannot or will not provide for every aspect of prescribed isolation because of lack of space, time, money, energy, or motivation. Occasionally, when a child has a genetic defect that cannot be alleviated, parents merely take simple precautions during his short life. When the child has a deficiency caused by a lifesaving medication or curable disease, parents can accept drastic changes more readily, as long as there is hope for relief in the future. Fortunately, most children have only mild immunodeficiencies that require such restrictions as avoiding children with colds, remaining home from school during influenza epidemics, and staying out of crowded areas.

The best efforts of the parents and the nurse will not prevent infections in the child with severe immunodeficiency. Infections respond normally to antibiotics, and the prompt recognition of early signs of immunodeficiency is essential. The infant usually will have difficulty in sucking and eating normal amounts for his size. He may require more sleep with drowsy waking periods, or he may be unable to sleep well. The older child may elect to stay in bed or take naps at unusual times. Report the usual signs of infection (fever, pain, loss of function, redness or warmth in an area, drainage, rashes, and so on) immediately. Since the immune defect may decrease or mask the inflammatory response, an infection can be advanced before signs and symptoms appear. Subtle changes in activity and mood may be initial changes in such cases, and the parents and child are usually the best judges of a problem. The physician usually will order a series of laboratory procedures to confirm suspicions.

Malnutrition

The child with any immunodeficiency is usually anorectic; this often causes malnutrition which, in turn, exacerbates the immunodeficiency. All of the techniques to encourage eating, mentioned in earlier chapters, should be used: offer small, frequent, colorful meals, treats brought from home, and a pleasant dining atmosphere that includes companionship; schedule treatments to occur well before or after mealtimes, and so on. A nutritionist can help plan a variety of foods for the child. If the child absolutely refuses to eat, do not overreact to this common behavior, since he may use not eating to manipulate you, family members, and staff. Hyperalimentation, a form of intravenous nutritional therapy (ch. 29), may be necessary in severe cases of malnutrition.

Altered Growth and Development

All chronic diseases affect growth and development to some extent and often retard them significantly. This is especially true of the child with immunodeficiency who requires protective isolation and numerous hospitalizations. Unfortunately, people who provide opportunities for learning also carry pathogens which threaten his life. Fresh air, too, carries pathogens, so only filtered and moisturized air is safe. Numerous acute and chronic infections retard the child's growth. As a result, he must often cope not only with lack of developmental skills but also with being smaller than his peers. Overprotection teaches a child that he obviously cannot take care of himself, yet parents must overprotect him if he is to live.

Increasing the child's responsibility for avoiding and recognizing infection is one way to improve his self-image. Whenever possible, let the child help you in decision making to show him and his parents his ability to participate in his own care. Explain to the child's parents why he needs to assume maximum safe responsibility for his own care and activities.

COMMON DIAGNOSTIC MEASURES

White Blood Cell Count with Differential

The *white blood cell count* (WBC) is the total number of white blood cells, or leukocytes, in a cubic millimeter (mm) of whole blood (see ch. 21). A low white count (*leukopenia*) indicates that the child does not have enough white blood cells to protect him from infection. If the count was previously normal (8,000 to 10,000) and drops to 4,000 or below, the child needs protective measures to prevent infection. The *white blood cell differential* specifies which type of leukocyte is deficient. For instance, a marked decrease in lymphocytes suggests a T-cell defect.

Biopsy

A *biopsy* of a lymph gland and/or bone marrow is a procedure used in differential diagnosis of immunodeficiencies. For example, if the lymph glands lack specific tissues that depend on the thymus for formation, the child may have a T-cell defect. Aspiration of bone marrow can reveal which cells are affected. Prepare the biopsy site by cleansing it with antiseptic solution according to physician's orders or hospital routine. Cover the site with a sterile dressing after the biopsy. Report any signs of infection to the physician immediately.

Biopsies for diagnosis of primary immunodeficiency in a fetus can be performed during pregnancy.

Once the diagnosis has been made, remember that the child has already been ill enough to scare his parents, and they may not be able to cope with further painful procedures immediately. Careful, repeated explanations usually reduce anxiety somewhat.

Immunoelectrophoresis

Immunoelectrophoresis is a method of measuring the amounts of individual immunoglobulins in serum. This process reveals a deficiency or absence of specific immunoglobulins, usually IgG (a deficiency which can cause hypogammaglobulinemia and or agmmaglobulinemia). This condition is usually related to B-cell defects.

COMMON TREATMENTS

Replacement Therapy

In most immunoglobulin deficiencies, the child is given intramuscular injections of human immune serum globulin (gamma globulin). The injection is given monthly in an outpatient setting for primary and secondary deficiencies. Phagocytic and complement disorders are treated by the regular infusion of these components.

Transplants

The child with a T-cell or a combined deficiency has a very poor prognosis without a *transplant* of bone marrow or thymus. A sibling is usually the best donor, although a wide search, if necessary, may yield another donor whose cells are compatible with those of the child. Since the body of a child with immunodeficiency lacks the normal rejection capabilities, transplants have a greater chance of being successful. Immunosuppressant drugs further the chance of acceptance by depressing any remaining rejection capabilities. Successful bone marrow transplants can bring about dramatic permanent immunological function.

Antibiotic Therapy

The child with an immunodeficiency responds normally to antibiotic therapy. In cases of severe deficiencies, the prompt administration of antibiotics on initial signs of infection is essential in preventing overwhelming infection leading to death. Continuous prophylactic administration may give the child more freedom to live normally, although the problem of resistant strains of microorganisms remains. Some antibiotics, such as chloramephenicol and actinomycin D, can be immunosuppressant and are therefore avoided. When you administer the antibiotic intravenously or intramuscularly, take extreme care to cleanse the site before puncturing the skin, and cover it with a sterile dressing if the deficiency is severe. Fortunately, most repeated parenteral injections of antibiotics are intravenous, and the child is spared the pain of various puncture sites.

COMPLICATIONS

Malignancies

The immune system recognizes and attacks foreign substances, including malignancies (see ch. 14). Pathophysiologists theorize that, although malignancies develop frequently, the normal immune system quickly destroys them except in rare instances. When the immune system is incompetent, tumors occur more often and grow more quickly. A child with a primary immunodeficiency is highly susceptible to malignancies, which further shorten his already short life expectancy. Immunotherapy as a possible cure for cancers is the subject of intense research (see ch. 20).

Chronic Infections

Chronic infections can affect various parts of the child's body. For instance, pulmonary infections can significantly decrease respiratory function and stunt the child's growth. Chronic upper respiratory infection often leads to sinusitis, mastoiditis, and many related problems. There is now some evidence that young adults who survived childhood with careful management may develop slow-acting viral diseases, such as hepatitis. Destructive changes from chronic infections give the child with immunodeficiency little chance of long life. If the deficiency is one that can be treated with replacement or transplant therapy, the prognosis depends on the anatomic changes caused by infection before the therapy began.

ALLERGY

Allergy is a broad term that covers abnormal, excessive immune responses to allergens (antigens). This common problem is worsened by numerous pollutants in the air, additives in food, and the frequent use of many medications. Also, since more atopic people are surviving to have children, heredity also plays a role in the increased incidence of allergy. Allergies may range from mild, transient symptoms to severely debilitating disease, and they are responsible for a major portion of acute and chronic illness in children. Many children on acute care units with ear, nose, throat, skin, gastrointestinal, and lower respiratory problems have underlying allergies.

The child with allergy has a chronic condition which cannot be cured but usually can be controlled (Figure 16–1). Although everyone tells the child that he will outgrow his allergy, it will only change as he gets older, and he must continue to control his allergy with various preventive measures and treatments, usually throughout his life. He also will have periodic acute illnesses that are directly related to the allergy. He and his family may need help in coping with symptoms and treatments. This complex situation always requires a team effort by physicians, social workers, therapists, and teachers, as well as nurses. Since the cost of adequate care is beyond the means of many families, the child with allegy may receive only intermittent treatment for acute phases.

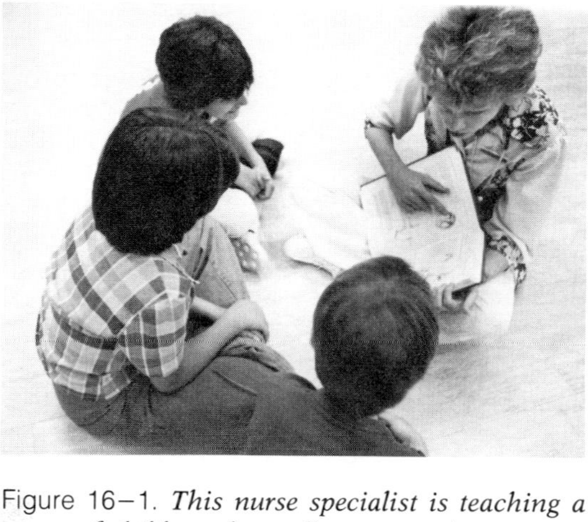

Figure 16–1. *This nurse specialist is teaching a group of children about allergy control.*

COMMON PROBLEMS, SYMPTOMS AND NURSING INTERVENTIONS

Antigen-Antibody Response

The child with allergy, regardless of the type, has to cope with antigen-antibody response. This process involves several chemical interactions resulting in inflammation, contraction of bronchial smooth muscle, and itching. *Histamine,* released from affected cells, is the primary factor in this reaction. The child's specific symptoms will depend on the location of his response. Antigen-antibody response (allergic reaction) of the skin results in edematous, pruritic skin that oozes at any point of weakness. A mucous membrane, on the other hand, swells with tissue fluid and begins to produce excessive mucus, obstructing passages, and providing an excellent medium for bacterial growth. When lungs are affected, there is tissue edema, excessive mucus is produced, and there is bronchoconstriction.

Nursing care of the child with an inflammatory response includes keeping the affected area cool and in a comfortable, elevated position. Remove excessive mucus whenever possible by suctioning, postural drainage, irrigation, and even wiping with a cool cloth. Cool, moist air will help to keep mucus in the respiratory tree liquid enough to be removed by coughing, suctioning, and nose-blowing. Too much moisture in the air, however, may overload the lungs with fluid that must be removed in addition to the mucus. Bronchoconstriction requires the usual techniques to combat respiratory distress (ch. 23) and prompt administration of bronchodilators.

Reduction or Elimination of Allergens

The best way to control allergy is to protect the child from agents that elicit an allergic response. This can be as simple as discarding all wool clothing or as impossible as removing all dust from a room. Allergens enter the body through mucus membranes and the skin or by parenteral routes (injection).

Inhaled, injected, and *contact allergens* enter through mucous membranes and skin. Inhalants include dust, pollen, mold, animal dander, and fumes of all kinds. Ingested allergens are foods, drugs, and a variety of animal parasites. Contactants include fibers, dyes, plants, cosmetics, topical drugs, metals in jewelry, and synthetics such as those used in shoes, belts, and so on. Usually injectables are medications, but they also include bee stings, snake bites, and other allergens introduced by trauma. Infectious microorganisms also cause allergic responses.

The child may be affected by a single allergen or by many different ones simultaneously. Apparently, the child with multiple allergies can tolerate exposure to some offenders without a noticeable response. Once the tolerance level is reached, however, a single additional allergen can elicit a severe reaction. Conversely, if all removable allergens are gone from the child's environment, he can usually tolerate the remaining allergies more successfully.

A child who is allergic to ingested allergens should have the known offenders eliminated from his diet. Parents and the child usually have a good idea of which foods cause the problem, unless there are too many allergens to identify. To test for food allergies, common offenders including milk and milk products, chocolate, eggs, nuts, wheat, and citrus fruits are removed from the diet and added one at a time every three or five days. If this process does not identify allergens, the child's diet is limited to a few foods that seldom cause allergic reactions. Then foods are added slowly until the child at least knows what he can eat. The infant's diet may be reduced to formula, and if no improvement occurs, he will be fed a hypoallergenic formula. Allergy to breast milk is extremely rare.

Contactant allergy is fairly easy to control in the child. Washing and rinsing clothing before the child wears it will prevent many allergic reactions to dyes. Cosmetics, jewelry, and topical drugs can easily be removed. Plants such as poison ivy or poison oak, on the other hand, can ruin outdoor play for the child who is sensitive to them. Yet this, too, can be avoided by his staying out of woods or wearing long pants and sleeves, followed by soapy showers after an outing. Contactants create more problems for adults who must touch allergens in occupations, such as hairdressing, horticulture, and various chemical plant duties. These people frequently must change their occupation to avoid the allergens.

Injectables usually are identified easily because of the puncture needed to inject the allergen. Parents and the child may not remember an injection immediately in the case of a delayed reaction, but they usually recall recent bee stings, snake or other animal bites, and injections of medication. Once it is known, a child's drug allergy must be recorded on his chart in the hospital, physician's office, and school or day care facility. The child should wear a tag and carry a card in his wallet warning of any severe injectable allergy. Avoiding stinging insects is frustrating for the child who enjoys playing outdoors. Since perfumes attract these insects, he should use only unscented soaps, lotions, and other skin preparations. Insect repellants offer some protection, but the child must learn to stay out of bushes and trees and to wear shoes, lightweight long pants, and long-sleeved shirts. These same precautions apply to other animal-injected allergies. He must stay away from the animals and their habitats. He also should keep any needed medication handy in case of an animal bite.

Inhaled allergens are probably the most difficult to control since they move freely with the air. Keeping air even relatively free from allergens is expensive and enormously time-consuming. Most effort is directed at keeping the sleeping area clean and closed from the rest of the house. Animal dander is controlled by removing all animals (including cats, dogs, gerbils, birds, hamsters, and so on) from the house and the immediate area. The child must not enter a pen or a place where animals are kept. Amazingly, many parents will not or cannot enforce these restrictions and will allow a cat, for example, to sleep with the wheezing child.

Mold elimination requires considerably more effort. Bathrooms must be scrubbed and dried regularly, and an antimold solution applied. A covering of polyethylene over the dirt under the house will decrease house mold. All plants and fish should be removed from the child's room. Dust is controlled by removing anything from the child's room that attracts dust, such as carpeting, drapes, ruffles on bedspreads or elsewhere, stuffed toys, books, etc. The remaining contents are wiped daily with a clean damp cloth and clean damp mop. An electric air filter in the room or on the furnace can also remove a large amount of dust. Pollens are part of house dust, and they also can be removed by these procedures. The many ways of removing inhalants are too numerous to list here and certainly too numerous for a normal family to carry out daily. Yet even the best efforts still do not protect the child from outside inhalants. Keeping his bedroom with a minimum of allergens usually provides noticeable relief of symptoms, however, and the results are worth the time and energy required.

Anorexia, Malaise

The hospitalized child with allergy often feels "bad" and has no desire to eat. When mucus flows continuously from his nose down the back of his throat, or when he has difficulty breathing, he cannot enjoy meals or active play. Relieving the symptoms by using various medications will improve the situation as will small, frequent, colorful meals eaten in the company of others. Brief rest periods throughout the day and a few play items at a time may also stimulate his interest. A change of scenery or, if he is hospitalized, food from home may help. But expect cranky behavior; the child often has good reason to be irritable, and you may not be able to alleviate his problems significantly. Try to accept the behavior without drawing undue attention to it.

Infections

The child with allergy is more susceptible to infection than is the well child. Edema weakens defense mechanisms by slowing circulation and the movement of immune components through tissues. Increased mucus provides a warm, moist medium that facilitates the growth of microorganisms. Edema and mucus easily close passages to lungs and sinuses, trapping microorganisms, which begin to multiply in this protected environment. Edema and mucus also hamper the action of cilia, the hair-like projections that move particles (including microorganisms) out of the respiratory tree.

Unfortunately, infections also elicit an inflammatory response, further increasing symptoms. Infections themselves seem to cause allergic responses, either by their inflammatory and irritative properties or by specific antigen-antibody reaction. When the child with allergy requires hospitalization, he often has to control a secondary infection as well as the alergy. Antibiotics and steroids may be prescribed concurrently (see common treatments).

Base your nursing care for these children on a combination of principles to treat infections, allergy, and the specific area affected (lungs, skin, etc.). Hydration is also necessary to liquefy thick, obstructive secretions. In addition to these complex demands, you have the difficult task, as always, of planning all interventions according to the child's age and stage of development.

Psychosocial Component

The allergic child with his family face all the problems accompanying chronic illness. An infant with severe allergies, for instance, is at increased risk for emotional problems. Allergic symptoms that disturb normal feeding and holding during infancy interferes with the very important infant-parent bonding process. Parents must also cope with a tremendous drain on their time, energy, space, and money—often when they are young, inexperienced, and broke. They become so concerned when allergies cause active illness that they try almost anything to prevent recurrences. The child, in turn, learns that his illness brings attention. The younger the child at the onset of his problems and the more severe the symptoms, the worse the emotional impact. This process seldom happens overnight, it can be so slow that the whole series of interactions are well ingrained before the parents seek help for the child's behavioral problems. Teachers may reinforce established patterns, since they often are afraid the child will have symptoms they are not prepared to handle at school. Even relatively minor allergies can lead to behavioral changes.

Todd, aged two, did not like to go to sleep at night. Too many interesting things were happening, and he didn't like to be isolated in his room. He had had a "runny nose" forever, it seemed to his mother; but one night at bedtime his father suddenly expressed concern about the copious drainage and cough and checked on Todd a couple of times. This happened a few nights, and soon Todd had respiratory difficulties each night resulting from the drainage. He even began to wake up in the middle of the night with them. His parents became anxious, exhausted, and irritated with Todd. Referral to an allergist led to a significant decrease of nasal discharge; yet the coughs, snorts, and sputters continued at bedtime and in the night. His parents were frantic. Something else must be wrong! They were not easily convinced of a psychogenic component, but they were willing to try anything. Once Todd was put to bed, they sat in the den and listened to his noises, fighting the temptation to go to him. When he started again during the night, he was allowed to sleep on a mat next to their bed. Slowly, his tricks subsided. Finally, after several weeks, they all were sleeping well.

Look for signs of manipulative behavior in the child hospitalized with an acute allergic condition. Put gentle but firm limits on this behavior. Give parents ample opportunity to talk about their frustrations in parenting. With a little guidance, they usually can pinpoint the interactional problem. You will not be able to solve these long-standing problems during one episode of illness; permanent resolution requires sustained teamwork. Referral to a community health nurse may provide all the support necessary, but family therapy in a mental health center may be required in extreme cases. Many parents' self-help groups are also springing up. Know what organizations exist relating to children's allergies, and give this information to parents *in writing* before the discharge of the child.

COMMON DIAGNOSTIC PROCEDURES

Data Collection

Data collection—taking a thorough account of the child and his family's past and present illnesses and symptoms—is an important part of diagnosing any condition, but is especially critical with allergy. An observant parent can list foods that probably cause skin eruptions or asthma attacks, times of year when symptoms are worse for the child, and many other possibly related aspects. Data gathering for a child with allergy is usually done in outpatient settings, using a guide with many questions about the child's home, neighborhood, school, environment, history of problems, and so forth. If you need to obtain this information while the child is in the acute care unit, parents may be defensive and resentful of long question-and-answer sessions. The usual emotions (anger, guilt, and fear) will be evident. Be sure to let the parents tell their story first, and then ask them questions about topics they did not discuss. Letting the parents talk often relieves their anxiety somewhat, and they are able to give a better account of their child and of the development of his allergic condition. This process also allows you to assess the parents' abilities to cope with both the stresses of their child's chronic illness and the present acute problem.

Skin Testing

Skin testing is a process used to identify specific allergins in which a diluted solution is either placed on a scratch or injected intracutaneously. A positive reaction (i.e., an inflammatory response or wheal) indicates that the substance is an allergen, although the substance occasionally causes no symptoms in the child. To further complicate matters, the child's skin does not always react to the allergen that is causing his problem. Skin testing is imprecise, but it does give the most information for the least money. The information provided by skin testing is interpreted in relation to a thorough history and other diagnostic procedures.

White Blood Cell Differential Count

The child with allergies has more eosinophils (eosinophilia) than the normal child, and this is determined by the white blood cell differential. Eosinophils normally comprise 2 to 3 percent of the total white count, but in the allergic child, eosinophils commonly constitute 10 to 20 percent of the total.

Smears for Eosinophil Identification

Smears to assist in the diagnosis of allergy are obtained from any secretory membrane and spread in a thin layer over a slide. The cells in an *eosinophil smear* are stained and viewed under a microscope. During most allergic reactions, eosinophils appear in secretions from the nose, eyes, lungs, and skin. This test is especially helpful in differentiating between allergic and infectious rhinitis.

Immunoelectrophoresis

Immunoelectrophoresis is a general test indicating levels of immunoglobulins. The child with allergies may have a marked rise in IgE. Since some children with allergies have normal or low levels, however, the allergist uses this test to support other data rather than for primary diagnosis.

Radioallergosorbent Test

The *radioallergosorbent test* (RAST) is a serologic test that measures IgE antibodies specific for substances, such as molds, pollens, and food. It may be used instead of skin testing to identify allergens to be eliminated from the child's environment or to prepare a hyposensitizing extract. It is especially useful for children for whom skin testing is not possible.

Joseph, aged four, was deaf. He had had upsetting experiences in a variety of health centers and developed an intense fear of all doctors and nurses. His allergist assessed his ability to cope with skin testing and discarded the idea. Joseph was able to tolerate a venipuncture for the RAST, which determined how the extract should be compounded.

RAST is also used to determine the effectiveness of hyposensitization by measuring specific IgE antibodies before and after a series of injections.

COMMON TREATMENTS

Hyposensitization

Hyposensitization (immunotherapy) is the process of decreasing the child's reaction to an allergen. The child is first tested for specific allergens either by skin testing or a RAST. Minute amounts of identified allergens are mixed to form an extract that is injected periodically in increasing amounts and strengths. This procedure lowers antibodies to the substances and stimulates the production of an antibody that blocks the offending antibody. The child's symptoms often lessen in six to twelve months. If the child shows no improvement after two years, however, hyposensitization is stopped. Often the child worsens after the injections are discontinued, indicating that they were more effective than originally recognized. Because of the uncertainty of this expensive, somewhat painful, and time-consuming process, however, it is prescribed only after other attempts at removing the allergen and treating symptoms have failed to provide adequate relief.

Occasionally, children on acute care units will need allergy injections, which are routinely given twice a week. The extract is injected subcutaneously in the upper outer arm, using a tuberculin syringe (Figure 16–2). The injection site is rotated to protect skin and underlying tissues. Most allergic reactions occur within 20 minutes after the injection, but some occur up to 24 hours later. Keep a tourniquet nearby to apply above the injection site if a severe reaction occurs. Benadryl is usually prescribed for local reactions, and epinephrine is used for systematic reactions (anaphylaxis). Severe reactions are rare, but since they do occur, ask the physician for specific instructions for treatment before you give the first injection.

Corticosteroid Therapy

Steroid therapy actually encompasses all treatment with adrenocorticosteroids, but

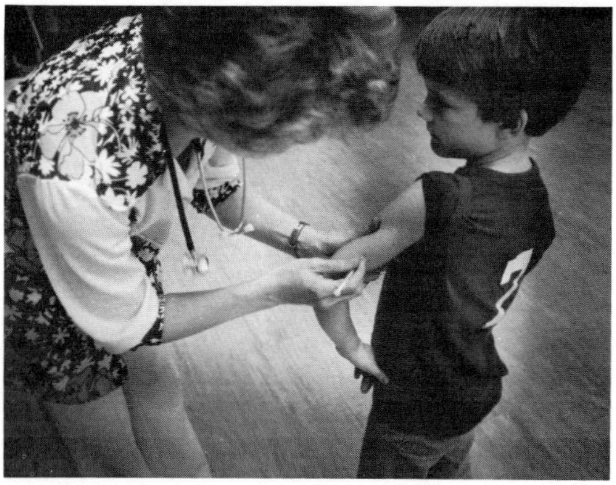

Figure 16–2. *After a few weeks of therapy, the child receiving allergy injections (immunotherapy) becomes accustomed to them and finds the process to be only a minor nuisance.*

this discussion covers only the glucocorticoids that are commonly called *corticosteroids* or simply *steroids* (see chs. 17 and 19). These hormones have an anti-inflammatory effect on the child and assist him in coping with physical and emotional stress. The body normally produces the hormones only as needed, but when corticosteroids are administered as medication, the possibility of *cushingoid appearance* (a moon face and fat on the back of the neck, the shoulders, and the hips), stunted growth, hyperglycemia, fluid and electrolyte imbalance, inability to fight infections, and other problems exist. The adrenal gland reduces its production of these hormones (adrenal suppression) when they are already present in the body as regular medications. Fortunately, except in extreme situations, these side effects do not usually occur in the child who is monitored carefully by a competent physician.

The child with allergy receives corticosteroids to reduce abnormal and/or excess immune reactions in the body. In addition to other anti-flammatory properties, steroids can be immunosuppressant by decreasing the number of circulating lymphocytes or eosinophils, shrinking lymph nodes and thymus, and depressing the production of immunoglobulins. Although these changes can dramatically improve the child's condition, physicians prescribe steroids cautiously because of the possible side effects. Experience and research have shown that large, short-term dosages or small, intermittent, long-term dosages usually produce few side effects. The child who is severely ill with an allergic condition (usually asthma but also rhinitis) often receives a large dose of corticosteroids for a short period of time. This therapy affords relief from symptoms that allows the body to rest briefly so that other medications can then control symptoms more effectively. If acute symptoms return, the child is given decreasing amounts of oral steroids every other day until the correct dosage is determined. The medication is taken in the morning to avoid adrenal suppression, since natural corticosteroid secretion increases in the afternoon. Once the decision is made to discontinue corticosteroids after long-term administration, the dosage is tapered off very slowly to allow the adrenal gland to adapt by increasing its production of the hormones.

The child who is receiving corticosteroids on the acute care unit runs the risk of masked infection and adrenal suppression. Adrenal suppression leaves the body vulnerable to such stresses as major illness and trauma, including surgery. The suppressed adrenal gland does not increase its production as it should in these cases, and additional corticosteroids must be administered to meet the body's need. Nursing care for him is similar to that of any other child who is immunodeficient. The child who has received long-term steroid therapy may remain immunosuppressed for a year or more after the medication has been discontinued. Always note prominently on the child's record past and present corticosteroid medications when you obtain admission data.

Cortiscosteroids are available in oral, parenteral, and topical preparations. The acutely ill child usually receives intramuscular or intravenous injections in divided daily doses; oral preparations are used in long-term therapy. Topical preparations, whether applied or inhaled, are absorbed in minute amounts by the body and have negligible systemic effect (Figure 16–3). Synthetic corticosteroids, such as prednisone, have been developed to create more active anti-inflammatory effects with less adverse reaction.

Bronchodilators

The three major *bronchodilators* (drugs used to relax constricted bronchi and bronchioles) are *epinephrine, theophylline,* and *ephedrine.* Know the actions and side effects of these bronchodilators well because they are used on any pediatric acute care unit. All stimulate the central nervous system, and can cause headaches, tachycardia, hypertension, anxiety, irritability, nausea, and vomiting. The child on these drugs requires close observation for signs of early toxicity, which may consist only of slight restlessness, irritability, or decreased sucking. The older child or parents can often recognize subtle warning signs quickly and alert you. (See Table 16–1 for a summary of these and other bronchodilators.)

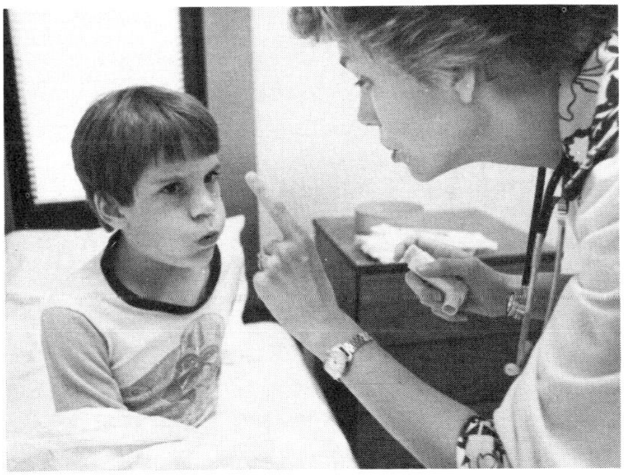

Figure 16–3. *Learning to inhale medications takes practice and patience.*

Epinephrine is a hormone used for immediate bronchodilating action, but its effects subside so quickly that the physician may need to repeat the dose every 20 minutes up to three times. Topical, inhaled, and long-acting injectable preparations are available. Epinephrine is not effective orally, so it is not an appropriate routine prophylactic medication. Many parents learn to give epinephrine injections if their child has asthma or a severe allergy to insect stings or unknown allergens. The injection, drawn into a tuberculin syringe, and usually given subcutaneously, is a 1:1,000 solution of regular epinephrine or a 1:200 solution of long-acting epinephrine (Sus-Phrine). Always check the strength of the solution, since a 1:100 solution for inhalation, infrequently prescribed for the child with bronchospasms, is also available and an injection of the drug in this strength can be fatal. Inhaled epinephrine is used with extreme caution, since a child may use it more often than prescribed for relief of symptoms. Adolescents have abused inhaled bronchodilators, and there have been instances of cardiac arrest.

Theophylline, the bronchodilator of choice for most children, acts directly on bronchial muscles. It works more slowly but lasts longer (six hours) than epineph-

Table 16–1. **Bronchodilators**

Name	*Administration*	*Usual Indications*	*Duration*
Epinephrine (adrenalyn)	Subcutaneous or intramuscular injection; inhalation	Acute asthma	Short (1 hour)
Epinephrine, Aqueous Suspension, (Sus-Phrine)	Subcutaneous injection	Acute asthma	Long (8–10 hours)
Theophylline	Oral, intravenous injection	Chronic or acute asthma	Long (6 hours)
Ephedrine	Oral	Mild asthma	Medium (4 hours)
Isoproterenol (Isuprel)	Inhalation, oral, injection	Acute asthma, home or school	Long (6–8 hours)
Ethylnorepinephrine (Bronkephrine)	Subcutaneous, intramuscular injection	Acute asthma, home or hospital	Long (6–8 hours)
Metaproterenol	Inhalation, oral	Mild asthma; usually given intermittently with other bronchodilators	Medium (4 hours)

rine, but side effects include central nervous system stimulation and gastric irritation. Theophylline is a potent diuretic, so the child must increase his fluid intake to replace the voided amount. The range between undertreatment and toxicity is narrow, and staying within this range is made more difficult by differing individual absorption and metabolism rates. The measurement of theophylline blood levels helps the physician to prescribe the correct dosage. Most children who regularly take oral theophylline to prevent bronchospasms develop mild toxicity from time to time, usually because they have deviated from their medication schedules. Aspirin or acetominophen helps relieve headache, and taking theophylline with meals helps minimize gastric distress. Decreasing or delaying the next dose will allow the body to recover from a mild overdosage. Intravenous theophylline is given on acute care units to children whose symptoms cannot be controlled with oral medications.

Ephedrine is a bronchodilator that is usually used in conjunction with theophylline. Physicians rarely prescribe this drug because of the restlessness and anxiety that frequently occur as a side effect. A combined preparation of theophylline and ephedrine often require the prescription of a mild sedative to counteract stimulation of the central nervous system.

All bronchodilators stimulate the central

nervous system, but they do so to varying degrees. When given together, bronchodilators can cause toxicity. When given alternately, two types of bronchodilators may provide increased relief of bronchospasms. For instance, metaproterenol, a relatively new drug, works very effectively in conjunction with theophylline for children who do not respond to theophylline alone.

Monitor vital signs carefully when administering any bronchodilators. Watch for nausea, vomiting, and restlessness. Unfortunately, the child may have to tolerate mild drug side effects to control his asthma, although these often disappear with time. Consult the physician when the medications cause sleeplessness, vomiting, headache, or marked emotional reactions.

Antihistamines

Antihistamines are medications that block the action of histamine released in an allergic response. To maintain continuous blocking action, they must be given regularly. If one type does not bring improvement, an antihistamine from another family may work, since each type has a different chemical base. Because antihistamines block the histamine effects of tissue edema, excess mucus production, itching, and so on, they have a drying effect. This property makes them particularly useful for nasal allergy (rhinitis) in which the child has a "runny nose," and skin manifestations, such as allergic welts (hives). Antihistamines are not used for pulmonary allergy (e.g., asthma, bronchitis) since they may thicken secretions in the lungs. They also have a mild sedative effect that helps the itchy, irritable child, but that can hinder the child who must go to school and stay alert. These side effects usually diminish with regular use.

Decongestants

Decongestants (sympathomimetics) are medications that shrink edematous membranes by constricting dilated blood vessels, thus decreasing the flow of fluid from blood vessels to tissues. Unfortunately, they also may cause anxiety, headache, nausea, and vomiting. Decongestants are frequently used in conjunction with antihistamines to provide relief, particularly from rhinitis. Decongestant nose drops have been overused in children, and have caused an immediate shrinking of the membranes, followed by a return of even worse symptoms (rebound effect). Most allergists do not recommend the use of decongestant nose drops at all; they find that oral preparations often bring relief for nasal congestion.

SPECIFIC ALLERGIC CONDITIONS

Eczema

Eczema (atopic dermatitis) is a skin disorder common to infants and young children who are born with a general tendency toward allergies. Characteristics include erythema, papular and vesicular eruptions, and edema with weeping, crusting, and scaling. The skin becomes hyperreactive not only to allergens and irritants but even to the touch. Itching is so severe that the child often rips open his fragile skin as he scratches. In later childhood, eczema is often followed by asthma and rhinitis. The child with eczema usually has a high serum IgE concentration, and this finding can help rule out nonallergic skin diseases,

Inhaled and ingested allergens are usually the cause of eczema. The infant may be obviously allergic to a specific food, such as cow's milk, eggs, or wheat, or he may not show a clear-cut allergy to anything. Once eczema appears, known offending allergens are removed from the child's diet and environment whenever possible. An elimination diet may be required to identify problem food; soy formulas are substituted when milk allergy is suspected. Clothing and linens should be soft cotton, washed in a mild soap. Diapers must be changed frequently, and the infant is cleaned carefully to curtail diaper rash, which can cause severe eczematous symptoms. The child's nails need to be cut as short as possible, since scratching is always a part of the cycle. Parents must avoid using wool, rough materials, perfumed fabric softeners, disposable diapers, and soaps that remove oil and cause further drying of the skin. The child should take infrequent baths and follow those with the application of oils, lotions, and ointments to seal in moisture. Topical steroid creams provide antiinflammatory effects when applied regularly. Antihistamines are prescribed to decrease the effects of histamine production and to produce mild sedation. Systemic antibiotics are given for secondary bacterial infections.

Most parents can successfully handle eczema at home if they have regular outpatient health services. The child with eczema on the acute care unit usually has a severe form of the disease because his parents have been unsuccessful in treating the disease at home. When the child is admitted, you must first remove potential allergens, and you may have to send home a security object if it is scratchy, straw-filled, or dirty. Soft, clean cotton blankets can be used as substitutes, although most toddlers are not satisfied with these, but stopping the itch-scratch-itch cycle is a priority. The physician may order restraints or simple bandaging of as much of the affected area as possible. Soaks, followed by ointment, are also often prescribed. A secondary infection (frequently the reason for admission) is treated with systemic antibiotics. Involve the child's parents throughout his hospitalization, and encourage them to accept increasing responsibility for their child's care as he improves so that they can continue the same routines at home. Refer the family to a home health nurse if you think they will need assistance in treating the eczema at home.

Allergic Rhinitis

The child with *allergic rhinitis* is plagued with sneezing; swollen, obstructed nasal membranes that cause him to breathe through his mouth; clear serous mucus flowing through the nasophraynx and the nares; sore throat in the mornings; and severe itching. He has dark, swollen circles under his eyes (Figure 16–4). Smears of nasal discharge will contain eosinophils. The child may have symptoms only during periods of pollination, or he may have them

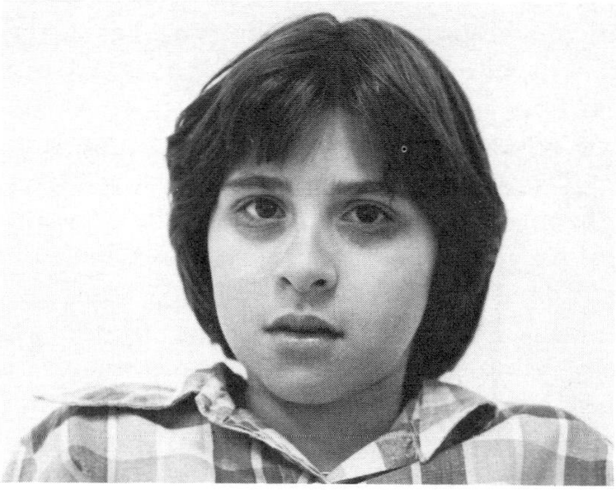

Figure 16–4. *This child has the typical facies of the allergic person: dark circles under the eyes and the open mouth of a mouth breather.*

year-round from constant allergens such as household dust. He frequently pushes the tip of his nose upward with the palm of his hand (an allergic salute) to relieve some of the itching and to open nasal membrane for breathing. Allergic rhinitis is treated with antihistamines, decongestants, hyposensitization by immunotherapy, and as much elimination of allergens as possible.

Complications of allergic rhinitis include serous otitis media, frequent upper respiratory infections, sinus obstruction, and bronchitis. The child may require hospitalization for treatment of these problems, especially for the insertion of polyethelene tubes into the tympanic membranes to relieve serous otitis media. More commonly, however, the child will receive treatment on an outpatient basis.

Asthma

Asthma is a chronic respiratory disorder (see ch. 23) characterized by bronchospasms (affecting the bronchioles and bronchi), mucosal edema, increased mucus production, and onverinflation of the lungs. It is diagnosed most frequently in preschoolers, but infants and school-age children also are found to have asthma. The disease may be extrinsic (caused by allergy) or intrinsic (caused by infections, cold, exercise, emotional upset, and unknown reasons). Asthma attacks may occur suddenly and result in severe bronchospasms limiting both inspiration and expiration. This reduced air flow is followed by edema of the bronchi and bronchioles and increased production of mucus, which further obstructs airways. Air passing through these narrow passages creates a wheeze. The child uses accessory muscles to increase his respiratory capacity. His heart and respiratory rates increase, cyanosis develops, and he suffers abdominal pain and coughing as he vigorously uses the diaphragm to increase vital capacity. Air is trapped in the alveoli beyond the bronchoconstriction and mucosal edema, resulting in reversible emphysema. Other asthma attacks may occur slowly, accompanied by mild coughing and wheezing which progressively worsens. The child may not have a strong "attack," and may wheeze and cough minimally and intermittently. Collectively, these different forms of asthma are responsible for a significant portion of chronic childhood illness. Although many children with asthma improve with age and treatment, they usually do not "outgrow" their allergy; it simply recurs with other symptoms.

In the past, asthma often was described as a psychogenic illness, implicating parents and their child rearing practices as the underlying problem. Today allergists and immunologists, who have researched the pathophysiological processes, generally discredit this notion. Emotional stress has a major impact on the child and his family in chronic illnesses, including asthma. The asthmatic child often learns to manipulate people with asthma attacks. Parents, in their attempts to prevent the terrifying attacks, give in to the child, then later become angry with him and themselves for the weakness. This inconsistency confuses the child, causing more stress and more asthma. Parents need a careful, repeated explanation of this phenomenon, with advice about how to prevent manipulation by the child. They may be forced to let the child experience an attack with a competent adult sitter while they go out for an evening. The sitter can administer treatments or even drive the child to the emergency room. This treatment may seem harsh, but it teaches the child that asthma is not something to be used to get his way, and that he can survive without his parents awhile. Some parents cannot or will not place limits on their child's behavior, and the resulting emotional component may be significant enough to require psychotherapy.

Asthma should be treated like other allergies: remove the offending allergen when possible, treat symptoms with specific medications, and hyposensitize with immunotherapy. Selecting the appropriate combination of medications, determining therapeutic dosage, and avoiding toxicity are difficult tasks which can be accomplished only with careful observation of the child by his parents and nurse. The physician may require the parents to increase or decrease medications (within specific limits) according to the child's symptoms, and the nurse must prepare the parents for this responsibility. The child with asthma usually requires a maintenance dosage of theophylline as a preventive measure and occasional doses of inhaled isoproterenol or metaproterenol for mild to moderate attacks. If these bronchodilators do not suffice, an inhaled steroid preparation can be added. Chromalyn sodium, another inhaled medication that prevents asthma with varying success, may be tried. If the child is not relieved with conventional drugs, systemic corticosteroids are then given. (Inhaled corticosteroids are usually more effective when they follow a course of systemic preparations.) Complications of chronic uncontrolled asthma are emphysema, decreased height and weight, and numerous respiratory infections.

Status asthmaticus is increasingly severe asthma that does not respond to epinephrine and theophylline. The child sticken with it requires intensive medical and nursing care in a critical care setting. He is usually dehydrated and acidotic, demanding immediate fluid and electrolyte correction. Appropriate intravenous medications include aminophylline (theophylline and ethylenediamene), antibiotics if indicated, and corticosteroids. Sedatives are avoided, unless absolutely necessary, since they may cause respiratory depression. The physician usually prescribes moisturized nasal oxygen, instead of a croup tent with nebulized oxygen, which may cause excessive wetting of the lungs. Vital signs, blood gases, serum theophylline levels, and pulmonary functioning are monitored frequently. Even after severe bronchoconstriction is improved, the resulting edema can still obstruct airways enough to cause death. An anesthesiologist or other respiratory specialist, should be consulted about the possibility of mechanical ventilation and remain ready to assist. Complications of status asthmaticus include atelectasis pneumothorax, pneumomediastenum, and asphixiation.

Most children hospitalized with asthma usually do not have status asthamaticus but do have severe enough symptoms to require intravenous therapy and monitoring. Expect an irritable, restless child. Watch for signs of toxicity from the bronchodilators. Many times the older child will recognize early signs of toxicity as such and will tell you when he has a headache, incipient nausea, or nervousness. Unfortunately, he may have to tolerate some side effects in order to prevent asthma. Parents may need a break from caring for the child during early hospitalization, since they are usually exhausted from caring for him at home. Increase their responsibility for treatments and medications as the child improves. Be sure that the parents know how to get immediate medical treatment for an asthma attack that is unresponsive to medications given at home. You cannot teach the parents of a hospitalized child exactly when the child needs medical attention, but in cases in which the physician's orders call for several medications to be given as needed, you can have them help you assess the child as his condition changes and as you make decisions about medications. Later you can encourage them to report the child's status and to request specific medications. Ideally, by the time of discharge, parents will have taken responsibility for their child's care, and you will be playing only a supportive role. The older child can participate in this process also. The family must still endure the process of going home and, ultimately, making decisions about whether to get help or to wait awhile in hopes medication will bring improvement. They also will have to recognize new signs of drug toxicity. Reassure them that observational and treatment skills will develop with experience. Reinforcement and support from a home health nurse can build their confidence in their abilities. The school nurse also can help parents and the child in coping with asthma.

Hives

Hives (urticaria) is a skin condition in which raised, erythematous, well-circumscribed lesions (welts) appear in small areas or over the entire body surface. It usually results from an allergic reaction but may be caused by cold or heat, emotional factors, or even pressure to the skin. Itching may be intense or may not even occur. Although hives usually disappear soon after they erupt, they may become a chronic condition. They often appear concurrently with other severe allergic reactions, such as anaphylaxis. Antihistamines are given for simple hives, and epinephrine is given for generalized welts and itching. As with all allergies, avoiding the allergen is the best treatment.

Anaphylaxis

Anaphylaxis is a severe, generalized, allergic response that may include laryngeal edema, urticaria, bronchoconstriction, or even circulatory collapse. The usual causative allergens are drugs (especially those administered parenterally), stinging insects, and foods. After the child's initial sensitization to the offending agent, subsequent contacts may cause increasingly severe and rapid reactions. Occasionally, anaphylaxis will follow as soon as the child's second contact with the allergen, but usually, children will begin with milder reactions which warn parents and professionals of danger. Allergens causing anaphylaxis must be avoided whenever possible, and hyposensitization is used to reduce the risk of accidental exposure. If the agent is unknown or if hyposensitization is not feasible, the child should be taught to take antihistamines and to inject epinephrine.

Anaphylaxis is a medical emergency that can occur at any time. Every hospital follows specific routines, directing the nurse in making decisions about emergency drugs and procedures. Be prepared; know the emergency routines and pediatric dosages. Be prepared to inject aqueous epinephrine 1:1,000 subcutaneously, and to start an intravenous infusion of anti-hypotensive agents to combat shock and of bronchodilators to assist in oxygenation. Begin oxygen support by mask, and be prepared to assist the physician in intubation of the child, if laryngeal edema is is severe.

AUTOIMMUNITY

Without any obvious explanation, a group infection, trauma, hormonal deviation, or poisoning, a group of similar inflammatory diseases cause destruction of body tissue. These diseases were once called "rheumatic diseases" because of the inflammation occurring in connective tissue of organs throughout the body. New techniques for studying antibodies, however, have led to the discovery that various strange antibodies, present in affected people's blood, were ruthlessly attacking the victims' own joints, hearts, skin, kidneys, brains, mucous membranes, and so on. Researchers have theorized that something (perhaps an infection, allergic reaction, or mutation) happens to the tissue, or even to a few cells, that leaves the affected areas different from the cells and tissues of the brain. The body's immune system reacts to these different tissues or cells as though they are foreign and vicious antibodies attack and destroy not only the changed cells but also the normal cells. This process is called *autoimmunity*. Sometimes, the process occurs because something foreign is touching a tissue (e.g., pollen in hay fever) or has been filtered by it (e.g., antigens filtered by the kidney), and the uninvolved tissue, an "innocent bystander," is attacked. Many unexplained diseases probably are caused by autoimmunity and the genetic defects that trigger the change in cells. The characteristics of some autoimmune conditions are summarized in Table 16–2.

COMMON PROBLEMS, SYMPTOMS, AND NURSING CARE

Inflammation

Inflammation caused by autoimmunity manifests itself by erythema, edema, warmth, loss of function, and pain. Mucus- and fluid-producing membranes overproduce and cause excessive drainage and fluid collections. Nursing care is specific to the affected tissues, organs, and systems, and the observable varied symptoms. The inflammatory process is usually intermittent, flaring up with the stress of infections, trauma, or emotional upsets, then subsiding.

The child with autoimmunity experiences complications that vary according to the organs attacked. For example, when the kidney is involved, fluid and electrolyte imbalance results. If a vital organ is constantly attacked because of repeatedly inflammatory episodes, it will cease to function, and the child will die. More commonly, the child with autoimmunity exhibits varying degrees of disability.

COMMON DIAGNOSTIC PROCEDURES

Tissue Biopsy

A biopsy of the tissues which are targets of the autoimmune process reveals clumps of antibodies, cells, complement and fibrinoid materials. Most autoimmune diseases do not require biopsy for diagnosis, however, since current clinical entities are well defined and laboratory methods are quite precise, but renal biopsy, puncture biopsy of the skin, and joint fluid aspiration may be necessary to rule out many other similar diseases.

Table 16–2. **Specific Autoimmune Conditions**

Disease	*Affected Organs and Tissue*	*Common Signs and Symptoms*
Rheumatic fever	Heart, joints, nervous system	Arthritis, fever, carditis, rash, chorea → sx which manifests snakelike movts
Juvenile rheumatoid arthritis	Joints, eyes (iris, ciliary body)	Pain, swelling, and degeneration of joints; visual impairment; photophobia
Systemic lupus erythematosus	Skin, joints, kidney, heart, nervous system, gastrointestinal tract, eyes	"Butterfly" rash, nephritis, carditis, seizures, vomiting, diarrhea, visual impairment
Glomerulonephritis	Kidneys, heart	Hematuria, proteinuria, oliguria, edema, hypertension, hematuria, fluid and electrolyte imbalance
Idiopathic thrombocytopenic purpura (ITP)	Platelets	Bleeding
Autoimmune hemolytic anemia	Erythrocytes	Anemia

Immunological Studies

Autoimmune diseases usually cause changes that can be measured by various laboratory procedures. Immunoelectrophoresis reveals increases in immunoglobulins. Rheumatoid factor, found in serum, reacts with immunoglobulins to form an immune complex. The *lupus erythematosus cell*, or *LE cell* (Figure 16–5), is a large white cell containing the by-products of an antigen-antibody reaction in which the antigen is the nucleus of all body cells. The actual antinuclear antibodies can be measured, as can the antibodies for streptococcal enzymes (via ASO titer), cytoplasm, and the the thyroid gland.

Complete Blood Count

The complete blood count in autoimmune disease is often abnormal; the white cell count is elevated and occasionally resembles leukemia, and anemia is common.

Other Tests

Numerous other laboratory procedures are useful in diagnosing autoimmune diseases with specific organ involvement. For

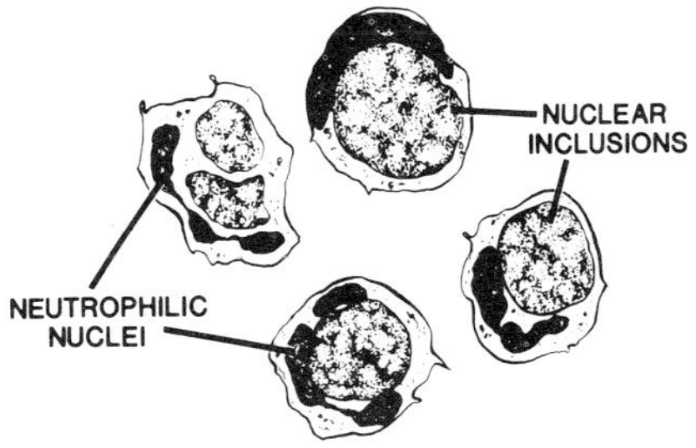

Figure 16–5. *The lupus eryhtematosus (LE) cell. The neutrophil has enclosed nuclear material from another cell.*

example, urine tests can help identify changes. Usually, no single test is sufficient for diagnosis since there are many common factors in the different forms. A combination of laboratory and clinical data lead to a diagnosis of specific autoimmunities.

COMMON TREATMENTS

Anti-inflammatory Medications

No medication will cure autoimmune disorders, but anti-inflammatory medications such as aspirin will decrease symptoms. The child must be closely monitored for side effects, however, and other medications substituted when necessary. Corticosteroids also are given during exacerbation, and doses are then decreased to prevent a rebound effect after the drug is discontinued. If maintenance therapy is required, doses of the lowest suppressive amount are given every other day.

Other Treatments

Other than anti-inflammatory therapy, treatment of autoimmune conditions is symptomatic. Kidney involvement, for example, is treated with fluid and electrolyte manipulation. Avoidance of stress is recommended, but a child must experience some stress if he is to develop normally. Extreme measures aimed at prevention of infection for children with autoimmunity may help to prevent some exacerbations, but such measures may hamper normal development. The ideal balance of protection and freedom is difficult for parents to achieve.

SUMMARY

The child with altered immunity faces a loss of his protective balance. A lack of immunity (immunodeficiency) leaves him vulnerable to many microorganisms, even those that live quietly in the well child's body. An excess of immunity (allergy) overwhelms his body with inflammatory processes. Misdirected immunity (autoimmunity) leads his body to attack itself. These conditions usually are chronic and their symptoms range from mild to fatal. Heredity (or at least the inherited tendency for the disease) is involved in most of these disorders. Medications have greatly improved the prognosis of the child with an immune deviation. Nursing care in critical and acute settings significantly increases the child's chance of survival during episodic illness. Nursing care in ambulatory settings provides support and education for the family. The on-going intensive research in immunology undoubtedly will continue to change the whole field of children's health care.

Bibliography

Bergner, M. and Hutelmyer, C. Teaching Kids How to Live with Their Allergies. *Nursing '76*, 8:11, 1976.

Bridgewater, S.C. et al. Allergies in Children: Recognition. *American Journal of Nursing* 78:614, 1978.

——— and Voigner, R.R. Allergies in Children: Teaching. *American Journal of Nursing* 78:620, 1978.

Carty, R.M. Some Facts about Allergy. *Pediatric Nursing* 3:7, 1977.

Collins-Williams, C. The Status of Immunotherapy in Children—What Are the Problems? *Annals of Allergy* 39:87, 1977.

Dharan, M. Immunoglobulin Abnormalities. *American Journal of Nursing* 76:1626, 1976.

Donley, D. L. Nursing the Patient Who Is Immunosuppressed. *American Journal of Nursing* 76:1619, 1976.

Dyer, B. Asthmatic Kids—Independence: One Giant Step. *Pediatric Nursing* 3:16, 1977.

Garh, S. *Laboratory Tests in Common Use.* New York, Springer Co., 1976.

Glasser, R.J. Autoimmune Diseases. *Nursing '77* 9:38, 1977.

Hawkins-Walsh, E. Drugs Used in the Treatment of Pediatric Allergy and Asthma. *Pediatric Nursing* 3:12, 1977.

Hill, M. Asthmatic Child or Asthma Expert? *Pediatric Nursing* 3:25, 1977.

Loebl, S., et al. *The Nurse's Drug Handbook.* New York, John Wiley & Sons, Inc., 1977.

McMillan, J. et al. *The Whole Pediatrician Catalog.* Philadelphia, W. B. Saunders Co., 1977.

Newton, D.W., et al. You Can Minimize the Hazards of Corticosteroids. *Nursing '77* 6:26, 1977.

Nysather, J.O., et al. The Immune System—Its Development and Functions. *American Journal of Nursing* 76:1614, 1976.

Tilkian, S.M. and Conover, M.H. *Clinical Implications of Laboratory Tests.* Saint Louis, C.U. Mosby Co., 1973.

Vaughn, V.C. and McKay, R.J. *Nelson Textbook of Pediatrics.* Philadelphia, W.B. Saunders Co., 1975.

Voigner, R.R. and Bridgewater, S.C. Allergies in Children: Testing and Treating. *American Journal of Nursing* 78:617, 1978.

SECTION THREE

Growth

CHAPTER **17**

Growth

BEHAVIORAL OBJECTIVES

After studying this chapter you will be able to:

- Describe normal growth.
- Explain how genes, hormones, and nutrients affect growth.
- Discuss the process of digestion.
- Discuss metabolism, explaining how protein, fats, carbohydrates, and vitamins are used by the body.
- Identify the glands that produce hormones and discuss the functions of the hormones.
- Discuss the effects of malabsorption, intestinal obstruction, and the stress of illness on growth.
- Explain the neoplastic process, contrasting malignant and benign growth.

TERMS AND CONCEPTS

Hormones
Calories
Metabolism
Anabolism
Catabolism
Proteins
Fats
Carbohydrates
Enzymes
Vitamins
Megavitamin therapy
Height age
Bone age
Neoplasm
Benign
Malignant
Metastasis
Grading
Staging
Typing

GROWTH

The child grows as cells enlarge, multiply, and divide. The attainment of additional motor and intellectual skills that results from cell differentiation and maturation constitute development. Growth and development are influenced by birth weight, genetic background, socioeconomic class, health state, and by the size of the family, the availability of food, and exposure to infections and parasites.

Growth is an increase in the size of the whole body or any of the body parts caused by an increase in cell number, cell size, or a combination of both. Growth is orderly and predictable; each body organ and system has its own unique growth pattern. Periods of rapid cell growth and differentiation are followed by periods of stability. The child's brain grows rapidly from the time of conception until the second year, when growth begins to decelerate. This is a period of rapid cell multiplication and increasing differentiation, during which the brain is especially vulnerable to the stresses of infection, trauma, or undernutrition; insults received at this time can produce permanent disabilities.

Genetic Influence on Growth

Genes determine the rate of growth and development as well as height at maturity. Some infants who are small at birth but who have the genetic capacity to attain a normal size show accelerated growth during the first six months of life; other infants who are small at birth do not catch up in growth during the first six months, continue to grow at a slower rate, and will be small as adults. The alleles that affect size at maturity and the pace of growth are located on the X and Y sex chromosomes. The female matures 10 percent faster than the male. Allowing for genetic differences, growth normally proceeds at an established rate. By one year of age, the infant is 50 percent longer than at birth and three times as heavy. Growth rate begins to decrease during the latter part of the first year, and a reduction in adipose tissue occurs. By eighteen months to two years, a consistent, slower pattern of growth is established. At this time the child's growth is characterized by a deceleration of linear growth and an acceleration of weight gain. This pattern continues until adolescence.

Hormonal Influence on Growth

Hormones direct growth by controlling the rate of chemical reactions inside cells, transporting substances through cell membranes, and secreting growth compounds; they are produced in glands that form a network called the *endocrine system.* The endocrine system is responsible for growth, maturation, reproduction, cellular functions, and the integration of body responses to stress (see Figures 17–1 and 17–2).

Adolescence begins when an increase in the secretion of chemical compounds called *hormones* occurs. Linear growth now accelerates, with peak growth occurring two to three years after the onset of adolescence. Females, having matured faster than males throughout childhood, began adolescence two years earlier, at the average age of ten.

Specific hormones contribute to adolescent growth and the appearance of secondary sexual characteristics. Females show breast, nipple, and areolae development. Pubic and axillary hair appear as the female's hips widen; the vaginal mucosa becomes thicker and pale pink. Peak height occurs at 12.1 years of age, and menarche usually begins by age 13.

The male matures more slowly, and the rate of growth is less predictable. The male's adolescence is heralded by the release of testosterone. Testical enlargement begins by ages nine to twelve and the penis increases in size. Pubic, axillary, and facial hair appears, and the release of hormones causes skin changes to occur (in both males and females), and this in turn causes acne. Linear growth accelerates, and the male's average peak growth occurs at 14.1 years of age. Vocal cartilage expands and the voice deepens. The number and strength of muscle cells double, muscular coordination is improved, and by eighteen most linear growth is completed.

Many hormones interact to facilitate and maintain growth. *Androgens,* produced in the adrenal gland, facilitate an increase in muscle cell size and number as well as an increase in bone mass, which results in increased linear growth. *Estrogens,* produced in the ovaries, increase lateral growth of the

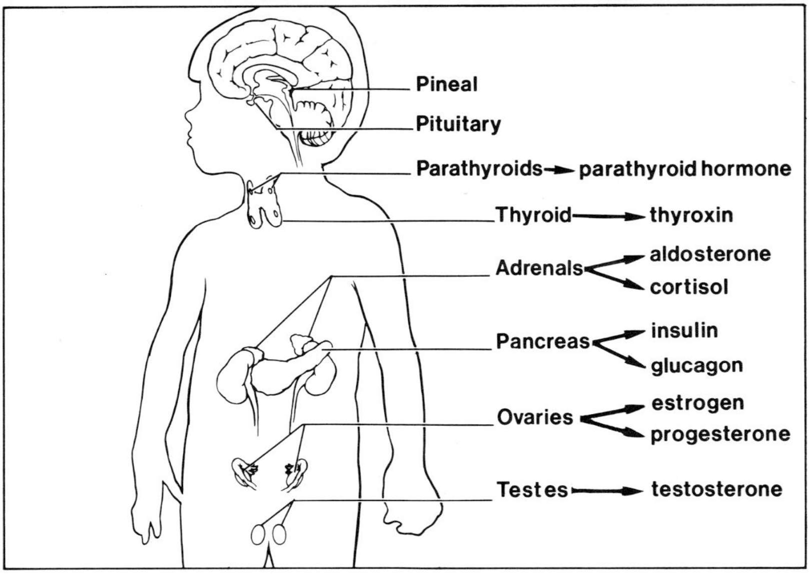

Figure 17–1. *Regulators of growth.* The endocrine network (Fig. 17-1) consists of glands that make, store, and secrete hormones. Hormones influence chemical reactions and regulate growth, metabolism, and reproduction. Certain hormones act on specific glands to stimulate additional hormones, while other hormones act directly on body cells. The rate of hormonal secretion is controlled by a negative feedback system; high blood concentrations of a hormone inhibit further secretion, and low blood concentrations stimulate secretion.

Seven glands secrete hormones. The *pituitary gland* has an anterior and a posterior section. The *anterior pituitary* produces hormones that stimulate other endocrine glands to secrete hormones; these are *thyroid stimulating hormone* (TSH), which stimulates the thyroid; *adrenocorticotropic hormone (ACTH),* which acts on the adrenal glands and reproductive gland stimulants; *follicle stimulating hormone (FSH), luteinizing hormone (LH),* and *interstitial-cell-stimulating hormone (ICSH). Prolactin,* a stimulant of breast milk secretion after childbirth, melanocyte-stimulating hormone *(MSH),* which influences skin pigmentation, and *growth hormone (GH)* are additional hormones secreted by the anterior pituitary. The *posterior pituitary* secretes two hormones: *antidiuretic hormone (ADH),* which facilitates water retention, and *oxytocin,* which stimulates uterine contractions during labor and delivery.

The *thyroid gland* secretes *thyroid hormone,* which regulates the rate of metabolism. Four *parathyroid glands* release *parathyroid hormone,* which helps to regulate blood calcium concentrations.

The *adrenal glands* consist of an outer cortext and an inner medulla. The *adrenal cortex* secretes *mineralocorticoid hormones* (e.g., *aldosterone*) that maintain a balance of blood sodium concentrations, and *glucocortoid hormones* (e.g., *cortisol*) that aid in the metabolism of proteins and fats, maintain normal blood pressure, and produce anti-inflammatory responses following stress. The adrenal cortex also secretes male hormones *(androgens)* and some insignificant amounts of female hormones *(estrogens).* The *adrenal medulla* secretes *epinephrine* and *norepinephrine,* hormones that increase body activity (i.e., raise the blood pressure and stimulate respiration and sweating) and prepare the body for a "fight or flight" reaction.

The *pancreas* secretes *insulin* and *glucagon.* Insulin promotes the transport and use of carbohydrates and fats. Glucagon increases blood glucose levels and is an insulin antagonist.

The *ovaries* produce *estrogen* and *progesterone* which influence female sexual characteristics, including fertility and menstruation. The *testes* secrete *testosterone,* which promotes fertility and other sexual characteristics in the male.

The *pineal gland* produces *melatonin,* which may influence ovarian hormone production; little is known about this gland.

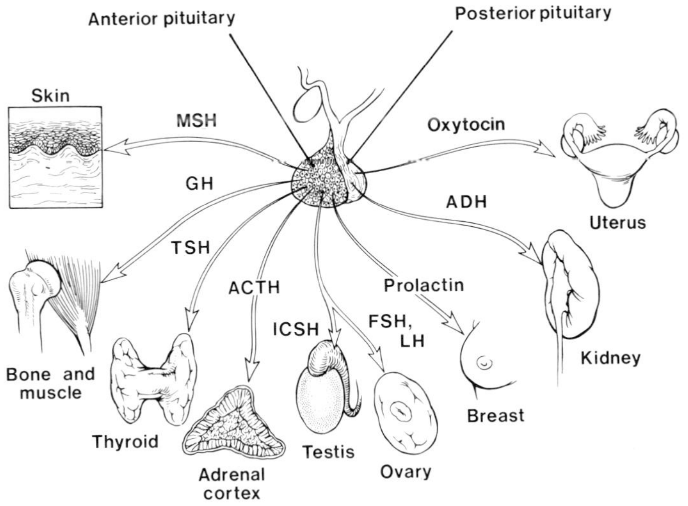

Figure 17–2. *Hormones produced by the anterior and posterior pituitary and their target glands.*

female pelvis and widen the hips. The pituitary gland produces a growth hormone that stimulates the release of *somatomedin* in the liver. Somatomedin is a growth hormone and is responsible for cell growth. However, somatomedin cannot produce growth without the help of estrogen and androgen.

NUTRIENTS FOR GROWTH

Nutrients are the chemical elements in food that are essential for growth. Unless the mother's nutrition is very poor, the fetus is able to obtain inadequate nutrition for fetal growth and development. After birth, however, the child must consume adequate nutrients if growth is to continue. To form and maintain tissue and to complete the reactions that sustain life within each cell, the child needs a regular supply of about 50 nutrients, including proteins, fats, carbohydrates, minerals, vitamins, and water. Complex biochemical mechanisms regulate the availability of nutrients and eliminate excesses in the urine, sweat and feces. If the nutrient intake is low and does not meet normal body needs, tissues and cells seek to conserve the limited supply by retaining nutrients for longer periods and by using more effective means to absorb nutrients from the intestines. If the dietary intake of nutrients continues to be inadequate, deficiency diseases occur; however, high concentrations of certain nutrients are equally hazardous and may be toxic. For example, excessive consumption of certain vitamins can result in *hypervitaminosis*.

Calories, Energy, and Metabolism

If cells are to function and grow, certain food nutrients must be consumed (see Figure 17–3). The energy content of food is measured in *calories*. *Metabolism* is the body's use of energy-containing nutrients. Metabolism consists basically of two func-

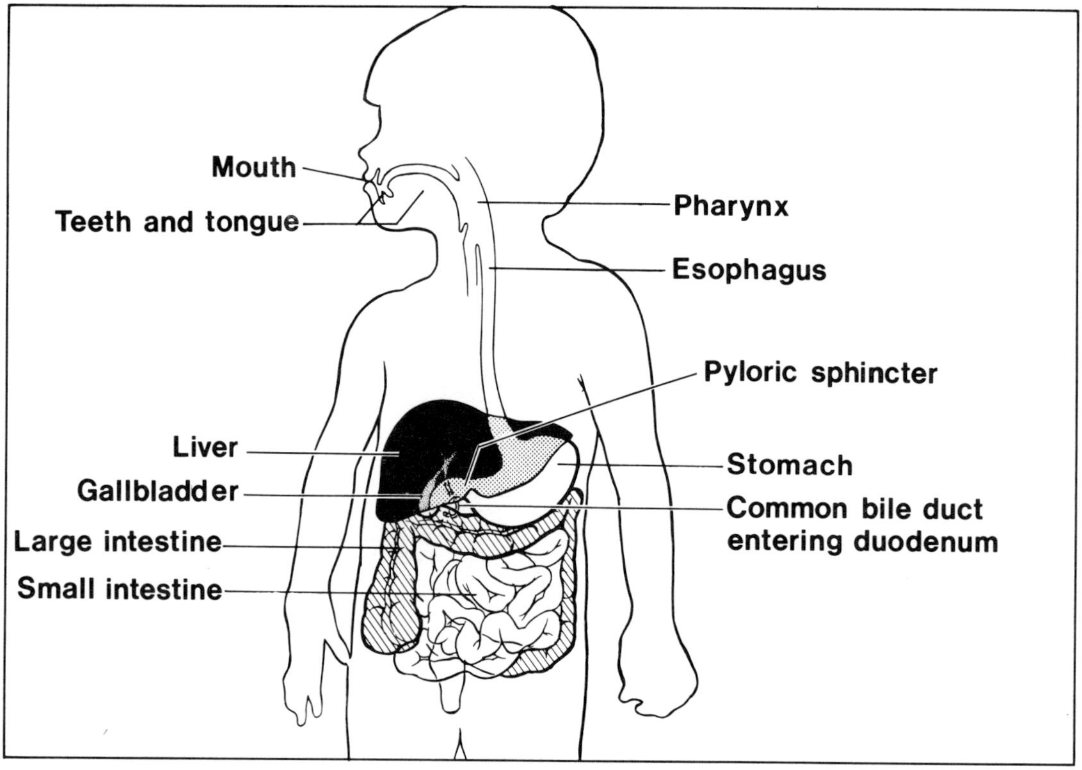

Figure 17–3. *Digestion. Digestion* is the changing of food into matter usable for metabolism. Digestion begins in the *mouth,* where chewing and secretions mix and degrade food. The food is cleared from the mouth by the swallowing action of the *pharynx* and transported to the *stomach* through the *esophagus.* Muscular contractions in the stomach act to mix, churn, and move the food into the *small intestine,* where additional mixing occurs. *Enzymes,* proteins that facilitate chemical reactions, and *bile,* a liver secretion released by the *gallbladder,* enter the *duodenum* of the small intestine by the *common bile duct* and act with intestional juices to further break down food nutrients. The degraded nutrients pass across the intestinal wall into the blood stream. Once in the circulation, nutrients are used in metabolism by the process of *catabolism* and *anabolism.* Catabolism is the breaking down of food molecules into simple compounds such as water and carbon dioxide; anabolism is the building up of food molecules into complex new compounds such as enzymes, hormones, and antibodies.

Leaving the small intestine, many nutrients enter the *liver,* a center for protein anabolism and catabolism. The liver makes new compounds, degrades and stores existing nutrients such as iron and vitamins, and detoxifies harmful compounds. The functions of the liver are so vital that if certain functions are impaired for a few days, death ensues. The *pancreas,* also vital to metabolism, empties digestive juices into the duodenum and secretes *insulin* and *glucagon,* which are used for carbohydrate metabolism.

The final stage of digestion is the accumulation of waste products in the *large intestine* where water is absorbed and digestive waste is expelled as feces.

tions, *catabolism* and *anabolism*. Catabolism is the breaking of molecules into smaller parts; anabolism is the building of large molecules by the combining of small molecules. The parts of a cell are continually being broken down and replaced with new molecules. Some molecules are replaced every few minutes, while others require years for replacement. As the molecules are broken down, energy is released, and the energy is used to maintain cell structure and function, to make molecules, and to transport materials; each process is essential for growth.

The energy needs of children differ according to age, body size and composition, activity, and rate of growth. Older children need more calories because of their larger size, but their energy need per unit of size decreases after infancy. If the diet is deficient in foods that provide energy, the child's growth is delayed and he loses weight. When food deficits continue, linear growth ceases and various disease may result (see Figure 17–4). If an excess of food is consumed, obesity results and the risk of disease increases. Three types of nutrients provide energy: *protein, fats,* and *carbohydrates*.

Proteins are made of *amino acids*, the kind, number, and arrangement of which determine the characteristics of the protein. At present, 24 different amino acids have been identified; they are classified as either essential (those that must be provided in the diet) or nonessential (those that can be synthesized by the body). Growth cannot proceed unless all essential amino acids are present, since the formation of new tissue depends on these substances. Amino acids are absorbed by the intestines, carried to the liver, and then distributed to the tissue, while excess amino acids are ex-

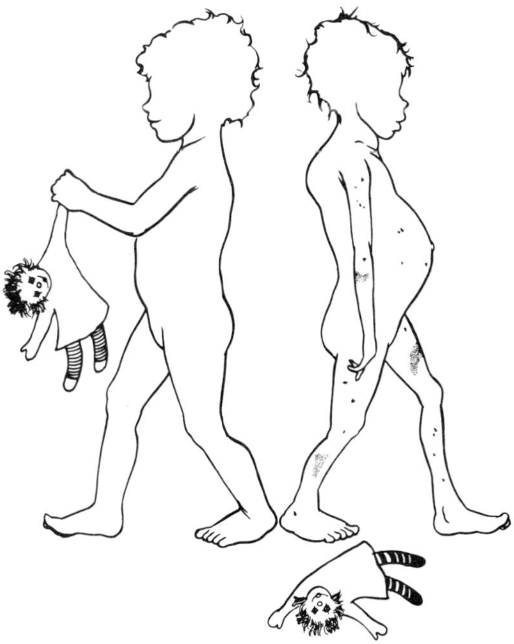

Figure 17–4. *The well-nourished child has shiny, glossy hair and a healthy scalp. The facial skin is smooth and moist; eyes are clear and bright, and the gums are firm and pink with no swelling or bleeding. The teeth are clean; no discoloration is present. Weight is normal for age; muscles are firm and well developed; and the posture is erect, with arms and legs straight and abdomen flat. The child's appetite is good, and bowel movements are regular. The child is active, alert, and shows attention span and behavior appropriate for age.*

The malnourished child has dull, brittle hair, greasy and scaly facial skin, and dry, possibly infected eyes. The gums are swollen and spongy; some teeth are missing and others have cavities. The child is overweight or underweight for height and age. The child's posture is poor; the shoulders are sagged, the back is humped, the abdomen is swollen, the legs are bowed, and the knees are knocked. Muscles are flaccid and underdeveloped. The child's appetite is poor; he is likely to have diarrhea or constipation. The child lacks energy and tires easily, and he seems listless and apathetic.

creted by the kidneys as urea. Alterations in the metabolism of individual amino acids result in diseases referred to as *inborn errors of metabolism,* such as phenylketonuria (PKU). Protein is needed for cell construction, function, and repair. Proteins are responsible for repairing wounds and forming scar tissue. In addition, special proteins maintain water balance and circulatory function. Cell walls are made of protein, as are *enzymes* (compounds that aid metabolism), *hormones,* and *antibodies*. Proteins in the blood act as buffers and react with acids and bases to maintain the neutrality of body fluids. Primary food sources of protein are milk, eggs, meat, fish, poultry, cheese, peas, beans, cereal, and nuts. Protein deficiencies cause growth retardation; if the deficiency is severe, it can cause edema, an enlarged liver, and behavioral changes. Fats, or *lipids,* are a concentrated source of energy; they provide 40 to 50 percent of the energy needed in infancy and childhood. Adipose tissue, which is composed of fats, serves as insulation against temperature changes and forms the body's membranous structures. Because fats are insoluble in water, they serve to transport vitamins A, D, E, and K, which are also insoluble in water. Fats in the body are derived from ingested meats and vegetables digested in the small intestine and absorbed in the blood. The fat derived from animal sources is called *cholesterol.* Most consumed fats are chemically classified as *triglycerides.* Fats are needed to produce vitamin D, certain hormones, and specialized tissue (e.g., the myelin sheath covering the brain). A deficiency of fat results in dry, thick skin and may retard neural development. Excessive fat intake may produce an increased number of fat cells, leading to obesity.

Providing the greatest portion of calories and comprising the largest part of the diet, carbohydrates produce cells and antibodies. Digested carbohydrates are used by the heart or brain or stored in the liver as *glycogen,* an important reserve of energy for all body systems. If carbohydrates are not available to the body, or if their utilization is altered, protein and fat are degraded and used for energy. Carbohydrates are provided in milk, breads, cereals, sugars, starches, and vegetables. Conditions such as diabetes mellitus may result if the metabolism of carbohydrates is altered. If the chemicals, such as enzymes, that are necessary for carbohydrate processing are not present in the intestines, diarrhea and malabsorption result. The protein contents of some common children's foods are listed in Tables 17–1 and 17–2.)

Vitamins

Vitamins are essential organic substances required, in small amounts, for the metabolism of amino acids, fats, and carbohydrates, and for the production of tissue, enzymes, and hormones. They are classified according to their solubility in fats or water. Since fat-soluble vitamins are absorbed and transported in lipids, the malabsorp-

Table 17–1. Approximate Protein Content of Milk and Other Foods Commonly Fed to Infants

Food	*Protein (gm/oz)*
Breast milk	0.3
Commercial formulas	0.5
Homogenized milk	1.1
High-protein infant cereals	9.9
Strained vegetable and meat dinners, e.g., vegetable and ham	1.1
Strained meat, e.g., beef	4.2

Table 17–2. Approximate Protein Content of Foods Commonly Fed to Children

Food	*Portion*	*Protein (gm)*
Egg	1	5.7
Hamburger	2-oz patty	15.4
Frankfurter	1	5.6
Chicken leg	1	12.2
Tuna	1/4 cup	11.5
Peanut butter	1 tablespoon	4.0

tion of fat may result in malabsorption of fat-soluble vitamins. Excesses of fat-soluble vitamins are not excreted but are stored in the body; this is especially significant because large stored reserves of Vitamins A and D are toxic. In contrast, water-soluble vitamins are not stored in reserves; excesses are excreted in the urine. If the diet contains adequate amounts of vitamins and the body absorbs them properly, no vitamin supplements are necessary. However, if certain foods are unavailable or cannot be tolerated, vitamin supplements may be necessary. (A list of vitamins and their corresponding food sources and deficiency states is presented in Table 17–3.)

Some vitamins are produced in the alimentary tract; others, especially the B vitamins, are not produced by the body. The intake of foods containing the latter group of vitamins is essential. Certain intestinal flora (microorganisms normally found in the intestines) can inhibit or alter the body's utilization of vitamins, causing deficiencies. In addition, various antimicrobial agents (e.g., neomycin) alter the absorption ability of the intestines and can cause malabsorption.

Although vitamins are popular symbols of health, widely advertised and consumed in great quantities, the administration of extra vitamins is justified only when a need is demonstrated; deficiency diseases are rare and need not be a concern if the child eats a typical American diet. Exceptions exist in infancy, when Vitamin D supplements are necessary if the child is drinking unfortified cow's milk; insufficient Vitamin D can cause rickets.

Controversy continues over *megavitamin therapy*, which entails the ingestion of large quantities of certain vitamins. The mass media have fostered the idea that the regular consumption of large amounts of some vitamins, particularly Vitamin C (abscorbic acid), decreases the incidence of colds and improves general health. The advocates of megavitamin therapy conclude that since metabolic reactions are completed by enzymes and many enzymes are derived from vitamins, a large dose of vitamin may favorably influence enzyme activity. Present theories about Vitamin C and the use of high dosages of other vitamins are highly speculative and must await further studies. Parents and health consumers frequently think that if a little is good, a lot is better. If your opinion regarding the use of supplemental vitamins is sought, bear in mind that present studies do not document the benefits of a megavitamin regimen.

MEASURING GROWTH

Three measurements are made to determine the child's overall growth pattern: length or height, weight, and head circumference. From birth until eighteen months of age, linear growth is usually measured with the child in a supine position. After that, height is measured with the child standing with shoes removed. Weight is measured with the child unclothed. Head circumference is measured from birth until

Table 17–3. **Vitamins**

Fat-Soluble Vitamins	*Dietary Sources*	*Deficiency Conditions*
A	Liver, milk, fat products, egg yolk, yellow fruits and vegetables, green vegetables	Night blindness. Prolonged deficiency causes dryness and thickening of the conjunctiva; corneal softening; and permanent blindness.
D	Fortified milk and margarine, eggs, cod-liver oil	Rickets
E	Green leafy vegetables, nuts, legumes, margarine	Hemolysis in the premature infant when mother's diet is deficient.
K	Green leafy vegetables, pork, liver	Bleeding disorders of varying severity, especially in the newborn.
Water-Soluble Vitamins		
B_1 (Thiamine)	Organ meats, milk, whole grain cereals, pork	Beriberi (peripheral nerve changes, edema, heart failure)
B_2 (Riboflavin)	Milk, cheese, organ meats, eggs, fish, green vegetables	Visual lesions (burning, blurring and itching); red lips, cracked mouth corners.
B_6 (Pyridoxine)	Meats, vegetables, whole grain cereals	Irritability, convulsions, muscle twitching
Niacin	Meat, fish, poultry, liver, peanuts, enriched cereals	Pellagra (a disease characterized by skin and gastrointestinal lesions, nervousness, and mental disorders)
Pantothenic acid	Widely distributed in foods	Fatigue, sleep disturbances, nausea
Folacin	Legumes, green vegetables, whole wheat products	Anemia, gastrointestinal disturbances, diarrhea, red tongue
B_{12} (Cobalamin)	Available only in animal foods (e.g., fish, eggs, milk, cheese, meat)	Pernicious anemia and neurological disorders
Biotin	Legumes, vegetables, meats	Fatigue, depression, nausea, dermatitis, muscle pains
Choline	Egg yolk, liver, grains	Not reported in man
C (Ascorbic acid)	Citrus fruits, tomatoes, green peppers, salad greens	Scurvy (degeneration of skin, teeth, blood vessels)

age two, the most critical period of head growth. To measure head circumference, place a nonstretchable tape firmly around the head, just above the eyebrows. (Illustrations of growth measurement techniques are presented in the Skills Manual.)

Growth measurements are recorded as percentiles for chronological age, from the third to 97th percentile. Frequently, the child's *height age* is requested; height age is the chronological age at which the child's stature represents the 50th percentile. For example, a ten-year-old boy with a height of 120 centimeters is below the 3rd percentile for his chronological age, however, his height is at the fiftieth percentile for six years and six months, thus his height age is 6.5 years. *Bone age,* another measurement used to assess growth, is bone maturation as revealed by x-ray photographs of the child's hand and wrist. Chronological age, height age, bone age, and mental age may be compared for a total growth assessment.

Recording growth values on a percentile graph identifies where the child ranks relative to all children of the same age and sex in the United States. When recording growth values, record the child's birth date, then carefully calculate age in years and months. Children with growth measurements between the 25th and 75th percentile are said to be developing normally. Measurements between 10 and 25 percent and 75 and 90 percent may or may not be normal depending on past and future measurements and genetic and environmental factors. Measurements above 90 or below 10 should be double-checked for accuracy and reported for further evaluation.

Growth assessment is a screening method, not a diagnostic procedure, because measurements alone do not reveal the cause of the deficiency. Growth is evaluated for each hospitalized child and used to identify children who are small for age or underweight for stature. Altered growth is a symptom of many chronic health problems.

GROWTH ALTERATIONS

A decrease or increase in growth may be a consequence of a problem inside or outside the body cells. Common problems affecting growth include an inadequate supply of nutrients (e.g., carbohydrates, fats, proteins, vitamins), a problem in digestion, or altered elimination. Alterations in hormonal secretion and effect can result in growth delays or uncontrolled, rapid growth. Frequent causes of growth alterations include nutrient supply problems, malabsorption, intestinal obstruction, and hormonal deviations.

Nutrient Supply Problems

Illness produces stress, which in turn causes an increased need for nutrients, especially protein. However, infection decreases appetite, thus reducing food intake at a time when the body requires additional proteins for antibody production. Acute illness can cause both a protein deficit and impaired body growth; chronic illnesses, such as heart defects and respiratory insufficiencies, may cause sluggish circulation and *hypoxia,* the inadequate delivery of oxygen to the cells. Without adequate oxygen, body cells cannot metabolize nutrients optimally, and impaired growth results. Children with chronic illnesses frequently suffer from delayed growth.

Other diseases can upset the metabolism of essential nutrients. For example, the body's optimal use of Vitamin D depends on the status of the liver and kidneys; if either organ malfunctions, the body's processing of Vitamin D is impaired, as is seen in some children with kidney disease who have skeletal abnormalities similar to those of rickets. Because the ill child usually does not want to eat, and the nutritional value of what he does eat may be impaired because of digestive or circulatory problems, growth may be altered by an inadequate delivery of essential nutrients to the body cells.

Malabsorption

Additional delivery problems occur in cases of malabsorption, which may result from inherited disorders, such as cystic fibrosis or celiac disease, or from an acquired condition, for example, intestinal or other infections, parasitic infestation, or trauma. In either event, the inadequate absorption of nutrients interferes with normal metabolism. Malabsorption is possible but unlikely if the child's growth, caloric intake, and stool output are normal.

Gastrointestinal Obstruction

Gastrointestinal obstructions are another cause of delayed growth. Obstructions occurring high in the gastrointestinal tract (i.e., in the duodenum or pylorus) cause vomiting, weight loss, and dehydration; lower intestinal obstructions (i.e., those of the colon) cause abdominal distension and difficulty in passing stools. Both cause growth delays due to nutritional deficiencies. Obstructions may be *complete* or *partial*. Complete obstructions must be corrected quickly or death may ensue, while some partial obstructions produce mild symptoms that are not only compatible with life but may go unrecognized and uncorrected. Common problems of intestinal malabsorption and obstruction and the appropriate nursing care approaches are discussed in Ch. 18.)

Hormonal Deviations

Some hormones have a rhythmic pattern to their secretion; others are secreted in response to blood levels of certain substances. Structural changes inside the glands, malfunctions of the secreting mechanisms, or failure of the body to respond to the hormone may be caused by inherited or acquired factors. Disorders of the endocrine network and subsequent aberrations in hormonal supply and usage are usually evidenced by a decrease or increase in secretion. Since hormonal changes cause alterations in metabolism, growth may be delayed or accelerated. (Specific problems, symptoms and nursing interventions of endocrine hyposecretion and hypersecretion are described in chapter 19.)

ABNORMAL GROWTH: NEOPLASMS

The rate of cell division and duplication is normally regulated by the body's need for cell replacement and repair. Uncontrolled cell division caused by impaired growth-controlling mechanisms may result in a *neoplasm*. The process of rapid, uncontrolled cell division is called the *neoplastic process*; the product, the neoplasm, is commonly called *cancer*. Cancer is not one disease but rather a group of diseases of unknown and probably multiple causes. Cancer can arise in all tissue composed of cells that can divide and proliferate.

A tumor is a mass or swelling; *most cancers are tumors, but not all tumors are cancerous*. Cancers are classified as *benign* or *malignant*. Benign cancers grow slowly, are enclosed in a capsule, and are thus isolated from surrounding normal tissue. Benign cancers are not a health threat unless their location permits undetected growth; for example, in the brain, a growing neoplasm exerts mechanical pressure, which is a major threat. The names of benign tumors are usually recognizable by the suffix *oma* added to the stem of the name of the tissue of origin. For example, fibroma is a benign tumor originating in the fibrous connective tissue.

Malignant neoplasms grow rapidly and are not usually limited by capsules. The suffix *sarcoma* indicates a malignant tumor arising in mesenchymal cells (connective tissue). For example, a lymphosarcoma is a malignant tumor of lymphoid tissue. Malignant tumors of the epithelial tissue frequently have the suffix *carcinoma* added to the name of the affected tissue of origin; thus, an adenocarcinoma is a malignant tumor of the glandular epithelium. Some names of tumors are eponymic (named after a person), for example, Hodgkin's disease.

Metastasis is the shedding of cancerous cells into lymphatic or blood vessels. The cells are then carried throughout the body and are capable of creating additional neoplasms. Because the lymph nodes act as temporary screens by catching and holding cells that break away from the original tumor, a high concentration of malignant cells is often found in lymph nodes. This is why a child with cancer frequently has enlarged lymph nodes.

Neoplasms are *graded* from I to IV according to the degree to which the neoplastic cells differ in organization and structure from normal cells. A grade I indicates minimal differentiation from normal; a grade IV signifies maximal variation. Neoplasms are also classified as belonging to one of four *stages* according to the extent of their growth and spread. Stage I indicates limitation of the neoplasm to the site of origin; Stage IV is widespread metastasis. Neoplasms of the colon are also *typed* as A, B, or C, according to the depth of penetration of the colon.

Neoplasms need nutrients, and they sustain themselves at the expense of normal cells, offering no useful functions in return. The child with cancer experiences pain, anemia, bleeding, and infection. (Common problems, symptoms, and nursing interventions for the child with cancer are discussed in chapter 20.)

SUMMARY

The child grows as body cells, nourished by proteins, fats, and carbohydrates, increase in size and number. Although directed by genetic background, growth is influenced by many forces inside and outside the child's body. Changes in the absorption of nutrients, an obstruction in the digestive tract, or a deficiency or excess of certain hormones affect growth. Alterations within certain cells allow for unrestricted growth and, therefore, for the appearance of neoplasms that demand nutrients at the expense of healthy cells. Stress from outside the body caused by acute or chronic disease, trauma, or parasites demands additional energy, but, because of the decrease in appetite that usually results, essential nutrients are not delivered to body cells, and growth is impeded.

Bibliography

Anderson, L., Dibble, M., Mitchell, H.S., Rynbergen, H.J. *Nutrition in Nursing*. Philadelphia, J.B. Lippincott, Co., 1972.

Anthony, C.P. and Kilthoff, N.S. *Textbook of Anatomy and Physiology*, ed. 9. St. Louis, C.V. Mosby Co., 1975.

Bishop, B.E. (ed.). Nutrition: A Subject Whose Time Has Come. *American Journal Maternal-Child Nursing* 2:85, 1977.

Brower, E.W. and Nash, C.L. Evaluating Growth and Posture in School-Age Children. *Nursing '79* 9:58, 1979.

Crouch, J.D. and McClintic, J.R. *Human Anatomy and Physiology*, ed. 2. New York, John Wiley & Sons, Inc. 1976.

Dansky, K. Assessing Children's Growth. *American Journal of Nursing* '77:1610, 1977

Guyton, A.C. *Textbook of Medical Physiology*, ed. 5. Philadelphia, W.B. Saunders Co., 1976.

Hegsted, M. Dietary Standards. *Journal of American Dietetic Association* 66:13, 1976.

Luke, B. *Case Studies in Therapeutic Nutrition. Boston, Little-Brown and Co., 1977.*

Maclaren, N.K. *Human Growth Hormone. American Journal of Diseases of Children* 127:906, 1974.

Mitchell, H.S., Rynbergen, H.J., Anderson, L., Dibble, M.V. *Nutrition in Health and Disease,* ed. 16. Philadelphia, J.B. Lippincott Co., 1976.

Pipes, P. *Nutrition in Infancy and Childhood.* St. Louis, C.V. Mosby Co., 1977.

Robinson, C.H. and Lowler, M.R. *Normal and Therapeutic Nutrition,* ed. 15. New York, MacMillan Co., 1977.

Scrimshaw, S.N. and Young, V.R. The Requirements of Human Nutrition. *Scientific American* 235:50, 1976.

Smith, D.W. *Growth and Its Disorders.* Philadelphia, W.B. Saunders Co., 1977.

Stare, F.J. and Williams, M. *Living Nutrition.* New York, John Wiley & Sons, Inc., 1977

Vaughan, V.C. and McKay, R.J. (eds.). *Nelson's Textbook of Pediatrics,* ed. 10. Philadelphia, W.B. Saunders Co., 1975.

Willard, K. *The Role of Citrus in Health and Disease.* Gainesville, University of Florida Press, 1976.

Williams, S.R. *Nutrition and Diet Therapy,* ed. 3. St. Louis, C.V. Mosby Co., 1977.

CHAPTER **18**

The Child with a Gastrointestinal Deviation

BEHAVIORAL OBJECTIVES

After studying this chapter you will be able to:

- Distinguish among vomiting, spitting up, regurgitation, rumination, projectile vomiting, and stercoraceous vomiting.
- Describe clinical manifestations of intestinal obstruction in the newborn.
- Plan the nursing care of a child with diarrhea.
- Name the procedures used to diagnose gastrointestinal problems in the child.
- Discuss reasons for gastric intubation in the child, including nursing responsibilities.
- Plan the nursing management of a child undergoing gastrointestinal surgery.
- Discuss nursing responsibilities for the child with each of the following: colostomy, ileostomy, esophagoscopy, and gastrostomy.
- Identify congenital anomalies of the gastrointestinal tract.
- Discuss nutrient deficiencies and dietary management of malabsorption syndromes common in the child.
- Describe infections of the gastrointestinal tract commonly seen in children.

TERMS AND CONCEPTS

Obstruction
Vomiting
Spitting up
Regurgitation
Rumination
Projectile vomiting
Stercoraceous vomiting
Nausea
Anorexia
Diarrhea
Constipation
Abdominal distension
Dehydration
Malabsorption
Noncaloric nutrient deficiencies
Esophagoscopy
Protoscopy
Sigmoidoscopy
Gastric intubation
Gavage feedings
Gastric lavage
Gastrostomy
Colostomy
Ileostomy
Anoplasty

Pyloromyotomy
Orchiopexy

INTRODUCTION

Gastrointestinal anomalies and diseases affect the growth of the child by interfering with his nutritional intake (i.e., the ability to ingest and utilize food), elimination, or both. This chapter discusses problems common to all children with gastrointestinal deviations, and nursing interventions for the alleviation of these problems. Diagnostic and therapeutic procedures are explained along with the nursing responsibilities for each. Specific conditions affecting the gastrointestinal tract, such as congenital anomalies, obstructions, malabsorption syndromes, and infectious processes, are discussed in Table 18–3, at the end of this chapter. Unique nursing management for each condition is offered.

COMMON PROBLEMS, SYMPTOMS, AND NURSING INTERVENTIONS

Obstruction

Obstruction refers to the partial or complete blockage, or the reversal, of normal intestinal flow. Conditions of the gastrointestinal tract that cause obstruction may be congenital or acquired. In either case, evaluation and treatment must not be delayed because vascular supply to the bowel may be compromised rapidly. Congenital conditions are treated as soon after birth as possible, while the newborn is in optimal condition. However, immediate surgery is contraindicated in certain instances (primarily in cases of pneumonia or prematurity, or when the effects of the lesion itself make surgery inadvisable) and is postponed until the infant is stronger.

Vomiting

Vomiting is the forceful ejection of stomach contents, usually accompanied by nausea. Vomiting occurring in the presence of abdominal distension is the classic sign of intestinal obstruction in the newborn and must be reported to the physician promptly. However, vomiting may be caused by a variety of other conditions ranging from benign and self-limiting problems to serious diseases. Irritation of the gastric mucosa caused by drugs and/or allergy to certain foods, increased intracranial pressure, or infection may all produce vomiting. Overdistension of the stomach with air or food is also a common cause of vomiting in infancy. Paroxysms of coughing, particularly in pertussis, may induce vomiting. Vomiting of bile or feces almost always indicates gastrointestinal obstruction. Generally speaking, symptoms of obstructions of the upper gastrointestinal tract are evidenced earlier than are those of lower obstructions.

Spitting up is the ejection of a small amount of milk that may occur immediately after feeding; the ejected matter does not smell sour because it does not reach the stomach before it is spit up. *Regurgitation* is the "overflowing" of a small amount of matter, accompanied by little effort or distress. The regurgitated material smells sour because it has reached the stomach. Regurgitation is usually caused by overfeeding or by the swallowing of excess air. Observe the mother carefully as she feeds her infant, noting the way she holds him, the position of the bottle, length of sucking time, and burping technique.

Each of these factors may contribute to gastric distension. The infant should be cuddled in a semi-upright position to keep any air bubbles in the upper segment of the stomach. For bottle-fed babies, the formula should always fill the neck of the bottle, thus preventing air from entering the stomach. Generally, 30 minutes is allowed for feeding an infant, but the sucking period itself should be limited to about 20 minutes; longer periods of sucking may contribute to regurgitation. Also, the mother of the infant who cries because of discomfort due to a distended stomach may interpret the crying as a sign of hunger, offer more food, and thus contribute to further distension. Encourage the mother to feed her baby at intervals of approximately four hours, and to bubble the baby, holding him upright and over the shoulder, for a few minutes after each feeding. The infant should be placed on his abdomen or right side after eating, although it may be necessary to place him in an infant seat for about an hour if vomiting is a problem. If the mother's feeding technique is ineffective, tactfully suggest the above measures.

Other measures that may help to alleviate regurgitation include using a nipple with a smaller hole, which permits some emptying of the stomach while the infant sucks, increasing the caloric content of the formula, so that less volume is needed to provide the necessary amount of calories, and decreasing carbohydrate intake (an excessive intake of carbohydrates delays emptying time and causes fermentation, which leads to irritation and vomiting).

Rumination is the voluntary regurgitation of stomach contents. It is usually seen in infants between 3 and 6 months of age and is regarded as a psychosomatic condition secondary to a stressful environment characterized by a lack of stimulation and a disturbed mother-child relationship.

Projectile vomiting is the ejection of stomach contents with such force that it travels several feet from the child. It is not usually associated with nausea. It is a symptom of increased intracranial pressure and high intestinal obstruction, such as in congenital hypertrophic pyloric stenosis.

Stercoraceous vomiting is the vomiting of fecal material and indicates a low intestinal obstruction.

The child who vomits may be put on an NPO regimen by the physician. If so, frequent mouth care is given to promote the child's comfort, and mouth care is always given after the child vomits. The infant who is NPO may be permitted to suck a pacifier to help meet his sucking needs, unless a pacifier is contraindicated.

Frequent, small sips of water are offered after the vomiting has subsided. The usual regimen is one tablespoon every fifteen minutes for one hour, then two tablespoons every 30 minutes for the next two hours. If the child tolerates the water, clear liquids are added, also at the rate of two tablespoons every 30 minutes. Fluids should be alternated to avoid electrolyte imbalance; colas, Kool-Aid, ginger ale, Gatorade, Coca-Cola syrup, gelatin water (made by adding twice the required amount of water), and bouillon all have different electrolyte compositions and are generally well tolerated. (See the Skills Manual for the electrolyte compositions of various fluids.) Carbonated beverages should be allowed to "flatten" (by leaving them uncapped) before being offered to the child who vomits. Cold fluids are not offered because they tend to cause muscle spasms that reactivate the vomiting. However, the child may be permitted to suck ice chips, which reduce the sensitivity of the taste buds and will warm before reaching the stomach.

Parents often find it difficult to restrict the child to small sips of liquids when he begs for a drink and seems very dehydrated. Explain that giving large amounts of fluids tends to make the child vomit more readily and that when he vomits, he not only loses the liquid, but valuable stomach contents (gastric juices and electrolytes) as well.

After a day on clear liquids, the child progresses to broth, clear soup, skim milk, crackers, and Jello, if tolerated (Table 18–1). A soft diet is offered on the third day, and, if the day's intake is retained, a regular diet is given on the fourth day.

Always chart accurately the amount, color, and character of the vomitus, as well as the child's activities immediately before vomiting. Did he have a paroxysm of coughing? Did he ingest food or medicine? If so, how long was the interval between the suspected cause and the onset of vomiting? This information is valuable to the physician in determining the cause and treatment of the vomiting. If the child vomits after taking an oral medication, estimate the amount of medication lost (the vomitus will be the color of the medicine) and notify the physician, who may wish to change the method of administration.

Your presence and touch are comforting to the child who is vomiting. Place your hand on his forehead to help brace him as he vomits. A cool washcloth on the forehead is often helpful. Place the child on his side or abdomen after a vomiting episode and stay with him to prevent the aspiration of vomitus. Place an emesis basin and box of tissues within reach of the older child. Offer mouth care after a vomiting episode.

Antispasmodics and antiemetics are often ordered, as are antibiotics, if necessary. Fluid and electrolyte balance is precarious in the vomiting child, and imbalances should be guarded against; Replacement via parenteral fluid is usually ordered. (See ch. 29 for discussion of imbalances and therapies related to vomiting.)

Nausea

Nausea often accompanies anorexia and may precede vomiting. Nausea may be caused by a noxious odor, an offensive sight, drug toxicity, emotional stress, or numerous other factors. Removing the stimulus may suffice; for example, if an unpleasant odor is the cause, increasing ventilation or spraying a disinfectant may help. A small amount of sugar, salt, or ice under the tongue, unless contraindicated, may reduce mild nausea. Diversion is another nursing measure that may alleviate nausea; merely changing the topic of conversation is helpful to some children.

Anorexia

Anorexia, the loss of appetite, is a common occurrence among persons who are ill, frightened, upset, or worried. Fostering adequate nutritional intake in the hospitalized child is an essential nursing intervention.

Learn from the parents which foods the child likes and dislikes. Encourage them to participate in solving the problem of their child's nutritional intake by having them bring favorite foods from home, but do not make them feel as though they are responsible for the child's total dietary intake. Arrange with the dietary department to provide midnight snacks, and see that your unit kitchen is well-stocked with peanut butter and jelly and milk shake ingredients.

In addition to offering foods the child

Table 18–1. **Diet for a Vomiting Patient***

Time	*Check off as Offered*	*Diet*
Every 15 minutes	First dose Second dose Third Dose Fourth dose Fifth dose Skip to ninth dose if vomiting has ceased Seventh dose Eighth dose	1 teaspoon Coca-Cola syrup
Every 15 minutes for two hours	Ninth dose	Sips 1 to 2 teaspoons of cold ginger ale or weak tea
	Tenth dose	Large swallows (1 to 2 tablespoons) of above; add hot bouillon soup
Every 20 minutes for two hours	Eleventh dose	Increase to one-quarter cup clear liquids; may add gelatin, pretzels, crackers, rice, or beef soup.
Every 30 minutes for four hours	Twelfth dose	One half cup clear liquids; also small amounts of boiled rice, finely ground hamburger, and a scant amount of butter to season
Every 30 minutes for 4 hours	Thirteenth dose	Cooked cereals and any soup except cream soups. Toast and jelly. No dairy products, oil, or fried foods.
Next 4 hours	Fourteenth dose	Full puree diet with small amounts of dairy products. Cook and mash all vegetables. No fried foods, oils, fats, or corn.

* A general plan to replace fluids and electrolytes. Offer everything on the diet, but do not force. The plan requires two days. Do not hurry it. Danger signs are high fever, pain, continued vomiting after six hours, no voiding in eight hours, and sleepiness, unless it is bedtime.

likes, other techniques can be used to promote adequate intake. If possible, let the child dine at a small table in the playroom with other children. If he must be confined to his room but can be out of bed, let him eat at a small table in his room, preferably with company (parents or nurse). Remove the plates from the tray to make mealtime seem more homelike. Ask the dietary department to send smaller portions on smaller, less imposing plates. Use juice glasses for liquids because they are small enough for a child to hold comfortably. Place a smiling face, star, or other stick-on on the bottom of the glass. When the glass is emptied, the child will be surprised by the decoration. If you alternate stick-ons, the child can look forward to a new surprise each day. Record the amount eaten and how the child tolerated the diet.

Elimination

Elimination problems accompany intestinal obstruction in infants and children. *Diarrhea,* an increase in the number and fluid content of stools, is a symptom of a variety of conditions, all of which cause intestinal irritation, either directly or indirectly. Viral, bacterial, or parasitic invasion of the gastrointestinal tract, infections of the urinary and respiratory tracts, antibiotic therapy, malnutrition, faulty diet, emotional disturbances, and allergy are all causes of diarrhea in the child. Diarrhea in the young child is serious because of his small extracellular fluid reserve. The increased peristalsis pushes the intestinal contents along so rapidly that there is not adequate time for absorption of fluids. Therefore, fluid loss is increased, and this presents a threat to the infant's relatively unstable water balance (see ch. 29). Dehydration ensues; its typical signs include tachycardia and dry mucous membranes, followed by signs of circulatory insufficiency, such as sunken eyes and fontanelles, pale or gray, cool skin, decreased blood pressure, oliguria with increased specific gravity; lack of skin turgor, and decreased temperature (unless infection is present). Because sodium and potassium are lost, the plasma volume decreases (water is lost with the sodium). Circulatory collapse and renal failure may occur, causing irreversible metabolic acidosis and death. Because the fluid volume deficit may occur rapidly, diarrhea of the infectious type is particularly dangerous; it is often fatal in infants and it can spread quickly through a newborn nursery. For this reason, infants with diarrhea are isolated until the cause of the diarrhea is determined and measures taken to prevent its spread. Assume the diarrhea is infectious until it is proven not to be. Good handwashing is the major precaution against the spread of infectious diarrhea and must be practiced by *all* who are involved with the child's care.

Diarrhea is classified as mild if the body weight loss is less than 5 percent. The child is usually treated at home and is given relatively large amounts of fluids infrequently (every two hours) (Table 18–2). Feedings tend to stimulate the *gastrocolic reflex*, which induces bowel movements when the child is fed; therefore, infrequent feedings are helpful. Lowering the fat content of milk may also be beneficial as is the substitution of glucose and electrolyte solutions for milk or formula feedings. Breast-

Table 18–2. Diet for Diarrhea Patient (if no vomiting is present)

First few hours or first day:
- Kool-Aid
- Very weak tea, slightly sweetened
- Jello water (Jello with two times the regular amount of water)
- Flat ginger ale, 7-Up, or watered-down Coca-Cola with sugar added

If child is hungry and crying for other food, try small amounts of the following, three or four times a day:
- Cream of wheat or rice
- Raw ripe bananas
- Cooked rice
- Boiled skim milk mixed half and half with water
- Dry toast and jelly
- Raw peeled apples
- Applesauce
- Jello
- Strained or junior baby foods are also acceptable for young children

If diarrhea worsens with this diet, discontinue solids and give only clear liquids for another day.

fed babies tend to develop diarrhea less frequently than do bottle-fed infants.

The infant with severe diarrhea loses 5 to 15 percent of his body weight and appears obviously ill. His temperature may range from 39.5° to 40.0°C (103 to 104°F), bowel movements are more frequent (as often as every few minutes), and the stools are expelled with force. They are green, or may contain mucus and blood. The goals of care are to restore fluid and electrolyte balance, establish renal function, and rest the gastrointestinal tract. Fluids are administered parenterally in an effort to meet these goals. Oral fluids are withheld for about 24 hours to rest the gastrointestinal tract and are resumed gradually as the infant demonstrates tolerance. Some physicians advocate giving glucose, water, and electrolytes by mouth as a supplement to the parenteral fluids, which are then administered for a longer period of time. The intravenous line is the child's lifeline and careful nursing care is necessary to maintain it (see ch. 29).

The infant with diarrhea is often seriously ill and demands meticulous nursing care. Good skin care is imperative. Skin breakdown adds to the infant's precarious state because it predisposes him to a secondary infection and the added stress of building new tissue. Bathe him only as necessary. Dry and air the skin folds to prevent the accumulation of excess moisture and microorganisms. Lubricate the skin to prevent cracking, paying special attention to bony prominences. Frequent change of position and the use of sheepskin and/or an eggshell mattress (foam rubber, weight-distributing mattress) helps to alleviate pressure and prevent bedsores.

The perineum is particularly susceptible to breakdown because the digestive enzymes in diarrheal stools irritate the skin. Change soiled diapers immediately. If the skin is not excoriated, wash gently with a mild soap and water and *pat* dry (rubbing may contribute to breakdown). A protective ointment such as zinc oxide is used to protect the skin from the stools. If the skin is excoriated, washing the buttocks may be especially painful. Try using a plastic squirt bottle to squirt a mild soap solution, such as Ivory liquid, on the child's buttocks. Rinse with clean water from a second bottle and gently pat dry. Exposing the area to air or light (from a gooseneck lamp with a 40-watt bulb positioned about 20 to 30 inches above the buttocks for 30 minutes) is helpful. Protective ointments are *not* used on excoriated areas because they hold bacteria in and provide a good culture medium on the wound itself. Take an axillary rather than a rectal temperature.

The child with diarrhea has less resistance to infection. Persons with colds or other illnesses can not be permitted to visit. Explain these factors to the family as you work with them in caring for their child. Encourage their participation in the child's care. Again, the infant who is NPO may use a pacifier to meet his sucking needs. Offer mouth care frequently. Hold and cuddle the child and offer extra age-appropriate stimulation. Remember that the child suffers numerous insults, such as "sticks" for blood studies and IV therapy, as well as restraints, pain, and restricted diet. He needs much love, warmth, and security. Diarrhea is particularly traumatic to the toddler who is learning to control his bowels. Let him know *you* know he is capable of doing that, but that his illness has caused his temporary lack of control.

Teddy, aged two and a half, suffered a three-day bout of diarrhea. He was completely bowel trained when the episode began and was extremely upset because his "stinky" would not "stay in." His nurse told him, "Teddy, I know you are a big boy now and you can go to the potty all by yourself and not mess your pants, but because you are sick your stinky comes out faster and sometimes you can't make it to the potty in time. That is OK. As soon as your tummy is better, your stinky will slow down, and you won't mess your pants anymore because you are a big boy." Teddy smiled and said, "Yes, I am big."

It is important to keep an accurate record of the child's intake and output. Because of the frequent liquid stools, it may be necessary to apply a urine-collection bag to the infant in order to separate urine and feces for more accurate measurement. The urine is usually scanty because of dehydration, and the specific gravity is high. Chart the amount, character, color, odor, and consistency of the stools, as well as the presence of mucus or blood (see Table 18–3). If a stool specimen is needed, place a piece of cellophane on the diaper; after the child defecates, transfer the stool to a specimen container, label it, and send it to the laboratory (See the Skills Manual).

Constipation, the irregular defecation of abnormally solid stools that are difficult to pass, may occur in a person of any age. A child may normally defecate once a day or once every three days, but as long as the stool is not hard and there is no difficulty in passing it, the child is not considered constipated. When taking the history, have the mother describe the child's stools in her own words. She may not understand that it can be normal to have a bowel movement less than once a day. Many people think that harmful substances are absorbed from the unpassed feces, and the child of such a family may be given enemas or home remedies to facilitate the passage of stools at least once a day.

When the child experiences real constipation, the pain associated with defecation may cause him to repress the urge to defecate next time. Feces accumulate in the rectum, the capacity of the rectum increases, and the urge to defecate is gradually diminished. Peristaltic contractions also become less powerful and cannot evacuate the feces. More water than usual is absorbed from the accumulated feces, and they become hard and dry. When the rectum is filled to its capacity, the child may have diarrhea or encopresis (the involuntary release of stool). Abdominal cramping may also occur.

Table 18–3. **Color and Character of Stools**

Probable Cause	*Color and Character*
Breast milk	Pale yellow, often green; large number of light yellow particles; pasty to loose consistency. Slightly sour, not unpleasant odor. Two to four per day.
Cow's milk	Paler, firmer, and smoother in consistency than stool of breast-fed infant. More unpleasant odor.
Drugs	
Iron	Dark brown or black
Achromycin	Reddish cast
Foods	
Beets, tomatoes	Red
Beans, spinach	Green
Cereal	Brown
Diarrhea	Green
Increased sugar	Loose, not greenish
Blood–digested	
High	Reddish brown or black
Low	Bright red (large amounts after intussusception)

Constipation may be caused by faulty eating habits, such as a lack of bulk in the diet, insufficient amounts of food to form fecal bulk, and a lack of fluids that causes the body to extract more liquid from the stools to meet its metabolic needs. Emotional disturbances may also result in constipation, but, in such cases, the treatment of the underlying emotional cause, although important in the long run, will *not* correct the physical problem of constipation. Finally, pathologic problems such as congenital aganglionic megacolon (Hirschsprung's disease) also cause constipation. A rectal examination will reveal hard stool in the rectum if constipation is present; however, no stool is usually palpated if the child has Hirschprung's disease.

Nursing management of the child who is constipated centers around improving his bowel habits. This process is often lengthier than toilet training because the child not only must learn new habits but must unlearn old ones.

Softening of the stool may be accomplished with the use of suppositories and small enemas until a new defecation routine is established. Stool softeners are administered orally, and the child is encouraged to defecate at the same time each day. The child, especially the preschooler and adolescent, sees the administration of enemas and suppositories as an intrusion. Always explain the necessity for the procedure, what you are going to do, and what you expect the child to do. Allow him to maintain his privacy as much as possible. Be calm, be gentle, and do not force the procedure on him. Ask someone to help you during the procedure to assure that he is properly restrained. Remember that physical restraints should be used only as a last resort. Gently helping the child to hold still and offering words of comfort and encouragement are frequently all that is necessary. (See the Skills Manual).

The physician will determine the type and amount of enema solution. Isotonic saline is most often used. Tap water enemas are never used because of the danger of water intoxication (see ch. 29). After administering the suppository or enema, hold the child's buttocks together firmly until the initial reflex urge to expel has passed, and encourage him to retain the medication for a short period.

If the child is to have enemas at home, show the parents the proper technique, and stress the importance of *not* using tap water. Saline enemas are available in prepared form, or they can be made by adding one teaspoon of noniodized salt to one pint of water. Remember to reinforce the instructions and make sure of the parents' understanding by having them repeat your instructions to you.

Abdominal distension is frequently seen in gastrointestinal anomalies and diseases. As stated earlier, it is a classic sign of intestinal obstruction in the newborn, when it is accompanied by vomiting. Abdominal distension may also be caused by excessive food or air intake.

The nurse's responsibility begins with recognizing distension, determining if vomiting is also present, and reporting these findings. If overfeeding or improper burping seems to be creating the problem, offer suggestions to the mother to correct the situation. Concentrating the formula (to more than the usual 20 calories per ounce) provides the needed nutrients without the volume; and burping after every one to four ounces, depending on the child's age, reduces the amount of air in the stomach.

Also, point out that crying causes the child to swallow air, as does thumb- or finger-sucking. If the baby cries excessively, burping him may help. A nasogastric or gastrostomy tube may be inserted into the stomach to relieve distension, especially if the child has gastrointestinal anomalies. Rectal tubes are not routinely used in children.

Dehydration

Dehydration is seen frequently in cases of gastrointestinal obstructions and diseases and is especially serious in the young infant. The infant's body surface area is greater in proportion to weight than that of the older child and adult; therefore, he has more skin, through which he loses a greater amount of fluid.

Fever increases the body's metabolic needs, and at the same time greatly increases water loss, and therefore depletes the body's stores of water and leads to dehydration. In diarrhea, the peripheral vessels constrict to conserve blood volume (thus decreasing the amount of insensible loss and sweat); this prevents the elimination of heat through the peripheral vessels, and unless the body fluid volume is restored, fever may result, or increase. Thus it is possible for a dehydration ⟷ fever cycle to develop (Figure 18–1).

Different types of dehydration, therapy, and nursing management are discussed in chapter 29. Strict intake and output records are kept, as well as a daily weight record. Fluids are offered frequently. Remember that water and clear liquids are easiest to digest, but offer the child his choice of liquids unless this is contraindicated by vomiting or diarrhea.

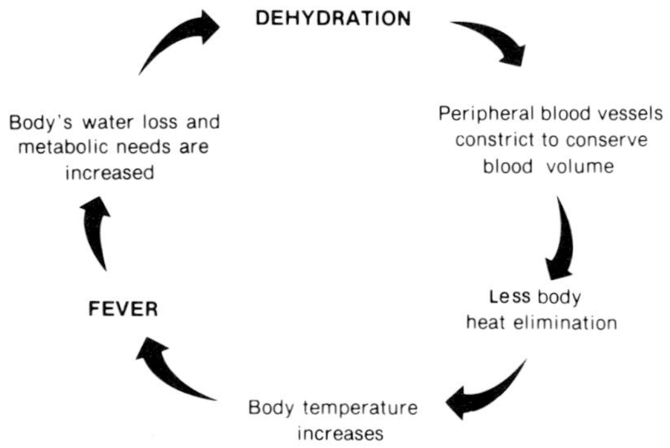

Figure 18–1. *The dehydration* ⟷ fever cycle.

Nutrient Deficiences

Nutrient deficiencies are commonly seen in cases of malformations and diseases of the gastrointestinal tract. Lack of proper intake (due to underfeeding, anorexia, NPO and so on) and faulty absorption of nutrients are among the causes of nutrient deficiencies. Failure to gain weight is often the first sign of a nutrient deficiency in the child. Typically, these infants or children will reach a plateau in weight gain, level off, and then lose weight. If treatment does not halt this progression, wasting of body tissues follows. The infant's sucking (fat) pads in the cheeks are the last to waste away, thus he may still be able to suck (and therefore survive) if nourishment is offered.

The severe syndromes of undernutrition are known as edematous and nonedematous protein-calorie malnutrition (PCM). Edematous PCM, or *kwashiorkor*, occurs when protein has been lacking in the diet for a long period of time. Nonedematous PCM, or *marasmus*, occurs when the child has had insufficient caloric intake, and is starved.

The child with kwashiorkor may have an adequate carbohydrate intake but lacks the necessary protein, as frequently occurs in underdeveloped countries where the staples are incomplete protein foods. Typically, the child is weaned from breast milk, which provides sufficient calories and protein, when his mother first discovers she is newly pregnant. The characteristic clinical findings are edema, wasting, irritability or apathy, poor muscle tone, silky hair that is unusually light in color, and skin lesions.

The malnourished child is in all cases a prime candidate for infection, particularly of the gastrointestinal tract. Antibiotics are not used prophylactically, but are prescribed as necessary when an infection has been positively diagnosed.

Proper feeding techniques are important in caring for the child who is losing or who has lost weight. Treatment is aimed at providing adequate nourishment as well as correcting the underlying cause. The physician will order intravenous and oral feedings as appropriate for the child's condition. A well-balanced diet for age, including extra nutrients of the type the child is lacking, is an important part of therapy. However, merely presenting the child with an adequate diet will not ensure that he will eat it. The nurse often must be innovative in getting the child to eat, as she must for the anorectic child. In addition, the weak and apathetic child who suffers from lack of nutrients presents a special problem. Frequently, intravenous fluids or total parenteral nutrition is necessary. Permit the child enough time to eat and ensure that mealtimes are pleasant.

Daily weights are necessary to help assess the child's response to nutritional therapy. Weigh the child at the same time each day and on the same scale. He should be naked or dressed in the same amount of clothes each time.

Skin care is important for the child with wasting of body tissues because the skin covering the bony prominences tends to break down. In addition, if the child is too weak to change position, the back of the head and heels may also become excoriated because of the constant pressure of lying down. Turning the child every hour is a necessity that will also help prevent pneumonia. Gently massage every area that is subjected to pressure with lotion after turning him. The edema that is present in some types of malnutrition is an excellent culture medium for bacteria and is another reason why skin care is important.

Secondary deficiencies, or *noncaloric nutrient deficiencies,* occur in association with other types of undernourishment. Either there is a lack of intake or, in the malabsorption syndromes, the child is not able to utilize the nutrients. The fat-soluble vitamins A, D, E, and K are stored in the body tissues. Along with Vitamin C, these vitamins are the most frequently deficient in diets in the United States. The child with fat malabsorption is given double doses of the fat-soluble vitamins to compensate for the increased loss in the stools. (See Table 17–3 for a summary of vitamin deficiencies.)

COMMON DIAGNOSTIC STUDIES

Good history taking is imperative in the diagnostic process. Ask the mother questions that will enable you to recognize characteristic symptoms. For example, for the infant with possible pyloric stenosis, ask: "How long has he been vomiting?" ("Three days") "When does he vomit?" ("Immediately after feedings") "Can you describe what happens when he vomits?"

("He just vomits his feeding. It is white and every time he vomits it is more forceful") "Is he sick in any other way?" ("No. He is even hungry right after he vomits and will take more feeding, but he vomits that too.")

Physical Examination

The physical examination will yield information important to the diagnosis of intestinal obstruction or malabsorption syndromes. The typical picture of dehydration with wasting is common. Of course, each defect, disease, or nutrient deficit will yield different clinical findings. For example, in intussusception, a sausage-shaped mass can be palpated in the abdomen; rebound tenderness is exhibited in appendicitis (pushing and releasing the right lower quadrant of the abdomen causes abdominal contents to shift and results in acute pain when the appendix moves); and an olive-shaped mass is palpable in pyloric stenosis.

Stay with the child during the examination, comforting him with an explanation of what is happening (age permitting), soothing words, and physical contact. Should restraint be necessary (as for a rectal exam), secure the child gently but firmly and continue to offer verbal support throughout the procedure.

X-Rays

X-ray studies are commonly ordered to aid in the diagnosis of obstructions of the gastrointestinal tract. In the diagnosis of esophageal atresia and trachoesophageal fistula (See Specific Conditions), a stiff rediopague 10–14 French catheter is passed through the nose toward the stomach. If resistance is met 9 to 13 cm from the nares, a diagnosis of esophageal atresia is made. A simple upright chest x-ray will then be taken to show the level of obstruction (the tubing will double back on itself, creating a U-shape), as well as the contour of the heart and gross vertebral defects; air in the stomach indicates a fistula between the esophagus and trachea. Abdominal x-rays will show the patency of the bowel and the distance between the rectal pouch and rectal sphincter in cases of imperforate anus; the infant is held upside down for a few minutes during this procedure (a Wangensteen-Rice or "upside-down" x-ray) to permit air to rise to the distal portion of the colon, thus outlining the rectum on x-ray. Barium is used to diagnose pyloric stenosis; the ingested barium will not pass readily through the narrowed pyloric lumen, resulting in a "string-like" appearance on x-ray, which is characteristic. Barium enemas are used in the diagnosis of Hirschsprung's disease (to outline the narrowed, nerveless portion and the proximal distended portion of the colon) and ulcerative colitis.

Biopsy

A rectal biopsy may be needed to aid in the diagnosis of Hirschsprung's disease, celiac disease, and others. In Hirschsprung's disease, a rectal biopsy will show the absence of ganglion cells. Biopsy of the large intestine may be obtained via simple suction biopsy to avoid general anesthesia in the very sick infant. Or, if a rectal biopsy is needed, general anesthesia is used and a section of muscle is taken with biopsy forceps. In suspected celiac disease, a nasogastric catheter may be passed and a suction biopsy performed. The child will be unable to swallow for a few hours after the biopsy. Place him on his abdomen or side, suction as necessary, and observe carefully for signs of respiratory distress.

Blood Studies

An evaluation of serum electrolytes and blood gases, in addition to routine laboratory procedures, are ordered for the child who suffers from dehydration. These studies show the state of the child's fluid and electrolyte balance as well as his acid-base balance.

Regardless of the diagnostic procedure employed, the parents (and the child, if he is not an infant) need explanations and support. Explain what will happen before, during, and after the procedure, as well as whether or not the child is likely to feel any pain. Many hospitals permit the parents to accompany the child to the x-ray room, or to carry the infant in their arms. If this is permissible, go with them and offer your support. Their involvement is healthy both for them and for the child and should be encouraged.

Endoscopy

Esophagoscopy is used in both diagnosis and treatment. In the child, it is most often used after surgery or lye ingestion to determine the extent of scarring and the presence of stenosis in the esophagus. The procedure is done under general anesthesia, and a normal diet is resumed after recovery.

Proctoscopy and *sigmoidoscopy* are used to visualize the bowel when Hirschsprung's disease, rectal polyps, or ulcerative colitis are suspected. Illuminated hollow tubes are used in these procedures. A flexible sigmoidoscope is used for viewing beyond the rectum. Biopsy and excision of rectal polyps can be done during this procedure. Anesthesia is seldom necessary, but clear and careful explanation of the procedure is imperative. The child should be made as comfortable as possible in whatever position is necessary (knee-chest or supine with knees abducted), and every effort to soothe and comfort him during the procedure should be made. Hold his hand, stand where he can see your face, and talk to him. Tell him that the discomfort will cease as soon as the procedure is over.

COMMON TREATMENTS

Therapeutic Nutrition

Therapeutic nutrition is employed in the treatment of nutrient deficiencies, whether due to obstruction, malabsorption, or inadequate intake.

Special Diets

Special diets are necessary for the child with a nutrient deficiency. For example, the child with Vitamin A deficiency will be offered foods high in Vitamin A, such as liver, carrots, and milk. The child with celiac disease will be restricted to a gluten-free diet for his lifetime. The child who is unable to absorb fats will have to ingest extra quantities of the fat-soluble vitamins (to compensate for the increased loss) or receive them in a water-soluble form. Constipation is another problem that requires a special diet, specifically, one that is high in roughage.

Engage the help of the dietician in preparing the child and his family for his special diet. Explain to the child in simple terms why the diet is necessary, which foods are permissible and which are not, and what to expect if the diet is not adhered to. If the child is to have some control over his diet and his health problem, he must know which foods are not permissible.

Barry, aged three, has celiac disease. He was offered a hot dog on a bun at a cookout. Knowing that bread and hot dogs that are not made entirely of meat give him abdominal cramps and diarrhea, Barry declined the hot dog. He went to find his mother to ask if "that's the kind of hot dog that's OK for me to eat."

Gastric Intubation

Gastric intubation may be necessary to obtain gastric secretions for diagnosis, to decompress the stomach before and after surgery, and to instill feedings or medication (See the Skills Manual for instructions on the insertion and management of nasogastric tubes). Preoperatively, decompression prevents vomiting and makes the intestines easier to handle during surgery. Postoperatively, the lack of peristalsis allows the swallowed air and gastric secretions to distend the stomach; this places tension on suture lines and on the diaphragm. Maintaining a patent tube is mandatory; if the tube is blocked, vomiting and aspiration may result. Levine (single lumen) tubes are used for medications and feedings; Salem-Sump (double lumen) tubes are used for suctioning and decompression. The smaller lumen (vent, or air, lumen) runs inside the larger lumen (drainage lumen) and provides a continuous airflow that controls the amount of suction at the gastric mucosa (See The Skills Manual). The physician will order a specific amount of irrigant to be administered. Irrigate the tubing, observe the child's reaction, note the contents returned, and chart your observations. The irrigating fluid is considered intake, and unless the exact amount is immediately aspirated, the irrigating fluid is charted on the intake/output record as intake. The child with nasogastric intubation is always on intake and output (I&O). If the nasogastric tube is used for decompression, it is left in place until gastrointestinal function returns, which is indicated by the passage of stools and flatus and by decreasing returns from the tube. After bowel sounds are heard, the tube is removed and small amounts of fluids are offered orally. If the tube is to be indwelling (either for gavage or decompression), change it every 48 to 72 hours, alternating nares. Frequent oral hygiene is necessary while the tube is in place. If intermittent feedings are desired, the tube is removed after each feeding.

Gavage feedings are used for the infant who is too weak to suck or too sick to tolerate oral feedings. Infants with gastrointestinal disorders, cardiac anomalies, and respiratory distress may require tube feedings, as may the child with burns or malnutrition. If possible, hold the child while administering the feeding, and permit him to suck on a pacifier; this helps him to retain the satisfaction that he associates with bottle feedings. If the infant cannot be held, place him on his right side or back, with his head and chest slightly elevated. Feedings must be administered slowly and must never be forced because forcing causes abdominal distension and regurgitation.

Gastric lavage may be necessary to decompress the stomach before or after surgery, to obtain gastric contents for diagnostic studies, or to remove ingested poisons.

Gastrostomy feedings may be necessary after gastrointestinal surgery to permit healing of the operative side. The gastrostomy tube is inserted surgically into the stomach through the abdominal wall and is held in place by purse-string sutures or tape. No dressing is used on the incision site, but zinc oxide, petroleum, or karaya gum powder or a heat lamp may be used to help prevent skin breakdown. The tubing is attached to a syringe for feedings and is elevated 10 to 12 centimeters (4 to 4¾ inches). The formula is instilled by gravity and is *never* forced. The infant is encouraged to suck a pacifier during the feeding in order to fulfill his sucking need, to relax him, and to permit him to equate the sucking with the relief of hunger. After feedings, the tubing is *not* clamped. It is elevated as for the feeding and covered with a sterile gauze square that acts as a safety and overflow valve should the infant vomit. It also allows air introduced during the feeding to bubble out and prevents gastric distension.

Total parenteral nutrition (TPN, or hyperalimentation) is used to supply protein and calories for the child who cannot be maintained otherwise. Ch. 29 includes a full discussion of TPN and the nurse's responsibilities in the care of the child.

SURGICAL INTERVENTION

A number of conditions affecting the growth of the child are incompatible with life and require surgical intervention. In general, the condition is repaired as soon as it is diagnosed; this lessens the child's chance of becoming dehydrated, malnourished, or emaciated, and improves his chances for successful surgery and recovery. Also, the better his overall physical condition, the less likely he is to contract an infection, which would complicate the pre- and postoperative course and increase the risk inherent in surgical intervention. Interference with intake and elimination caused by congenital anomalies or surgical procedures may have serious psychological consequences for the child. All surgery on the gastrointestinal tract will involve some degree of restriction of oral intake and may affect bowel function and elimination.

Surgical Procedures

A *cervical esophagostomy* is done in cases of esophageal atresia, in which the esophagus dead-ends in a blind pouch. The lower (pouch) end of the esophagus is externalized on the left side at the base of the neck, allowing oro- and nasopharyngeal secretions to drain to the outside. This procedure is performed when the infant is not in condition to withstand definitive surgery.

Immediately after surgery, a catheter is placed in the esophageal opening (stoma) for a few days to permit drainage. After the catheter is removed, a soft piece of absorbent material is placed over the stoma to absorb secretions. Because saliva is not irritating, excoriation does not occur if good care is given to the surrounding skin and the absorbent material is changed regularly. A thin layer of zinc oxide or petroleum jelly may be used to protect the skin.

The infant is fed via a gastrostomy. In addition to the pacifier given during gastrostomy feedings, the child is "fed" glucose water or formula (which drains out through the stoma) to accustom him to the hunger-suck-swallow-relief of hunger cycle. If this is not done, he will have to relearn to eat, a lengthy process at best.

Thoractomy tubes (for chest drainage) are used when the thoracic cavity has been entered during surgery. Nursing management for the child with chest drainage is discussed in Ch. 22.

An *ostomy* is the surgical creation of an opening. It is usually temporary, permitting definitive surgery at a later date when the child has grown and may be better able to tolerate the often complex procedures involved in corrective surgery. The type of ostomy created depends on the type of defect or intestinal condition.

A *colostomy* is an opening on the abdomen for the evacuation of feces. It may have a single *stoma*, or opening, such as when the sigmoid colon is involved, or it may be double-barreled, or looped, as when the transverse colon is opened. A sigmoid colostomy with a single stoma is usually permanent. A transverse colostomy (double barreled or loop) is used in the correction of Hirschsprung's disease, rectal atresia, and imperforate anus. The proximal portion is the drainage fistula, and the distal portion is the mucus fistula.

An *ileostomy* is an opening into the ileum (the distal portion of the small intestine). Often used in the treatment of ulcerative colitis, it is also used for the neonate with necrotizing enterocolitis, meconium ileus, and Hirschsprung's disase. Drainage from an ileostomy is typically more fluid than drainage from a colostomy.

The obvious difference between an adult and infant stoma is the size of the stoma itself and of the surrounding abdominal area. Some infants as small as 1.1 kilograms (2.5 pounds) may have a colostomy; obviously a standard appliance will not fit such a small area.

Until the operative incision has healed, great care must be taken to avoid contamination. A dry sterile dressing is placed over the operative site while the stoma itself is left uncovered at least until peristalsis returns, and the child begins passing stools (about 24 hours). Never place one large dressing over both the incision and the stoma. Antibiotic therapy and daily wound cultures are initiated when wound contamination is suspected. Restraining the child is necessary to prevent him from kicking or bumping the fresh stoma, which will bleed easily.

Irrigations, which help regulate the bowel movement, are not routinely used for the infant or small child with a colostomy. Dilations may be necessary however, to check for bowel stenosis, to widen the stomal lumen, and to encourage the passage of stool. The first few dilations are performed by the surgeon because of the danger of possible perforation of the bowel and excessive trauma to the stoma. Care must be taken to prevent crusting of the stoma caused by excessive drainage. Saline soaks alternated with gauze saturated with petroleum jelly, which is changed when soiled, may be used to help keep the stoma soft.

Skin care to prevent excoriation around the stoma consists of keeping the skin clean and dry. Until the stoma is functioning, no dressing is necessary, but inspection of the site for signs of irritation or inflammation is a necessity. After about 24 hours, peristalsis returns, and the child begins to pass stools through the stoma. The zinc oxide and tissue paper technique is most effective in protecting the skin around the stoma from drainage (see the Skills Manual). It has the advantage of being absorbent and non-irritating and can be adapted as the infant grows by varying the size of the tissue square and adding extra layers of tissue as needed for absorbency. The tissue dressing can be used until the child can be fitted with a pediatric stoma bag. In addition, this technique is simple and can be learned easily by parents. Excessive diarrhea or liquid stools contribute to skin breakdown. Exposing the area to air and a heat lamp every four to six hours is beneficial but often not possible because of the frequency of bowel movements.

When using a collecting appliance, make a tight seal around the stoma to prevent leakage onto the skin. Apply a diaper to help hold the collection bag in place. Change the bag every 24 hours at bath time if it is secure, and no leakage is noted. Weigh the infant while the bag is removed to obtain an accurate weight.

Careful explanation to the parents (and to the child if he is old enough) is necessary before surgery. Reiterate the physician's explanation of why the ostomy is necessary, and what can be expected after surgery. Assure the parents that they will be taught how to care for the child. After surgery they may be hesitant to touch or hold the child for fear of hurting him. Encourage them to gradually begin to care for him; they may begin simply by offering their hand for him to grasp, and graduate to holding and feeding him. They will need support as they try to accept the change in his body and learn to tolerate and then care for his ostomy. Assess their readiness to learn by observing their verbal and nonverbal responses during a regular ostomy dressing change. Explain in simple terms what you are doing. Re-explain during the next dressing change, gradually including the theory behind each step. Permit them to help fold tissue or apply the zinc oxide. Gradually, as they gain confidence, they will be able to perform the entire procedure.

The child with an ostomy, particularly an ileostomy, requires dietary instruction. Low residue foods—lean meats, liver, hard boiled eggs, rice, cottage cheese, cooked cereals, gelatins, simple sugars, clear soups, orange juice, and some cooked vegetables—are most easily tolerated. Highly seasoned or spicy foods are usually avoided, as are cabbage, onions, turnips, whole kernel corn, nuts, coconut, raisins, and berries with seeds; these foods are more likely to cause diarrhea or the formation of gas.

SPECIFIC CONDITIONS

Cleft Lip and Palate

Cleft lip and cleft palate, common congenital anomalies occuring in 1 out of every 800 births, result from incomplete fusion of the maxillary and premaxillary processes and/or palatal processes in intrauterine life (see Figures 18–2 and 18–3). These defects may occur together or as separate entities. Cleft lip is more common in males; cleft palate is seen twice as often in girls than boys. About 25 percent of the cases suggest familial tendencies. The cleft lip may appear as a simple notch in the lip or may extend to the nose, causing the naris to be flattened. Cleft palate may affect only the soft palate or it may involve the hard palate, nose, and alveolar ridge. Clefts may be unilateral or bilateral.

Initial nursing management is directed towards the parents. The birth of a less-than-perfect baby is always a shock to the parents, who must then grieve for the beautiful baby they dreamed of and lost. An obvious defect of the face is often more shattering than is the news of a more serious but unobservable defect. Parents feel a tremendous amount of guilt and wonder what they did to cause such a tragedy. It is hard for them to accept the fact that they have "created" this imperfect infant. They

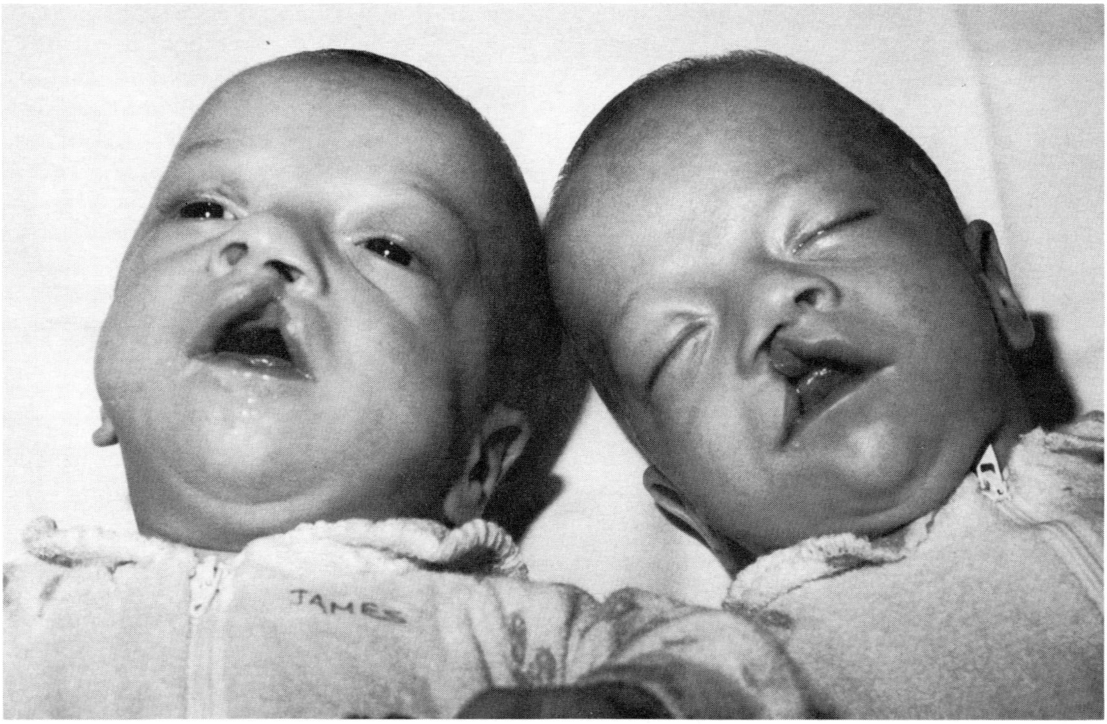

Figure 18–2. *Unilateral cleft lip in twin boys.*

may have trouble accepting the baby and will be ashamed for family and friends to see him. Understanding and reassurance are imperative in working with the family; allow them to express their feelings, to question, to cry, to be angry. Be present when the physician discusses the steps necessary for correcting the defect and the long-term care. Leave them alone for a while to assimilate the information, and return a short time later to answer questions and to reiterate what the physician has told them.

An interdisciplinary cleft palate team routinely cares for the child. Because of the usual involvement of the upper gum and teeth, and problems with hearing and speech, the orthodontist, otolaryngologist, speech therapist, and audiologist are needed in addition to the pediatrician, plastic surgeon, and nurse. Treatment and prognosis depend on many factors, among them the skill of the surgeon, the quality of nursing care, and most importantly, the extent of the defect.

Cosmetic repair of the lip is done early to alleviate some of the problems parents are faced with in showing and caring for their new baby. Many parents find it difficult to show the baby to relatives and friends, who may be shocked at the child's appearance and are unable to offer the usual compliments. The parents themselves may have difficulty in cuddling and caring for their

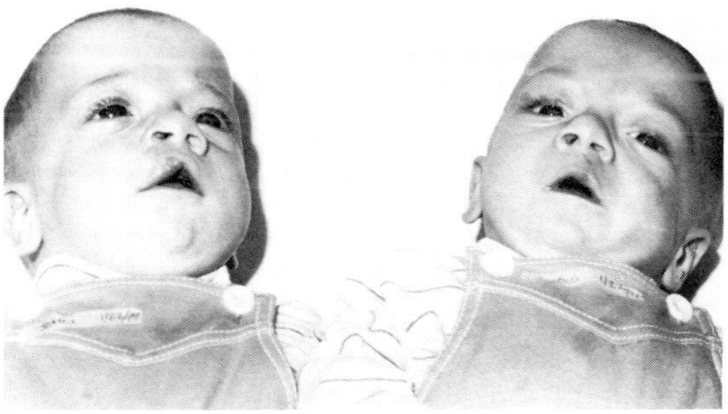

Figure 18–3. *The twins pictured in Figure 18–2* are shown here after surgery.

baby. Some surgeons repair the lip in the first 48 hours in full-term healthy infants. Others follow the "rule of tens," waiting until the baby weighs 10 lb., is 10 weeks old, and has 10 grams of hemoglobin.

Cleft palate repair is done between twelve and eighteen months of age, to allow for optimal growth of the palatal processes, and to alleviate the problem before the child's speech patterns develop. Earlier repair may damage teeth buds.

The child with a cleft lip and an intact palate does not usually require special feeding devices because his tongue pushes the nipple against his palate to create suction. The child with a cleft palate is not able to form this vacuum and has difficulty with feedings. Several devices may be employed to assist the child in taking formula. A long, soft lamb's nipple, a "premie" nipple with an enlarged hole that allows the formula to drop out when the bottle is inverted (but not so fast that it chokes the baby), or a Beneflex nurser are all effective. Also, a commercial baby bottle that utilizes a plastic bag to contain the formula may be used. Simply enlarge the hole on one side of the hard plastic bottle and compress the bag with your index finger to express the milk (see the Skills Manual). Instruct the mother to hold the baby nearly upright and to feed him slowly and burp him often because he swallows a lot of air. Explain that the formula is likely to return through the nose (hence the upright position) and teach her to watch for respiratory distress. Permit her to take full responsibility for the child's care for two or three days before discharge; this will give her time to adjust to the demanding feeding regimen while the nurse is available to help or take over.

If the child with a cleft palate begins to speak before the palate is repaired, the parents should encourage good speech habits by speaking slowly and clearly to the child. *Never* mimic or make fun of the gutteral sounds he makes.

Prior to surgery for repair of the lip or palate, the child is accustomed to the restraints and feeding methods that will be necessary postoperatively. After repair of the lip, the infant will be restrained on his back for several days to keep him from lying on the suture line or touching it with his hands. Placing him in an infant seat and moving him to the site of activities will provide variety. He will not be permitted to suck in order to avoid putting stress on the suture line. Feed him with a 10 cc syringe attached to a short length of feeding tube. Position the tubing to the back and side of his mouth, being careful not to touch the suture line: (See Skills Manual). Do *not* let him suck. This method of feeding is slow and frustrating to the hungry infant who wants to suck. He tires easily and swallows an excessive amount of air. Burp him frequently and cuddle him during the feeding. If the child is allowed to feed this way before surgery, he will be somewhat accustomed to it and feeding will be easier after surgery. Similarly, the older child must be able to drink from a cup before surgery. He must be reminded both verbally and with the aid of restraints not to put his hands (or toys) in his mouth. After feedings, rinse the child's mouth with small amounts of clean water to cleanse the suture line.

Care must be taken to keep the suture lines clean and free from tension. A Logan bar is used over the lip repair to prevent tension on the suture line. Anticipate the child's needs and give him plenty of TLC and cuddling to keep him from crying postoperatively. It may help to place him in the center of activity and give a mild analgesic for pain. Cleanse the suture line gently with applicators soaked in hydrogen peroxide to prevent crusting of dried blood and secretions, which leads to scar formation. Some surgeons prefer to use a topical antiobiotic ointment to prevent crusting and local stitch sepsis. Take care not to place stress on the suture line while cleaning it (see the Skills Manual).

Because the child with a cleft lip is a mouth breather, he will need frequent mouth care preoperatively, and he may find breathing difficult after repair of the cleft. A mist tent helps to alleviate respiratory problems. Gently suction the child's nose and mouth with a soft catheter to remove blood, mucus, and saliva. Observe for signs of respiratory distress and hemorrhage.

Tonsillitis, adenoiditis, and otitis media frequently accompany cleft palate. Care should be taken to recognize and treat these infections early to prevent complications resulting from them.

Because of the danger of hemorrhage after surgical repair of the palate, bleeding and clotting times are determined preoperatively. Some oozing is to be expected; turn the child on his side to permit the blood to drain out. Do not suction because this may cause more bleeding. Keep the child in a humidified environment (by using a tent, mask, or humidifier) for several days to help liquify the secretions.

Fluids are given orally several hours after surgery. The child is not permitted to put *anything* in his mouth; feed him with the side of a spoon or a cup. As with the child who has had a cleft lip repair, straws are forbidden and the child must be reminded verbally, and with the aid of restraints, not to put his hands or toys in his mouth. Rinse after feedings of other than clear liquids with clean water to cleanse the suture line. Swallowing is painful and the child may drool. Offer a mild analgesic to alleviate pain. If a gauze pack has been used to help control bleeding, the surgeon will probably remove it three days postoperatively.

The child with a cleft palate must undergo several hospitalizations for repair of the defect and will have outpatient dental and orthodontic treatment for many years. The cleft palate team coordinates therapies in order to provide the best possible care.

Esophageal Atresia

Esophageal atresia (EA) and *tracheoesophageal fistula* (TEF) occur (very often together) in about 1 in 2,500 births and are among the most common congenital anomalies that cause respiratory distress and/or death. Heredity is not believed to be a factor in these defects; a systemic insult to the embryo is thought to be the cause. Esophageal atresia with or without fistula commonly occurs in association with other defects, especially those involving the cardiac, genitourinary, and vertebral systems, as well as defects of the lower gastrointestinal tract such as duodenal atresia and imperforate anus. Other visible anomalies are seen in 50 percent of the cases and 35 percent are premature. Maternal hydramnios (an excess of amniotic fluid) is very frequently associated with high obstructive gastrointestinal lesions, which prevent effective fetal swallowing and absorption of amniotic fluid. Hydramnios is a factor in 85 percent of infants with esophageal atresia. It may be a precipitating factor in premature delivery.

The three types most often seen are shown in Figure 18–4. Type A, esophageal atresia (complete obstruction) with distal tracheosophageal fistula, accounts for about 87 percent of cases. Early symptoms, caused by the atresia, are drooling and hypersalivation. Swallowed secretions that cannot pass to the stomach accumulate in the blind pouch from where they constantly bubble over from the nose and mouth. Saliva is aspirated, and the respirations sound coarse. Diagnosis can be made within the first few hours of life if physicians and nurses are alert to these early signs. Air enters the stomach through the fistula, distending it, and gastric juices flow backward up the fistula from the stomach to the trachea, compounding the risk of penumonia.

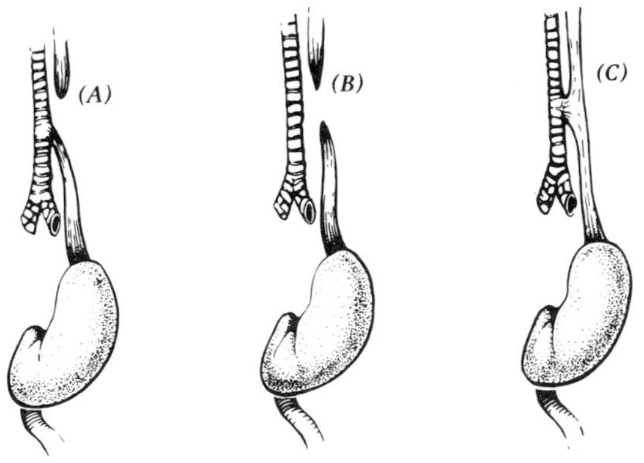

Figure 18–4. *(A) Tracheoesophageal fistula with atresia. The esophagus ends in a blind pouch, and the trachea connects to the lower esophagus and stomach via a fistula. This is the most common type of esophageal anomaly, occurring in 87 percent of cases. (B) Esophageal atresia without fistula. Both upper and lower ends of the esophagus end in blind pouches. (C) Tracheoesophageal fistula without atresia (H-type). The trachea and esophagus connect via a fistula.*

Type B, isolated EA without fistula, is characterized by excess saliva bubbling over into the child's mouth and nose, as in type A. Because there is no fistula with the trachea, no air enters the stomach; the abdomen is therefore not distended, and there is no danger of reflux of gastric juices into the trachea. Pneumonia can arise from a spillover of secretions and feedings from the blind pouch of the esophagus into the upper end of the trachea.

Type C, tracheosophageal fistula without atresia, is more difficult to diagnose because the symptoms are not as clear. Classic symptoms are coughing and choking during feedings and recurrent bouts of pneumonia.

Division of the fistula and direct suturing of the esophagus is the ideal treatment for TEF with atresia (Type A) and is employed if the infant is full-term and has no other serious anomalies, and if the two ends of the esophagus are close together. The survival rate in such cases is about 100 percent. The mortality rate and nursing difficulties increase if the baby is premature, has other defects, if the diagnosis is delayed, or if the esophagus cannot be sutured during the first operation. Gastostomy (to decompress the stomach) is the most important aspect of preoperative management because it is the only way to ensure the lowest incidence of gastroesophageal reflux leading to chemical pneumonitis.

The infant with esophageal atresia without fistula will have a gastrostomy for feedings and a *cervical esophagostomy* whereby the upper end of the esophagus is externalized at the neck to allow for drainage of saliva, which can cause pneumonia if aspirated. At a later date, when the infant has gained weight and is stronger, a colon transplant is performed to link the ends of the esophagus. An alternative method is to keep the baby in a prone position (to prevent pneumonia) with the gastrostomy; this makes the esophagostomy and subsequent colon transplant unnecessary. Type C is corrected by means of early surgery to divide the fistula.

Nursing care unique to the baby with esophageal atresia includes positioning him with head and chest elevated to prevent the reflux of gastric juices into the lungs. Placing the incubator pad in a reverse Trendelenburg position is an effective way to elevate the infant's head and chest; an alternative is to place the infant in an infant seat, but be sure to strap him in and place blanket rolls on either side to prevent slumping. Frequent nasopharyngeal suctioning is important and is facilitated by the use of a small sump tube inserted into the blind esophageal pouch and attached to low suction.

Postoperatively, suctioning the nasopharynx is the most important aspect of nursing care. If early respiratory distress is not recognized and treated, the infant will rapidly become exhausted. Use a small, soft plastic catheter inserting it carefully so that you do not disturb the suture line. Chest drainage via a water seal tube removes air and blood from the chest cavity. (Water seal drainage is discussed in ch. 22).

When oral feedings are begun, the infant will usually want more milk than his esophagus can handle. Feed him slowly with a medicine dropper. While you refill the dropper, he has adequate time to swallow. Always have suction available when feeding the infant.

If an esophagostomy has been done, care is taken to keep the irritating saliva away from the skin. Absorbant gauze pads are used over the opening, and a diaper is tied loosely around the neck to soak up the secretions. Gastrostomy feedings will continue after surgery until the esophagus is repaired at a later date.

A leak at the site of an anastomosis is the most serious postoperative complication. If the chest tube has been removed, tension pneumothorax will develop; if not treated promptly, this condition leads to respiratory distress and death. A leak often necessitates a second operation and is a serious setback. Be alert to any changes in vital signs and report them at once. Strictures are common after surgery and are prevented and/or treated by dilatations. The baby with a stricture will have difficulty swallowing and may aspirate.

Diaphragmatic Hernia

A *diaphragmatic hernia* is a surgical emergency. When the diaphragm fails to fuse properly to the abdominal wall, the stomach, intestines, spleen, and liver may herniate into the chest. Swallowed air distends the stomach and encroaches on the lung of the affected side (usually the left), and forces the heart toward the opposite side. The right lung becomes compressed and severe oxygen deprivation results.

Symptoms vary with the amount of abdominal contents displaced into the thoracic cavity and with the degree of lung compression. Rapid, labored respirations, and cyanosis usually develop on the first day of life and progress in severity unless diagnosed promptly. The empty abdomen is scaphoid, and there are no breath sounds on the affected side. The apical heartbeat will be heard further to the right in the usual case. X-rays will show the intestines in the thorax. Early repair is indicated, and time is of the essence; the most common cause of preoperative death is a delay of surgical repair.

Nursing care unique to the infant with a diaphragmatic hernia includes placing him with head and chest elevated and turned to the affected side to allow for maximum expansion of the unaffected lung and to minimize compression of the heart. Prop up the child with a blanket roll. Administer oxygen as necessary and have sodium bicarbonate on hand; both are used to combat the acidosis resulting from anoxia.

Postoperatively, the infant may have respiratory distress for several days until the compressed lung fully expands. Change his position frequently, aspirate the nasopharynx as necessary, and observe for changes in respiration. Chest drainage via a water seal tube is used until the lung is fully expanded. A nasogastric tube is used until peristalsis returns, and the abdomen is flat.

The mortality rate for diaphragmatic hernia is about 25 percent due to associated anomalies of the heart, lung, and intestine.

Intestinal Obstructions

Intestinal obstructions may be caused by intrinsic lesions such as atresia or stenosis, or by extrinsic compression, as in malrotation of the midgut. Atresia (complete obstruction) or stenosis (narrowing or partial obstruction) occurs most often in the duodenum and least often in the colon.

Malrotation of the intestine occurs when the intestines do not complete their normal shift across the peritoneal cavity during intrauterine life. A *volvulus*, or twisting, of the small intestine is associated with malrotation in a large percentage of the cases. The duodenum is compressed and obstructed (Figure 18–5).

The most important sign of intestinal obstruction is bilary, ("green") vomiting. It is characteristic because these obstructions occur below the ampulla of Vater, where bile enters the duodenum. Other signs are abdominal distension and failure to pass stools. Infants with a high obstruction will have upper abdominal distension. An obstruction in the ileum or colon produces a hugely distended abdomen. Failure to pass meconium within the first 24 hours of life almost always indicates intestinal obstruction. However, an infant with atresia or stenosis may initially pass a small amount of putty-like stool; the infant with a partial obstruction may pass normal-looking stools.

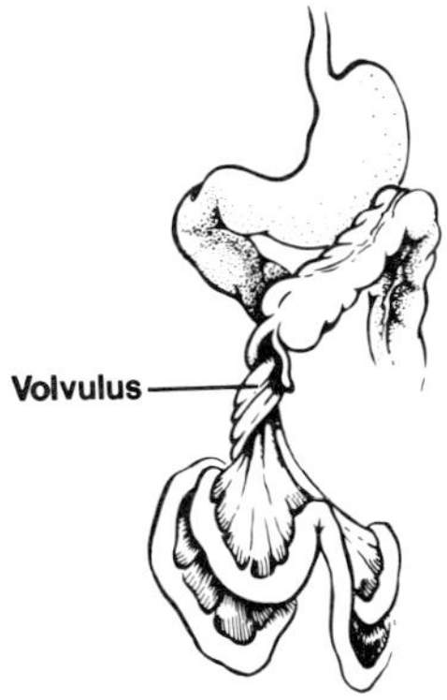

Figure 18–5. *Malrotation of the intestine with volvulus.*

During surgery, the atresia will be resected and the bowel sutured together. For low obstructions, a temporary ileostomy may be done, bypassing the obstruction. Postoperatively, vomiting and aspiration must be prevented. Place the baby on his side and suction the nasopharynx as needed. A nasogastric or gastrostomy tube will remove swallowed air and secretions until peristalsis returns.

Stools and drainage from tubes and fistulas are measured and recorded; fluids are replaced to maintain fluid and electrolyte balance. Diarrhea may be a problem after surgery because the infant may not have enough bowel to absorb nutrients. As was mentioned earlier, frequent liquid stools are irritating to the skin because of the digestive properties of the enteric juices. Expose the perineum to air, cleanse it frequently and cover it with zinc oxide or aluminum paste.

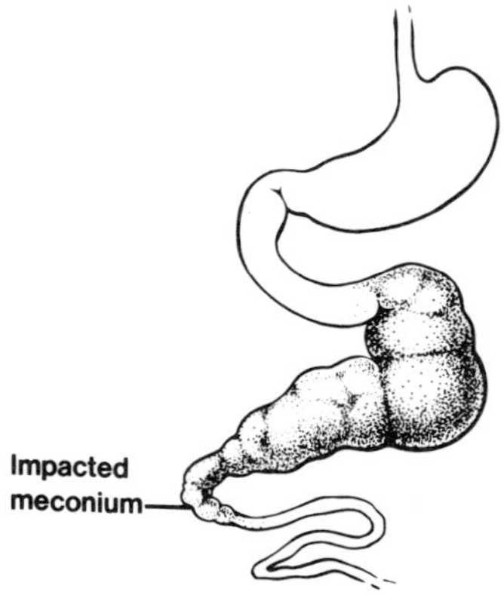

Figure 18–6. *Meconium ileus. Note the dilated ileum above the impacted meconium.*

Meconium Ileus

Meconium ileus occurs when puttylike meconium accumulates in the terminal ileum, completely obstructing the lumen (Figure 18–6). The ileum above this point dilates and hypertrophies in an attempt to move the meconium. The infant vomits thick, dark green material. The abdomen is distended and firm, and loops of bowel can be palpated through the abdominal wall. Enemas of sodium diatrizoate (Gastrografin) are used to liquify the meconium and to stimulate bowel peristalsis. If this fails, surgery is performed to remove the thick meconium. An ileostomy is often done to facilitate cleansing of the lower bowel with irrigations. Postoperatively, pulmonary infection and obstruction are the greatest hazards. Meticulous attention is paid to care of the respiratory tract and prophylactic antiobiotics are given routinely. Pancreatic enzyme supplements are given with feedings. Most infants with meconium ileus survive surgery but have severe cystic fibrosis and later succumb to pulmonary complications.

Imperforate Anus

An *imperforate anus* is caused by an arrest in the development of the anus, lower rectum, and often the urogenital tract. The most common types are: 1) a skin membrane over the anus, 2) an imperforate anus with rectovaginal fistula in girls, and 3) high rectal atresia with urinary tract fistula in boys (Figure 18–7).

Inspection in the delivery room may reveal the imperforate anus, but, in some infants with a deep anal dimple, the diagnosis may not be made until the nurse attempts to take a rectal temperature. Girls with a low rectoperineal fistula may pass stool and therefore the diagnosis may be overlooked. If a boy has no obvious anal opening, save his urine for the physician to examine. If it is tinged with green

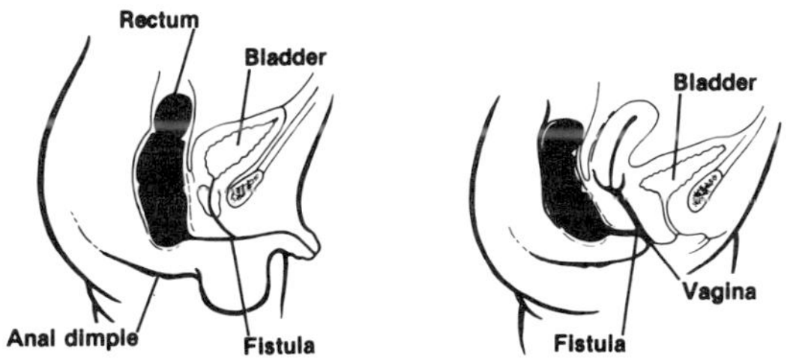

Figure 18–7. *Imperforate anus. The rectum ends much lower in the female (shown on the right) and can be reached via a perineal approach.*

meconium, a fistula exists between the rectum and urinary tract. A small lead marker is taped to the perineum or barium paste is applied and the infant is x-rayed in the upside-down position (Wangensteen-Rice x-ray). Gas will rise to the level of the rectal pouch, and the distance between the pouch and perineum can be measured.

Infants with imperforate anus are checked for other defects, particularly esophageal anomalies. Anal stenosis is corrected by simple dilation using Hegar dilators. The anus is gradually enlarged to a size sufficient to allow daily digital dilation by the mother. Imperforate anal membranes are also treated this way after the membrane is punctured with a hemostat or scalpel.

Perineal *anoplasty* (repair of the anus) is done for low pouches with low vaginal fistulas. The fistula is divided and the rectum is sutured to the anal sphincter. After anoplasty, the perineum is exposed to air and kept meticulously clean. Stool is washed away with a syringe and warm sterile saline, and the perineum is gently patted dry with absorbant cotton.

Higher rectal pouches (more than 1.5 centimeters from the anus) and fistulas require a temporary colostomy. Definitive repair by means of an abdominoperineal pull-through is performed later.

The mortality rate in cases of imperforate anus varies from 10 to 20 percent. The higher rate is usually associated with higher pouches, other anomalies, and prematurity. Fecal impactions often occur for a year or two because some affected children lack sensation and the normal urge to defecate.

Omphalocele

An *omphalocele* is a herniation of the abdominal viscera through the umbilical ring. (Color Plate 4). It is usually covered with a thin translucent sac. A *gastroschisis* is a herniation without a sac, and may occur either below the umbilical ring or adjacent to it, with a bridge of skin between the umbilicus and the defect. These two defects occur in 1 out of every 6,000 births. Other congenital anomalies are commonly found.

A major preoperative problem in infants with omphalocele or gastroschisis is hypothermia. They are placed in an incubator, and the sac or viscera is covered with sterile saline sponges. A nasogastric tube is passed to decompress the abdomen. If possible, the viscera is restored to the abdominal cavity. However, the cavity may not accommodate large defects without elevation of the diaphragm and respiratory distress. Closure of the skin and subcutaneous tissue is often necessary to permit gradual replacement of the organs.

An alternate treatment is to paint the intact sac with 2 percent aqueous mercurochrome, thus protecting it from infection. An eschar will form and will gradually be replaced with new skin. Definitive surgery is delayed with this procedure.

A temporary synthetic covering is sometimes used to cover the viscera, whether or not there is an existing sac. A covering of Silastic, sutured to the edges of the abdominal wall to cover the viscera, is tightened gradually to reduce the mass within the abdominal cavity. A sterile environment in an isolette is a necessity for affected infants. The survival rate is presently 70 to 90 percent; deaths occur more frequently in cases complicated by associated anomalies and prematurity.

Pyloric Stenosis

Pyloric stenosis is characterized by hypertrophy and hyperplasia of the pyloric muscle at the bottom of the stomach. The muscle forms a tumor the size of an olive which restricts the lumen of the pylorus and delays or prevents emptying of the stomach (Figure 18–8). Pyloric stenosis occurs in 1 out of every 200 live male births, most often in first-born males, and is rare in blacks. There may be some familial tendencies, but the exact cause is unknown.

The infant, usually in good health, begins to vomit his feedings at about three weeks of age. As the obstruction worsens, the vomiting becomes projectile, often traveling three or four feet. The vomitus does not contain bile because the obstruction is above the ampulla of Vater. Immediately after vomiting, the infant seems hungry and will eat again; no nausea is associated with the vomiting episodes. Reverse peristaltic waves are visible during the feeding and just prior to vomiting. These muscle contractions move from left to right and are called "rolling of balls." Diagnosis is made on the basis of history, visible reverse peristalsis, palpation of an olive-shaped tumor in the abdomen, and a "positive string-sign" on x-ray. After a barium meal, x-rays will reveal barium in the stomach and a "string" of barium leaving the stomach through the narrowed pylorus. After the x-ray, empty the barium from the stomach with a nasogastric tube to prevent aspiration, and place the infant on his side.

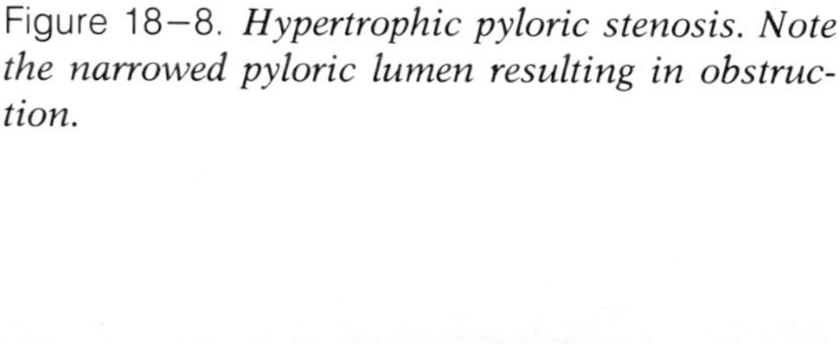

Figure 18–8. *Hypertrophic pyloric stenosis. Note the narrowed pyloric lumen resulting in obstruction.*

The infant with pyloric stenosis may be dehydrated and emaciated if diagnosis is delayed. He may exhibit the typical appearance of a "withered, little old man" because of the loss of subcutaneous tissues and fluids. He is susceptible to pneumonia and other infections. He will have to be hydrated and his electrolyte balance must be restored before surgery. When his mucous membranes are moist and his cry is lusty, he is ready for surgery.

A Fredet-Ramstedt *pyloromyotomy* is a simple and effective treatment for pyloric stenosis. Under general anesthesia, an incision is made through the abdomen to visualize the pylorus. A superficial incision is made into the muscle, which is then spread down to, but not through, the mucosa. The lumen can then expand outward through the muscle as the child feeds. Skin sutures are taken, and the infant is fed in 4 to 24 hours, at the discretion of the surgeon. Feedings are gradually increased from a small amount of glucose water to full-strength formula according to the child's tolerance. Prevent contamination of the wound with feces and urine by applying the diaper below the wound.

Intussusception

An *intussusception* is the invagination, or telescoping, of one part of the intestine into another, causing intestinal obstruction (Figure 18–9). It is most commonly found at the ileocecal valve. Intussusception occurs most often during the first two years of life and more often in boys than in girls. The affected infants are usually healthy and well nourished. Often, no organic cause of the defect is found, although recent studies have shown viral enteritis to be a probable factor. Spasm of the intestine, in which peristaltic waves push the area of spasm into the more distal intestine, is thought to be another cause. Occasionally, an inverted Meckel's diverticulum or a polyp can start the invagination.

The history of intussusception in infants and children is usually classic. A well-nourished, healthy male infant under one year of age is playing happily. He is seized with severe abdominal cramping and cries out in pain. He turns pale and draws his legs up; his abdomen is rigid. After the pain subsides, he returns to his play, only to have another episode shortly afterward. Vomiting follows, along with the passage of "current jelly stools," mostly consisting of blood and mucus. The infant becomes listless, pale, and shocky.

A diagnosis is made on the basis of a history and physical findings. A sausage-shaped mass can be palpated in the upper right quadrant of the abdomen, and the lower right quadrant is empty because the cecum has invaginated into the ascending colon. X-rays confirm these findings.

If the child is in shock, IV fluids, electrolytes, and blood are given as needed. A nasogastric tube is passed to suction the stomach and prevent vomiting. Barium enemas may be given to reduce the invagination by hydrostatic pressure unless signs of peritonitis are present, then immediate surgery is performed to resect a portion of the bowel. Death rarely occurs from intussusception unless gangrene or peritonitis is present secondary to delayed diagnosis and treatment.

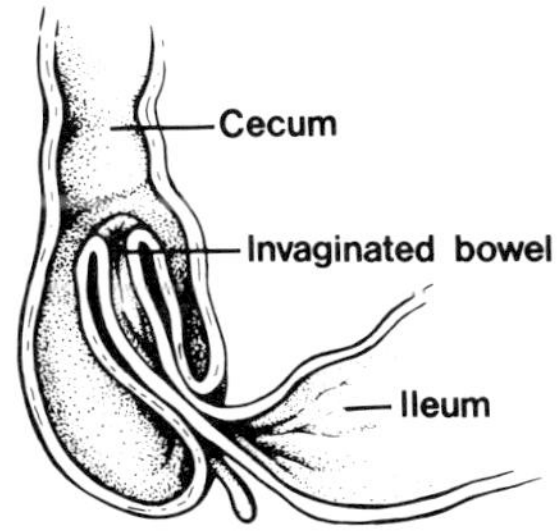

Figure 18–9. *Intussusception. The distal portion of the bowel has invaginated into the cecum.*

Meckel's Diverticulum

Meckel's diverticulum, a defect of embryonic development, is an outpouching on the terminal ileum. The child may be asymptomatic or may have intestinal obstruction, perforation, and peritonitis or bleeding. Bright red blood is seen in the feces rather than in vomitus because this defect is low in the intestine.

Observation of the child's vital signs and amount of blood lost in the stools are vital to the diagnosis since x-rays do not reveal a Meckel's diverticulum. Observe the child carefully for skin color, pulse, blood pressure, and color of stools. Blood transfusions are required if the child goes into hypovolemic shock.

Biliary Atresia

Congenital atresia of the bile ducts is not easily diagnosed. Clay-colored stools, seen in the adult with jaundice, may go unnoticed in the infant because his stools are often colored in the diaper by deeply pigmented urine. Liver function tests do not differentiate between biliary atresia and neonatal hepatitis. If biliary atresia goes undetected for two months occlusion of the bile ducts occurs, and the liver will be permanently damaged. During an exploratory laparotomy, the liver is biopsied, and the bile ducts are x-rayed. If a bile duct is found, it is sutured to the small intestine; if not, there is no satisfactory treatment and the infant will not survive.

Observe and record the color of all stools. Save them for the physician to examine. Skin itching is relieved with a soothing skin cream or calamine lotion. To prevent excoriation caused by scratching, trim the fingernails and/or apply mittens. Liver damage lowers the child's resistance to infection, and pneumonia is a constant threat. This should be guarded against by turning the child frequently and suctioning as needed.

Hirschsprung's Disease

Congenital *aganglionic megacolon*, or *Hirschsprung's disease*, is a congenital absence of parasympathetic ganglion cells in variable lengths of the colon (Figure 18–10). Recent studies have shown that sympathetic fibers are also absent. The affected colon is in a constant state of tonic contraction, as is the internal anal sphincter. The bowel proximal to the aganglionic portion gradually dilates and becomes hypertrophied as the peristaltic waves try to propel stool into the contracted aganglionic segment. Intestinal obstruction results, the severity being directly related to the length of the aganglionic segment.

Hirschsprung's disease affects males four times as often as females and whites three times as often as members of other races. The incidence is 1 in 5,000 births, and associated birth anomalies may be present. The diagnosis can be based on history alone; in less severe cases, diagnosis may be delayed until later childhood. The newborn will show signs of an intestinal obstruction: lack of meconium, distended abdomen, and vomiting of bile or fecal material. He is difficult to feed, becomes dehydrated, and loses weight. He may develop "overflow diarrhea," usually caused by a secondary enterocolitis. Stools are rarely spontaneously expelled, and they are pellet-like or "ribbon-like." The older child will be malnourished, with wasted extremities and a large feces- and gas-filled abdomen that encroaches on the diaphragm, causing breathing difficulties.

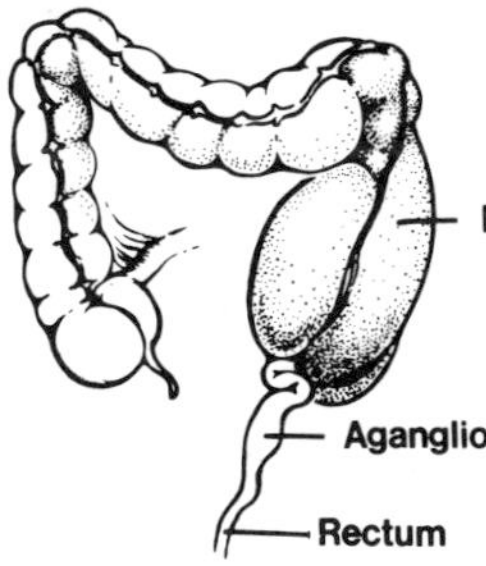

Figure 18–10. *Hirschsprung's disease (congenital aganglionic megacolon). The bowel is markedly distended above the aganglionic section.*

Death in Hirschsprung's disease is usually caused by a severe enterocolitis, perhaps arising from fecal stagnation and an overgrowth of bacteria, leading to severe bowel irritation and diarrhea. Hypovolemic shock and death may occur within 24 hours. The symptoms are the same as for any other gastoenteritis, except that the watery or bloody diarrhea is profound and rapidly progressive. Teach the mother to be alert for it and to seek medical attention at once. Treatment includes replacement of fluids and electrolytes intravenously and emptying the colon.

Hirschsprung's disease may be confused with chronic constipation, however, a careful history and physical exam will differentiate between the two (see Table 18–4). A barium enema will show the narrowed aganglionic segment and the hypertrophied intestine proximal to it. Rectal biopsy usually is not necessary, and intra-abdominal biopsy can be done to confirm the diagnosis at the time of colostomy or corrective surgery.

Treatment regimens prior to definitive surgery at six to twelve months of age vary; some surgeons advocate a prompt colostomy in the neonate and some use conservative therapy consisting of daily colonic lavage to empty the colon. (see the Skills Manual). The absorptive surface is tremendously increased in the greatly distended colon. Tap water must not be used for colonic lavage because of the risk of water intoxication and convulsions caused by cerebral edema. Saline or skim milk (made with powder to drinking strength) is safe to use. The colon will have to be cleansed before surgery, and the same technique of colonic lavage is employed until the return is clear. Be careful not to tire the child. It may be necessary to lavage twice a day for several days rather than risk wearing the infant out.

If the child has a colostomy or ileostomy, watch for a *water ring* on the dressing. This indicates a loss of fluid. The definitive surgical intervention is an abdominoperineal pull-through, where the aganglionic segment is resected and the normal bowel pulled down and sutured to the anus.

Postoperative nursing care consists of protecting the perineal area. No rectal temperatures are taken, and the crib should be so labeled. Cleanse the bloody drainage

Table 18-4. **Differences Between Hirschsprung's Disease and Chronic Constipation**

Hirschsprung's Disease	*Chronic Constipation*
Constipated from first day of life; history of problems in moving bowels.	Some difficulty with passage of stools; during infancy a painful fissure may develop, causing withholding of stool *or* traumatic toilet training resulting in psychogenic constipation.
Chronically ill; abdomen distended with gas and feces.	Flat abdomen in spite of stool retention because gas escapes normally.
Small stools; never encopretic because state of tonic contraction of internal sphincter prevents involuntary leaking of stool around an impaction.	Passes enormous stools; encopresis during the day and night.
Rectal exam reveals empty rectum; internal sphincter tight.	Enormous rectum; frequent bulging of stool at the anus.
Barium enema demonstrates narrow aganglionic segment.	No aganglionic segment; greatly dilated rectum or huge fecal impaction at anus.

or dark mucus from the anus with warm water and cotton balls. Pacififers, stroking, and sedation are all necessary for the relief of pain and the promotion of comfort. In three to four days, the child will pass stools which will not only hurt, but will surprise him (remember that he is not used to having a normal bowel movement). Teach the mother to recognize, and avoid for a while, those foods that increase the number of stools. Some degree of perineal excoriation usually occurs because the child's perineum is not accustomed to fecal contamination. In addition to the routine care for such problems, sitz baths may also help. Complications include pelvic abscess, adhesions resulting in intestinal obstruction, and prolonged paralytic ileus.

Other Anomalies

Inguinal hernia, hydrocele, and *undescended testicle* are associated anomalies. By the seventh month of intrauterine life, the testicle normally descends from its position near the kidney down through the inguinal canal into the scrotum. As it descends, it carries with it a peritoneal sac that normally seals off at the abdominal ring. If this sac fails to close, the intestine may descend into the inguinal canal, forming an *inguinal hernia*, or it may fill with fluid and form a *hydrocele*. If the intestine becomes trapped in this hernia it is *incarcerated*, and strangulation of the intestine may occur as the blood supply is compromised.

Descent of the testicle may be arrested at any time during intrauterine life, and it will not be present in the scrotum at birth. However, it may continue to descend and reach the normal position by four to five years of age. *Cryptorchidism* or undescended testicle is always associated with a hernia.

Unless strangulation occurs, these anomalies may be asymptomatic. When the child cries, a soft lump may be palpated in the groin; it recedes when he relaxes. A firm lump accompanied by vomiting and abdominal distension suggests intestinal obstruction. Local tenderness and edema at the site indicates strangulation but may be overlooked until the infant cries from pain. A painless scrotal lump that does not recede when the child lies down indicates a hydrocele. If the testicle has not descended, it may be palpated in the inguinal canal, and the scrotum on the affected side is empty and smaller than normal.

Hydroceles and inguinal hernias are repaired surgically. Since hydroceles are not as potentially dangerous as hernias, however, surgery may be delayed for several years. Incarcerated hernias call for emergency surgery. While preparations are being made for the operation, a short trial of Trendelenburg position is tried in an attempt to reduce the hernia. Pad the child's ankles and tie his feet to the foot of the bed to prevent him from sliding to the head of the bed. Sedate him as ordered with small doses of a narcotic or rectal barbiturates. Observe and record vital signs. A reduced urine output accompanied by tachycardia and hypotension suggests fluid loss from vomiting and impending shock. Do *not* push on the intestines to help reduce the hernia. If it does not reduce within an hour, surgery is performed.

Cryptorchidism is corrected before the child starts school. The testicle will be damaged by body heat if left in the inguinal canal beyond this time, resulting in sterility if the cryptorchidism is bilateral.

Postoperatively, a diaper is placed over the genitalia to keep the incision dry. Do not pin it over the incision. After hernia repair, the child can ambulate. After *or-*

chiopexy (fixation of the undescended testicle in the scrotum), a traction suture may stabilize the testicle and scrotum to the thigh and ambulation is not permitted until it is removed.

An *umbilical hernia* results from a weakness or imperfect closure of the umbilical ring. The size of these asymptomatic hernias of the intestine varies, and incarceration is very rare. Most umbilical hernias close spontaneously, therefore repair is postponed until the age of three or four.

MALABSORPTION SYNDROMES

Secondary Lactase Deficiency

Secondary lactase deficiency is common and may develop after any disease that damages the epithelium of the small intestine. The child suffers from a transient malabsorption of lactose, the disaccharide present in human and cow's milk. Gastroenteritis is the most common cause of lactose intolerance in infancy. Therapy requires the elimination of all dairy products from the diet for a period of a few days to a few months. The parents are instructed to read the labels on food products to identify foods containing lactose. Formulas well-tolerated by affected infants are Isomil and ProSobee, neither of which contains lactose.

Cystic Fibrosis

Cystic fibrosis (CF) of the pancreas (mucoviscidosis) is the most common lethal genetic disease of childhood as well as the most common cause of chronic malabsorption in children in the United States. It is transmitted as an autosomal recessive trait and occurs most often in whites, occuring once in every 1,000 to 2,000 live births. Although this disease is ultimately fatal, 50 percent of affected children now survive beyond the age of twenty-five.

CF is an inborn error of metabolism in which there is a generalized dysfunction of the exocrine glands. Lack of a mucolytic (mucus-liquifying) enzyme causes mucus-secreting glands of the body to produce a thick, tenacious mucus which, in turn, causes obstructions, mainly in the pancreatic ducts and bronchi. Pancreatic enzyme deficiency causes abdominal distension and cramping as well as steatorrhea (fatty stools), evidenced by greasy, bulky, foul-smelling stools. The child is unable to utilize fat in the diet. For this reason, fat-soluble vitamins are not absorbed and must be given in a water-miscible preparation to prevent deficiencies. Pancreatic enzymes (such as Viokase), are given with meals and the child is placed on a low-fat diet. Viokase comes in powder, tablet, and capsule form. For infants and small children who have difficulty swallowing, use the powdered form, mixing it with a sweet food to disguise the taste. Do not mix with warm foods. Add the powder just before feeding to minimize decomposition, and feed the preparation at the beginning of the meal to ensure intake. Dosage varies with the child. The criterion of adequate replacement is a decrease in steatorrhea and diarrhea and a decreased food intake. The dosage is increased to stimulate maximum improvement in growth. Overdosage causes constipation but is rare because of the unpleasant odor and taste of the preparation. If the regimen does not bring about a decrease in steatorrhea and diarrhea, a milk-free diet is begun.

Rectal prolapse may occur secondary to the large, bulky stools and also as a result of the vigorous coughing that accompanies pulmonary infections in the child. With the increased longevity of the CF child, recent studies have recognized sterility in the male and reduced fertility in the female, both complications of the thick mucus secretions.

A diagnosis of cystic fibrosis is based on four factors: family history, increase in electrolyte concentration in sweat, lack of pancreatic enzymes, and chronic pulmonary disease. Meconium ileus occurs in about 10 percent of children with CF. Iontophoresis of pilocarpine HCI with quantitative chloride analysis (sweat test) is a simple and reliable test for cystic fibrosis. Questionable levels of chloride are 50 to 60 mEq per liter and 60 mEq per liter is diagnostic; sodium levels are about 10 mEq higher. Duodenal contents are examined for pancreatic enzyme activity, and the stools are checked for the absence of trypsin and for fat content. Chest x-rays and pulmonary function tests reveal chronic lung disease.

The nurse must carefully observe, record, and report the character of the child's stools to aid the physician in diagnosing and managing cystic fibrosis. Nursing assessment of the child's respiratory status is most important to his well-being and is an integral part of daily care and parent-child teaching. Over 90 percent of the mortality and most of the morbidity stemming from CF is caused by pulmonary infection and obstruction. The treatment and nursing management of respiratory problems are discussed in Ch. 23.

Treatment for pulmonary involvement consists of the prevention of infection and the control of disease. Antibiotics are given as indicated by deep throat culture. Intermittent aerosol therapy is used to deliver small amounts of medication or water (to liquify secretions) to the lower respiratory tract. Medications used are decongestants, bronchodilators, antibiotics and mycolytic and/or anti-inflammatory agents. Drugs that suppress the cough reflex are never given to the CF child. Aerosol therapy is followed by postural drainage in 12 different positions; clapping for one to two minutes in each position is followed by vibrating during five exhalations (see the Skills Manual). Encourage coughing after each segment and if the cough is productive, repeat the therapy for that segment. Regular exercise and deep breathing are to be encouraged.

Celiac Disease

Celiac disease or *gluten-induced enteropathy*, is the second most common cause of malabsorption in children. In addition to heredity, a variety of non-specific stresses, such as infections and emotional upsets, may initiate or aggravate symptoms. The symptoms are not manifest until after the introduction of cereal into the diet, usually at six months of age. The presence of gluten (a protein found in wheat, rye, oats, buckwheat, and barley) causes changes in the mucosa of the small intestine, resulting in malabsorption of fats. The child is likely to have repeated bouts of diarrhea associated with respiratory infections and accompanied by vomiting. There may be severe diarrhea, or the stools may be bulky, frothy, and foul-smelling (because of the undigested fat). In a few cases, the child is constipated. Weight loss and emaciation with wasting of the extremities is common. The child is apathetic and anorectic and may develop hypoproteinemia and nutritional edema. Anemia and deficiencies of the fat-soluble vitamins are common.

Diagnosis is based on history, physical appearance, presence of steatorrhea (fat in stools), biopsy of the jejunum, and evidence of improvement on a gluten-free diet. Complete fecal collection is done for a period of 72 hours, and the fat content is analyzed. A nasogastric tube is passed to obtain a biopsy of the jejunum; if celiac disease is present, the intestinal villi will be typically flattened. Gastrointestinal symptoms, anorexia, apathy, and negativism will all improve dramatically on a gluten-free diet. Nursing management centers around the effects of the gluten-free diet on the child. Observe, record, and report the character of his stools, his behavior, and general physical reaction to each new food. Your observations are invaluable in the diagnosis and treatment of this disease.

Treatment consists of a gluten-free diet and the avoidance of infections and excessive psychological stress. Explain to the parents the importance of reading labels on food products, and be sure they understand which foods are prohibited. Monosodium glutamate is derived from grain as are "hydrolized vegetable protein" and most instant coffees. Ice cream, canned soups, and some salad dressings contain flour as a stabilizer, and are therefore prohibited, as are luncheon meats and hot dogs that are not labeled "all meat." Allowable flours are those made with rice, corn, soy beans, potatoes, and gluten-free wheat. Rice and corn cereals, nuts, cheeses, corn and potato chips (made without monosodium glutamate) are gluten-free. Cookbooks for the child with celiac disease are available; some are listed in the bibliography for this chapter.

If the child has periods free of overt symptoms while ingesting gluten, he and his parents may have difficulty in adhering to the demanding and expensive gluten-free diet. However, a return to a gluten-containing diet will result in recurrence of the flat intestinal villi with resultant symptoms.

ELIMINATION PROBLEMS

Gastroenteritis

Gastroenteritis is an inflammation of the stomach and intestines resulting in diarrhea, abdominal cramping with increased passage of gas, nausea, and vomiting. The cause may be viral, bacterial, or psychological, and the disease ranges from mild to severe. Recall that all diarrhea in young children is assumed to be infectious until proven otherwise. Viral diarrhea is usually self-limiting and mild. *Escherichia coli* is commonly the causative agent in bacterial diarrhea and may occur in epidemic proportions. Projectile vomiting and explosive, green, liquid stools are usually the presenting symptoms. The child dehydrates quickly and is extremely ill. Until stool cultures are negative, isolation procedures are strictly followed. *Salmonella* or *Shigella* are bacterial organisms causing a mild diarrhea in young children. These organisms are spread in contaminated food, such as eggs, milk, shellfish, and meat, and also by direct contact with household pets. The presence of these organisms must always be reported to the local health department.

Intractable Diarrhea

Chronic, intractable diarrhea of infancy is characterized by its severity and a duration of at least two weeks. This disease affects infants less than three months of age and results in malnourishment, weight loss, and wasting. It seems to be self-perpetuating and is often unresponsive to formula changes or antibiotic therapy. Treatment consists of breaking the vicious cycle by resting the bowel while curing the underlying cause. Total parenteral nutrition is used to alleviate nutritional deficiencies and to supply maintenance needs.

Neonatal Necrotizing Enterocolitis

Neonatal necrotizing enterocolitis is diffuse intestinal necrosis accompanied by sepsis and often followed by perforation, peritonitis, and death. It is an acquired condition of premature infants weighing less than 1,500 grams who have sustained significant perinatal stress. Ninety percent of these cases occur before 10 days of age. There is soft abdominal distension with retention of gastric secretions that are clear at first, then bile-tinged. Occult blood is lost in the stools. Localized erythema and hardness of the abdominal wall over the necrotic area indicates possible perforation of the intestines. The untreated baby deteriorates rapidly, showing signs of sepsis: thermal instability, lethargy, metabolic acidosis, jaundice, disseminated intravascular clotting (DIC), and, finally, death. Thrombocytopenia is common. The exact cause is not known, but the present theory is that the causative organisms are normal bowel flora.

Diagnosis is based on the typical physical findings and blood, throat, and stool cultures for Escherichia coli, Klebsiella, Enterobacter, and Proteus. X-ray shows nonspecific intestinal distension without mechanical obstruction.

Prompt recognition and treatment is necessary if the baby is to survive. Nasogastric suction, IV fluids, and systemic antibiotics are begun before signs of sepsis are noted. Peripheral parenteral hyperalimentation is used for nutritional support. Metabolic acidosis and electrolyte imbalances are corrected. The infant is given a re-examination including x-rays every 6 hours. If perforation occurs, immediate surgery is done to resect the necrotic and perforated intestine. Postoperatively, the infant may have a gastrostomy to decrease the risk of aspiration. Peripheral hyperalimentation is maintained until sepsis is controlled. The infant will have a temporary ileostomy until he is fully recovered and shows significant weight gain.

The nurse's responsibility begins with early recognition, observation, and reporting. Care of the child with peripheral parenteral hyperalimentation or total parenteral nutrition (TPN) is discussed in ch. 29.

Appendicitis

The peak incidence of *appendicitis* is found in patients 15 to 21 years of age. Unless the appendix has ruptured, the surgical removal is a simple procedure. However, if rupture and peritonitis occur, the child may be critically ill for several weeks.

If a child complains of abdominal pain, appendicitis should be considered. Pain beginning around the umbilicus that settles in the right lower quadrant of the abdomen (McBurney's point) and is accompanied by anorexia and vomiting is indicative of appendicitis, although many diseases mimic this inflammation.

After surgery the child is placed in Fowler's position to permit peritoneal exudate to drain to the lower part of the abdomen. Be alert for fever, abdominal distension and vomiting, which often follows a perforation. Plan the child's care to conserve his energy and improve his nutritional status.

SUMMARY

Gastrointestinal deviations affect the child's growth by interfering with nutrition, absorption, or elimination. Some anomalies are life-threatening and require immediate surgery in the newborn period. Other conditions, such as the malabsorption syndrome, are chronic and require life-long therapy. All of these deviations may cause psychological problems for the child and his family. Patience, understanding, and meticulous nursing care are necessary if the child is to conquer his anomaly, learn to live with it, and achieve his ultimate potential.

CLINICAL APPLICATION

Tony K., two months old, is brought to the unit in his mother's arms as an emergency admission. His diagnosis is pyloric stenosis. Mrs. K. states that the doctor wants to operate on Tony but that he said Tony was not in good condition for surgery. The physician plans to spend several days improving Tony's condition before operating. Tony will be your patient for the next week.

1. Explain Tony's clinical symptoms. How can you tell that he is not in good condition for surgery?
2. Mrs. K. states, "I don't understand what Tony has. Why is he sick? I didn't think you operate on somebody just because he vomits. That doctor thinks I don't take good care of Tony. He said Tony was not in good shape." Why does Mrs. K. feel the way she does? What feelings are evident? What do you say, and why?
3. Design a plan of care for Tony, including pre- and postoperative care.

Bibliography

Adkins, J.C. and Kiesewetter, W.B. Imperforate Anus. *Surgical Clinics of North America* 56:379, 1976.

Ament, M.E. Malabsorption Syndromes in Infancy and Childhood, part II. *Journal of Pediatrics* 81:867, 1972.

Ashcraft, K.W. and Holder, T.M. Esophageal Atresia and Tracheoesophageal Fistula Malformations. *Surgical Clinics of North America* 56:299, 1976.

Connors, M. Ostomy Care: A Personal Approach. *American Journal of Nursing* 74:1422, 1974.

Copeland, L. Chronic Diarrhea in Infancy. *American Journal of Nursing* 77:461, 1977.

Davidson, M. Diarrhea, in Rudolph, A.M. (ed.) *Pediatrics*, ed. 16. New York, Appleton-Century-Crofts, 1977, p. 990.

Fochtman, D. and Raffensperger, J.G.: *Principles of Nursing Care for the Pediatric Surgery Patient*, ed. 2. Boston, Little, Brown & Co., 1976, p. 1.

French, A.B.: *Low Gluten Diet with Tested Recipes*. Ann Arbor, Michigan, University Hospital.

Gross, L. Ostomy Care: A Letter to Parents. *American Journal of Nursing* 74:1427, 1974.

Jones, K.M.: Love and Lavage: The Urgent Needs of Children with Hirschsprung's Disease. *Nursing '78* 8:33, July 1978.

McCreery, M. Diet: First-line Defense against Celiac Disease. *Registered Nurse* 39:50, 1976.

Perman, J.A., and Watkins, J.B. Malabsorption Syndromes and Intestinal Disaccharidase Deficiencies, in Gellis, S.S. and Kagan, G.M. (eds.). *Current Pediatric Therapy*. Philadelphia, W. B. Saunders Co., 1978, p. 234.

Roy, C.C., Silverman, A., Dubois, R.S.: Gastrointestinal Tract, in Kempe, C.H., Silver, H.K., O'Brien, D. (eds.). *Current Pediatric Diagnosis and Treatment*, ed. 4, Los Altos, California, Lange Medical Publications, 1976, p. 414.

Schnaufer, L. Hirschsprung's Disease. *Surgical Clinics of North America* 56:349, 1976.

Sheedy, C.B., and Kafetz, N. *Cooking for Your Celiac Child.* New York, Dial Press, Inc., 1969.

Thorbjarnarson, B. Intussusception. *Hospital Medicine* 11:58, 1975.

Touloukian, R.J.: Neonatal Necrotizing Enterocolitis: An Update on Etiology, Diagnosis, and Treatment. *Surgical Clinics of North America* 56:281, 1976.

Wrenn, E.L.: Omphalocele and Gastroschisis. *Surgical Rounds* 1:12, 1978.

CHAPTER **19**

The Child with a Hormonal Deviation

BEHAVIORAL OBJECTIVES

After studying this chapter you will be able to:

- Identify the metabolic changes that follow hormonal overproduction and relate common symptoms to alterations in physiology.
- Identify the metabolic changes that follow hormonal underproduction and relate common symptoms to alterations in physiology.
- Construct a nursing care plan for a child with a disorder caused by a hormonal deficit, offering a rationale for the nursing interventions.
- Construct a nursing care plan for a child with a disorder resulting from a hormonal excess, offering a rationale for the nursing interventions.

TERMS AND CONCEPTS

Hormonal excess
Hormonal deficit
Hormonal replacement
Acidosis
Polyuria
Polydipsia
Ketoacidosis
Renal threshold for glucose
Clinitest 5-drop, 2-drop, 1-drop
Fasting blood glucose
Oral glucose tolerance test
Radioactive iodine uptake
T^3 and T^4 serum assay
Vanillylmandelic acid
17-ketosteroids
Insulin
Atrophy
Hypertrophy

Jim, aged twelve, is five inches shorter than his seven-year-old brother. Jim's size, immature features, and childish voice cause his peers and adults to treat him as if he were a young child. Although tests document that he is of above average intelligence, Jim is a poor student and has repeated two grades. Jim has insufficient amounts of growth hormone.

Five-year-old Julie has an enormous appetite but continues to lose weight. She has begun wetting the bed at night, and yesterday her mother smelled a strong, fruity odor on Julie's breath. Today Julie lies on the couch, complaining of a stomach ache and breathing rapidly as if "hungry for air." Fearing Julie has ingested a household cleaning agent, her mother calls the poison control center. Julie lacks insulin hormone.

Debbie is a tall, slender, sixteen-year-old who is teased about her protruding eyeballs and wide-eyed stare by her peers. Previously an honor roll student, Debbie cannot concentrate and appears nervous and fidgety in class. Always popular and surrounded by friends, recently Debbie has been unable to get along with her classmates or family. Although Debbie has a good appetite, she continues to lose weight. Debbie has an excess of thyroid hormone.

Both Jim and Julie have a hormonal deficit, while Debbie has an excess of a hormone. Each child has a deviation from normal hormonal secretion and function. Chapter 17 discussed hormones, their sites of secretion, and their effects. Review Figures 17–1 and 17–2, studying the production sites and target gland of each hormone.

The best way to understand a hormonal deviation is to remember that the symptoms of deviation can be explained by the metabolic actions of the hormone. Hormonal disorders usually occur because of *excessive* or *deficient* hormone production. When a hormone is overproduced, the physiological responses to that hormone also increase. Conversely, when a hormone is underproduced, the physiological responses decrease accordingly. Variations from normal hormonal production almost always cause a change in energy metabolism, growth, responses to stress (such as infection or trauma), and the chemical balance within the body.

An excess of hormone may develop from overproduction by a gland, abnormal production of hormones by tissue outside the gland (for example, a neoplasm), or inadequate excretion of the hormone from the body. Deficiencies can arise from a congenital absence of the hormone or destruction of the gland resulting from trauma, an immunological response, or surgical removal. Frequently however, the source of the hormonal imbalance is unknown. Hormonal deviations cause metabolic changes which lead to noticeable alteration in weight, height, and rate of maturation. Most children with a hormonal deviation experience some undesirable changes in appearance, which, in turn, frequently lead to emotional problems.

The changes that result from hormonal deviation can be illustrated by a study of hyperthyroidism and diabetes mellitus. *Hyperthyroidism* results from thyroid overproduction; diabetes mellitus results from insulin deficiency. The metabolic alterations and subsequent physiological changes typical of these disorders demonstrate the problems encountered by the child with a hormonal deviation.

COMMON PROBLEMS AND NURSING INTERVENTIONS

Hormonal Excess

Hyperthyroidism

Excessive thyroid secretions create widespread effects, the most obvious of which are accelerated fat, protein, and carbohydrate metabolism.

When extra protein is burned to meet the body's demand for energy, more nitrogen is excreted. A negative nitrogen balance may develop and lead to muscular weakness and wasting of muscle mass; the child becomes fatigued easily. As extra fats are burned to meet body needs, weight is lost, and although the child has a large appetite, he continues to lose weight. The accelerated metabolism causes an increase in growth, but the growth is premature; the child's bone ends will close before he reaches his maximum potential height.

Frequently, when too much of one hormone is produced, it speeds up the metabolism, thereby requiring extra amounts of other hormones. In this instance, the increased rate of metabolism also requires more insulin. The added insulin secretion causes abnormally quick rises and falls in blood glucose.

Correspondingly, the increase in metabolism raises oxygen consumption. Extra heat is generated as more energy is produced. Superficial capillaries dilate to disperse heat through the skin. The child's skin feels warm and moist, especially in the palms and soles. The child perspires easily and prefers less clothing and cooler temperatures.

As the blood vessels dilate, both peripheral blood flow and heart output increase; the child's blood pressure and pulse increase. More blood also flows to the brain, and when this response is added to the others the child becomes hyperactive, irritable, nervous, and restless. He has difficulty concentrating in school. Hand and tongue tremors may make writing and speaking difficult. The child is frequently labeled a behavior problem; and teachers will report that he has a short attention span, fidgets, and is not getting along with other classmates. He has jerky eyelid movement, and his eye balls protrude (*exophthalmos*), resulting in a staring, bright-eyed look. The child fatigues easily, yet his mind is so active that he has trouble sleeping (*insomnia*) despite physical exhaustion.

Physical changes caused by thyroid overproduction develop slowly, usually over several months. The family frequently attributes the alterations in growth and personality to the child's age and accompanying stage of development. Once the hormonal problem has been diagnosed, parents often feel guilty and inadequate, blaming themselves for not seeking medical attention earlier.

Assure parents that subtle changes in personality and body build are difficult for anyone to recognize, especially parents who see the child daily. Emphasize that the child's hyperactive behavior results from the increased amounts of thyroid hormone and that these personality changes will be alleviated with medication and the restoration of normal thyroid secretion. After several weeks of medication, the child's metabolism will return to normal. Since the hyperactive behavior and exhaustion are most distressing to parents, plan a quiet, destimulating environment to help calm the child. Suggest routine naps with a 15- to 20-minute quiet period of story reading or music before the nap. It is good to restrict visiting, television, and other sources of stimulation during this period,

Another consideration for the child with a hormonal excess is nutrition. As his metabolism rate increases, the child needs extra calories and protein. Offer high protein snacks such as cheese or peanut butter with crackers, and milk shakes, and provide extra calories and nutrients at each meal. Supplemental vitamins also may be necessary.

The child's altered body image should be discussed frankly with him and his family. Exophthalmos, for example, may not recede, but the eyes will not enlarge further once therapy begins. Suggest the adolescent use shaded glasses or tinted lenses to eliminate the self-consciousness about eye shape.

The extra heat body generated by the increased metabolic rate creates a need for less clothing and bedcovering to help cool the child. Because perspiration also increases changing the child's underclothes frequently will help maintain skin integrity and minimize skin breakdown resulting from maceration. Ask the child if he feels warm, feel his skin, check his temperature, and then adjust his clothing and the room temperature accordingly.

Explain to the family that hormonal excess is corrected in one of two ways; sometimes both treatments are necessary. The first method is *surgery:* the whole gland or part of the gland responsible for overproduction can be surgically removed. For the child with hyperthyroidism, removal of the entire gland is a *thyroidectomy* and removal of part of the thyroid is a *subtotal thyroidectomy.* A successful subtotal thyroidectomy eliminates thyroid excess but leaves enough of the gland to secrete sufficient amounts of thyroid hormone. When the entire gland is removed, *hormonal replacement* is necessary; and in the case of a thyroidectomy, thyroid must be taken for life.

The second method of treating hormonal excess is *medication.* The child may be given a medication that interferes with hormonal production by blocking or destroying the tissue that produces the hormone. For hyperthyroidism, Tapazole and propylthiouracil are commonly used to suppress the formation of thyroxine. The medication is needed for an indefinite period, often for years, after which time the child is gradually weaned from the drug and his thyroid function is reevaluated.

Although this discussion has highlighted the child with hyperthyroidism, the changes in metabolism and accompanying alterations in growth and body image described also are typical of children with other hormonal excesses.

Whenever a hormone is overproduced, metabolism almost always increases, frequently causing extra secretions of other hormones to meet the added metabolic needs. Nutritional deficits and growth alterations are common as the child tries to satisfy increased body demands for energy. Body image and personality frequently change as metabolic deviations become apparent. Treatment involves surgical removal of part or all of the gland or use of medications to suppress hormone production. Hormonal replacement may be required for years or for a lifetime.

Hormonal Deficit

Diabetes Mellitus

Changes in metabolism also become apparent when a hormonal deficit is present. The child with diabetes mellitus has a deficiency of insulin that initiates metabolic alterations. Most body cells need insulin to convert glucose into energy. When the lack of insulin prevents glucose from entering the cells, glucose accumulates in the blood stream and eventually spills into the urine (*glycosuria*). Excess glucose in the blood acts to pull fluid from cells; the extra water is excreted in the urine at frequent intervals (*polyuria*). The fluid loss causes dehydration and excessive thirst. The child tries to compensate by consuming extra liquids (*polydipsia*), but he is unable to keep pace with the large fluid losses. Dehydration becomes more severe as sodium, potassium, and bicarbonate are lost in the urine. Bicarbonate, for example, is a buffering agent, and without sufficient bicarbonate, acids accumulate in the body, resulting in the condition known as (*acidosis*). Since many life-sustaining chemical reactions can occur only within a narrow acid-base range, acidosis is very serious and needs immediate correction.

Fats normally travel in the blood as fatty acids which are converted by the liver to *ketones,* an acid. Insulin helps to stimulate the conversion of fatty acids to triglycerides rather than to ketones, and by so doing aids in keeping the critical acid-base balance normal. When glucose cannot be used for energy, the body uses proteins and fats instead, and the necessary balance is disturbed. This results in large amounts of ketones in the blood, a condition that increases the acidosis and leads to nausea, vomiting, and further dehydration. Acidosis decreases cardiac output and lowers blood pressure. The child's body tries to correct the mounting acidosis by increasing the burden of the kidneys and lungs. Respirations become faster and deeper, thus more carbon dioxide leaves the blood, helping to reduce the acidosis. The kidneys increase the excretion of certain chemicals in an effort to decrease acidosis. For a short time the body is able to compensate; then, the increasing ketones, resulting acidosis, and accompanying dehydration worsen. The child has large amounts of ketones and glucose in the urine and blood. He is dehydrated. Dry skin and mucous membranes, flushed cheeks, and sunken eyeballs characterize the child. He is in a state of *ketoacidosis* (acidosis caused by accumulated ketone bodies). If the child does not receive insulin and fluids immediately, he will become comatose and may die.

The child may be diagnosed at any point after the insulin deficiency begins, and the severity of his symptoms are directly related to the duration of insulin deficiency. Although a few children are diagnosed and begin treatment after minimal illness, most children arrive at the hospital following two to three weeks of weight loss, increased appetite, polydipsia, and polyuria; and some children (10 to 20 percent) are not diagnosed until they become acidotic or comatose.

To restore normal carbohydrate, protein, and fat metabolism, the child is given rapid-acting insulin. To correct the dehydration and imbalances of acids, bases, and salts, intravenous fluids are administered. Insulin is given as separate injections or as a continuous intravenous infusion. The exact dosage of insulin is calculated according to body weight. Blood glucose levels are analyzed often, and the insulin is increased or decreased according to the amount of glucose in the blood. Before insulin can be delivered to the waiting tissue, depleted blood volume must be replaced. For this reason, as well as for correcting the dehydration, special fluids are infused. Glucose is given as part of the fluid mixture although too much unused glucose contributed to the acidosis, since with insulin available body cells are now ready to use glucose for energy. If adequate glucose is not supplied, the cells will continue to use fats and proteins, thereby increasing the acidosis.

During the treatment of ketoacidosis, the child is vulnerable to complications of overhydration (receiving too much fluid), hypoglycemia (lack of glucose), and fluid imbalances. Carefully monitor blood pressure, level of consciousness, intake and output, and urine and blood levels of glucose and ketone. When ketones are cleared from the urine and the child is rehydrated, he will be alert, feel well, and most probably be hungry.

Ketoacidosis is usually corrected in 12 hours. Once treatment begins, the child improves dramatically. The use of insulin, diet, and other care needed for the child with diabetes mellitus is discussed later in this chapter.

Diabetes mellitus is only one example of hormonal insufficiency. Other deficiencies are treated similarly: the child must be given the hormone his body is not producing adequately. The daily administration of the hormone, dosage regulation, and recognition and care of any ensuing complications are family responsibilities. Family roles and relationships change, and the chronic illness creates its stress within the family. Also, the hormonal deficit frequently alters growth, causing a delay in skeletal growth and sexual maturity. These setbacks may be partially, but usually not totally, corrected. The child's body image and self-concept change as others relate to him differently; he is no longer a "normal" child. Because of the hormonal deficit, he is at great risk to complications during infection, trauma, or other stresses. With his hormonal system impaired, he cannot provide the exact regulation needed during periods of added stress and metabolic demand. In short, when any hormone is deficient, changes occur in metabolism, growth, chemical balance, and response to stress.

COMMON DIAGNOSTIC STUDIES

Glucose Measurements

Screening and diagnostic tests for alterations in carbohydrate metabolism, such as occurs in diabetes mellitus, measure glucose in the urine and blood.

Urine Tests

Urine tests are relatively simple because they require no advanced preparation and can be completed quickly with a chemically treated paper or tablet. The amount of glucose spilled into the urine (*glycosuria*), depends on the *renal threshold for glucose,* that is, the point above which glucose is no longer reabsorbed by the kidneys but rather excreted. The normal renal threshold for glucose is 160 to 180 mg/100 ml of blood, but many diabetic children have a fasting blood sugar of 200 or 250 mg and register a negative urine test for glucose. A particular child may have a *high* renal threshold for glucose, and blood glucose levels must exceed 250 mg before glucose is measured in the urine. Another child with diabetes may have a *low* renal threshold (160 to 170 mg). When this child's blood glucose reaches 200 mg, glucose is spilled into the urine. Thus, a negative urine test does not mean normal or small amounts of glucose in the blood, nor does glycosuria always indicate high glucose in the blood.

Urine glucose is always tested prior to a meal using a second voided specimen, so that fresh urine is evaluated instead of urine that has been in the bladder for several hours. For a second voided specimen, have the child empty his bladder. Then 20 to 30 minutes later ask the child to void again, and test this specimen. Since it is difficult for anyone to urinate twice in one hour, it may help to have the child drink a half glass of water after the first voiding and then engage in some active play.

Several different products are available for testing for glycosuria; each has an accompanying color chart, which is compared to the tested urine for indication of glucose content. The variety of testing materials can cause confusion because the color chart for each testing method is different. Some tests indicate the amount of glycosuria as the symbol +; other tests are recorded as percentages. Two or three different systems may be used within the same hospital, and it is essential to record the type of testing method used on the chart.

Clinitest 5-Drop

The Clinitest 5-drop kit includes a test tube, dropper, and Clinitest tablets. The test is made by mixing five drops of urine and ten drops of water in a dry, clean, test tube and adding one Clinitest tablet. The mixture is observed for at least 15 seconds for color changes. The color is compared to the chart accompanying the test kit and the amount of glycosuria recorded. Color changes occur quickly; and if the reaction turns orange, even though the test reverts to blue or green, record the value for orange. This reaction is called "pass through" or "burn through" and indicates a large amount of glucose in the urine.

Clinitest 2-Drop and 1-Drop

The 2-drop and 1-drop Clinitest methods can indicate glucose concentrations up to 10 percent. To make the 2-drop test, place ten drops of water in a dry test tube, add two drops of urine, and one Clinitest tablet. After 15 seconds, compare the color of the urine solution to the Clinitest 2-drop color chart. If the maximum 5 percent, orange, reading is present or if "pass through" occurs, the 1-drop test should be done.

To do the Clinitest 1-drop test, place eleven drops of water in a clean, dry test tube and add one drop of urine. After adding one Clinitest tablet, compare the reaction to the 2-drop color chart. Multiply the result by two to correct for dilution; that is, if a 3 percent result occurs, 6 percent is recorded. Always record the highest value obtained. For example, if the 1-drop test indicates 4 percent (2 percent doubled), record the original 5 percent concentration shown in the 2-drop test.

The 2-drop and 1-drop tests are used to measure glucose content in a portion of a large urine collection. The portion is called an *aliquot* and enables a measurement to be made of the amount of glucose lost in a 24-hour period without doing a test on each voiding. To test an aliquot, collect all urine voided during a set 24-hour period in one container. Then make a Clinitest 2-drop test. To apply the results of the aliquot test to the total urine collection, multiply the volume of urine (in milliliters) by the glucose percentage (in decimals). This equals the number of grams of glucose spilled, and hence the number of calories the child lost in the urine. A child who voids 1200 milliliters of urine in 24 hours and shows 1 percent glucose with a 2-drop Clinitest, has lost 12 grams ($1200 \times .01 = 12$). Since 1 gram of glucose equals 4 calories, the child has lost 48 calories during the 24-hour period. A child voiding 1200 ml but with an 8 percent glucose has lost 96 grams or 384 calories—a big difference. The amount of glucose lost in the urine helps to determine the amount of insulin needed for the child with diabetes mellitus.

Because the Clinitest 5-drop color chart is different from the Clinitest 2-drop color chart, take care not to interchange the testing methods and color charts. Avoid touching the test tube during the chemical reaction because the heat can cause a burn. The Clinitest tablets are poisonous and must be stored out of the reach of young children —preferably in a dry, dark place, to minimize spoilage. Touching the tablets with a wet hand adds moisture and begins the chemical reaction; therefore, drop the tablet directly from its foil wrapper or container into the test tube. False positive reactions from Clinitest methods occur if the child is taking certain drugs, including Keflex, Keflin, salicylates, Vitamin C, or penicillin.

Enzyme Tape and Strips

Enzyme Testape and Clinitest enzyme strips offer fast measurement of urine glucose. They are convenient and easy to use, especially when the child is away from home on a trip or at school. These methods are only sensitive to low levels of glucose;

none indicate glucose concentrations higher than 2 percent. The enzyme determinators are dipped into urine and compared with a special color chart.

Acetone Test

Acetone is one of the ketone bodies that is easily measured in the urine. The amount of acetone in the urine indicates how the body is using—or not using—glucose. To test for acetone, place one drop of urine on a Acetest tablet and watch for color changes. A color chart comes with the tablets. Acetone also can be measured with Ketostix and Acestix, which are dipped in urine and observed for the change in color. Ketones are present in the urine when the child is using fats for energy because glucose is unavailable, and acetone should be checked in the child with glycosuria, continued vomiting, weight loss, and prior to surgery. The presence of acetone signals a metabolic problem.

Blood Tests

The *fasting blood glucose* (commonly called FBS, or fasting blood sugar) is drawn in the early morning after six to eight hours without food. Normal fasting glucose levels are 60 to 120 mg of glucose per 100 ml of blood. Higher levels indicate inadequate glucose usage. A postprandial (after meal) blood glucose test is drawn two hours after the child eats a prescribed amount of carbohydrates. Within two hours after a carbohydrate load, sufficient insulin should have been excreted to reduce the blood glucose to normal. Both the FBS and two-hour postprandial tests are only screening devices and may indicate an abnormality in glucose metabolism.

The *oral glucose tolerance test* (OGTT) is used for a more sensitive measurement of the child's ability to maintain a normal blood glucose level. For the OGTT, the child must eat a normal diet for at least three days prior to the test. Naturally, if the child is ill, such as with acidosis, the test cannot be done. Certain drugs including hormones, hypoglycemic agents, and diuretics are likely to influence the results; therefore, these drugs need to be discontinued at least three days before the test. For eight hours prior to the test, no food is permitted, although water is permitted. After the fasting, blood is drawn, and the child receives an oral glucose preparation; the dosage is based on his body weight. If the child vomits the glucose during the first hour, the test is canceled and rescheduled. Blood is drawn 30 minutes after the glucose load and at 30-minute intervals thereafter for three hours. The child may not have food during the test, but may drink water. It is difficult for a child to go from dinner until the following noon without food, and games, crafts, TV, and stories should be used to help pass the time.

Thyroid Tests

Two principal hormones are made in the thyroid: *thyroxine* (T_4) and *triiodothyronine* (T_3). Several tests measure the amount of these hormones in the body.

Radioactive Iodine Uptake

For the thyroid gland to make thyroxine (T_4) and triiodothyronine (T_3), sufficient iodine must be consumed in the diet and available in the body. The radioactive iodine (I^{131}) uptake study measures the amount of iodine the thyroid gland can absorb. For six to eight hours preceding the test, the child has nothing to eat or drink. He is then given a solution containing radioactive iodine (I^{131}). After ingesting the iodine, the child can have a regular diet. After twenty-four hours, the amount of I^{131} absorbed by the thyroid is measured by a scanning machine. Excessive accumulations of I^{131} indicate overproduction by the gland; conversely, small accumulations indicate a hypoactive thyroid gland. If the child vomits following ingestion of the solution, record the time and tell the physician.

T_3 and/or T_4 Serum Assay Tests

The total amount of thyroxine (T_4) and triiodothyronine (T_3) in the blood can be measured by the highly reliable T_3 and T_4 serum assay tests. Only a small sample of the child's blood is extracted for these tests.

Protein-Bound Iodine (PBI)

In the test for protein-bound iodine (PBI), a blood sample is drawn and studied for the iodine that is normally attached to serum proteins. A change from normal values indicates overproduction or underproduction of the thyroid gland. If the child has consumed a large amount of a cough medicine containing iodide shortly before he is tested, the PBI may be abnormally elevated.

Adrenal Function Tests

Vanillylmandelic Acid Test

Vanillylmandelic acid (VMA) is a metabolic product of both epinephrine (Adrenalin) and norepinephrine (noradrenalin), that is excreted in the urine, and can be measured to assess adrenal medulla function. For the VMA test, all urine voided during a 24-hour period is placed in a collection bottle containing a preservative. The bottle is kept in the refrigerator. For two days prior to the collection period, all tea, chocolate, and fruits should be removed from the diet since these foods are likely to give a false positive result.

17-Ketosteroids

Adrenal androgens, which are responsible for male secondary sexual characteristics and the presence of auxiliary and pubic hair in females, are excreted into the urine as 17-ketosteroids. To measure 17-ketosteroids, all urine voided for 24 hours is collected and kept in the refrigerator. No dietary restrictions are necessary for this test; in fact, the family frequently collects the specimen at home, bringing it to the laboratory for analysis. In a female's urine, the amount of 17-ketosteroids indicates the amount of adrenal androgen production, while the male's urine provides only a partial indicator, since androgens are also produced in the testes. Excessive androgens produce secondary male sexual characteristics in girls (*virilism*) and enhanced masculinization in boys.

COMMON TREATMENTS

Although surgery, radiation, medication, and hormonal replacement are all used to treat children with hormonal deviations, hormonal replacement is the most common therapy. This section focuses on the principles of hormone replacement, using insulin as an example.

Hormone Replacement

Insulin is a major hormone which regulates carbohydrate, fat, and protein metabolism. Insulin acts in the liver, fat tissue, and muscle to aid glucose use, stimulate the formation of glycogen (a complex sugar), and suppress glucose production.

Types of Insulin

There are three types of insulin: *short-acting,* such as Regular and Semilente insulins; *intermediate,* including NPH, Lente, and Globin; and *long-acting,* such as PZI and Ultralente. Notice in Table 19–1 that each type of insulin has a specific appearance, onset of action, peak effect, and duration of action. Each type is available in three concentrations: U–40, U–80, and U–100. *Concentration* means the amount of insulin per milliliter of liquid. U–40 Lente insulin has 40 units per ml; U–80 Lente has 80 units per ml, making it twice as concentrated. Each concentration of insulin has an accompanying marked syringe (see Figure 19–1).

The most frequent error in insulin dosage is caused by mismatching syringe and concentration. A U–40 bottle of insulin, for example, must be used with a U–40 syringe. Another important principle is that a unit of insulin always remains the same amount. For example, if a child needs 20 units of regular insulin, you can use U–40, U–80, or U–100 Regular insulin and withdraw 20 units with the appropriate syringe. Some insulin syringes have a U–40 scale on one side and a U–80 scale on the other. This is confusing for everyone; a single marked syringe is preferable. Eventually, U–100 insulin will replace U–40 and U–80 concentrations, providing a standard insulin concentration.

Children with diabetes mellitus usually are treated with an intermediate-acting insulin that lasts 24 hours. Sometimes a short-acting insulin, such as Regular, is combined with the intermediate insulin for added insulin effect during the morning. If added insulin is needed during the evening and night, a second injection of intermediate insulin (perhaps with the addition of short-acting insulin) is given before dinner. The insulin type and dosage prescribed varies according to the child's age, weight, activity, health (illness and stress necessitate added insulin), and development. Preferably the family should understand the different types, action, and concentrations of insulin. When the family is knowledgeable about insulin options, they can help the physician in determining dosage regulation.

With the exception of Regular insulin, which can be given intravenously and subcutaneously (SC), all insulins are given subcutaneously. Insulin remains potent for 36 months when refrigerated and 18 to 24 months at room temperature. Children

Table 19–1. **Types of Insulin**

Type	*Appearance*	*Effect Begins (in hours)*	*Peak Effect (in hours)*	*Duration of Effect (in hours)*
Regular	Clear	½–1	2–4	5–7
Semilente	Cloudy	½–1	2–4	12–16
NPH	Milky	2–4	8–12	24–28
Lente	Cloudy	2–4	8–12	24–28
Protamine zinc (PZI)	Cloudy	4–8	16–24	36+
Ultralente	Cloudy	4–8	14–24	36+

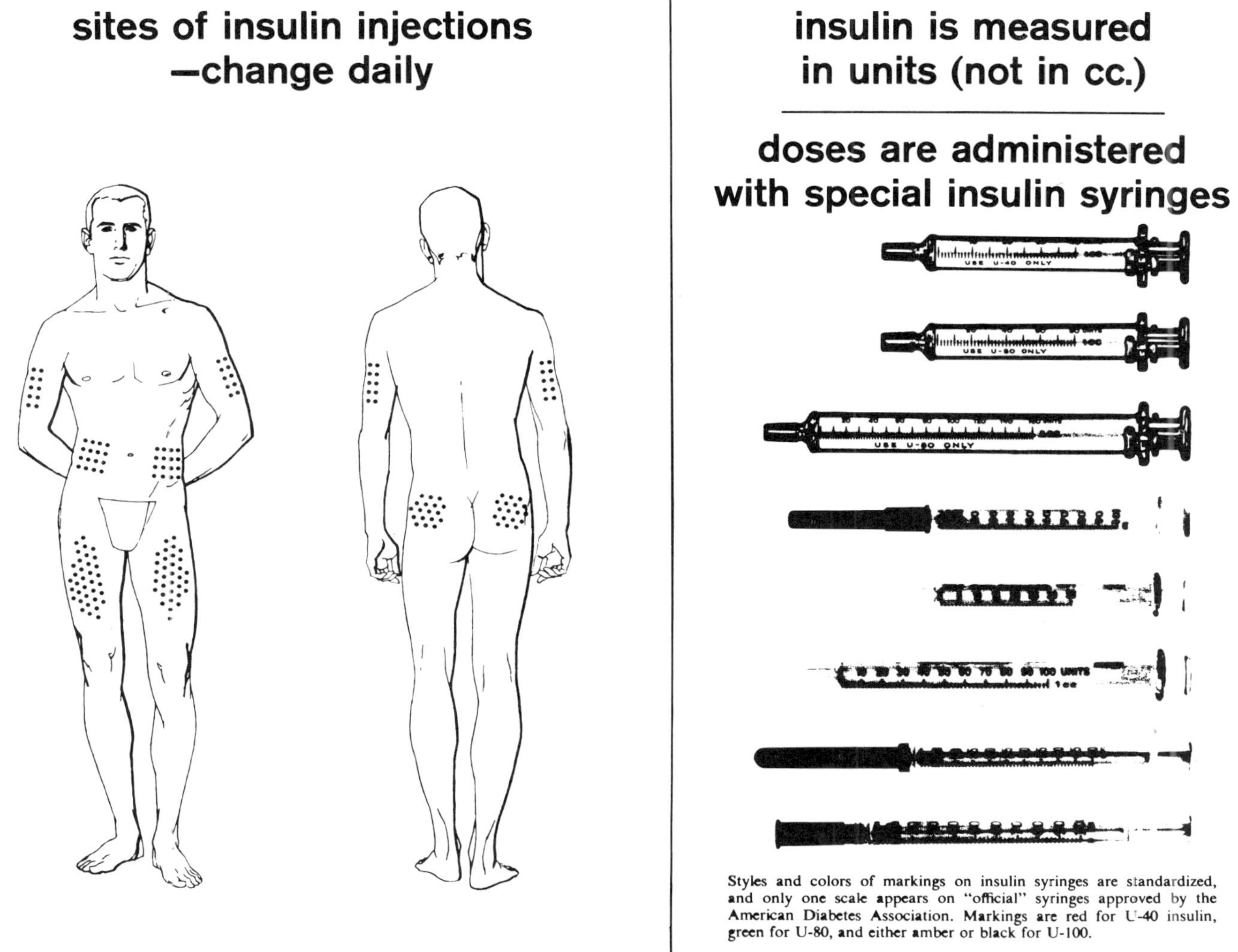

Figure 19–1. *Insulin: injection sites and measurement.* (Courtesy, Eli Lilly and Company)

using insulin daily can leave it at room temperature; however, if insulin is used only intermittently, as in hospitals and clinics, it is best to keep it refrigerated. Insulin needs protection from intense light and temperature extremes, and while it should not be kept on a window sill, subject to direct sunlight, it can be stored safely in a medicine cabinet. If you are ever unsure about the potency of a bottle of insulin, examine the color. Regular and Globin insulins are clear; the other types are cloudy but free of clumps or aggregations.

Insulin Administration

The mechanics of insulin injection are the same as for any injectable medication (see Figure 19–2). Since insulin is injected every day, however, site rotation is very important. If sites are not rotated, subcutaneous skin *atrophy* or *hypertrophy* may occur at repeatedly used injection sites. Atrophy may begin as a slight dimpling of the skin and progress to extensive and disfiguring pitting of the subcutaneous tissue. Although atrophy does not impair the effectiveness of the insulin, disfigurement can be embarrassing and traumatic for the child. Hypertrophy looks like a spongy mass of fibrous and avascular scar tissue at the injection site, and commonly occurs on the anterior and lateral thighs. If insulin is injected into a hypertrophied area, absorption is slow and incomplete. The hypertrophied area becomes anesthetized, and since the child feels little discomfort when injecting into this area, the site may be preferred and used repeatedly—increasing the problem. Both hypertrophy and atrophy can occur in the same child; in fact, children seem more likely than adults to have both atrophy and hypertrophy.

Rotating the injection site provides both the best prevention and therapy. The same site should never be used more than once a month. Site rotation charts can easily be made by sketching a figure with numbers corresponding to days of the month noted on the arms, legs, thighs, abdomen, and buttocks. If today is the tenth, then the child finds the number 10 on the figure and uses the corresponding site on his body for the injection. Make sure everyone assisting or giving the child's insulin injection knows the rotation system. At each injection, record the site used on the child's chart.

When ready to draw up insulin, gently rotate the bottle in your palms both to warm the insulin (if it has been in the refrigerator), and to mix a cloudy insulin. Never shake insulin. If a short-acting insulin is to be mixed with an intermediate insulin (for example, Regular and NPH), always draw up the short-acting insulin first. Then add the intermediate insulin to the syringe. This sequence avoids any accidental mixing of intermediate insulin with the rapid-acting insulin, which needs to be kept pure for its rapid-action time to remain constant. If some of the short-acting insulin accidently enters the intermediate bottle, however, it does not change the effect of the immediate insulin.

When giving an insulin injection, pinch, or bunch up the skin with one hand. Then, with the syringe in the other hand, enter the skin at a 90° angle. Insert the needle the entire length to ensure deposit of the insulin into the subcutaneous tissue. Draw back on the plunger to make sure you are not in a vein (blood will appear if you are). Although an insulin injection may seem like two steps (withdrawing and injection) it actually involves over twenty steps (Figures 19–3 and 19–4).

When teaching families about insulin,

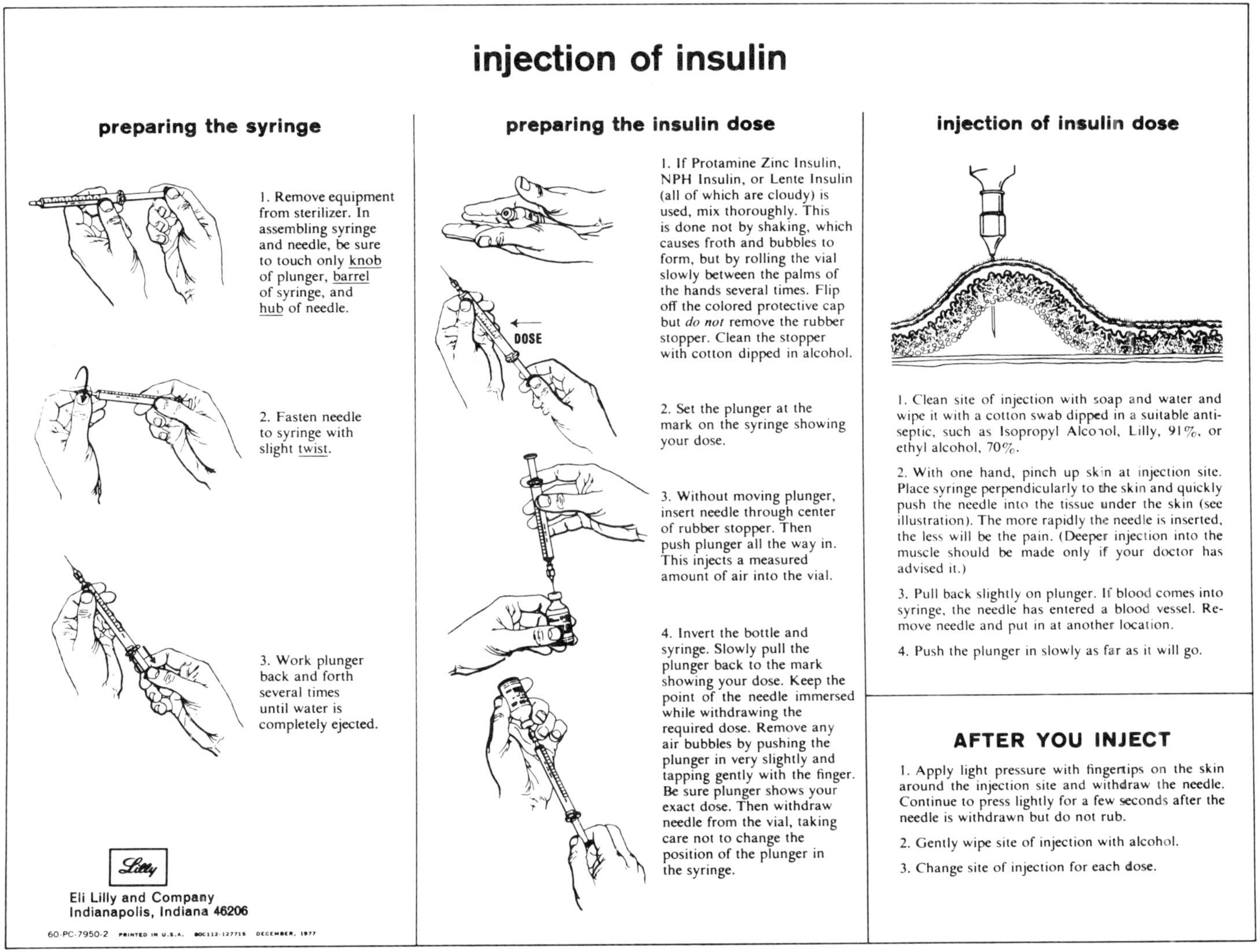

injection of insulin

preparing the syringe

1. Remove equipment from sterilizer. In assembling syringe and needle, be sure to touch only knob of plunger, barrel of syringe, and hub of needle.

2. Fasten needle to syringe with slight twist.

3. Work plunger back and forth several times until water is completely ejected.

Eli Lilly and Company
Indianapolis, Indiana 46206

60-PC-7950-2 PRINTED IN U.S.A. DOC112-127719 DECEMBER, 1977

preparing the insulin dose

1. If Protamine Zinc Insulin, NPH Insulin, or Lente Insulin (all of which are cloudy) is used, mix thoroughly. This is done not by shaking, which causes froth and bubbles to form, but by rolling the vial slowly between the palms of the hands several times. Flip off the colored protective cap but *do not* remove the rubber stopper. Clean the stopper with cotton dipped in alcohol.

DOSE

2. Set the plunger at the mark on the syringe showing your dose.

3. Without moving plunger, insert needle through center of rubber stopper. Then push plunger all the way in. This injects a measured amount of air into the vial.

4. Invert the bottle and syringe. Slowly pull the plunger back to the mark showing your dose. Keep the point of the needle immersed while withdrawing the required dose. Remove any air bubbles by pushing the plunger in very slightly and tapping gently with the finger. Be sure plunger shows your exact dose. Then withdraw needle from the vial, taking care not to change the position of the plunger in the syringe.

injection of insulin dose

1. Clean site of injection with soap and water and wipe it with a cotton swab dipped in a suitable antiseptic, such as Isopropyl Alcohol, Lilly, 91%, or ethyl alcohol, 70%.

2. With one hand, pinch up skin at injection site. Place syringe perpendicularly to the skin and quickly push the needle into the tissue under the skin (see illustration). The more rapidly the needle is inserted, the less will be the pain. (Deeper injection into the muscle should be made only if your doctor has advised it.)

3. Pull back slightly on plunger. If blood comes into syringe, the needle has entered a blood vessel. Remove needle and put in at another location.

4. Push the plunger in slowly as far as it will go.

AFTER YOU INJECT

1. Apply light pressure with fingertips on the skin around the injection site and withdraw the needle. Continue to press lightly for a few seconds after the needle is withdrawn but do not rub.

2. Gently wipe site of injection with alcohol.

3. Change site of injection for each dose.

Figure 19–2. *Preparing the insulin injection.* (Courtesy, Eli Lilly and Company)

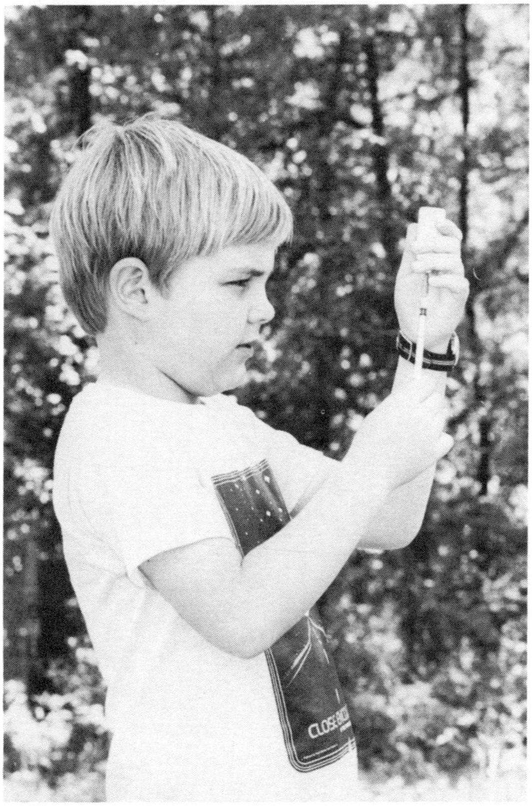

Figure 19–3. *This child is in a summer camp for diabetic children where he learns self-care skills.*

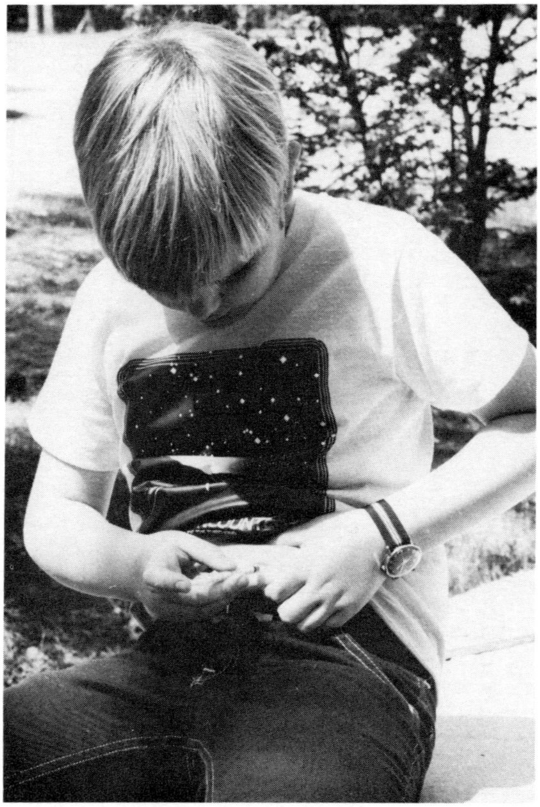

Figure 19–4. *Self-administration of insulin; this can be accomplished only after the child has learned more than 20 steps in preparing the injection.*

begin by discussing the different types and concentrations available. Then explain how insulin is stored and mixed. Discuss site rotation, how to inspect for and recognize atrophy and hypertrophy, and the equipment needed (syringe, needle, cotton balls, alcohol, and insulin) before you teach the actual injection technique.

Teaching Families about Hormonal Deviations

Of course, insulin is not the only hormone replaced in children who have a hormonal deficit. Table 19–2 shows that antidiuretic hormone, vasopressin, thyroid, and steroids are all administered for hormonal disorders. Whenever a hormone is administered, the effect of the hormone must be considered, and the child and his parents should be informed about the desired action of the hormone. This will help parent and child determine if sufficient amounts of hormone are being replaced. They should be aware of the frequently dangerous side effects of excess hormonal replacement, such as hypoglycemia which results from too much insulin. Equally important are signs of hormone insufficiency. Because children are growing, their metabolic and related hormone needs continuously increase. Regular increases in hormone because of growth are normal and essential.

Physical and emotional stress affect hormonal needs and an increased dosage frequently is necessary during illness. For example, when a child with diabetes has an infection, his temperature and metabolic rate increase, and his body needs extra glucose and more insulin to use the glucose. Whenever a diabetic child is ill, the family should notify the physician so the insulin dosage can be adjusted. Usually insulin is adjusted by a percentage, not by a set number of units, and the child who normally injects 20 units of insulin will probably need a 10 to 20 percent increase (up to 22 to 24 units) during a cold, flu, or other illness. A percentage increase is always much safer than a set number of units, which may be too much for one child and far too little for another.

Children with a hormonal deviation should carry identification stating their name, address, phone number, and what emergency measures are necessary if they act or look ill. The school teacher, scout leader, baby-sitter and others who spend time with the child need to understand his disorder. Understanding avoids erroneous assumptions and unnecessary limitations.

Identification, emergency care, and hormonal regulation can seem very frightening to the family whose only previous experience with illness was with a cold or flu. Most hormonal disorders are chronic and demand lifelong medication. Families are expected to perform a wide array of procedures skillfully. There are no days off from insulin injection or thyroid administration. The child is different. His activities and diet need more attention; and when he is ill, his medications may require regulation and special care. The long-term nature of the disorder, coupled with the possibility of acute and chronic complications, can produce chronic anxiety for the entire family. Often it is the nurse who repeatedly instructs, reassesses the health status, and coordinates a teaching and support plan for the child and family.

Each child, regardless of age, needs to understand his disorder. The toddler may only need to know that he takes a special medicine every day to stay well. The preschooler can understand more about how the medicine helps keep his body healthy. The four- to five-year-old child is eager to help in daily procedures. The preschool child's participation in suitable tasks, such as matching the urine test to the color chart, or holding the alcohol swab for the injection should be encouraged. By school age he can take responsibility for some of his care. The six-year-old can complete his urine tests alone. By age eight or ten, most children have the fine motor coordination to learn self-injection (with parental supervision, of course). By adolescence, the diabetic can assume responsibility for his disorder, using his parents as consultants.

Although limitations and precautions are continually repeated to families, the nurse sometimes forgets to emphasize all the child *can* do because of treatment. Stress the positive effects of treatment as well as the precautions. It is helpful to make a "worry" and "no-worry" list for the family. If diet, exercise, and skin care are no different for the child with a hormonal disorder than the non-affected child, then say so on your "no-worry" list. Planning the future for the child with a chronic disorder is often crucial for family integrity. If parents have a positive attitude—and if people who

Table 19–2. Common Conditions of Hormonal Imbalance

Condition	*Definition*	*Treatment*	*Special Nursing Considerations*
	Increased Hormone Secretion (Hypersecretion)		
Cushing's syndrome	Overproduction of cortisol by the adrenal cortex or as the result of long-term steroid therapy. Signs of excess cortisol include slowing of growth; redistribution of fat to the face, shoulder, and trunk; loss of muscular activity, and hypertension. (These features are referred to as cushingoid appearance.)	If a tumor exists, surgical removal is attempted; if no tumor is found, the pituitary is irradiated since the pituitary secretes ACTH which stimulates the adrenal glands to secrete cortisol. If a major portion or all of the adrenal gland is removed, oral replacement cortisol is needed for life.	
Giantism	Excessive secretion of growth hormone causing rapid longitudinal growth. Without treatment the child may grow 8 feet tall. After linear growth is completed, growth hormone hypersecretion leads to thickening of bones and soft tissue, causing enlargement of the hands and feet, a condition called *acromegaly*. As the excessive secretion continues, the child becomes easily fatigued, weak, and lethargic. The skin is coarse and oily. The head size increases and leads to signs of increased intracranial pressure (See Ch. 27).	If a tumor exists, surgical removal is recommended; if no tumor exists, irradiation may be used to reduce the production of growth hormone.	Encourage good nutrition to meet increased body demands. Plan high protein snacks and extra calories with each meal.
Hyperthyroidism (Graves' disease)	Excessive secretion of thyroid hormone. Most common among adolescent females, un-	Oral drugs that block the production of thyroid hormone, such as methimazole (Tapazole) and	Monitor the child for possible toxic reactions to the drug treatment, such as skin rash,

	common in children, and rare among infants. Symptoms develop slowly over a 6- to 12-month period. Metabolism increases, resulting in a rapid pulse, forceful heartbeat, and elevated systolic pressure. Weight loss is accompanied by appetite increase. The thyroid gland is enlarged, visible, and palpable. The patient is nervous and "jumpy" and sleep, gross body movements, and concentration are disturbed. A wide-eyed stare and protrusion of the eyes (exophthalmos) are common.	propylthiouracil. If drugs do not correct the secretion, most or part of the thyroid may be surgically removed. Following surgery, thyroid hormone replacement may be necessary.	itching, fever, pain, or swelling. Instruct the family to report early signs of possible postsurgical infections, including skin lesions, a sore throat, or fever.
	Decreased Hormone Secretion (Hyposecretion)		
Adrenogenital syndrome (Congenital adrenal hyperplasia, CAH)	An inherited deficiency, leading to a deficient secretion of *hydrocortisone* and an excessive production of *androgens*. Both hormones are produced in the adrenal gland. Without sufficient hydrocortisone, the child cannot respond adequately to the stress of infection, surgery, or trauma. Excessive production of androgens causes rapid bone growth and sexual maturation. Females with CAH have fetal enlargement of the clitoris and labia that, at birth, may be mistaken for male genitalia. However, the uterus, tubes, and ovaries are completely normal. Males with CAH ap-	Replacement hydrocortisone, which must be continued for life, usually is given IM to the infant and young child (to ensure exact intake and predictable results) and orally to the older child. Plastic surgery is indicated for girls with an enlarged clitoris or closed labia. Children deficient in aldosterone must take extra salt in their diet. A salt-retaining hormone, such as desoxycorticosterone acetate (DOCA), is given to infants as a monthly injection or placed under the skin in pellets that last about a year. By age one, most children can discontinue DOCA and be given a	Counsel parents that CAH is an autosomal recessive condition. Each child of carrier parents has a 25 percent chance of inheriting this disorder. Instruct parents to report early signs of illness such as sore throat, cold, or fever so that changes in hydrocortisone dosage can be made. An emergency exists when the child is pale and cool (signs of shock), has vomited repeatedly, or is unconscious. At these times the child must immediately receive intramuscular hydrocortisone sodium succinate (Solu-Cortef). Teach parents how to give the intramuscular injection and tell them to inject the Solu-Cortef

(continued)

Table 19–2. *(Continued)*

Condition	*Definition*	*Treatment*	*Special Nursing Considerations*
	pear normal at birth but have rapid genital growth with an adult-size penis and scrotum by age two or three. One-half of all infants with CAH have a deficiency of aldosterone, the salt-retaining hormone. These infants have a poor appetite, vomit frequently, and fail to gain weight. The sodium loss causes dehydration, shock, and death. All children with CAH have high levels of 17-ketosteroids (the breakdown product of androgens) in their urine.	high oral salt intake and/or daily Florinef Acetate (fluorocortisone acetate), an oral salt-retaining hormone. CAH children are in danger of collapse or death under such stress as surgery, trauma, or illness, because more hydrocortisone is needed. At these times hydrocortisone dosage must be increased three to four times. For emergencies, a rapid-acting injectable hydrocortisone is given.	while someone else calls the doctor. Stress that the Solu-Cortef may save the child's life and will not harm him if given unnecessarily. Recommend that an ampul of Solu-Cortef be kept in the automobile and home medicine cabinet for emergency use. Reassure the parents of a girl needing plastic surgery that normal sexual function and appearance can be expected because her internal organs are not affected. Parents need help in overcoming guilt feelings and fear about their child's abnormal genitalia.
Sexual ambiguity	Incomplete development of external genitalia structures at birth, occurring in one of every 1,000 births. Most common cause of sexual ambiguity in the female is the adrenogenital syndrome (discussed above); other causes include genetic changes, enzyme defects, and hormonal deficit. Types of sexual ambiguity include: *female pseudo-hermaphrodites:* females with some male characteristics; *male pseudo-*	Gender assignment one to four days after birth, using a karyotype (See Ch. 3). Hormone replacement as needed. Surgery to remove structures not congruous with gender, and construction and/or enlargement of needed structures.	Parents are grieved and anxious. Explain to parents that the child's sex organs were not completely developed. Use and help parents understand proper terminology of the genitalia, such as *clitoris, labia majora* and *scrotum.* This will help parents explain the child's problem to relatives and friends. Parents are distressed to hear the term *intersex* or *pseudo-hermaphrodite* and these diagnostic terms should

	hermaphrodites: males with some female characteristics; *intersex:* a child with both ovarian and testicular tissue.		be used only for charts and medical conferences. Assure parents that the child will not grow up with abnormal sexual desires because parents frequently confuse the term *hermaphrodite* with *homosexual.* If sterility is predicted, it is better for the child to grow up with this knowledge than to discover it later.
Diabetes Insipidus: Neurogenic	A lack of antidiuretic hormone (vasopressin), normally secreted in the hypothalamus and stored in the posterior pituitary, which may be caused by a lesion, tumor, or injury to the posterior pituitary. The kidney is unable to concentrate urine, and large amounts of water are lost, and the urine is pale or colorless and very dilute. The specific gravity is 1.001 to 1.005 (normal 1.010 to 1.015). Because of water loss, the child is thirsty and may drink 4 to 40 liters of water in a single day (1 to 2 liters is normal). The child loses weight and is febrile, dehydrated, and constipated.	Surgery, if a tumor is causing the hormone deficiency. When the cause is unknown, intramuscular vasopressin (Pitressin Tannate) in oil, administered every one to three days, will control the symptoms; dosage depends on daily number, volume, and specific gravity of urinations, as well as amount of fluid ingested.	Until the child has a normal urine output, all liquids consumed and urine excreted are measured and recorded. Carefully pour all liquids into a measuring cup, read the amount at eye level, and record it. Although a specific gravity and measurement are done on *each* voiding during hospitalization, one to two measurements a day are sufficient for pitressin regulation when the child returns home. Help the parents to set up a recording system. During hospitalization, assess hydration daily by noting and recording the child's skin turgor, thirst level, body temperature, and body weight. Pitressin administration is very difficult because the hormone is suspended in an oil base. To

(Continued)

Table 19–2. *(Continued)*

Condition	*Definition*	*Treatment*	*Special Nursing Considerations*
			administer Pitressin: place the ampul in warm water; shake the ampul vigorously to mix the brown vasopressin granules; *Quickly* withdraw the correct dosage; Inject before the vasopressin granules separate. Inform parents that additional pitressin is needed after vomiting or diarrhea and remind them to report illness quickly.
Nephrogenic	A sex-linked disorder affecting males. Here, the problem is in the kidney, which cannot respond to vasopressin, the antidiuretic hormone. The symptoms are the same as those of neurogenic diabetes insipidus.	No specific treatment. Child is given enough water to prevent dehydration and maintain serum osmolality. Diuretics, such as hydrochlorothiazide and ethacrynic acid, are used in combination with a restricted sodium intake to reduce urinary volume and increase urinary concentration. Proper nutrition is crucial.	
Juvenile diabetes mellitus	Acute insulin deficiency resulting in the inability to metabolize carbohydrates because the pancreas cannot produce sufficient amounts of insulin. The exact cause is unknown. Signs of insulin insufficiency are polydipsia, polyuria, and loss of body fat. Acute ketoacidosis	Replacement Insulin. Dietary Restrictions: *Free Diet*—A diet well balanced in all essential nutrients, containing little or no artificial food stuffs, but including nutritious snacks such as crackers and cheese, fruit, or a sandwich at mid-morning, mid-afternoon,	A teaching program that includes information, demonstrations, and supervision of the following: *Urine testing*—how and when to collect and test urine for sugar and acetone; recording the results. *Pathophysiology*—location and function of the

	is common before diagnosis. Complications include diabetic ketoacidosis and hypoglycemia.	and bedtime; *Exchange Diet*—A prescribed system of food lists categorized according to carbohydrate, protein, and fat content. The child is allowed a certain number of selections from each list; certain foods from one list can be "exchanged" for foods from another list.	pancreas; changes caused by lack of insulin. *Insulin*—types, concentrations, actions, and effects; site rotation and skin inspection; equipment for an injection; injection techniques; mixing two insulins in the same syringe. *Hypoglycemia*—signs; first aid, including how to use glucagon. *Ketoacidosis* signs. *Illness*—notify physician; test each urine for sugar and acetone; continue insulin dosage; have the child take sips of ginger ale or Coca-Cola syrup if nauseated.
Pituitary dwarfism	Deficiency of growth hormone, causing slow growth, extreme shortness, and physical immaturity first noticed at two or three years of age although his body proportions are normal. Secondary sexual characteristics fail to develop.	Intramuscular pituitary growth hormone (from human cadavers) is injected two to three times a week. Maximum growth occurs during the first year of treatment. If deficiencies exist, replacement of thyroid hormone and/or adrenal steroids are necessary.	Short stature creates a psychological problem that increases as puberty approaches and self-concept and vocational desires solidify. Use vocabulary and play interactions appropriate for the child's age, regardless of his physical appearance. Teach the family how to administer the intramuscular injections of growth hormone.
Hypothyroidism:	Deficiency of thyroid hormone.		
Congenital (cretinism)	The infant appears normal at birth because he has been supplied thyroid from his mother, but signs of thyroid deficiency develop within a few weeks or months following	Thyroid is given in graduated dosages until the maximum that does not produce symptoms of overdosage is reached. Thyroid must be taken for life. The child must	*Normal* brain growth during the first six months depends on sufficient amounts of thyroid hormone. If the child is hypothyroid during this period, he is likely to have

(Continued)

Table 19–2. *(Continued)*

Condition	*Definition*	*Treatment*	*Special Nursing Considerations*
	birth. Signs of congenital hypothyroidism include dry skin, constipation, low temperature and pulse, pallor, and feeding problems (the child feeds slowly and chokes easily). The infant sleeps a lot, is sluggish when awake, and has a hoarse cry. All physical, motor, mental, and sexual development is retarded.	also consume adequate amounts of Vitamin D to prevent rickets, because thyroid causes rapid bone growth.	permanent mental defects. Instruct parents to recognize the side effects of thyroid overdosage: rapid pulse, weight loss, vomiting, diarrhea, irritability, and elevated temperature.
Acquired (juvenile hypothyroidism)	Lack of thyroid causes a delay in growth and development. The child looks pudgy and immature. Heart rate is slow and pulse pressure low. Poor circulation leads to skin pallor, coolness, and dryness. The child acts sluggish, and his tendon reflexes are slow.	Oral thyroid hormone for life.	Teach parents the side effects of thyroid overdosage (See above). Increased growth that follows thyroid treatment needs added Vitamin D and calcium in 3 to 4 glasses of milk every day. Offer high protein foods and snacks plus extra calories to meet the child's increased metabolic needs. These children are prone to tooth decay and should brush after each meal. Sweets should be restricted, and regular dental care is essential.
Hypoglycemia	Hypoglycemia (low blood sugar) is a symptom of a larger problem (e.g., diabetes mellitus), never a disorder by itself. An infant of low birth weight is	Intravenous glucose followed by carbohydrates is given to newborns; the older child receives intramuscular glucagon, which changes glycogen into	Never offer liquids with added carbohydrates to a child who is incoherent; use injectable glucagon. Follow all glucose treatments with food. If the

	hypoglycemic if his blood sugar (BS) is less than 20 mg/100 ml. The full-term baby, at least three days old, is hypoglycemic if his BS is less than 30 mg/100 ml. For the older child, a BS less than 50 mg/100 ml is hypoglycemic. Signs of hypoglycemia in the infant include irritability, eye rolling, sweating, twitching, jitteriness, cyanosis, and seizures. The older child has pallor, sweating, distured behavior (i.e., headaches, irritability, and negativism), rapid pulse, seizures, and even coma. Hypoglycemia most often occurs in newborns, with particularly low birth weight babies and infants of toxemic or diabetic mothers.	glucose. (This treatment is ineffective in the newborn because his glycogen stores are small.) The child also should be given five or six feedings daily of a diet high in protein and carbohydrates.	child is ill and anorectic or vomiting, offer him liquids high in carbohydrates. The blood glucose level can be tested quickly with Dextrostix (a specially treated paper strip). Drop one drop of blood from the heel of a newborn, toe of an infant, or finger of a child on to the Dextrostix. Wait 60 seconds, then rinse the Dextrostix with water, and match the color on the Dextrostix to those on the chart on the outside of the Dextrostix container.
Hypoparathyroidism hypocalcemia	A deficiency of parathormone, which most commonly occurs during the first two to three days after birth. The child has a low calcium level of 5 to 7 mg/100 ml (normal is 10 to 12 mg/100 ml) which causes muscle pain and cramps, resulting in numbness, stiffness, and twitching of the hands and feet—a condition called *tetany*. Convulsions with loss of consciousness may occur, and hypoparathyroidism is frequently mistaken for epilepsy.	Emergency care for tetany is intravenous calcium gluconate. Replacement treatment is oral Vitamin D and supplemental calcium. Delay in treatment may result in permanent physical and mental impairment.	Have emergency equipment at the bedside in case laryngospasm and the need for intubation.

(Continued)

Table 19–2. *(Continued)*

Condition	*Definition*	*Treatment*	*Special Nursing Considerations*
Addison's disease (chronic adrenal cortisol insufficiency)	A lack of cortisol, aldosterone, and androgens—hormones made in the adrenal cortex. The child suffers muscle weakness, anorexia, and loss of weight and may have hypoglycemia and convulsions. Cortisol is essential for normal stress responses to surgical stress, trauma, or infection. A lack of *aldosterone* causes increased losses of water and salt in the urine, leading to hypotension. *Androgen* deficiencies cause loss of axillary and pubic hair.	Replacement therapy with oral cortisol and an aldosterone analogue.	Prompt medical attention for infection and special care for minor surgery, such as a tooth extraction is essential. The minor stress of an infection can cause an *adrenal crisis*. Signs of adrenal crisis include cool, clammy skin; a febrile pulse; and low blood pressure. Immediate hormonal replacement is needed for survival.

continually assess, teach, and care for the medical needs of the child are optimistic and truthful—the child will view his disorder as a challenge instead of a burden.

Clinical Application

"Why did you do it? Why, John, why?" John, an only child, is fifteen and has been a diabetic for two years. He was admitted yesterday in diabetic ketoacidosis after not taking his insulin for three days. Following intravenous fluids and insulin, John's vital signs are stable. He is alert but refuses to talk to anyone.

John's mother remains at the bedside, pleading for an answer as his father paces the floor. Grandparents enter the room as you prepare to give John's morning NPH and regular insulin. Suddenly, John's mother says, "Stop. Your syringe is marked U−40, and John uses only U−80."

> Discuss the difference between U−40 and U−80 insulin, offering an explanation of the term *concentration*.

Following the injection, the grandmother asks why an injection is necessary. Her brother, aged seventy-five, has been a diabetic for twenty years and only takes pills.

> You explain that the oral hypoglycemic agents are used to stimulate the pancreas to secrete added insulin; however, in children the pancreas does not respond to produce sufficient amounts of insulin or insulin that is effective. That's why children need insulin injections.

John quickly eats his breakfast and asks for a second tray. His mother responds by telling John that one serving is sufficient, and if he eats more he will get fat.

> You recognize that John has many demands for increased food intake. He is in puberty and experiencing rapid body growth. In addition, he has been unable to use glucose since stopping his insulin. Now, with insulin available, body cells are eager for glucose to restore normal metabolism.
> Explain John's need for extra nutrients to his mother. Include an explanation of how insulin works and the changes that occur when John's body lacks insulin.

The grandmother asks why John's food is not measured and selected from exchanged lists.

> Knowing John is on a "free diet," explain what this means. Contrast the free diet to an exchange plan.

At 11:30 P.M. John tests his urine, and the result is 2 percent. "Bad!" exclaims his father. "See, that's what happens when you eat too much." His father asks why the percent sign is used instead of the + sign which is on their urine chart at home.

> Explain what 2 percent sugar means, discussing individual differences in the kidney's ability to spill or reabsorb sugar. Discuss the different tests for glycosuria, reviewing how each test is done and the type of information yielded. Lastly, explain why 2 percent glucose is not necessarily "bad."

After his parents and grandparents leave for lunch, you tell John that he seems very unhappy and that you are concerned about him. Spend the next 20 minutes with him and the time can be used to talk, play cards, or whatever he chooses. John asks if you can get an order to keep his family out of the room. He continues that his parents and grandparents continually nag him about diet, urine tests, food amounts, and exercise. He is angry at them and his "dumb diabetes." He decided to stop taking his insulin to "see what would happen."

You comment that diabetes requires a lot of time for urine testing, injections, diet, and all the care necessary to stay feeling good. It is natural to get tired and angry at the routine. His parents are concerned and worry about him, and that causes them to be anxious and seem to be always checking on him. You offer to talk to John and his parents together to review the basics of diabetes, emphasizing what needs to be worried about (for example, insulin dosage, illness, and hypoglycemia) and what need not be a concern (second helpings of food, a positive urine sugar, and so on). His parents return from lunch and are eager to review diabetic care.

Since John will be hospitalized three more days, you decide to spend 1 hour daily with the family, 30 minutes in the morning and 30 minutes in the afternoon. Construct a teaching plan that reviews the physiology of diabetes, causes and signs of uncontrolled diabetes (hypoglycemia and ketoacidosis), insulin dosage and regulation, urine tests and records, and diet planning. Offer guidelines for care on sick days and insulin regulation when activity and diet vary. How will you assess the present understanding level of John and his parents in each topic? List questions that will aid in an assessment.

How will you present the teaching material; in what order? How can you evaluate their understanding of the material you teach? How do the special emotional and physical needs of the adolescent affect your teaching plan? (This is a good time to review normal adolescent behavior in chapter 8, identifying the conflicts and concerns of the adolescent).

The next morning John is to receive 10 units of Regular insulin and 25 units of NPH insulin. Since John will continue on this new dosage, it is necessary for him to learn how to mix and self-administer the insulins.

Write a teaching plan, listing each step you want to demonstrate.

During your 20-minute sessions with John, he continues to express feelings of being overly protected and unnecessarily restricted by his parents and grandparents. He feels angry and inadequate. Deciding John and his family need a therapeutic opportunity to discuss feelings about the problems of living with diabetes, you refer them to a family nurse therapist. The weekly sessions are very helpful, and after three months the therapy ends with John assuming the major responsibility for his diabetes.

Bibliography

Brimblecombe, F. and Barltrap, D. *Children in Health and Disease,* ed. 1. London, Balliere Tindall, 1978.

Fonville, A. Teaching Patients to Rotate Injection Sites. *American Journal of Nursing* 78:880, 1978.

Garber, R. The Use of a Standardized Teaching Program in Diabetes Education. *Nursing Clinics of North America* 12:375, 1977.

Gardner, L. I. (ed). *Endocrine and Genetic Diseases of Childhood and Adolescence,* ed. 2. Philadelphia, W.B. Saunders Co., 1975.

Gellis, A. and Kagan, B. *Current Pediatric Therapy*, ed. 8. Philadelphia, W.B. Saunders, Co., 1978.

Guthrie, D. Diabetic Children: Preparing Them to Live, in *Managing Diabetes Properly*. Horsham, Pa., Intermed Communications, Nursing '77 Books, 1977.

Guthrie, D. and Guthrie, R. Diabetic Ketoacidosis. *Nursing '78* 8:55, 1978.

Hill, S. The Child with Ambiguous Genitalia. *American Journal of Nursing* 77:810, 1977.

Hobdell, E.F. Growing Up Without Growing: The Child with Growth Hormone Deficiency. *American Journal of Maternal-Child Nursing* 2:298, 1977.

Krueger, J. and Ray, J. *Endocrine Problems in Nursing*. St. Louis, C.V. Mosby Co., 1976.

Lundin, D. Reporting Urine Test Results: Switch from + to %. *American Journal of Nursing* 78:878, 1977.

McFarlane, J.M. Congenital Adrenal Hyperplasia. *American Journal of Nursing* 78:1290, 1976.

———. The Child with Diabetes Mellitus. *Pediatric Nursing* 1:6, 1975.

Moses, A. Diabetes Insipidus and ADH Regulation. *Hospital Practice* 13:37, 1977.

Parks, J. Endocrine Disorders of Childhood. *Hospital Practice* 12:93, 1977.

Schaefer, C. and Millman, H. *Therapies for Children*. San Francisco, Jossey-Bass Publishers, 1977.

Slater, N. Insulin Reactions to Ketoacidosis: Guidelines for Diagnosis and Intervention. *American Journal of Nursing* 78:875, 1978.

Small, D. A Patient Education Program. *American Journal of Nursing* 78:889, 1978.

Spencer, R.T. *Patient Care in Endocrine Problems*. Philadelphia, W.B. Saunders Co., 1973.

Steele, S. *Nursing Care of the Child with Long-Term Illness*, ed. 2. New York, Appleton-Century-Crofts, 1977.

Steiner, M. *Clinical Approaches to Endocrine Problems in Children*. St. Louis, C.V. Mosby Co., 1970.

Walesky, M. Diabetic Ketoacidosis. *American Journal of Nursing* 78:872, 1978.

Wolfe, L. Insulin: Paving the Way to a New Life. *Nursing '77* 7:38, 1977.

CHAPTER **20**

The Child with Cancer

BEHAVIORAL OBJECTIVES

After studying this chapter you will be able to:

- Discuss immunosuppression and myelosuppression, identifying the accompanying health problems.
- Discuss infection in the child with cancer, stating the prophylactic, acute, and continual nursing care needed to prevent and control infection.
- Discuss bleeding problems in the child with cancer, stating prophylactic, acute, and continual nursing care measures to prevent and control bleeding or hemorrhaging.
- Explain the use of noninvasive and invasive studies for diagnosing neoplasms, listing nursing interventions for each.
- Contrast the use of surgery, chemotherapy, radiotherapy, and immunotherapy as cancer treatments explaining when each is used, the desired effect, common side effects, and nursing interventions.
- Make a teaching plan explaining common diagnosis and treatment to the child with cancer, and his family. Discuss ways to promote understanding by both child and adults.

TERMS AND CONCEPTS

Immunosuppression
Myelosuppression
Lymphocytes
T Lymphocytes
B Lymphocytes
Erythrocytes
Platelets
Petechiae
Ecchymoses
Invasive test
Noninvasive test
Bone Marrow Aspiration
Biopsy
Chemotherapy
Induction
Maintenance
Remission
Relapse
Cyclic therapy
Central nervous system prophylaxis
Intrathecal
Alopecia
Radiotherapy
Radiosensitive
Radioresistant
Immunotherapy
Pheresis
Leukopheresis
Bone marrow transplant
Laminar air flow

Although cancer in children is relatively rare, it is the second ranking cause of death in children between one and fourteen years of age. Approximately 6,700 children will be diagnosed with cancer this year; of these, over 2,000 will die. In each child, the cancer causes uncontrolled cell growth. As the cancerous cells grow, they demand space and food, robbing healthy cells of needed nutrients and halting their normal growth. Cancer cells multiply quickly and can push into surrounding tissue or migrate to distant body sites. They interrupt the child's normal growth, energy, and health, and he loses weight and is constantly tired.

The space demanded by cancer cells may crowd out normal body cells and leave the child susceptible to infection, bleeding, and anemia. Small pathogens once quickly destroyed are now left to multiply and create infection. Each small cut or sore is a possible infection site. Normal controls that prevent bleeding are impaired, tears in blood vessels are left unmended, and bruises dot the child's body. He suffers nosebleeds and anemia—insufficient delivery of oxygen to his body cells—and cell functions are impaired. If cancer cells intrude on vital organs and body control centers, the child may have difficulty seeing, walking, thinking, and caring for himself.

Pressure on vital organs, suppression of the immune system, and failure of the bone marrow are all problems of children with cancer. This chapter is concerned with the problems of a suppressed immune system, *immunosuppression,* and suppressed bone marrow, *myelosuppression*. The problems of infection, bleeding, and anemia—as well as the nursing care that can prevent or minimize these problems are discussed. Specific diagnostic terms and procedures are explained, as are the major treatments used for cancer—surgery, chemotherapy, radiotherapy, and immunotherapy—and the accompanying nursing care interventions used to treat their side effects. Table 20–1 lists common childhood cancers, defines them, and outlines both treatment and special nursing considerations.

COMMON PROBLEMS AND NURSING INTERVENTIONS

Immunosuppression

All malignant conditions are immunosuppressive, and the suppression allows common, usually harmless pathogens present in the body to become potentially destructive. Of course, cancer is not the only condition that can depress the immune system; certain congenital abnormalities, malnourishment, alcoholism, and drug abuse may also cause immunosuppression. (Specific terms, general functions, and common alterations of the immune system are discussed in chapters 14 and 16.)

Lymphocytes, important to the immune system and commonly affected in childhood cancers, are made in the bone marrow. One group of lymphocytes, the *T lymphocytes,* travel from the bone marrow to the thymus where they mature and directly destroy pathogens or recruit other leukocytes (such as neutrophils or monocytes) to kill pathogens. A second group of lymphocytes, the *B lymphocytes,* also originate in the bone marrow, but they migrate to the spleen, lymph nodes, or other peripheral lymphoid tissue where they change appearance and act as antibodies against specific antigens. Neoplastic growth,

Table 20–1. Common Malignant Neoplasms in Children

Neoplasm	*Definition*	*Treatment*	*Special Nursing Considerations*
		Malignant Solid Tumors	
Brain and Central Nervous System			
Astrocytoma	A common type of brain tumor. It occurs in the cerebrum, cerebellum, thalamus, optic chiasm, and pons. Growth is slow and symptoms are insidious; frequently, increased intracranial pressure is the only early change.	Surgical removal and radiotherapy if the tumor is not completely removed.	See Ch. 27, noting behaviors and nursing care for increased intracranial pressure. Observe for these signs before and after surgery. A portion of the child's head is shaved before surgery. After surgery, position the child on the unoperated side with the bed flat or slightly elevated. Carefully note how much body movement the child is allowed; the physician may request the child's head and neck be moved as a single body part. The child may be comatose or lethargic for several days after surgery because of brain irritation and edema. Prepare the child and family for lethargy, facial swelling, and possible ecchymoses around the eyes. Observe the dressing for drainage, and report extent, color, and location of seepage.
Medullo-blastoma	A fast-growing tumor, usually located in the cerebellum, that causes a rapid increase in intracranial pressure, blockage of spinal fluid, and severe, sudden symptoms.	Surgical removal, with postsurgical radiation and chemotherapy.	
Glioma	A tumor which occurs almost only in children. Brain stem gliomas involve several cranial nerves.	Radiotherapy is used for temporary reduction of the tumor mass. Surgery usually is not done because respiratory and cardiac centers are located in the brain stem.	
Neuro-blastoma	A tumor of sympathetic nervous tissue occurring anywhere on the craniospinal axis, but frequently in the region of the adrenal glands. Metastasis results from transmission through the lymphatics and blood to the liver, bone, and lymph nodes.	After surgical excision of the tumor mass, radiotherapy and/or chemotherapy may be given.	Begin oral fluids with small sips, observe for nausea and vomiting. Vomiting increases intracranial pressure and is best minimized. Carefully regulate intravenous fluid infusion;

			overinfusion increases intracranial pressure. A decrease in respirations, pulse, or instability of body temperature, and vasomotor abilities indicates progressive tumor growth and brain stem compression.
Kidney			
Nephroblastoma (Wilms' Tumor)	Tumor of the kidney; the most common intraabdominal tumor of childhood.	Nephrectomy with postoperative radiotherapy to the abdominal cavity, and chemotherapy according to the stage of the tumor.	The prognosis is better here than for any other malignant neoplasm in childhood. Children have a 90 percent survival rate for localized tumors. Even with metastasis, long-term survival is possible. After surgery, measure and record fluid intake and output carefully.
Bone			
Osteogenic sarcoma	Tumor of the bone usually involving extremities, such as femur, tibia, or humerus.	Immediate amputation of affected extremity with postsurgical chemotherapy to prevent metastasis.	An amputation is mutilating, and it is very difficult for the child or his family to accept. Offer your time, support, and understanding. After amputation surgery, observe the child for hemorrhage every 15 minutes for four hours then every hour for 24 hours. The stump is bandaged with a pressure or rigid plastic dressing to prevent edema. Place a large tourniquet at the bedside to wrap around the limb if hemorrhage begins. The child may experi-

(continued)

Table 20–1. *(Continued)*

Neoplasm	*Definition*	*Treatment*	*Special Nursing Considerations*
			ence "phantom pain" at the site of the amputation. This is real pain and a normal sensation following amputation surgery. Acknowledge the pain, and offer the child analgesics. Teach him how to walk with a crutch in the hospital and arrange for a prosthesis fitting schedule.
Ewing's sarcoma	A non-osseous sarcoma usually arising from a trunk bone (a rib, scapula, or vertebra) or extremity bone (the femur, tibia, fibula, or humerus); usually metastasizes to other bones or to the lungs.	Radiotherapy and chemotherapy to destroy the tumor yet maintain useful function of the affected area.	
Eye			
Retinoblastoma	A rare congenital tumor of the eye arising in the retina. Although present at birth, it may not be detected until years later. Once this slow-growing tumor breaks through the globe, it metastasizes to the bone marrow, lymph nodes, and liver.	If the tumor is extensive, enucleation of the affected eye. Chemotherapy and radiotherapy if vision can be preserved.	Visual loss causes developmental problems. Refer to Ch. 10 for common problems and nursing care interventions for the child with a perceptual deviation.
Connective tissue			
Rhabdomyosarcoma	A common tumor of soft tissue which can occur anywhere in muscle tissue, but is frequently	Surgical excision, if possible. If not, radiotherapy and chemotherapy are used to re-	Recurrences are likely two years after the initial diagnosis. Prognosis is better when the

	found in the head and neck and especially in the orbit, sinuses, nasopharynx, and middle ear. The tumor, which can be spotted by the swelling but is not tender, metastasizes by direct invasion or by the bloodstream to bone, bone marrow, and the lungs.	duce the tumor size until surgery can be done.	malignancy is localized and for children under seven.
	Leukemias and Lymphomas		
Leukemias			
Acute lymphocytic (ALL)	A malignant proliferation of immature lymphocytes (leukocytes formed in the lymphatic tissue) that accounts for 85 percent of all leukemias in children.	Induction with chemotherapy; prophylactic chemotherapy to the central nervous system; radiotherapy; maintenance chemotherapy.	To the layman leukemia frequently means death in a few weeks. Correct this misconception; current treatments, especially for ALL, offer a five-year survival for 50 percent of the affected children. Children that survive five years have a 50 percent chance of a continual indefinite disease free state.
Acute myelocytic (AML)	A malignant proliferation of granulocytes, (leukocytes formed in the bone marrow) which accounts for 10 percent of leukemias in children.	Induction with chemotherapy; maintenance chemotherapy; immunotherapy.	Explain the use of chemotherapy, radiotherapy, and immunotherapy, offering nursing interventions for side effects. Prognosis is poor since children usually survive only six months after diagnosis.
Lymphomas			
Hodgkin's disease	A proliferation of lymphocytes and the appearance of large multinucleated Reed-Stern-	Depending on the stage of the disease, radiotherapy and/or chemotherapy are used.	Nursing care needs are essentially the same as for children with leukemia. The incidence

(continued)

Table 20–1. *(Continued)*

Neoplasm	*Definition*	*Treatment*	*Special Nursing Considerations*
	berg cells. Frequently occurring in the adolescent, the lymph glands contain solid tumors, causing the glands to become enlarged and firm. As the disease spreads, the bone marrow, lungs, liver, bone, and kidneys may become affected. The disease is staged from I to IV.		of Hodgkin's disease increases during adolescence—a period of changes in body image and sexuality. The treatment is long-term, and definite plans are difficult to make. The adolescent is removed from peer group activities at a crucial time. Allow ample opportunities for the teenager to discuss his fears, anger, and the unfairness of having a chronic disease.
Lymphosarcoma	Solid tumors in multiple lymph nodes. The Reed-Sternberg cell is absent. Lymph nodes enlarge quickly but painlessly. Lymphocytes seem arrested in development at an immature stage.	Surgical excision with postsurgical radiotherapy and/or chemotherapy.	

medicines or treatments that suppress bone marrow function, or interference with the development and function of lymphocytes can suppress the normal activity of the child's immune system, making him more prone to infection.

Myelosuppression

In addition to leukocytes, the bone marrow makes *erythrocytes,* the cells that carry oxygen, and *platelets,* bodies that aid in controlling bleeding. Both erythrocytes and platelets emerge from the bone marrow as finished products. When the bone marrow does not make a sufficient number of erythrocytes—either because the bone marrow is filled by cancer cells or because treatment has depleted the marrow's cell-making ability—the child cannot produce enough erythrocytes to carry oxygen and nutrients, and he becomes anemic. Effects of anemia include weight loss, fatigue, and pallor. Erythrocytes also pick up waste products from body cells, and a decrease in their production causes an accumulation of nutrient waste. One such waste product is *uric acid*, which in large quantities can precipitate in the urinary tract and kidneys, causing obstruction, oliguria, and renal failure. This condition is called *hyperuricemia* and is treated prophylactically with such drugs as *allopurinol* (see Table 20–2).

A deficiency of platelets is called *thrombocytopenia* and can result in unchecked bleeding of the gums, nose, and gastrointestinal tract. Multiple bruises, seen as *petechiae* (purplish-red pinpoint spots caused by intradermal or submucosal hemorrhages) and *ecchymoses* (large hemorrhagic areas) may appear on the skin.

Cancer and the drugs and treatments used to control it can suppress the immune system, leaving the child at increased risk to infection. In addition, the neoplastic process may invade the bone marrow, altering normal cell production, causing simultaneous myelosuppression. Cancer treatments can further depress bone marrow function. The combination of immunosuppression and myelosuppression result in infection, bleeding, and anemia. Preventive care and immediate first aid interventions for each of these major health problems will be reviewed below.

Infection

Nonbacterial infections are the major cause of illness and death in immunosuppressed children with cancer. Common viral infections, such as varicella (chickenpox), herpes zoster (shingles), and measles, become serious problems for the immunsuppressed child.

Chickenpox, for example, causes a 7-percent mortality rate in immunosuppressed children. Hepatitis, pancreatitis, and meningoencephalitis are complications of chickenpox that affect these children, and parents should report any exposures to chickenpox immediately. The hospital admissions office must be extremely careful to investigate if there has been a recent exposure to chickenpox. The severity of chickenpox may be lessened if immunosuppressive therapy, such as specific drugs and radiation, are stopped at the time of exposure so that the immune system can rebound and respond to the varicella virus.

Thirty percent of immunosuppressed children who contract shingles from herpes zoster die—usually from pneumonitis. Measles, another common childhood infection, also can be fatal. Since the immune system cannot respond normally, no live vaccines, such as those for measles, rubella,

Table 20–2. **Common Drugs Used to Treat Pediatric Malignant Neoplasms**

Drug name	*Route*	*Use*	*Possible Side Effects*	*Special Nursing Considerations*
Adriamycin	IV	Rhabdomyosarcoma Neuroblastoma Osteogenic sarcoma Wilm's tumor Reinduction and maintenance of ALL Hodgkin's Disease Lymphomas	Nausea and vomiting Fever Stomatitis Alopecia (loss of hair) Red urine (not hematuria) Bone marrow depression Cardiac toxicity in cumulative doses Tissue necrosis at infusion site if drug infiltration occurs	Antiemetics before treatment Antipyretics Soft diet; oral hygiene Support body image change Observe for bleeding and infection Check apical pulse for irregularities See Vincristine
Allopurinol	PO	To inhibit production of uric acid and accompanying problems.	Liver toxicity Fever Nausea, vomiting, and diarrhea	 Antipyretics Antiemetics Maintain fluid intake of at least 3,000 $ml/m^2/day$ to prevent renal problems; the drug is excreted only by the kidneys.
L-asparaginase	IV	Induction, reinduction of ALL	Hypersensitive reactions, danger of anaphylactic shock Pancreatitis Anorexia Hypotension Lethargy Fever Convulsions Chills and fever Clotting abnormalities Hyperglycemia Liver damage	Have Benadryl, epinephrine, and resuscitation equipment at the bedside; stay with child constantly Assess blood pressure Conserve energy Antipyretics A reaction may occur at any time during any part of the therapy. Observe for changes in blood pressure, pulse, respirations, skin color, and body tempera-

				ture; for signs of hives or rash; for complaints of stomach pain, chest pain, headache or blurred vision, restlessness, nausea, or vomiting.
5-azacytidine (5-AZACR)	IV	AML induction and maintenance	Bone marrow depression Nausea and vomiting Dermatitis Liver toxicity	Observe for infection and bleeding Antiemetics, small frequent feedings, bland diet
Cyclophosphamide (Cytoxan)	PO IV	Induction and maintenance of ALL Neuroblastoma, osteogenic sarcoma Rhabdomyosarcoma Wilm's tumor Ewing's sarcoma Retinoblastoma	Hemorrhagic cystitis Liver dysfunction Bone marrow depression Immunosuppression Alopecia Nausea and vomiting Mucous membrane ulcerations	Keep well hydrated, note I&O Observe for hematuria Observe for infection and bleeding Support body image change Antiemetics Oral hygiene
Cytosine arabinoside (Cytosar)	IV IM SQ IT	AML induction and maintenance ALL maintenance (sometimes) Reinduction CNS prophylaxis	Severe nausea and vomiting Diarrhea Bone marrow depression Immunosuppression Stomatitis Liver toxicity	Antiemetics prior to treatment, I&O, added hydration Observe for infection or bleeding Oral care
Dactinomycin (Actinomycin D, Meractinomycin Lyovac Cosmegen)	IV	Wilm's tumor Rhabdomyosarcoma Ewing's sarcoma Neuroblastoma	Stomatitis, Mucositis Nausea, vomiting, diarrhea Abdominal pain Alopecia Acne Bone Marrow depression	Soft bland diet, oral hygiene Antiemetics, antidiarrheals Support body image change Support body image change Observe for bleeding and infection

(Continued)

Table 20–2. *(Continued)*

Drug name	*Route*	*Use*	*Possible Side Effects*	*Special Nursing Considerations*
			General malaise, lethargy	Conserve energy
			Fever	Antipyretics
			Tissue necrosis at infusion site if drug infiltration occurs	See Vincristine
Daunorubicin (Daunomycin Rubidomycin Cerubidine)	IV	Induction AML	Severe tissue necrosis at site if drug infiltrates	See Vincristine
			Pain along vein during and immediately following infusion	Apply moist heat
			Bone marrow depression	Observe for infection and bleeding
			GI ulcerations; stomatitis	Oral hygiene
			Abdominal pain, nausea, vomiting	Antiemetics
			Diarrhea	Antidiarrheals
			Alopecia	Support body image change
			Fever	Antipyretics
			Skin rashes	
			Red urine with first voiding after infusion	
Imidazole Carboxamide dimethyltriazino (DIC DTIC)	IV	Neuroblastoma	Nausea, vomiting	Antiemetic before treatment
			Headache, malaise	Added fluids for hydration
			Liver toxicity	Observe for infection and bleeding
			Bone marrow depression	
			Burning sensation when injected	
6-mercaptopurine (6-MP, Purinethol)	PO	ALL maintenance	Skin blisters and ulcers at, above, or below site of infusion	See Methotrexate
			Bone marrow depression	Observe for infection and bleeding
			Anorexia, nausea, vomiting	Antiemetics, small frequent feedings

			Stomatitis	Oral care
Methotrexate (MTX, Amethopterin)	PO IV IT IM	Osteogenic sarcoma ALL maintenance and reinduction ALL CNS prophylaxis	Oral ulcers, gingivitis Sore throat Nausea, vomiting, diarrhea Liver damage	Oral hygiene, anesthetics for numbing Antiemetics, small frequent feedings, I & O, guaiac stools
			Kidney damage	(Drug *cannot* be given to children with reduced kidney function since MTX is only eliminated by the kidneys)
			Menstrual problems	Be supportive of sexual concerns
			Reduced sperm	
			Bone marrow depression	Observe for infection and bleeding
			Skin blisters and ulcers at, below, or above infusion site	Apply ice to skin blisters for 10 min after the infusion. Keep area clean; cover ulcers
			Headache, drowsiness, blurred vision	Provide for safety
Prednisone	PO	Induction and maintenance of ALL and AML	Increased appetite and weight gain	Plan nutritious meals; avoid junk foods
			Fluid retention, muscle wasting	Salt restriction
			Immunosuppression	Observe for infection and bleeding
			GI ulcerations, gastric ulcers, or complaints of "stomach burning"	Good oral hygiene Antacids
6-thioguanine (6-TG, Thioguan)	PO	AML induction and maintenance	Bone marrow depression	Observe for infection or bleeding
			Nausea, vomiting	Antiemetics
			Diarrhea	Antidiarrheals

(Continued)

Table 20–2. *(Continued)*

Drug name	*Route*	*Use*	*Possible Side Effects*	*Special Nursing Considerations*
			Stomatitis	Oral care
			Because of possible teratogenic effects, avoid during first 3 months of pregnancy	Assess if adolescent is pregnant
Vincristine (Oncovin)	IV	Induction and maintenance of ALL and AML Wilm's tumor Rhabdomyosarcoma Neuroblastoma Ewing's sarcoma Retinoblastoma Osteogenic sarcoma	Neuromuscular disorders, such as leg weakness, muscle cramps, foot droop, weak hand grasp, hand tremors	Provide for safety
			Obstipation or constipation	Stool softeners or laxatives
			Alopecia	
			Tissue necrosis if infiltration occurs	Use one needle to withdraw, a second to inject. Prior to injection, use a saline flush. Inject slowly, follow with saline flush. If infiltration occurs, inform physician and apply ice packs for 24 hours or until swelling is gone; then moist heat for 30 minutes every 2 hours until inflammation is gone

Key:
ALL Acute lymphocytic leukemia
AML Acute myelocytic leukemia
IM Intramuscular
IV Intravenous
SQ Subcutaneous
IT Intrathecal
PO Per os (by mouth)
I&O Intake and output

mumps, smallpox, and polio, are ever administered to the immunosuppressed child.

A viral pneumonia, caused by Pneumocystis carinii, is a major cause of illness and mortality in children with altered immune responses. Such children need special nursing care, especially for the hypoxia, which is more severe with this pneumonia than it is with others. The nurse must be alert to signs of pneumonia and should notify the physician of even a slight cough. Indeed, all respiratory infections are more dangerous for the immunosuppressed child; even common colds last longer than usual. If antibiotics are used to treat these infections, overgrowth of certain microorganisms may occur—such as Candida (monilia) in the mouth, genitals, or anus—necessitating the use of additional medication to treat the side effects.

Common bacterial infections—especially Pseudomonas, Escherichia coli and Proteus—are also a problem for the child who is immunosuppressed. Simple preventative measures can protect these children from these troublesome infections. For example, a frequently overlooked preventative, effective against all types of pathogens, is frequent hand washing by the child, family, and all persons working with the child. Furniture and equipment should be damp dusted with a disinfectant solution because dry dusting can disperse rather than remove pathogens. Humidifying the air also helps to reduce microorganisms; pathogens laden with moisture drop to the floor and die. Disposable equipment, such as individual thermometers changed daily, also helps. Although controlling dust and humidifying the air may not seem like nursing interventions, each can prevent infection and can be easily employed by parents when the child returns home.

Intact skin and mucous membranes are a child's first defense against infection, but the skin and mucous membranes of the child with cancer are assaulted by drugs and surgery, deprived of nutrients, and bombarded with radiation. Daily routine hygiene for the skin, oral mucous, and rectal-perineal areas can preserve and maintain their function. Working with the family and child, establish a simple daily care plan for total body hygiene that can be continued at home.

Oral Hygiene

Suggest that the child use a soft toothbrush, further softened in warm water, for teeth brushing after every meal. The soft bristles will help to keep delicate gum tissue intact. Frequent sprays and oral irrigations of saline or mouthwash also will help to keep the mouth fresh and clean. If mouth sores appear, toothbrushing should be discontinued, and cotton-tipped applicators, or other soft swabbed material should be used to clean the teeth and gums. Lemon and glycerin swabs will freshen the mouth. If the mouth ulcers are mild, warm sodium bicarbonate rinses can be used; if bleeding occurs, diluted one-half strength hydrogen peroxide rinses can be substituted. For severe mouth ulcers, rinsing with a solution of two ounces water, two ounces hydrogen peroxide, and two ounces mouthwash every two to four hours will cleanse the lesions and debris. If the child will not tolerate the hydrogen peroxide solution, use water alone, since the goal is cleaning and debridement to promote new tissue formation. Local anesthetics, such as Xylocaine or Chloroseptic, may be applied directly on the sores with cotton swabs. Straws, small colorful cups, or a chart with stars or smiling faces can be used to encourage the young child to pursue the oral irrigations and care.

All care for severe mouth ulcers must be done around the clock. With intensive oral care, mouth ulcers can be cured in four to eight days. Teach the child and his family to examine the mouth daily; using a flashlight, they should look for redness, white patches, or ulcers. If the child is home and mouth ulcers appear, the family should notify their physician or clinic immediately. Seemingly small abraded areas can quickly become major infections, hence the need for prompt action. Mouth ulcers are painful, and the child may refuse all food until he receives some relief. Because adequate protein, calories, and vitamins are essential to normal immune system functioning, and a well-nourished child is better able to tolerate chemotherapy and radiotherapy, a plan that encourages food consumption must be devised (see ch. 18). Cool drinks, soft bland foods, and frozen liquids, such as popsicles, offer numbing comfort to mouth sores and provide needed hydration. Mycostatin suspension may be prescribed for oral care.

Rectal-Perineal Care

The rectal and perineal areas are also prone to infection and need to be checked daily for redness or fissures. There should be a careful plan for keeping the rectal area clean, beginning with routine, gentle, cleansing after each bowel movement. A soak in a warm tub of water is cleansing, soothing, healing, and can provide a stimulating water play experience for the child. A sitz bath followed by use of a bedside heat lamp can help to heal rectal abrasions. Antibacterial ointments applied after the cleansing will also help. Undergarments need to be changed daily. Avoid taking the child's temperature rectally. Parents are usually most comfortable taking an axillary temperature, especially if the child is young. Evaluate the parents' home equipment. Review the use and care of a thermometer; proper positioning and holding of the child; methods for reading and recording temperatures, time, and whether it was an oral or axillary temperature (See the Skills Manual). A temperature of 38°C (100°F) or higher in a child with cancer requires medical attention.

Skin Care

The skin also provides protection against infection. Unfortunately, the child with cancer requires repeated blood studies, diagnostic procedures, intravenous infusions, and drugs that assault his skin and provide sites for possible skin infection. Minimize these multiple procedures as much as possible by coordinating various studies. For example, if a daily blood sample is needed and the continuous infusion site is to be changed, arrange the two activities so that the child receives only one needle puncture. Families quickly become familiar with procedures and schedules. Elicit family support in requesting that whoever will do a venipuncture wait a few minutes while materials are brought to the bedside for the infusion site change. Before each venipuncture, cleanse the skin with alcohol. If continuous intravenous infusions are used, the needle site is changed every three days, and all tubing is changed daily. Because of the child's increased tendency to bleed, rotate infusion sites, and apply prolonged pressure for at least five minutes after each venipuncture. Avoid intramuscular injections. When an intramuscular injection is necessary, choose the smallest gauge needle possible, and apply local pressure for five minutes after the injection. Incision into veins for fluid infusion, such as in cutdowns is rarely used, because it increases the potential for infection and bleeding and destroys veins needed for future treatments. Lotions and creams should be used to prevent dry skin. Fewer complete baths, less soap, and the addition of bath oils to the water also protect the skin. Prolonged contact with moisture macerates the skin, and wet or soiled linens, diapers, or clothes need changing as soon as possible.

If the child is confined to bed, massage those areas prone to pressure sores with alcohol. Solid tumor masses frequently exert pressure on overlying mucous membranes, causing ulceration, bleeding, or both, and may result in infection. Since tumors can obstruct organ drainage, predisposing that organ to infection, the location and accompanying pressure of cancerous masses must be considered.

Sunburn is another hazard for the immunosuppressed child because a burn can promote infection. Apply a commercial sunscreen and dress the child in protective clothing when he is going outside. Superficial infections on the skin like boils or canker sores need protection from trauma, a thorough cleansing, and treatment with antibiotic ointments. If the infection shows signs of spreading (such as increased edema, erythema, pain, or exudate), a physician should be notified. The child with a low leukocyte count is not only less resistant to invading organisms but also less able to form pus; therefore, look for other signs of infection, such as localized redness, streaks, swelling, or complaints of discomfort and tenderness. Keep the child's nails short to discourage scratching because even small skin abrasions can invite infection. If open lesions appear, cleanse them with Betadine, and cover them with gauze material that will not stick to the lesions. Antibiotics are usually given.

Danger Signs

Any infection in the child with cancer may lead to an overwhelming sepsis. He must be observed closely and any sign of sepsis should be reported immediately. Sudden changes in vital signs, lethargy, confusion, skin changes or lesions, decreased urinary output, or acute abdominal pain (which may mean an internal abscess has ruptured) are all danger signs. If a child with a low leukocyte count who is free of fever and who is not on antibiotics, suddenly develops a fever, he is most probably septic, and must be treated with high dosages of broad spectrum antibiotics, and perhaps adrenal steroids. Blood cultures must be done. If, during any infection or treatment, the child's leukocyte count falls below 1,000, the child is usually placed in isolation.

Initially these preventive and acute care measures for infection seem overwhelming and frightening, especially to parents who will care for their child at home. Thoroughly explain to the family the reasons for preventive and immediate care of infections, and ask them for suggestions on measures to prevent infection. The hospitalization period gives the parents and child a chance to learn and practice mouth and skin care. Together they can develop ways to make the child more comfortable, can practice taking temperatures, and can learn how to look for possible infection. The hospitalization period can help the family to cope with and accept the chronic needs of a child with cancer.

Bleeding and Hemorrhage

Megakaryocytes (platelets), which are formed in the bone marrow, function to control bleeding by mending torn blood vessels and halting bleeding (See Ch. 21). Platelets live only 10 days, and if their production is impaired, as it is in the myelosuppressed child, bleeding and hemorrhage become daily concerns. The child with a low platelet count is termed *thrombocytopenic* and needs special prophylactic care. Tree climbing, swinging, bike and skateboard riding, and other potentially dangerous activities must be stopped temporarily until the platelet count rises. Platelet concentrates are available for infusion, but these are best reserved for active bleeding.

Prevention of bleeding is the most beneficial aspect of nursing care. While he is hospitalized, the child can be protected from falling out of bed by a bed rail. Intramuscular injections should be avoided, if possible. When they are necessary, select the smallest gauge needle possible and apply firm pressure to the site for five minutes following the puncture. If restraints are required during a procedure, support the child's extremities to avoid trauma. Catheters and drainage and suction tubes must be handled carefully to prevent mucosal bleeding. If the skin or mucosa are broken, quickly begin the preventive care discussed above.

When bleeding occurs, reassure the child and family that it can be controlled. Apply local pressure to control the bleeding, using care not to interfere with clot formation. Teach the child and parents how to control nosebleeds, by pinching the nostrils gently until the bleeding stops. If the child bleeds at puncture sites, apply a pressure bandage and watch closely for signs of hemostasis. For bleeding at any site, keep the area clean at all times since blood provides an excellent medium for the growth of pathogens. For oral or rectal bleeding, give care as discussed under infection. Hemorrhaging is a real threat to children with cancer. Check the skin daily, looking for petechiae, ecchymoses, bruises, or frank bleeding. Test stools, urine, and vomitus for the presence of blood. Be aware of the child's daily blood counts to anticipate a bleeding episode, such as a nosebleed.

Anemia

Red blood cells, or erythrocytes, carry oxygen and nutrients to body cells and remove waste products from them. If too few erythrocytes are produced in the bone marrow, the child is anemic. The anemic child suffers from hypoxia, a deficiency of oxygen to the cells. He is fatigued and tires easily. (A complete discussion of erythrocytes is presented in chapter 21; chapter 24 discusses the problems of anemia and resulting hypoxia. Refer to these chapters for specific nursing measures which apply to the child with cancer who is also anemic.)

Anemia can be treated with transfusions of packed red blood cells, but they usually are reserved for severe anemia cases. Parents need repeated explanations about why their anemic child will not be as active as other children. Stress that naps and rest periods are necessary to conserve his energy for eating and other important activities. If the child remains in bed, his position should be changed frequently to prevent pressure sores from developing. Since children frequently curl up in the fetal position to sleep, the child with an enlarged lymph node or tumor in the head or neck area must be watched carefully. Respiratory obstruction can occur if his sleeping position exerts pressure on the neoplastic mass and a change in position may be necessary.

COMMON DIAGNOSTIC TESTS AND NURSING IMPLICATIONS

Physical Examination

Many solid tumors are first felt by parents as they bathe and play with their child; the child himself may feel an unusual lump; or a physician may notice a mass during a routine physical examination. If neoplastic growth is suspected, blood tests are done to study the number, size, and appearance of the blood components. Cerebrospinal fluid may be examined for pressure and the presence of any cancerous cells. An *electroencephalogram,* a test that determines the electrical activity of the brain, can help to localize a possible brain tumor.

Although blood studies, a physical examination, and symptoms of pain, fatigue, bruises, nosebleeds, and weight loss may indicate a neoplasm, they are not conclusive evidence. Radiographs and a sample of cellular material are used for a final diagnosis of cancer.

Radiographs

X-rays are used to show bone masses, bone destruction, or metastic lesions on the bone. If a neoplasm in the cranium is suspected, the skull is x-rayed to look for areas of calcification or sutures that have separated. Separated sutures indicate increased intracranial pressure and the possibility of a tumor mass. Unfortunately, the machines used for radiographic diagnoses are frequently large and look frightening. Because a medical team may be hurrying to diagnose the child, so therapy can begin, sometimes no one takes the time to prepare the child and parents for the procedure. Each family needs information on the name of the x-ray procedure, why the study is necessary, what information the test will yield, and how the child will feel after the procedure. Often you will need to explain this information several times, using descriptive words and drawings to identify parts of the body affected during and after the study. Since many x-ray studies do not require the child to be sedated, parents may be able to accompany him to the tests. Verbal reassurance during a procedure comforts the child, furthering his cooperation and ability to comply with necessary behavior. Common radiographic studies are described in Figure 20–1.

Bone Marrow Aspiration

The child with leukemia will have many bone marrow aspirations. The bone marrow not only confirms the diagnosis of leukemia but also warns of a relapse and verifies a remission. Explain to the child and his parents that the bone marrow is the origin and growth site of blood cells. You can compare the marrow to a factory where products are made and then distributed for use. A bone marrow aspiration is the extraction of a sample of bone marrow tissue. The aspiration is usually taken from the iliac crest (hip bone), and the aspirated cells are microscopically studied.

One effective approach to help families understand the size, shape, and function of blood cells is to use a microscope and stained slides of erythrocytes, leukocytes, and platelets. This factual approach takes time but can eliminate the fear and accompanying anxiety of misunderstood information.

No special preparation is necessary for a

Figure 20–1. **Common Invasive and Noninvasive Radiographic Studies for Cancer**

Invasive Procedures

Brain Scan. A radioactive substance is injected intravenously and does not penetrate normal tissue; however, heavy concentrations are found when brain lesions are scanned by machine.

Cerebral Angiograph. Dye is injected into an artery or vein, and x-rays are taken as the dye flows through the blood vessels of the cerebrum. The pictures are studied for masses in the blood vessels or defects in the vessels themselves. Following this procedure, observe for neurological complications: seizures, transient loss of vision, or hemiplegia. Observe the injected site closely for thrombus, hemorrhage, or hematoma. Evaluate any change in intracranial pressure and level of consciousness.

Lymphoangiograph. Dye is injected into the lymphatic system. X-rays are used to look for size and structure of lymph nodes.

Myelogram. Air or a contrast material is injected into the subarachnoid space by a lumbar puncture. X-rays are then taken to look for lesions, masses, dislocation or fracture of the spinal cord. Following the test, keep the child flat in bed, offer fluids, and observe for changes in intracranial pressure.

Pneumoencephalogram. Air is injected into the cerebral spinal fluid of the spinal cord. As air fills the ventricles and the subarachnoid space, x-rays are taken to look for structural abnormalities of the brain. After the procedure, place the child flat in bed and observe for signs of increased intracranial pressure (See Ch. 27). Check vital signs frequently and offer fluids.

Ventriculogram. Air is injected into the lateral ventricle through the anterior fontanelle. X-rays are taken of the ventricles of the brain to look for a lesion, or mass. After the procedure, place the child flat in bed, take his vital signs, and watch closely for change in intracranial pressure. Offer fluids.

Noninvasive

Echoencephalography (ultrasonograph). High frequency sound waves are used to project tissues of various thicknesses and properties. For example, the ventricles can be outlined. A two-dimensional picture, which can be photographed for a permanent record, is shown on a screen. No special preparation is necessary; there is no discomfort and no special care or complication. The procedure can be repeated frequently to record any change in the size of a structure.

Computerized Axial Tomography (CAT). Special electronic devices are able to determine small differences in tissue density. The machine is rotated 180° around the child's head, and readings are taken at different angles. As in the echoencephalography, a picture which can be photographed for a permanent record appears on a screen. Both benign masses (such as abscesses or cysts) and malignant lesions can be detected. No special preparations are necessary. A tomography can also be taken of specific organs at various depths to determine the exact location of a lesion.

bone marrow aspiration except to immobilize the child. He should lie on his stomach, and the area should be swabbed with a local anesthetic. When a large needle is inserted, the child will feel pressure as the sample is removed. The entire procedure lasts two or three minutes. At the conclusion of the procedure apply firm pressure to the site and offer a bandage. If you can help the child to develop a positive attitude during the first aspiration, he will be able to tolerate future aspirations with minimal physical and psychological trauma.

Biopsy

A *biopsy* is the removal of a small piece of tissue for microscopic examination. Although it is more commonly done in adults than in children, occasionally a whole lymph node or a portion of a node is extracted for biopsy study. Evidence of cancer that has spread into the lymphatic system is evaluated by a *nodal biopsy*. It is relatively easy to take a biopsy of lesions of the head and back because of the easy accessibility of the area. During a biopsy, a thin needle is inserted and a portion of the tissue is removed. The child is given a sedative or analgesic before the procedure. Carefully immobilize the child, applying restraints if needed (See the Skills Manual). As you hold the child firmly, reassure him and discuss the progress of the procedure. Apply pressure for five to ten minutes after the biopsy.

Classification and Staging

After diagnostic tests, the neoplasm is classified and staged. *Classification* is the anatomical and histological description of a neoplasm. *Staging* describes the extent of neoplastic involvement and is done by x-ray, biopsy, or surgery.

Numerous tumor classification and staging systems have been developed; however, many lack consistency and result in confusion about treatment. The most widely used system of staging involves the use of the letters *T* (tumor), *N* (node), and *M* (metastasis). The addition of the letter *O* to the letters indicates no abnormal growth. Thus, *TO* means no evidence of primary tumor, *NO* means the regional lymph nodes are not abnormal, and *MO* indicates no evidence of distant metastasis. Numerical subscripts are added to the letters to show the degree of growth. The figures T_1, T_2, T_3, show a progressive increase in the tumor size and involvement; N_1, N_2, N_3, mean increasing abnormality of regional lymph nodes; and M_1, M_2, and M_3 indicate degrees of distant metastasis.

COMMON TREATMENTS AND NURSING IMPLICATIONS

Following diagnosis, the physician will prescribe a program of treatments based on the place of origin and tissue type of the neoplasm, as well as the present location, size, and extent of the cancer. Treatments include surgery, chemotherapy, radiotherapy, immunotherapy, transfusions, and bone marrow transplant.

Surgery

Surgery is used to remove a primary tumor mass; to determine the extent of the neoplasm (e.g., a nodal biopsy), or to reduce pain and discomfort, as a palliative. Surgery can be used to remove some, but not all tumor masses (see Table 20–1). In preparing the child with cancer for surgery, explain the surgical procedure, including the location, anatomical part affected, and the exact postsurgical appearance. Inform the child and his family where dressings will be placed, what care will be necessary, and what equipment will be needed. Be present when the physician explains the surgical procedure so that you can repeat the information to the child and his parents as often as needed. Changes in body image, especially if a limb amputation or eye enucleation is necessary, may be sudden. Frequently, the child is rushed to surgery, leaving his family in a state of shock and confusion. Information, reassurance, and hope that the surgery will improve the quality of the child's life is most supportive and important during this stressful period.

As with any child following surgery, the immediate nursing responsibility is to monitor the airway. Intubation irritates the respiratory tract and causes the child's bronchial secretions to increase; the smaller the child, the more difficult the problem. If an endotracheal tube is used for more than four hours, a child may develop laryngeal edema. Decadron is frequently used to reduce spasms, which can increase dangerously without warning. Postoperative sedation is limited because a child's crying is the best indicator of full lung expansion, and sedation is one of the most common causes of lung collapse in the young child. Explain these facts to parents, emphasizing that crying and movement aid lung expansion.

A slowing of the pulse rate is the first indication of airway obstruction, occurring before noisy respirations or the color changes of cyanosis. Explain to the child and his family the need for turning, coughing, and deep breathing (see ch. 2). All normal postsurgical care routines are used for the child with cancer.

Fluid balance and *infection* present special postsurgical considerations for the child with a neoplasm. Fluid needs following surgery are based on a corrected weight measurement that allows for loss of tumor or limb mass. When an organ or node is removed, fluid and serum frequently move into the empty space. This shift in fluid is referred to as *third space fluid loss*. Because of it, children may require plasma replacement during the first two or three postoperative days. Signs indicative of third space fluid loss are:

1. An increase in pulse rate.
2. A decrease in blood pressure.
3. A falling central venous pressure (CVP). The CVP is a measurement of the vascular volume and heart pumping action on the *right* side of the heart. The CVP is measured by inserting a catheter through the superior vena cava into the right atrium. A *rising CVP* means the heart is overloaded, as it is in heart failure and pulmonary edema. A *falling CVP* indicates decrease in blood volume (hypovolemia).
4. A falling urinary output.

Urinary output falls after any surgery but should return to normal, unassisted, within 24 hours. The kidneys are very sensitive to blood volume changes, so urinary output is measured hourly. Output per day should measure two-thirds of the total fluid intake.

The child with a neoplasm may be immunosuppressed; therefore, be alert for signs of infection or bleeding following surgery. A fever of 103° F the night after surgery is most likely caused by atelectasis (a collapsed lung) or pneumonia. Fever that develops during the first two or three postoperative days usually results from upper respiratory or urinary tract infections. A temperature elevation four to five days postoperatively is probably caused by wound infection or an internal abscess. Infection may be difficult to detect, especially if the child is receiving immunosuppressive therapy. The only indicators of infection may be lethargy, weakness, disinterest in play, or lack of crying. The first 48 hours following surgery are crucial and require close observation.

Chemotherapy

The goal of chemotherapy is to destroy cancerous cells and to return bone marrow function to normal. Frequently, several chemotherapeutic drugs are used—some with a very specific action, others which have a broad, general effect. For example, vincristine destroys cells only during division, while prednisone only kills cells as they make and secrete compounds. Other chemotherapeutic drugs, such as Cytoxan, are general and destroy body cells at any stage of development. By using a combination of drugs, physicians can destroy cancerous cells during all phases of growth. Table 20–2 lists commonly used chemotherapeutic agents, their route of administration, the type of neoplasm they are used to treat, possible side effects, and specific nursing actions that minimize discomfort. The greatest problem with chemotherapy is that it also destroys the child's healthy noncancerous cells. For this reason, treatments must be spaced far enough apart to give the bone marrow time to replace destroyed cells. The exact timing of chemotherapy is crucial, as is its administration and the recording of side effects. The appearance of side effects provides guidelines for continuing or changing the chemotherapy schedule. Chemotherapy works best to decrease the cancer cell population when used in conjunction with surgery, radiation, or immunotherapy. Terms used in the chemotherapy regimen for the child with leukemia are explained in Figure 20–2.

Chemotherapy dosages are calculated according to the child's body surface area and expressed as milligrams per square meter of body surface area. This differs from body weight dosages which are written as milligrams per kilogram of weight. Exact height and weight measurements are used to determine the body surface area in square meters.

Weight loss is a common side effect of chemotherapy, and the child must be weighed daily so that changes in dosage calculation can be made. When weighing a child, use the same scale, same time of day, and, if possible, same amount of clothing. Have a second person weigh the child too, and compare the two results. If a discrepancy exists, reweigh the child. A height measurement is needed only once a month.

Children with cancer frequently receive high dosages of steroids such as prednisone, and the steroids often cause fluid retention and an increase in appetite. For this reason, the chemotherapy dosages must be calculated according to presteroid weight. If dosages are based on steroid weight, a grave overdosage may occur. Primary nursing responsibilities during chemotherapy include 1) accurate measurement of the child's weight; 2) exact measurement and administration of chemotherapy; 3) observation and recording of drug reactions or side effects.

Intravenous Chemotherapy

A danger of intravenous chemotherapy is leakage (infiltration) from the needle or vein into surrounding tissues, causing tis-

Figure 20–2. **Induction, Remission, Maintenance: What They Mean**

Induction is the first step of chemotherapy aimed at reducing the leukemic cell population. If, after induction, the cancerous cell population is sufficiently reduced so that the child is free from the signs and symptoms of leukemia and his bone marrow is producing and functioning adequately, a *remission* is achieved. This is a happy day and an important accomplishment. At the initial diagnosis of leukemia, most children have about one trillion leukemic cells. For remission, the leukemic cells must be reduced to one billion or less; this is a thousand-fold reduction that frequently takes four to six weeks of induction therapy.

Maintenance therapy is the continuation of drugs to reduce the leukemic population still further. Often several drugs are used during induction and maintenance. The rotation of drugs is called *cyclic therapy*, and it is almost always used in caring for children with leukemia.

Relapse is the reappearance of leukemic cells in the bone marrow or peripheral blood. The appearance of leukemic cells in the cerebrospinal fluid is a *central nervous system (CNS) relapse*. With the exception of prednisone, the antileukemic drugs do not affect the central nervous system (CNS): hence leukemic cells can invade the CNS, multiply, and cause a CNS relapse. To prevent a CNS relapse, the cranium is irradiated, and methotrexate is injected into the spinal canal. This process if called *intrathecal methotrexate*. Both irradiation and intrathecal methotrexate are done as CNS *prophylactic care*.

Therapy cessation is the stopping of all medications, which takes place if the child remains in continuous, complete remission for a certain time period. Therapy may also be stopped at a terminal stage of the child's illness.

sue necrosis. When giving periodic intravenous chemotherapy, be sure the needle is in the vein. Insure patency by rinsing the vein with sterile saline both before and after administering the drug. If an infiltration occurs, apply ice packs to the site for 24 hours, and follow with moist heat for 30 minutes every 2 hours until the inflammation is reduced. If necessary, alternate heat and ice after the first 24 hours for pain relief. When continuous intravenous chemotherapy is given, check the infusion site frequently for patency and skin integrity. Carefully assess for signs of infiltration (see the Skills Manual).

Side Effects of Chemotherapy

Side effects of chemotherapy may occur soon after the drug is administered, or may appear weeks later. Since children frequently continue to receive chemotherapy drugs at home, parents must be aware of possible side effects and have a home care plan prearranged.

Nausea and vomiting are common side effects of many anticancer drugs. Antiemetics, such as Compazine or Phenergan, can minimize nausea, if they are given before the chemotherapy, although they tend to make the child sleepy. Another method is to administer the nauseating drug in the evening so that the child sleeps through the hours of greatest discomfort. If this approach is used, the child should sleep on his side to minimize the possibility of aspiration if he should vomit; an emesis basin and call cord should be within easy reach, and the child should be observed frequently during the night. When nausea and/or vomiting do occur, try offering the child small sips of flat cola, apple juice, fruit punch, gelatin, water, or broth. Keep a record of the amount of vomitus and show the family how to measure and record the amount and color. These are important observations that parents and child will need to record at home, and it is important to teach them and give them practice in fluid measurement during the child's hospitalization. Prolonged or delayed nausea may indicate that the medication should be withheld or the dosage reduced. When the child is vomiting frequently, observe his urine, if it becomes dark, the child needs additional fluids. Whenever urine is not a light amber color, consult a physician.

Alopecia, hair loss, is a side effect of many chemotherapeutic agents. Prepare the child and family for its occurrence, emphasizing that the hair will grow back, although it may change its color or texture. The scalp needs frequent shampooing to prevent cradle cap, a scaly scalp condition. If cradle cap develops, use a lubricant to soften and remove the scaling tissue. Suggest cutting long hair short so that the child can adjust to a gradual change in appearance. The child and his parents will be anxious about when the hair will begin to shed, and they should be reassured that the hair loss will be gradual.

Once the hair is lost, the child and family learn to cope with the baldness very quickly. Since attractive wigs are now available, offer assistance in obtaining a wig. Boys frequently prefer a cap, while girls may choose to rotate colorful scarves with a wig. The hair will begin to grow back in one to two months, usually a shade darker than it was.

Several chemotherapeutic drugs may decrease the gastric motility, causing *constipation* and *obstipation*. Begin giving the child stool softeners at the first sign of difficulty, but do not use laxatives and enemas unless they are absolutely necessary. Diarrhea, another common gastric disturbance, may also occur. Keep a record of the number and amount of diarrhetic stools, rating the color and checking for blood and large amounts of mucus. If diarrhea occurs, discontinue giving the child fruits and fruit juices, since they have a laxative effect, and increase the child's fluid consumption (see ch. 18).

Anorexia is a frequent side effect of chemotherapy and may be related to nausea and vomiting or to oral bleeding and irritation. It may also be a separate occurrence (see ch. 18).

Certain drugs have characteristic side effects. For example, prednisone tends to increase the child's appetite and causes him to gain weight. It gives him a feeling of fullness and tightness in the abdomen. Since he is also likely to prefer salty foods, his salt intake may have to be restricted to minimize fluid retention. Food restrictions usually are not appropriate, but the family should be helped to plan menus that avoid junk foods and satisfy hunger with more nourishing foods.

Vincristine, another common chemotherapeutic drug, causes changes in the peripheral nervous system, including weakness of the hands, feet, and legs. The child's hands may droop from the wrist, his feet may droop from the ankles. He may feel numbness or tingling of the toes and fingers. Discuss these possible changes with the child and his parents, since most children taking vincristine notice some temporary weakness and increased fatigue.

When cyclophosphamide (Cytoxan), another common chemotherapeutic drug, is broken down, the byproducts can irritate the bladder and cause sterile hemorrhagic cystitis. To minimize exposure of the bladder to the chemical irritants, offer the child many fluids and have him empty his bladder frequently after receiving the drug, including at least once during the night. If cyclophosphamide is given daily, continue both the high fluid intake and the nightly voidings.

Everyone caring for the child receiving chemotherapy must be aware of the special needs and possible side effects of the treatments. Help parents decide what aspects of the diagnosis, care, and possible side effects of treatment they wish to discuss with the child's scout leader, teacher, baby sitter, or significant others who spend a great amount of time with the child.

Although it is not a side effect, another common problem of chemotherapy is the oral consumption of the drugs. Some of the medicines are bitter, and the child may refuse to take the drug, or he may swallow and then immediately regurgitate it. Parents become frantic and frustrated, fearing the immediate return of symptoms if one dosage is missed. Reassure parents and suggest that they mix the drug in fruit, peanut butter, chocolate syrup, or ice cream. These foods disguise the taste and make the drug easier to take. Always be honest with children; tell them when you are going to mix the medicine with food, and ask them what food they want to be used.

Radiation

Radiation disrupts the chemical bonds necessary for cell division, growth, and survival. Body cells, both malignant and normal, are most susceptible to radiation when they are dividing. Radiation is administered externally or internally and is measured as *electron volts (eV)*. *Kilovolts (KeV)* are used to measure low energy radiation; *megavolts (MeV)* measure high energy. *External radiation therapy* is most commonly used for children and is administered by directing radiation to an area *on* or *in* the child's body. *Internal radiation therapy* involves placing an isotope inside a body cavity or tissue. Both types of radiation therapy are used to cure the primary neoplasm and, as a palliative measure, to reduce pain, discomfort, and drainage. Radiation therapy, or *radiotherapy*, is used as an adjunct to chemotherapy, surgery, or immunotherapy.

The amount of radiation is divided into daily or weekly doses because large single doses would cause irreparable damage to normal as well as to tumor cells. The time between doses is as important as the amount of radiation. Although normal body tissue repairs faster than neoplastic cells, if the period between treatments is too long, the tumor cells will also repair. The dosage and time period between treatments is carefully regulated to provide maximum destruction to the cancerous cells while maintaining an adequate number of healthy cells.

Malignant tumors are classified according to their *radiosensitivity* or *radioresistance*. A *radiosensitive tumor* is destroyed by dosages of radiation well tolerated by the surrounding normal tissue. A *radioresistant tumor* can be eradicated by radiation but the required dosage is too toxic for the surrounding tissue. Malignant cells in the hematopoietic and lymphatic tissues are very radiosensitive; however, neoplasms in the connective tissue are radioresistant.

Radiotherapy attempts to deliver a maximum dose to the tumor and a minimal dose to the surrounding normal tissue. Sometimes, however, normal cells are damaged. The damage is usually acute, but lasts only until the end of treatment or for a short period afterward.

Side effects of radiotherapy relate to the body area irradiated. Radiation therapy to the head and neck commonly causes ulcers in the mouth and pharynx; while irradiation to bones depresses the bone marrow and reduces blood cell production. Radiation therapy affecting the digestive tract may cause loss of appetite, vomiting, and diarrhea.

When caring for a child receiving radiotherapy, carefully discuss the purpose of the radiation therapy with the family. Explain that colored markings are used to outline the area on the child's body to be irradiated; these markings should not be washed off. Discuss the importance of good nutrition to maintain the child's weight and to help speed tissue repair. Since nausea and vomiting are common side effects of radiotherapy, assess the child's food likes, dislikes, and meal times. Using this information, try to plan menus with high protein and carbohydrate content but with a minimum of fat and residue. Foods, such as baked or mashed potatoes, white breads, puddings, ice cream, diced carrots or beans, creamed soups, soft cooked eggs, applesauce, and gelatin usually are tolerated best. Avoid serving tough fibrous or whole sliced meats, frankfurters, shrimp, lobster, cheese, spices, fried eggs, coarse breads or rolls, and raw fruits and vegetables. Depending on the child's intake, a low-residue, easily absorbed dietary supplement may be prescribed to maintain fluid and nutritional intake. It is especially important that the child drink more to compensate for fluid losses resulting from vomiting and diarrhea. Nursing interventions for the side effects of diarrhea, oral ulcerations, and bone marrow depression with possible infection and bleeding were discussed earlier in this chapter.

Skin reactions are unique to radiotherapy. No matter where the neoplasm is located, skin epithelial cells are constantly dividing and in the path of radiation, and thus are especially liable to assault. Skin reactions vary from mild erythema to severe blistering and skin sloughing. If a skin reaction occurs, it will begin three to six weeks after the start of radiation. The skin becomes red, dry, and scaly—a "dry reaction." As therapy continues, blisters may form and burst, forming ulcers that expel serum. This is a "wet reaction." If a wet reaction occurs, the child is given a rest from therapy. Home-prescribed creams, ointments, or deodorants should not be applied to the areas being treated. Similarly, the child must avoid wearing restricting garments that can cause further irritation. Keep the red, blistered, or weeping areas dry at all times. It is best for the child to wear cotton garments next to the skin because they absorb moisture. Cornstarch also can be used to absorb the wetness. The affected skin can be washed with a mild soap and patted dry. The skin should not be exposed to direct sunlight, however, because of the danger of sunburn.

Advise the family not to use heating pads, hot water bags, or compresses on the child. They should also avoid perfumes, powders, or ointments containing alcohol, which can dry the skin. Baby oil can be applied as needed for dryness. In each case, the goal is to maintain skin integrity and minimize possible infection. After radiotherapy is completed, the child can resume bathing and the normal use of lotions and powders.

Immunotherapy

Immunotherapy is based on the premise that since the immune system can recognize and react to foreign organisms that cause infection, it may be stimulated to respond and react to cancerous cells. In order for the immune system to work against neoplastic growth, however, the body must recognize a neoplasm as different, and to be different the neoplasm must have antigens not found in the child's body. Such specific antigens do exist in human neoplasms, and immunotherapy acts to stimulate the immune system to recognize and destroy the neoplastic cells.

Stimulants used to challenge the immune system include microorganisms, prepared compounds, and altered neoplastic cells. Immunotherapy is usually done in conjunction with other previously discussed treatments. The timing of immunotherapy is crucial. Because the neoplastic process (like radiotherapy and chemotherapy) can be immunosuppressive, immunotherapy works best when there are as many healthy cells as possible available to respond to the stimulation.

The primary danger of immunotherapy is enhancement. *Enhancement* means the promotion, or enhancement, of neoplastic growth as a result of overstimulation of antibody production and the presence of large amounts of circulating antigen-antibody complexes.

When the child is considered for immunotherapy, his immune system response is evaluated. The T and B lymphocytes are measured and examined for their proliferation capacity. Exact laboratory tests exist for these measurements. Skin patch tests can be used to evaluate the ability of the T cells to respond to a stimulus. Frequently, a nurse gives the skin test, following a definite procedure, and explaining to the family how to care for the site and when to read the test. Immune evaluations are done before the initial immunotherapy, after remission, and at other appropriate intervals of three to six months. It is important that the child's system be free from cytotoxic drugs during these evaluation periods.

Immunotherapy is classified as specific or nonspecific. *Specific immunotherapy* focuses on the tumor, and the general immune capacity of the child may not be affected. Specific immunotherapy uses substances related to, or products of, the tumor such as killed tumor cells from the patient or from another person with a similar tumor. Tumor cells that have been altered in vitro, rendering them more immunogenic, may be used.

Nonspecific immunotherapy stimulates the overall immune response to enhance the child's ability to respond to the neoplasm. Nonspecific immunotherapy uses materials that have no antigenic relation to the tumor, but which increase the general immune ability of the child. Microorganisms used for nonspecific immunotherapy include bacillus Calmette-Guérin (BCG), the methanol-extractable residue of BCG (MER), and Corynebacterium parvum, (c. parvum). Bacillus Calmette-Guérin is a form of living bovine tubercle bacillus—a compound that has been used for many years to immunize persons against tuberculosis. It is a potent agent capable of increasing the recipient's immune response to a wide variety of tumor-specific antigens. BCG may be injected directly into the tumor nodules or intradermally at sites distant from the tumor. Both MER and Corynebacterium parvum are nonspecific stimulants which promote immunity and antibody production.

Immunotherapy affects neoplastic cells only, destroying new lesions—some of which are so small that they are not yet noticeable. By doing so, it prevents new growth and further spread of the neoplasm. Immunotherapy may be effective in reversing the immunosuppressive effects of the neoplastic process itself and of chemotherapy and radiotherapy.

Both specific and nonspecific immunotherapy is further subclassified as active, passive, or adoptive. *Active immunotherapy* uses vaccines prepared from the child's own tumor cells or from cells from a similar tumor. The vaccines are given to induce specific immunity against cancer antigens. *Passive immunotherapy* is the administering of the product of an immune reaction that has occurred in one person to another person. For example, the transfusion of sera containing antibodies is passive immunotherapy. *Adoptive immunotherapy* is the transfer of the means for a prolonged specific immune response to a recipient's immune system. An example is the use of *transfer factor,* a leukocytic extract which, when administered, can transfer skin reactivity to specific antigens. For example, transfer factor prepared from the lymphocytes of a person designated positive by a skin test can transmit the positive person's reaction when given to a person whose skin test originally showed a negative reading.

Immunotherapy is relatively new, and its use is expanding. When working with children receiving immunotherapy, be aware of the different agents used to stimulate the immune system. Find out if the material contains tumor cells or a potentially allergic substance. Does it contain a live organism that may be infectious? Both the nature of the material and the expected result need to be explained to child and his family. Ask the immunologist whether or not to expect an immediate hypersensitivity reaction or toxicity. Ascertain the procedure to be followed for giving the immunotherapy and any special precautions needed for protecting the child, his family, or the staff. How will the immunotherapy interact with other therapies the child is receiving? The unknown always creates anxiety and fear. Conveying information on immunotherapy simply and thoroughly provides reassurance and support—and the continual partnership between staff and family—needed for optimal care.

Transfusions

The child with cancer frequently has too few erythrocytes, leukocytes, and platelets—a condition called *pancytopenia*. The cause may be the neoplastic process and the concommitant suppression of the immune system and bone marrow, the effects of chemotherapy or radiotherapy, or a combination of these forces. Regardless of the reason, when his vital blood components are reduced, the child is liable to infection, hemorrhage, and severe anemia. A blood transfusion can replenish the child's supply of normal blood cells. Unfortunately, parents frequently consider a blood transfusion a last resort reserved for the dying child. This is not true; blood transfusions can improve the child's health by offering a donor's blood cells to resist infection or carry oxygen until the child's own supply can be replenished.

A successful transfusion depends on crossmatching of blood products for compatability. The child's and donor's specific cell characteristics, such as the bloodtype and antigens, must be matched. Unmatched blood products trigger an immune reaction, causing characteristic symptoms of apprehension, severe headache, restlessness, chills, or fever. The reactions will occur soon after the transfusion begins if unmatched products are present. Transfusions and the immediate nursing care are discussed in chapter 24.

Transfusions may contain only one blood product, such as erythrocytes, or a combination of erythrocytes, leukocytes, and platelets, as in whole blood. The process of separating blood into its individual parts and removing selected components is called *pheresis*. *Pheresis* can be done manually or by an elaborate machine process. Pheresis machines can separate the components of a donor's blood and remove only the needed cells, such as leukocytes; the remaining blood can be returned to the donor. Pheresis permits repeated donations of blood by the same donor. *Leukopheresis* is the process of separating leukocytes from the donor's blood; the remaining blood is returned to the donor. Special procedures are necessary for the preparing both the donor and the receiver when pheresis is used.

A complication of any transfusion is the development of antibodies. The child's blood may form antibodies against antigens carried on the donor's blood components. When this occurs, the child's antibodies recognize a donor's foreign antigens, and the donated blood components are destroyed within minutes after transfusion. Close typing and crossmatching is required to guard against antibody-antigen reactions. Chapter 21 presents a complete discussion of blood types.

Bone Marrow Transplants

A *bone marrow transplant* is the intravenous infusion of bone marrow from a donor into a recipient. Children qualifying for a bone marrow transplant must meet certain criteria developed by the treatment center, and then must submit to vigorous preliminary radiation and chemotherapy prior to the actual infusion of the bone marrow. Careful monitoring and special care are important before, during, and after the bone marrow infusion. Although it is rare with proper immunosuppressive therapy prior to the transplant, the child may reject the transplanted bone marrow.

The biggest problem affecting a successful bone marrow transplant is *graft-versus-host disease* (GVHD). When marrow is transplanted, the marrow graft produces lymphocytes that can recognize the recipient (host) as foreign, and, instead of the receiving child rejecting the transplant, the donated marrow rejects the host. GVHD occurs in 70 percent of children receiving a bone marrow transplant. The skin, liver, and gastrointestinal tract may be affected, each in varying degrees of severity. Although immunosuppressive drugs are used to prevent and minimize GVHD, many children have a reaction and some die because of it.

Laminar Air Flow Units

The child with cancer frequently becomes dangerously susceptible to infection because of the immunosuppressive effects of his neoplasm and the treatments he receives. Reverse isolation measures may be necessary to protect the child from pathogens. Another more elaborate form of reverse isolation is the *laminar air flow unit*. These rooms or units filter all entering air, removing bacteria and moisture-bound viruses. A constant *onward* flow of air circulates into the unit. All food, linen, toys, and other items entering the laminar flow unit must be specially prepared and sterilized. Elaborate procedures are also followed for all persons entering the unit.

Children with cancer and children with other immunological deficiencies have benefited from this pathogen-free environment. The technical and economic problems of operating a laminar air flow unit are immense, as are the potential psychological problems of being isolated for long periods of treatment. The units are rare in small communities, but are becoming increasingly common in urban areas.

Going Home

After what seems like an endless period of treatment in the hospital, the child with cancer goes home to outpatient and home therapy. If his condition permits, the child will return to school. Discharge can be a very frightening time as parents try to recall their child's medication; clinic revisit schedule; the home first aid for nausea, vomiting, nosebleeds, constipation, and so on. If parents have participated in the giving, monitoring, and recording of care in the hospital, they are more confident of their ability to care for their child at home.

Each family needs additional verbal reassurance and *written* instructions about 1) when each medicine is to be given; 2) some simple first aid measures for each common side effect of therapy; and 3) most important, what symptoms signal a needed call or visit to a medical care facility. Provide phone numbers and alternative names to call if a certain physician or nurse cannot be reached. Coordination with community medical personnel is especially important. Review discharge planning (see ch. 2), making sure each item is covered before the child's departure. Carefully review the clinic routine and what parents should expect when they return for laboratory work, treatments, and procedures, such as a bone marrow aspiration.

Parents need continual support in the care of a child with cancer and assurance that their child can and should follow a normal routine. Discipline is as important after the diagnosis as before. If the child is excused from chores, catered to, and made to feel different, he may be convinced that he is going to die or that his parents feel guilty. Each child needs love and discipline. A child without limits is frustrated and unhappy; he does not learn how to cope with each new stage of his illness and therapy.

The role and behavior of the mother and father tend to be different. The mother usually makes the daily or weekly trips to the clinic for care, gives the medicines at home, and offers first aid for side effects. Frequently, mothers befriend other mothers during clinic waits and discuss their child's illness, treatments, and prognosis. When a child dies, all mothers soon know. Death is considered as a real possibility for the child and the mother, since both are intimately involved with the disease every day. In contrast, the father is at work and not involved in day-to-day care management. He is more removed from the illness and can easily deny its existence as he watches his child at play. He can believe there is no cancer.

This difference in roles and perception of the disease often causes communication problems between husband and wife. Parents may find it difficult to talk—the mother wanting to share her feelings of loneliness and frustration while the father seeks to deny the problem. If he discusses the illness it is an admission of its existence, so he refuses to talk. Added stress is placed on family relationships already burdened with financial and time constraints.

Be aware of the parents' feelings, and assure them that their depression, denial, and guilt are normal. The family is in stress, and all its members need extra support and help. Frequently, groups of parents will meet to discuss problems and share concerns, experiences, and questions about their children's treatment, care, and prognosis. Through group support, families gain a better sense of mastery and understanding of their feelings and can then become more involved with the child's and other family members' feelings, accomplishments, and frustrations.

After all, some children with cancer die, but many others recuperate and go on to lead normal lives. Yet long years of treatment, pain, and frustration test everyone's patience and integrity. Families may grasp for sure cures or painless methods of treatment. They will hear about hundreds of unproven, some possibly dangerous, cures for cancer. Miracle drugs that offer a cure for all cancers, recipes and food regimens that guarantee a prevention and cure of cancer, occult techniques of trances and rituals, various injectable concoctions—these are all part of the thriving business of cancer quackery. Families turn to unproven miracle cures because they fear pain, body mutilation, the unknown, and most of all death. For many people cancer means death. Even when parents have not listened to claims of miracle cures initially, uninformed friends and relatives can convince a family to experiment with various forms of cancer quackery.

Be aware of what different "miracle cures" are offered in your community and listen to patients, peers, friends, and relatives as to what myths are circulating about cancer diagnosis, treatment, and rehabilitation. Offer correct information whenever possible. When unproven methods of cure are offered in a community, report them to the health department, local medical society, or cancer society. Lastly, provide the family with what the quack cures offer—time to listen, a sense of dignity today, and hope for tomorrow. Be present to listen, offer understanding, and provide dignity. Assist and support the family during those long painful treatments.

Some children with cancer will die, sometimes after an unanticipated relapse following several healthy months or years. This is very difficult for the health staff and family to accept. Children and adolescents with terminal cancer may spend their last weeks or days in the hospital, or they may be cared for at home or in special hospitals, termed *hospices*. *Hospices* care for people who are dying; these centers offer comfort, concern, and support. They seek a peaceful death, one free from all pain, if possible. Although previously reserved for adults, hospices now often admit adolescents.

Children taken home to die need a special supportive relationship between the health staff and their families. Offer the parents written instructions for comforting and caring for pain and hemorrhage, which are likely terminal complications. If possible, help them to feel free to call and discuss concerns, problems, and frustrations at any time of the day or night. If families are provided with home care as a choice, thoroughly discuss this option with the family, making sure the whole family desires this choice and will accept the accompanying responsibility. It is important that the family does not feel pressured into the decision. Children usually prefer to die at home surrounded by familiar persons and favorite toys, pets, and music. Most children who die at home have peaceful deaths, frequently nestled in their parents' arms. Families feel strengthened by the experience, feeling they offered love and peace to their child.

SUMMARY

The child with cancer houses an uncontrolled growth that alters normal body functions. Because his immune system is impaired, the child is liable to major infections and life-threatening illnesses. If the neoplasm grows in the bone marrow, the production of erythrocytes, leukocytes, and megakarocytes is impaired. Without sufficient bone marrow products and a functioning immune system, nutrients cannot be delivered to and waste cannot be gathered from body cells. The child loses weight, is anemic, and is fatigued. Torn blood vessels bleed easily and may hemorrhage. Infections loom with every pathogen, and families must take stringent precautions to ensure health. Major treatments of chemotherapy and radiotherapy kill cancerous cells but also destroy normal healthy cells, causing the child's bone marrow and immune systems to be suppressed even further. Radiotherapy and chemotherapy cause nausea, vomiting, and diarrhea, making it hard for the child to consume the nutrients vital for new cell production and tissue growth. Hair is shed, skin becomes blistered and dry, and with surgical scars and repeated test and treatments, the body image is changed. Everyone knows when a child has cancer.

During treatment, care must focus on the quality of the child's life. Careful planning can prevent and minimize nausea and vomiting. Persistent support and creativity can entice a child to eat needed protein, and body image changes can be incorporated into a positive self-concept.

New noninvasive diagnostic means make repeated examinations less painful and frightening; there are no side effects. Immunotherapy stimulates the child's own defense mechanisms into action against the cancer, and bone marrow transplants and laminar air flow units offer additional hope and means for treating cancer. With preventive measures and close attention to bleeding and infection sites, major complications can be minimized and the child's immune defenses and blood cells can be protected until they have been reestablished and health has been restored.

Some children with cancer die; but many others attend school, play, grow, and make death wait.

CLINICAL APPLICATION

"But tomorrow is my birthday, I'm not going to the doctor." Mrs. B. had been concerned about Kelly's lack of appetite, fatigue, and pallor for several weeks. However, with four school-age children, she was used to temporary changes in activity and eating habits. But now, because of Kelly's persistent fever and so much illness in the neighborhood, Mrs. B. had made a doctor's appointment for ten-year-old Kelly. Kelly sat reading a comic as the doctor told her that additional tests were needed to determine the cause of her fever, and that she must be admitted to the hospital that afternoon.

Kelly was quickly admitted to the children's unit and left crying as Mrs. B. hurried home to make arrangements for her other three children who were due home in an hour. Later that evening, Mr. and Mrs. B. were told that Kelly had leukemia, and that chemotherapy and radiotherapy were necessary for treatment. As you enter the room the next morning, Mrs. B. is staring out the window as Kelly sleeps. You say "Good morning" and Mrs. B. dissolves into tears.

> Identify the known stresses now confronting the B. family. Select two stresses—perhaps the diagnosis, unanticipated hospitalization, fatigue, or uncertainty—and list nursing interventions for each.

You tell Mrs. B. that leukemia is a frightening condition. There are so many medicines and special words used to discuss leukemia that it is normal to feel confused and scared. You offer to reexplain to the parents the meaning of leukemia, the purpose of chemotherapy and radiotherapy, and the expected results of each. Mr. and Mrs. B. listen, asking several questions. As you finish, they ask how they can explain leukemia to Kelly's siblings, who are five-, seven-, and nine-years-old.

> With the parents' help, form a teaching plan for the siblings using illustrations and descriptive words to explain leukemia, the needed treatments, and possible effects of treatment. Kelly begins induction with prednisone, vincristine, and Cytoxan. Explain to the B.'s why these drugs are used for induction, and describe their expected effect and possible side effects. Anticipating nausea and vomiting, anorexia, and further bone marrow depression with possible infection, bleeding and anemia—list specific nursing care interventions that can prevent and minimize these side effects.

Kelly gains weight and has a cushnoid appearance after taking prednisone. Having also lost her hair, Kelly is being teased by siblings and other children about her appearance.

> What information about the school-age child may help the B.'s and Kelly cope with the teasing? Offer suggestions for how to tease back. What verbal support will encourage a positive self-image, helping Kelly through these temporary changes in physical appearance?

Following induction, Kelly is to receive central nervous system prophylaxis with cranial irradiation and intrathecal methotrexate.

> Using simple, hand-drawn illustrations, explain how intrathecal drugs are administered and the expected effect.

Kelly returns to school, receiving maintenance therapy of 6-MP, methotrexate, and Cytoxan.

> Prepare a home care plan for the B.'s, listing each maintenance medication, the possible side effects, and home first aid measures for those side effects. Since the bone marrow and immune system may continue to be depressed, what precautions for infection and bleeding should the family take?

Several months later Mrs. B. phones to ask about a wonder diet that is a cure for cancer. The treatment is expensive and must be ordered in the mail.

Offer a response.

Kelly has been in remission for three years, and all treatments have stopped. Now thirteen, Kelly has learned to play the guitar, is enjoying her fifth year of ballet, and hates science but enjoys literature. Kelly is a healthy adolescent who feels good about herself and others.

Bibliography

Bingham, C.A. The Cell Cycle and Cancer Chemotherapy. *American Journal of Nursing* 78:1201, 1978.

Bloomquist, L.M. and Lewis-Hunstiger, M. J. To Care for the Child at Home: Discharge Planning for the Child with Leukemia. *Cancer Nursing* 1:303, 1978.

Bouchard, R. and Owens, N.F. *Nursing Care of the Cancer Patient,* ed. 3. St. Louis, C.V. Mosby Co., 1976.

Brewis, E.L., Robertson, H., House, F. Nursing Children under the Laminar Flow: A Boy with Leukemia. *Nursing Times* 73:1154, 1977.

Brewis, E.L., Robertson, F., House, F. Practical Aspects of Nursing Children under the Laminar Flow. *Nursing Times* 73:1120, 1977.

Burkhalter, P.K. Cancer Quackery. *American Journal of Nursing* 77:451, 1977.

Burkhalter, P. and Donley, D. (eds). *Dynamics of Oncology Nursing.* New York, McGraw-Hill, 1978.

Burns, V. Cancer Chemotherapy: A Systemic Approach. *American Journal of Nursing* 8:57, 1978.

Dietz, K. Radiation Therapy. *Cancer Nursing* 2:129, 1979.

Dodd, M.J. Theoretical Bases of Immunotherapy. *American Journal of Nursing* 79:310, 1979.

Donley, D. Nursing the Patient Who Is Immunosuppressed. *American Journal of Nursing* 76:989, 1977.

Elliott, C.S. Radiation Therapy: How You Can Help. *Nursing '76* 6:34, 1976.

Fochtman, D. Malignant Solid Tumors in Children. *Pediatric Nursing* 2:11, 1976.

Foley, G. and McCarthy, A.M. The Child With Leukemia: The Disease and Its Treatment. *American Journal of Nursing* 76:1108, 1976.

Greene, T. Current Therapy for Acute Leukemia in Childhood. *Nursing Clinics of North America* 11:3, 1976.

Isler, C. Immunotherapy. *RN* 39:35, 1976.

Jo Clapp, M. Psychosocial Reactions of Children with Cancer: A Program for Rehabilitation. *Nursing Clinics of North America* 11:73, 1976.

Leahy, I., St. Germain, J., Varricchis, C. *The Nurse and Radiotherapy: A Manual For Daily Care.* St. Louis, C.V. Mosby Co., 1978.

Martinson, I. Parents Help Each Other. *American Journal of Nursing* 76:1121, 1976.

McCalla, J.L. Immunotherapy: Concepts and Nursing Implications. *Nursing Clinics of North America* 11:59, 1976.

Miller, S.A. The Oncology Nurse and Chemotherapy. *American Journal of Nursing* 77:989, 1977.

Peterson, B.H. and Kellogg, C.J. *Current Perspectives In Oncologic Nursing,* vol. 2. St. Louis, C.V. Mosby Co., 1978.

Pilapil, F. and Studva, K.V. Cancer Chemotherapy. *Cancer Nursing* 1:153, 1978.

Rossman, M., Slavin, R., Taft, E. Pheresis Therapy: Patient Care. *American Journal of Nursing* 77:1135, 1977.

Stagner, S.A. and Wood, A. The Child With Cancer on Immunosuppressive Therapy: Implications for Nursing. *Nursing Clinics of North America* 11:21, 1976.

Tenczynski, J. Leukopheresis: The Process. *American Journal of Nursing* 77:1133, 1977.

Van Scoy-Mosher, M.B. Chemotherapy: A Manual for Patients and Their Families. *Cancer Nursing* 1:234, 1978.

Voors, B.B. Pneumocystis carinii in the Immunosuppressed Child. *Cancer Nursing* 2:15, 1979.

Walker, P. Bone Marrow Transplant: A Second Chance For Life. *Nursing 77* 7:24, 1977.

Zimmerman, S., Cohen, T., Diekman, R., Calvo, C., Hangstenfer, M. Bone Marrow Transplantation. *American Journal of Nursing* 77:1311, 1977.

SECTION FOUR

Oxygenation

CHAPTER **21**

Oxygenation

BEHAVIORAL OBJECTIVES

After studying this chapter you will be able to:

- Discuss the structure of the heart, describing the blood flow of the systemic circulation and the pulmonary circulation, identifying the special valves, muscles, and vessels that aid circulation.
- Describe the electrical conduction system of the heart and identify the structure that acts as the pacemaker of the heart.
- Explain the pressure differences within the heart during fetal circulation and the changes that normally occur at birth.
- Compare the causes and diagram the circulation pattern of a right-to-left and left-to-right shunt.
- Describe the production and functions of erythrocytes and platelets.
- Explain respiration, discussing how air is conducted into the lungs and diffused through the blood.
- Explain the function of partial pressure of gases in the pulmonary and systemic circulations.
- Define hypoxia, comparing ischemic hypoxia, hypoxic hypoxia, and anemic hypoxia.

TERMS AND CONCEPTS

Atria
Ventricles
Pericardium
Pulmonary circulation
Systemic circulation
Cuspid valves
Anastomosis
Sinoatrial node
Stenosis
Coarctation
Reticulocytes
Oxyhemoglobin
Carbaminohemoglobin
Polycythemia
Bilirubin
Prothrombin
Fibrinogen
Thrombin
Fibrin
Thrombosis
Antithrombin
Fibrinolysin
Agglutinins
Lymphatics
Pulmonary bronchi
Bronchioles
Alveolar ducts
Alveolar sacs
Alveoli
Tidal volume

Partial pressure
Blood pH
Ischemic hypoxia
Hypoxic hypoxia
Anemic hypoxia

Circulation is the movement of blood through vessels. Blood, a mixture of cells and fluid, is ejected from the heart and thrust into one of two waiting circuits that transport nutrients and retrieve waste from body cells. Pressure differences within the heart and the two circuits promote the exchange of oxygen and carbon dioxide. This chapter focuses on normal circulatory structure and function. The structure of the heart, circuits, and blood determine circulatory function. When changes occur in structure or production, function is immediately altered and health is jeopardized.

THE HEART

Layers of muscle form the heart and divide it into four chambers; two upper cavities called *atria* and two lower *ventricles* (Figure 21–1). The lower border of the heart forms a blunt point known as the *apex*. The *apical heartbeat* is heard by placing a stethoscope directly over the apex. Before age two, the apical heartbeat is heard in the fourth left interspace outside the mammary line. After age two, the apical beat is usually in the fifth interspace within the mammary line. Heart boundaries determine heart size and are age-related. Since a change in heart size accompanies certain heart diseases, heart boundaries are usually noted and charted during an examination of the heart.

The heart is covered by a loose-fitting sac called the *pericardium*. The pericardium attaches to the large vessels emerging from the top of the heart but does not attach to the heart itself. Consisting of a sac of tough fibrous tissue on the outside and a smooth, moist membranous covering next to the heart, the pericardium forms a snug jacket that offers the heart protection against friction. If the pericardium becomes inflamed, a condition called *pericarditis* results; fluid or pus accumulates in the pericardial space, and friction and rubbing can occur, hampering the action of the heart. The wall of the heart consists of three layers of tissue: the *epicardium* or outer layer, the *myocardium* or middle layer, and the *endocardium* or innermost layer (Figure 21–2).

The myocardium forms the bulk of the heart wall and contains special cardiac muscle that contracts to squeeze blood through the heart chambers into circulation (Figure 21–3). Blood is directed from the heart into two different paths. One path takes deoxygenated blood to the lungs where it is resaturated with oxygen and returned to the heart; this is the *pulmonary circulation*. A second circuit takes oxygenated blood to all body tissue; this is the *systemic circulation*. In order for circulation to occur, both the pulmonary and systemic circulation must be operating (Figure 21–4).

Four sets of valves are important to circulation. Two of these valves are located inside the heart between the atria and ventricles; the remaining two are inside the great vessels that leave the heart. The *cuspid valves* operate the opening between atria and ventricles (atrioventricular orifices). The cuspid valve at the right atrioventricular opening is the *tricuspid valve*. The cuspid valve on the left side is the bicuspid valve, usually referred to as the *mitral valve*. To remember which side is tricuspid and which mitral, remember that the letter *m* is close to the letter *l*; the *m*itral valve is on the *l*eft side. The letter *t* is close to the letter *r*; the *t*ricuspid valve is on the *r*ight side of the heart. Both cuspid valves *permit* blood to flow from the atria into the ventricles and *prevent* blood from flowing back up into the atria from the venticles. The cuspid valves permit only *one-way blood traffic*. Of the two remaining valves, one is located in the pulmonary artery and one in the aorta. Each prevents a backflow of blood.

Three types of vessels carry blood within the body: *arteries, capillaries,* and *veins*. Arteries carry blood away from the heart. Small arteries are called *arterioles*. The alternate expansion and recoil of an artery creates a *pulse*. The pulse is felt wherever an artery lies near the skin surface; for example, the radial pulse is at the wrist and is easily felt, as is the temporal artery at the outer side of the eye. Capillaries deliver

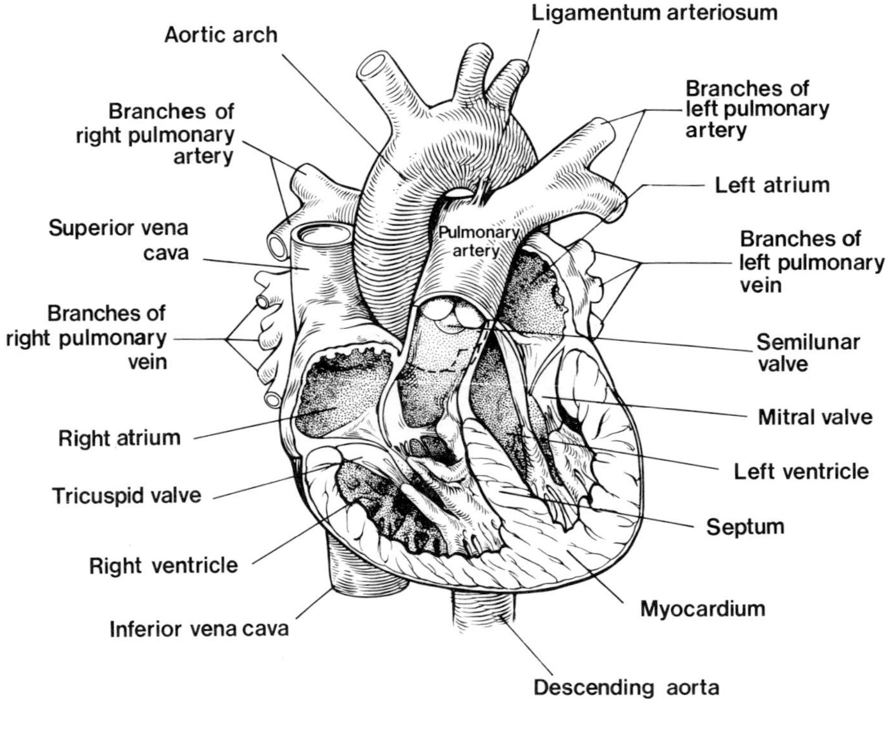

Figure 21–1. *The Heart. Blood returns to the heart via the superior and inferior vena cava. Entering the right atrium, the blood passes through the tricuspid valve into the right ventricle. The blood is ejected through the pulmonary (semilunar) valve into the pulmonary arteries through the lungs. Returning by the pulmonary veins, the oxygenated blood enters the left atrium, passes through the left atrium and mitral valve into the left ventricle. The blood is ejected through the aortic valve into the aorta and out into the systemic circulation.*

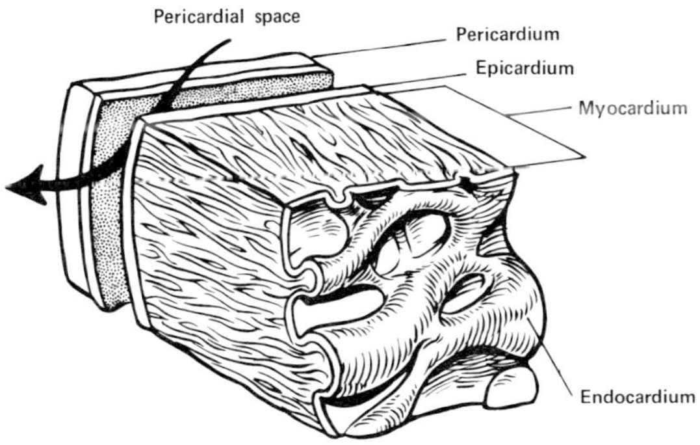

Figure 21–2. *Three layers of tissue comprise the heart wall: the endocardium, the myocardium, and the epicardium. Between the epicardium and the pericardium is the pericardial space.*

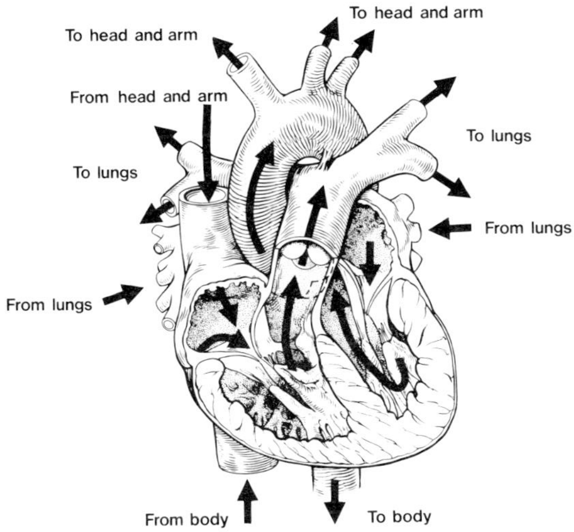

Figure 21–3. *Normal circulation.*

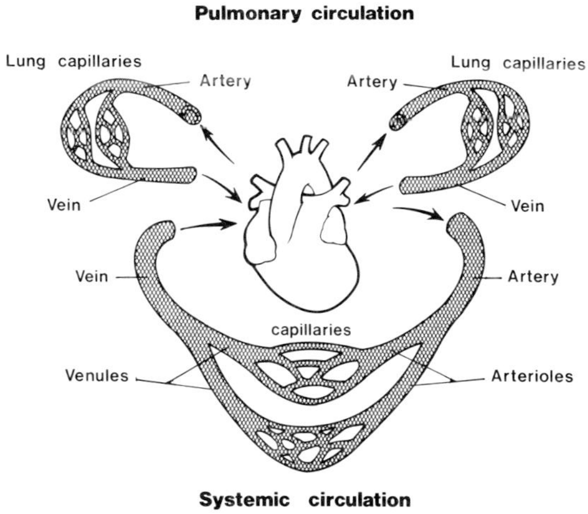

Figure 21–4. *The systemic and pulmonary circulations oxygenate the body.*

oxygen and nutrients to individual cells and pick up waste products. Capillaries carry blood from arterioles to *venules*, which are small veins. Veins carry blood back to the heart. Due to their different functions, arteries, capillaries, and veins look different. Arteries have strong vascular walls, and blood flows rapidly in their lumen to the tissues. Capillaries function to exchange fluid and nutrients between the blood and interstitial spaces. Thus capillary walls are very thin and permeable by small substances. Veins collect blood. Since the pressure is low as blood returns to the heart, veins are thin-walled; however, veins can contract or expand, thereby storing small or large amounts of blood, depending on the body's needs.

In order to pump blood into circulation, the heart needs oxygen, nutrients, and the removal of waste products. Blood is circulated to the heart muscle by two small vessels, the *right* and *left coronary arteries*. The largest amount of blood going to the heart is delivered to the myocardium of the left ventricle, since the left ventricle does the most work and thus needs added oxygen and nutrients. Unfortunately, only a few anastomoses exist between the branches of the coronary arteries; an *anastomosis* is a branch that bridges a part of an artery to a more distal part of itself or another artery. Similar to detours, anastomoses can provide alternate paths for blood flow if a main route is obstructed. Since there are few anastomoses between coronary arteries, a potentially dangerous situation exists: if one of the larger coronary artery branches is obstructed (for example, by a blood clot), adequate amounts of blood cannot reach the heart muscle. Without oxygen the heart muscle cannot pump. Cardiac muscle deprived of oxygen becomes *ischemic*, i.e., lacking oxygen. Ischemic tissue cannot function, and if it is not oxygenated quickly, cell death occurs.

Special tissue enables the heart to pump blood. This tissue forms structures that conduct impulses necessary for heart muscle contractions. The *sinoatrial node (SA node)*, called the "pacemaker," initiates impulses that travel throughout the muscle fibers of both atria at regular intervals. The impulses are further conducted by additional nodal tissue that stimulates the ventricles to contract. It is the SA node that initiates heartbeats and sets the pace of contractions. Artificial pacemakers electrically stimulate the heart to contract. These artificial pacemakers maintain a steady heart rate and allow a person with a damaged heart to live for many years; however they *cannot* speed up or slow down the heart beat.

The nodal tissue generates small electrical currents in the heart. This current is dispersed throughout the surrounding tissue and can be measured on the surface of the body and recorded on an *electrocardiograph* (EKG) as an *electrocardiogram.* An electrocardiogram is a graph of the heart's impulses shown as electrical impulses. The electrical impulses cause the heart muscle to contract and create the pressure needed to move the blood through the valves. The heart's contraction is called *systole* and its relaxation is called *diastole*. The pressures that occur at the times of contraction and relaxation are measured on a *sphygmomanometer* and are referred to as *blood pressure*. The systolic blood pressure is the force of the blood pushing against the artery walls when the ventricles are contracting; the diastolic pressure is the force of blood when the ventricles are relaxed. Systolic pressure relates to the force of the *left* ventricular contraction, and the diastolic pressure relates to the *resistance* of the blood vessels. The diastolic pressure is considered more important because it indicates the pressure or strain to which blood vessel walls are constantly subjected.

The two atria contract at the same time. As they relax, the two ventricles contract and then relax. The entire heart does not contract as a whole; rather, as one part relaxes, another part contracts, producing a "milking" action that moves blood from chamber to chamber, then out into the body. The characteristic sounds made as the blood is pumped through the chambers can be heard with a stethoscope. Abnormal sounds may indicate a malfunctioning valve. A *murmur* is an abnormal heart sound and usually indicates an improperly functioning valve, frequently caused by incomplete closing or narrowing of the valve opening.

Pressure Differences Within the Heart

The muscle, tissue, chambers, and valves of the heart could not pump blood unless pressure differences existed within the heart itself. Pressure provides the force necessary to propel blood through the body. If changes in heart structure that affect these different pressures occur, heart functions change.

Blood saturated with carbon dioxide and oxygen enters the right atrium. The pressure in the right atrium is low, only 2 to 4 millimeters of mercury (mm Hg). From the right atrium blood moves into the right ventricle, then through the pulmonary arteries to the lungs. The pressure increases in the pulmonary arteries to between 20 and 25 mm Hg. Blood is saturated with oxygen in the lungs and then moves into the left atrium. The left atrium has a pressure of 8 to 10 mm Hg. A huge change in pressure occurs as the blood leaves the left atrium at 8 to 10 mm Hg and enters the left ventricle, where the pressure is 100 to 110 mm Hg. This drastic increase in pressure is needed to force blood into the systemic circulation.

During fetal circulation (Figure 21–5) the fetal lungs are collapsed and do not function because the placenta supplies all needed oxygen. Since the lungs are collapsed, there is resistance to any pulmonary circulation, thus *high pressure* exists in the right ventricle and right pulmonary artery. Simultaneously, the aorta and left ventricle meet little systemic resistance, as there is *low pressure* on the left side of the heart. The pressure differences between the right and left sides of the normal child's heart are *reversed* during fetal circulation, and so, therefore, is the oxygenation process.

The umbilical vein carries oxygenated blood from the placenta to the fetus. When this vein arrives at the fetal liver, it divides, allowing half of the oxygenated blood to bypass the liver by passing through the *ductus venosus* and into the inferior vena cava and heart chambers.

A second small connecting lumen, the *ductus arteriosus,* shunts blood away from the nonfunctioning lungs into the aorta and out into the systemic circulation. This is a very efficient way of delivering blood to the fetus and is made possible by the pressure relationships. Higher pressures in the right

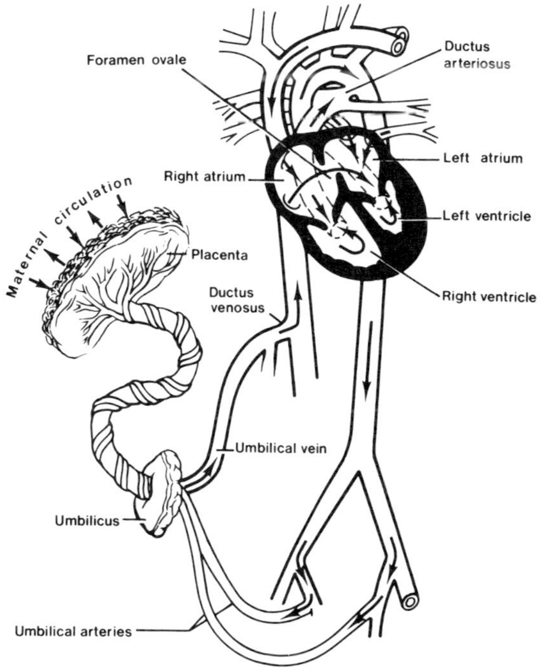

Figure 21–5. *Fetal circulation. Blood enters the fetal heart from the umbilical vein. The blood then enters the right atrium and is pumped through the foramen ovale into the left atrium. From the left atrium the blood goes to the left ventricle, then into the aorta and out to the upper extremities and head. From the superior vena cava, blood returns to the right atrium, into the right ventricle, and into the main pulmonary artery. At this point most of the blood passes through the ductus arteriosus into the aorta where it mixes with blood from the left ventricle. The blood then circulates to the lower extremities, abdomen, and pelvis. The blood returns to the placenta through the umbilical arteries.*

ventricle and pulmonary artery shunt blood toward the aorta, where pressure is lower. At birth, the umbilical cord is cut and the supply of oxygenated blood from the placenta is suddenly stopped. The ductus venous occludes, the lungs expand, and pressure in the pulmonary arteries falls to a level equal to the pressure in the aorta; the blood flow through the ductus arteriosus ceases. The pulmonary pressure continues to fall until, at about two weeks of age, the ductus is obliterated and a pressure of 25 mm Hg is established in the pulmonary arteries. If the open ductus arteriosus does not close, blood is passed from the aorta into the pulmonary arteries. A *left* to *right* movement of blood occurs because the higher pressure is on the left side of the heart and the lower pressure is on the right side.

A third bypass route present during fetal life is the *foramen ovale,* which allows blood entering the right atrium from the placenta to pass directly into the left atrium and out the aorta into the systemic circulation. After birth, the entire right ventricular output enters the pulmonary vessels, causing a rise of pressure in the left atrium that closes the foramen ovale. If the opening does not close adequately, blood will move from the higher pressure in the left atrium to the lower pressure in the right atrium, similar to an open ductus arteriosus. Abnormal openings within the heart are called *shunts;* shunts are classified as left-to-right or right-to-left.

Left-to-Right Shunts

When blood passes from the left to the right side of the heart, the left side has an increased work load because blood is moving in two directions (Figure 21–6). Part of the blood is sent from the left side out into the body while another portion passes through

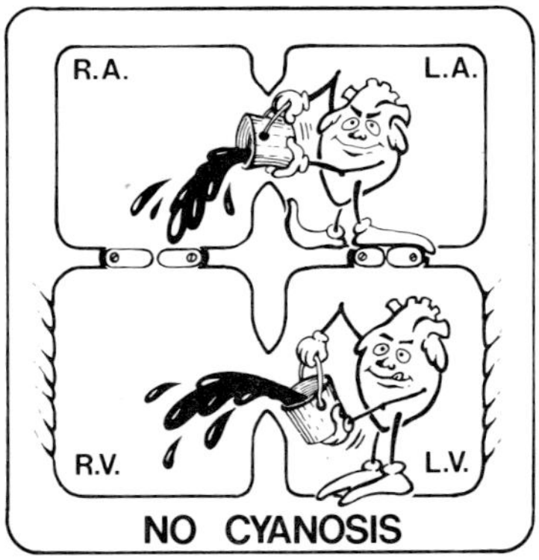

Figure 21–6. *Left-to-right shunt.*

the abnormal shunt opening into the right side and recirculates to the lungs. Since the blood that flows to the body is saturated with oxygen, no *cyanosis* occurs; left-to-right shunts are therefore referred to as *acyanotic* conditions. However, the right side of the heart must accept an increased amount of blood that is then passed on to the lungs. The added blood volume in the pulmonary veins can cause increased resistance and pressure. Thickening and narrowing of the lumens causes further stress on the heart, less blood flow to the body, and congestion in the lungs. (Heart conditions that cause a left-to-right shunting of blood are pictured and described at the end of ch. 22.) If a left-to-right shunt is present and pressure on the right side equals that on the left side of the heart, blood flows in *both* directions, from right to left and from left to right. Cyanosis may occur if the blood flow is sufficiently desaturated; however, cyanosis is less likely and less severe than in a right-to-left shunt.

Right-to-Left Shunts

Blood can also flow through an abnormal opening from the right side of the heart to the left. Right-to-left shunts happen when the pressure in the pulmonary circuit is *higher* than the pressure in the systemic circuit (Figure 21–7). Since deoxygenated blood is on the right side, the passage of this blood into the left side without first having traveled to the lungs means some deoxygenated blood will be sent to the systemic circulation, resulting in cyanosis. Several different types of heart abnormalities can cause shunting of blood from the right to left (See ch. 22).

Obstructions

Other types of defects occur in valves and vessels of the heart. These defects may occur with or without abnormal shunting of blood. For example, disease, trauma, or infection may damage the heart, causing narrowing or compression of the walls of a vessel, referred to as *stenosis* and *coarctation,* respectively. If valves do not seal correctly, they are said to be incompetent and may cause blood to seep backward in the wrong direction. Valves may be stenosed and/or incompetent. Frequently, several of these abnormalities of abnormal shunting, vessel stenosis or coarctation, and incompetent valves may appear in the same child. An example of such a combination of defects is *tetralogy of Fallot,* which includes four abnormalities of the heart. Common structural abnormalities of the heart, descriptions, treatments, and unique nursing considerations are discussed in chapter 22.

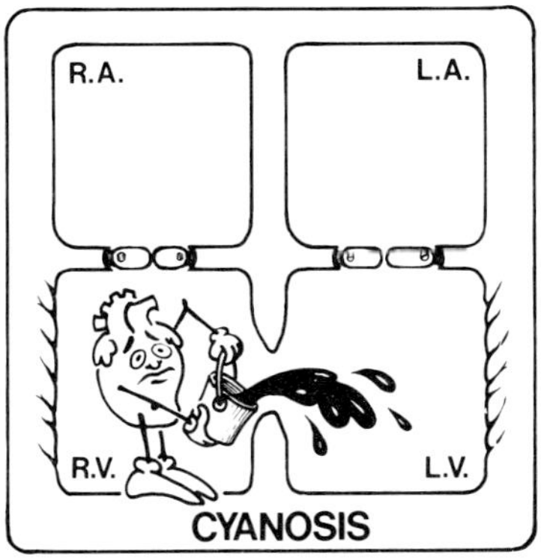

Figure 21–7. *Right-to-left shunt.*

THE BLOOD

Blood is the body's intertransportation system. Blood picks up food and oxygen through the processes of digestion and oxygenation, then makes deliveries to waiting cells. Waste products are collected by the blood and delivered to certain organs for removal from the body. Hormones and enzymes also enter the blood and are transported from one site to another. Each of these transportation functions is possible because of the unique constituents of blood; blood is made of *plasma,* a fluid, and three major kinds of cells: *erythrocytes, leukocytes,* and *platelets*.

Erythrocytes

Erythrocytes (Figure 21–8) deliver oxygen and pick up carbon dioxide. They are the most numerous of the formed blood cells. The erythrocyte is a flexible disk that can pass through the tiniest capillary. Erythrocytes are made in the bone marrow. The rate of erythrocyte production is called *erythropoiesis*. Erythropoiesis is measured by a *reticulocyte count; reticulocytes* are newly formed erythrocytes.

Packed inside each erythrocyte are millions of molecules of a compound called *hemoglobin*. Made of chains of amino acids, *three* types of hemoglobin function to transport oxygen. *Fetal hemoglobin* (HbF) predominates intrauterine life until shortly after birth when it is gradually replaced with *hemoglobin A* (HbA). Hemoglobin A makes up 95 percent of the hemoglobin in

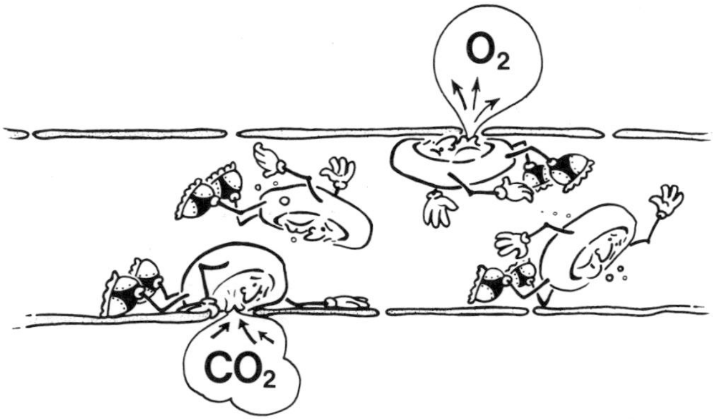

Figure 21–8. *Erythrocytes.*

persons over one year of age. Small amounts of *hemoglobin A_2* (HbA_2), an additional hemoglobin, and fetal hemoglobin account for the remaining five percent (Figure 21–9).

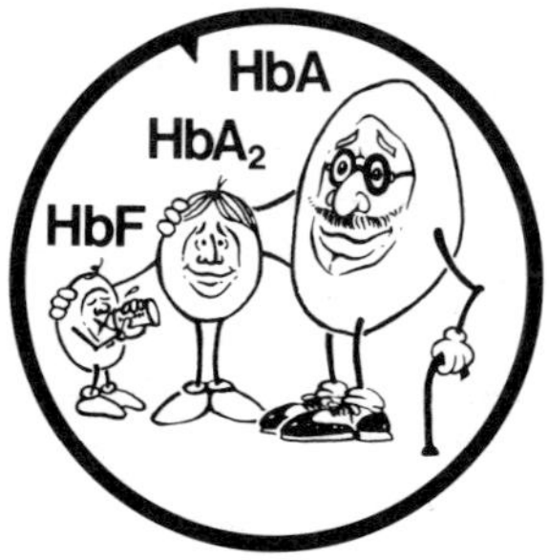

Figure 21–9. *The three types of hemoglobin.*

Hemoglobin is made of two parts; *heme* and *globin*. Heme is a pigment made with iron that gives blood its red color, and globin is a protein made of hundreds of amino acids. The heme and globin combine to form a molecule of hemoglobin. Several thousand molecules of hemoglobin are contained in each erythrocyte. Hemoglobin has a unique quality: it can unite with oxygen molecules in the lung to form *oxyhemoglobin* that is then delivered to every cell. As the oxygen is delivered, carbon dioxide is picked up and unites with the hemoglobin to form *carbaminohemoglobin*. Changes in the composition of hemoglobin can occur; for example, if one substitution of a single amino acid occurs, an abnormal hemoglobin results. These abnormal hemoglobins are called *hemoglobinopathies*. Some hemoglobinopathies cause health problems, but most do not. One form of abnormal hemoglobin is sickle hemoglobin, in which one amino acid is substituted for another. This change results in an abnormal reaction between the sickle hemoglobin molecules when oxygen is released to waiting cells. Upon deoxygenation, the normally smooth, flexible, disk-shaped erythrocyte is changed into a rigid, rough-textured, crescent-shaped cell. The problems of sickle hemoglobin are discussed in chapter 24.

Sufficient amounts of *Vitamin B_{12}*, *folic acid*, and *iron* are essential for adequate production of erythrocytes (Figure 21–10). If these nutrients are not supplied because of undernutrition, malabsorption, obstruction, or other growth problems, the bone

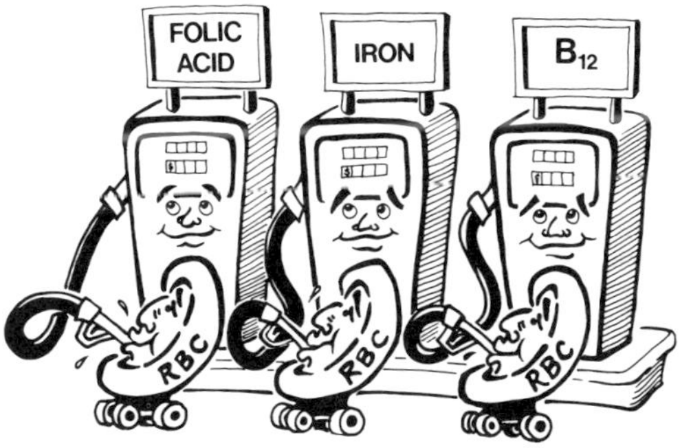

Figure 21–10. *Folic acid, iron, and Vitamin B12 are essential for erythrocyte production.*

marrow cannot produce enough erythrocytes and the child becomes *anemic*. Anemia can also be caused by an increased rate of destruction of the erythrocytes arising from infection, a neoplasm, radiation, drugs, or structural changes in the erythrocyte that may be either inherited or acquired. The opposite condition, an increased amount of hemoglobin, is termed *polycythemia*.

The life span of one erythrocyte is about 120 days. Special cells in the lining of the blood vessels and in the liver and spleen phagocytose erythrocytes. During phagocytosis, iron is separated from the hemoglobin and a pigment called *bilirubin* is made. When the amount of bilirubin is elevated, the sclera, mucous membranes, and skin may become *jaundiced* (yellowed), resulting in a condition termed *icterus*. Both iron and bilirubin are transported to the liver. Iron is temporarily stored and bilirubin is excreted as bile. The iron is eventually reduced to make new hemoglobin.

One of the most frequently used tests for evaluating the quantity of erythrocytes is the *hematocrit,* which is the volume of red cells in whole blood. For example, a hematocrit of 30 means that in every 100 milliliters of whole blood there are 30 milliliters of blood cells and 70 milliliters of fluid plasma. (Average pulse rates and normal hematologic values during infancy and childhood are shown in Tables 21–1, 21–2, and 21–3.)

Leukocytes

Leukocytes function as part of the body's defense system against pathogens (Figure 21–11). Leukocytes are a varied group of nucleated cells that do not contain hemoglobin. Each leukocyte has the unique ability to move out of capillaries by squeezing through the intercellular spaces of the capillary wall. In contrast, erythrocytes and platelets function only within the blood vessels. Once in the tissue, leukocytes phagocytose, ingest, and digest injurious particles; they are the body's surveillance system against pathogen invasion.

Platelets

Platelets, or *thrombocytes,* are formed in the bone marrow. They live for only 10 days but

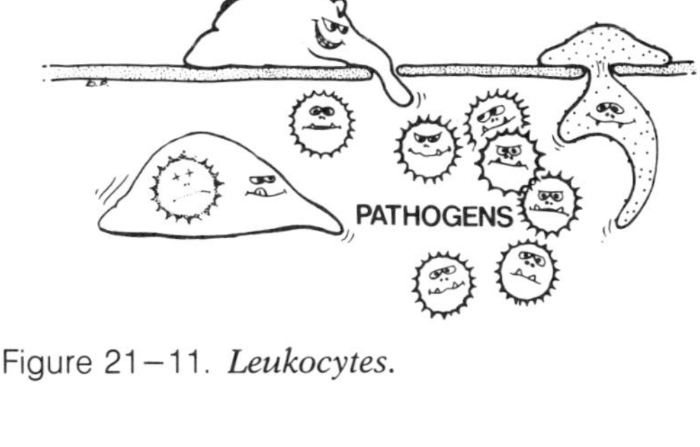

Figure 21–11. *Leukocytes.*

Table 21–1. **Average pulse rates at rest**

Age	*Lower Limits of Normal*		*Average*		*Upper Limits of Normal*	
Newborn	70		120		170	
1–11 months	80		120		160	
2 years	80		110		130	
4 years	80		100		120	
6 years	75		100		115	
8 years	70		90		110	
10 years	70		90		110	
	Girls	*Boys*	*Girls*	*Boys*	*Girls*	*Boys*
12 years	70	65	90	85	110	105
14 years	65	60	85	80	105	100
16 years	60	55	80	75	100	95
18 years	55	50	75	70	95	90

From Vaughn, V.C., III and McKay, R.J., Jr. *Textbook of Pediatrics,* ed. 10. Philadelphia, W.B. Saunders Co., 1975. Used by permission.

serve as vital components of the blood clotting mechanism, which stops bleeding and prevents the loss of body fluid.

Coagulation is the process of blood clotting. Coagulation must occur swiftly when a vessel is cut or ruptured if blood loss is to be minimized. Conversely, coagulation must not occur when it is not needed because clots can plug up vessels and deprive cells of nutrients and oxygen. Coagulation is a rapid process of events that begins with the appearance of a rough spot in the lining of a blood vessel, such as in the cut edge of a vessel. Within one to two seconds, clumps of platelets adhere to the rough portion of the blood vessel and begin to release a variety of substances that accelerate coagulation. Some of the released substances are called *platelet factors*.

As the platelet factors and other substances are released, two important proteins, *prothrombin* and *fibrinogen,* are converted to other substances that help form the clot. Both prothrombin and fibrinogen are made in the liver. It will be recalled that the liver takes food nutrients and remakes them into specific compounds needed by the body. It is that process, anabolism, that produces prothrombin and fibrinogen. However, for anabolism to occur, Vitamin K must be available in the liver. Vitamin K is absorbed from the intestines and cannot be made by the body; thus, a Vitamin K deficiency causes a dangerous lack of fibrinogen and prothrombin. During coagulation, prothrombin changes to *thrombin* and the thrombin converts fibrinogen to *fibrin,* which looks like fine threads tangled together. Blood cells catch in the entanglement and a clot begins. (See Figure 21–12.)

Another factor that hastens clotting is an abnormally slow flow of blood. Immobility, for example, can cause a slower blood flow

Table 21–2. Hematologic Values during Infancy and Childhood

Age	Hemoglobin gm/100ml		Hematocrit %		Retic-ulo-cytes %	WBC/mm³ %		Neutrophils %		Lympho-cytes %			
	Mean	Range	Mean	Range	Mean	Mean	Range	Mean	Range	Mean (Relatively Wide Range)	Esosinophils % Mean	Monocytes % Mean	Nucleated Red Cells /100 WBC
Cord blood	16.8	13.7–20.1	55	45–65	5.0	18,000	9–30,000	61	40–80	31	2	6	7.0 3–10
2 weeks	16.5	13.0–20.0	50	42–66	1.0	12,000	5–21,000	40		48	3	9	0
3 months	12.0	9.5–14.5	36	31–41	1.0	12,000	6–18,000	30		63	2	5	0
6 months –6 years	12.0	10.5–14.0	37	33–42	1.0	10,000	6–15,000	45		48	2	5	0
7–12 years	13.0	11.0–16.0	38	34–40	1.0	8,000	4500–13,500	55		38	2	5	0
Adults													
Female	14	12.0–16.0	42	37–47	1.6	7,500	5–10,000	55	35–70	35	3	7	0
Male	16	14.0–18.0	47	42–52									

From Vaughn, V.C. III and McKay, R.J., Jr. *Textbook of Pediatrics*, ed. 10. Philadelphia. W.B. Saunders Co., 1975. Used by permission.

Table 21–3. **Hematologic Values**

Determination (whole blood unless otherwise indicated)	*Age/Sex*	*Normal Value*
Hematocrit (vol%)	Newborn	44–64%
	Neonatal	35–49%
	Infant	30–40%
	Child	31–43%
	(Thereafter Male, Female)	40–54%
		37–47%
Hemoglobin	Newborn	14–24gm/100ml
	Neonatal	11–20gm/100ml
	Infant	10–15gm/100ml
	Child	11–16gm/100ml
	(Thereafter Male, Female)	14–18gm/100ml
		12–16gm/100ml
Hemoglobin, fetal (Hb F)	Newborn	40–70% of total
	Neonatal	20–40% of total
	Infant	2–10% of total
	Thereafter	1–2% of total
Nucleated RBC's	Cord	250–500/mm^3
	Day 1	200–300/mm^3
	Day 2	20– 30/mm^3
	Thereafter	0
Osmotic fragility 50% hemolysis		0.44–0.40%NaCl
		0.5 –1.5% NaCl
Platelet count	Premature	100–300 000/mm^3
	Newborn	140–300 000/mm^3
	Neonatal	150–390 000/mm^3
	Infant	200–473 000/mm^3
	Thereafter	150–450 000/mm^3
Red Blood Cell Count (RBC)	Newborn	4.8–7.1 million/mm^3
	Neonatal	4.1–6.4 million/mm^3
	Infant/Child	3.8–5.5 million/mm^3
	Thereafter Male, Female	4.6–6.2 million/mm^3
		4.2–5.4 million/mm^3
Blood Indices		
MCH	Newborn	32–34 $\mu\mu$g
	Thereafter	27–31 $\mu\mu$g

Table 21–3. *(Continued)*

Determination (whole blood unless otherwise indicated)	*Age/Sex*	*Normal Value*
MCV	Newborn	96–108 μ^3
	Thereafter	82–91 μ^3
MCHC	Newborn	32–33%
	Thereafter	32–36%
Reticulocyte count	Newborn	2.5–6.5% total RBC
	Neonatal	0.1–1.5% total RBC
	Infant	0.5–3.1% total RBC
	Thereafter	0–2.0% total RBC
Sedimentation Rate (ESR) (uncorrected)	Newborn	0–2mm/hr
	Neonatal/Puberty	3–13mm/hr
	Adult: Male	10–15mm/hr
	Female	15–25mm/hr
White Blood Cell Count (WBC)	Newborn, total	9,000–30,000/mm^3
	%neutrophiles	≃ 61%
	%lymphocytes	≃ 31%
	1 week, total	5,000–21,000/mm^3
	%neutrophiles	≃ 45%
	%lymphocytes	≃ 41%
	4 week, total	5,000–19,500/mm^3
	%neutrophiles	≃ 35%
	%lymphocytes	≃ 56%
	6–12 month total	6,000–17,500/mm^3
	%neutrophiles	≃ 32%
	%lymphocytes	≃ 61%
	2 year total	6,200–17,000/mm^3
	%neutrophiles	≃ 33%
	%lymphocytes	≃ 59%
	Thereafter. total	5,000–10,000/mm^3
	%neutrophiles	≃ 60%
	%lymphocytes	≃ 30%

From Vaughn, V.C. III and McKay, R.J., Jr. *Textbook of Pediatrics*, ed. 10. Philadelphia, W.B. Saunders Co., 1975. Used by permission.

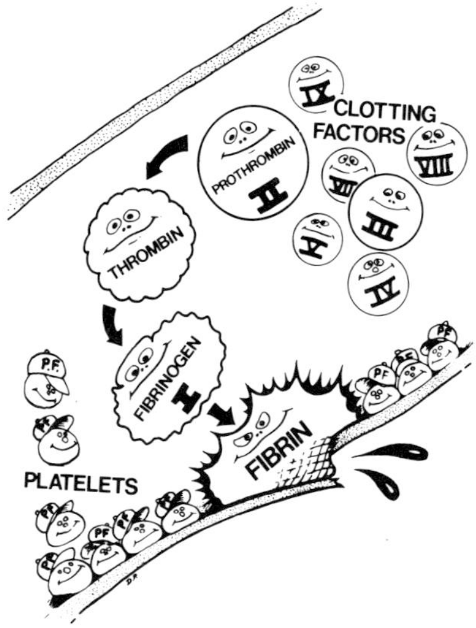

Figure 21–12. *Coagulation.*

and clotting may occur. This type of clot is called a *thrombosis*. Once a thrombosis is formed, it can grow larger because platelets inside the fibrin web disintegrate and release additional material, causing more clotting. If the thrombosis is dislodged (by trauma, movement, drugs, or other causes) and moves from its original site to another part of the body, it is termed a *thrombotic embolus* or *embolus*. An embolus can occur at any site in the body; it is a serious occurrence because it can obstruct blood flow, thereby depriving tissue of oxygen.

Another important substance in the blood is *antithrombin,* which opposes thrombin and the continual formation of a clot. In the presence of antithrombin, coagulation is halted. The final step in coagulation is the presence of the enzyme *fibrinolysin* which causes the fibrin web to dissolve and the clot to resolve. If the child does not have sufficient numbers of platelets, or if the platelets formed do not contain a necessary clotting factor, the child bleeds easily and is at risk for excessive fluid loss. Various bleeding problems, as well as alterations in coagulation, are discussed in chapter 25.

Blood Types

Blood types are named according to the kind of antigen present on the erythrocyte's membrane. For example, blood type A means antigen A is present on the erythrocyte's membrane, and blood type B means antigen B is present. There are four common blood types: *A, B, AB,* and *O.* In blood type O, neither antigen A nor antigen B is present (Figure 21–13).

In each person, plasma never contains antibodies against the antigens present on its own erythrocytes because the antibodies would destroy the cells. However, plasma *does* contain antibodies against the antigens *not present* on the erythrocytes. For example, a child with blood type A has antigen A present on the erythrocytes; the plasma contains anti-B antibodies but does not contain anti-A antibodies. *Anti-A and anti-B antibodies* are called *agglutinins,* which are chemicals that can cause cells to stick together in clumps. Agglutinins can cause serious effects, since they may plug small vessels and deprive cells of oxygen and nutrients.

The danger in giving a blood transfusion is that antibodies in the plasma of the receiver may agglutinate with the donor's erythrocytes. If, for example, type A blood were transfused into a person with type B blood, the anti-A antibodies in the receiver's blood would agglutinate the donor's type A erythrocytes (Figure 21–14). Therefore, before blood is transfused it is *crossmatched,* meaning the receiver's blood

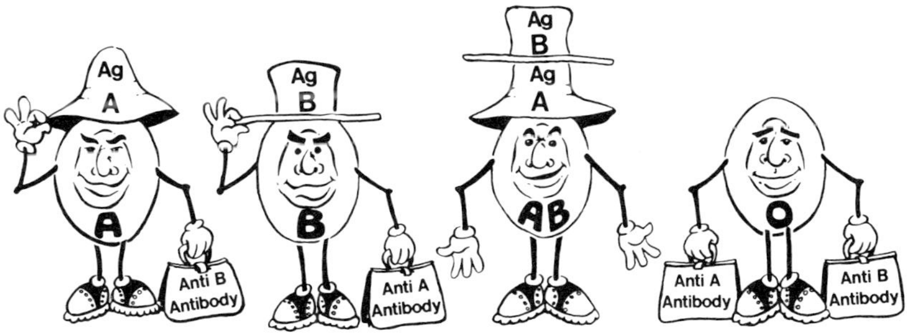

Figure 21–13. *Blood types.*

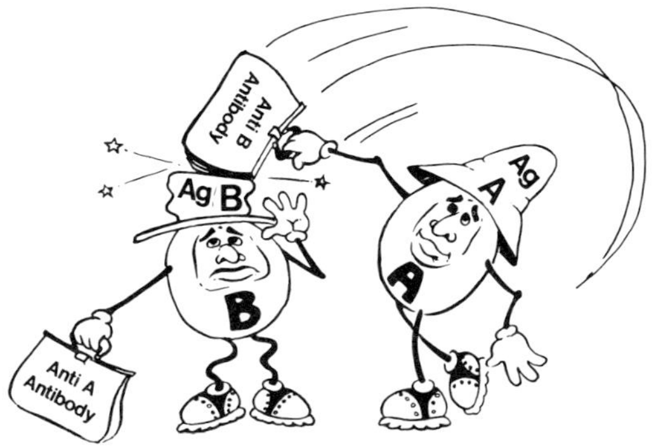

Figure 21–14. *Transfusion of incompatible blood types.*

is mixed with the donor's blood and observed for agglutination of the donor's erythrocytes (see ch. 24.)

Blood Plasma

Plasma is the liquid part of the blood; it is whole blood minus its cells. Plasma is a clear, straw-colored fluid consisting of 90 percent water and 10 percent *solutes*. The majority of the solutes are proteins. These proteins consist of three main kinds of compounds: *albumins, fibrinogen* and *globulins*. Plasma proteins are essential for body functioning. For example, prothrombin (an albumin) and fibrinogen are essential for clotting, and globulins are important to immunity; circulating antibodies are modified globulins.

All of the plasma proteins contribute to normal blood viscosity, blood osmotic pressure, and blood volume. Since the anabolism of plasma proteins takes place in the liver, injury, disease, or infection affecting the liver may decrease the production of these valuable plasma proteins.

Lymph

Lymph, derived from blood plasma, is composed of salts, glucose, lipids, and water. Lymph enters a network of vessels called the *lymphatic system*. As muscles contract and relax the lymph is pushed through lymph vessels called the *lymphatics*. *Lymph nodes* are filter sites that cleanse the lymph as it passes through the vessels. Lymph nodes also contribute to the production of lymphocytes and plasma cells. The lymphatic system functions to return water and proteins from the interstitial fluid to the blood. Proteins can return to the blood only through the lymphatics. Thus, if the lymphatics are blocked, the blood protein concentration level falls, and fluid imbalance can result.

THE PULMONARY CIRCULATION

Circulation is the flow of blood through vessels. As discussed earlier, blood flows through the systemic circulation and the pulmonary circulation. Blood circulates through these two circuits because of pressure differences within the heart and between the heart and the two circulations.

The pulmonary circulation oxygenates blood. *Oxygenation* is the delivery of oxygen from the lungs into the blood. Blood circulates from the heart to the lungs where gases are exchanged; oxygen is picked up and carbon dioxide is delivered. The blood then returns to the heart and is circulated to the body where oxygen and carbon dioxide are exchanged within each body cell. The conduction of oxygen into the lungs and the subsequent exchange of gases across membranes into the blood constitutes *respiration.* Respiration consists of several processes, the first being conduction of the oxygen into the lungs.

The nose warms, moistens, and filters air, "examining" it for substances that may be irritating to the lining of the respiratory tract. Passing the nasal tunnels, air passes through the *pharynx.* From the pharynx, air enters the *larynx,* or voice box. In addition to causing membranes called vocal cords to vibrate, producing the voice, the larynx functions to protect the airway against the entrance of solids or liquids during swallowing. Air then arrives at the *trachea,* or wind pipe, a lumen that funnels air in and out of the lungs. Obstruction of this passage for even a few minutes can cause death due to *asphyxiation,* a lack of oxygen. The lower end of the trachea divides into two *pulmonary bronchi,* the right (or primary) bronchus being slightly larger and more vertical than the left bronchus. Both bronchi enter the lungs and immediately divide into smaller branches called *secondary bronchi.* The secondary bronchi further divide into small *bronchioles.* The bronchioles subdivide into smaller and smaller tubes, terminating in tiny branches that divide into *alveolar ducts.* These alveolar ducts end in *alveolar sacs;* the walls of the sacs consist of numerous *alveoli* (see Figure 21–15). Gases are exchanged in the alveoli.

If any of the structures that conduct air into the lungs and alveoli become obstructed by structural changes, accumulated secretions, or spasms, oxygenation is

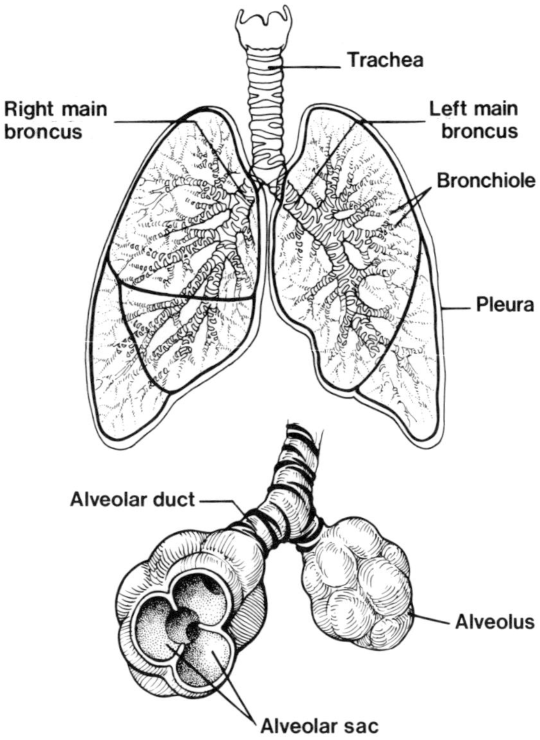

Figure 21–15. *Air travels from the trachea through the bronchi to the grapelike alveolar sacs, where gases are exchanged through the thin walls of the alveoli.*

restricted, and the child has a respiratory disorder.

The Lungs

The *left lung* is divided into two lobes, *upper* and *lower*. The right lung is divided into three lobes, the *superior, middle,* and *inferior*. The inside of each lung houses the tubes that conduct air to the alveoli. A layer of *visceral pleura* covers the outer surfaces of the lung and adheres to them. The space between the lung tissue and the pleura is called the *pleural space*.

The lungs distribute air and exchange gases. Air is conducted from the nose toward the alveoli, where carbon dioxide and oxygen are exchanged by the alveoli and surrounding blood capillaries. The alveoli have very thin walls, as do the blood capillaries; when these two tissue-thin surfaces interface, gases are exchanged and oxygenation occurs.

The *thorax*, or chest, moves during respiration; it becomes larger during *inspiration* (when air moves into the lungs) and smaller during *expiration* (when air moves out of the lungs). Inspiration and expiration occur because of pressure differences. When the atmospheric pressure is greater than the pressure within the lung, air moves into the lung (inspiration), and when pressure in the lung is greater than the pressure in the atmosphere, air moves out of the lung (expiration). The volume of air moved in and out of the lungs and the volume remaining in the lung must remain normal if adequate gas exchange is to occur between the alveoli and the capillaries.

Several terms are used to describe the volume of air exchanged in the lungs. The amount of air exhaled after a *normal* inspiration is *tidal volume* (TV). The amount of air that can be forced out of the lungs after normal expiration is *expiratory reserve volume* (ERV). *Inspiratory reserve volume* (IRV) is the amount of air that can be forcibly inspired over and above a normal inspiration. The amount of air that *cannot* be forcibly expired is *residual volume* (RV). *Vital air capacity* is the sum of TV + ERV + IRV and is the largest volume of air one can move in and out of the lungs. Vital capacity is affected by excess fluid in the pleural covering of the lung, and by structural or disease conditions that affect the inspiration and expiration ability of the lungs.

The Partial Pressure of Gases in the Blood

Air is made of gases; respiration is the exchange of these gases between alveolar air and venous blood that flows through the lung capillaries. The diffusion of gases from alveoli to capillaries to body cells occurs because of a difference in partial pressures. *Partial pressure* is the pressure exerted by any one gas in a mixture of gases or in a liquid; the letter *P* is used for partial pressure. The symbol of the gas being measured follows the *P*; for example "PO_2" refers to the partial pressure of oxygen. The word *tension* is frequently used to mean partial pressure; *P* is the symbol used, regardless of which term is used.

The partial pressure of alveolar air is *greater* than the partial pressure of venous blood entering the lung capillaries; this difference makes oxygenation possible. Gases diffuse from a *higher pressure* to a *lower pressure;* thus oxygen moves from a partial pressure of 100 mm Hg in the alveolar to a partial pressure of 37 mm Hg in the venous blood that enters the lung capillaries. Simultaneously, the partial pressure of carbon dioxide in the venous blood entering the lung capillaries is higher than the PCO_2

in the alveoli; thus carbon dioxide diffuses from the higher partial pressure in the venous blood to the lower partial pressure in the alveolar sacs. If the pressure difference between alveolar air and venous blood changes, oxygenation is affected. For example, at high altitudes the PO_2 of alveolar air is reduced, so less oxygen can diffuse through the blood. When the functioning surface area of the alveolar-capillary membranes is reduced, such as during infections or following structural changes that obstruct gas diffusion, less oxygen enters the blood. Structural changes in the respiratory system immediately affect oxygenation. A general rule that applies to all body sites is the relationship of structure to function: *when structure changes so does function.*

THE SYSTEMIC CIRCULATION

In the *systemic circulation,* the exchange of gas between the arterial blood and the tissue is accomplished by diffusion; the gases move from a higher pressure to a lower pressure. Interstitial PO_2 is much lower than arterial PO_2, and intracellular PO_2 is much lower still than interstitial PO_2; the oxygen therefore diffuses from a higher pressure in the blood to a lower pressure inside the cells. Carbon dioxide also diffuses, but the pressure differences are *opposite.* Large amounts of carbon dioxide accumulate when body cells complete their work cycle, resulting in very high intracellular levels of PCO_2. Interstitial PCO_2 is also high but not as high as intracellular PCO_2; venous PCO_2 is lower still. Like oxygen, carbon dioxide diffuses across the cell membrane into the tissue, then across capillary walls into the venous circulation.

Blood pH

The symbol pH denotes the acid-base balance of the blood according to the blood's concentration of *hydrogen* (H^+) *ions.* The *greater* the concentration of H^+ ions, the *more acid* the blood and the *lower* the pH value. The *less* the concentration of the H^+ ions in the blood, the *more alkaline* the blood and the *higher* the pH value. The pH scale runs from 0 to 14; pH7 is neutral. For the pH to remain normal, the hygrogen ion concentration must be kept in balance. Even a slight alteration in pH can cause major changes in the rate of cellular chemical reactions.

Excess hydrogen ions can be buffered by hemoglobin, but the actual elimination of hydrogen ions is dependent on the kidneys. Since the kidneys expel hydrogen ions, the kidneys also must be able to alter their function and decrease hydrogen ion excretion if a deficit of hydrogen ions occurs in the body. Adequate kidney function is central to a normal acid-base balance in the body. (Chapter 29 further discusses fluid balance and the acid-base relationship.)

When insufficient oxygen is delivered to the tissue and body cells, the resulting condition is *hypoxia.* Various changes within the body can cause hypoxia; the following examples typify three types of hypoxia, and chapters 22 through 24 focus on these changes in greater detail.

John, a thin, underweight-for-age three-year-old, is pulling a wagon when he suddenly stops, squats with his knees touching his chest, and gasps for air. John's heart has several structural defects. It cannot pump adequate amounts of oxygenated blood to the body; John suffers from *ischemic hypoxia.*

Ten-year-old Mark has not been eating normally for several days; he is lethargic and has had an unproductive, dry, hacking cough for two weeks.

Last night his temperature suddenly rose to 103_F. Today he lies under a mist tent, holding his chest as he coughs, taking short, shallow breaths; Mark has pneumonia. His lungs are obstructed with pathogens and secretions, and adequate amounts of oxygen cannot pass from the alveolar sacs to the capillaries. Mark has *hypoxic hypoxia,* a reduced amount of oxygen available for circulation to the body cells. Hypoxic hypoxia is caused by resistance or obstruction of the airway arising from disease, infection, or structural changes that decrease the amount of oxygen diffusing through the circulation.

Five-year-old Jane sits watching the other children at play. She tires easily at vigorous play and needs to rest frequently. Jane has a hereditary disorder that affects her hemoglobin. Jane's hemoglobin causes her erythrocytes to change from their normal round shape to an elongated crescent shape when oxygen is released. These malformed erythrocytes can no longer carry sufficient amounts of oxygen to body cells; Jane has *anemic hypoxia.* Children with anemic hypoxia have insufficient numbers of oxygen-carrying erythrocytes, or the hemoglobin inside the erythrocytes is altered or reduced.

SUMMARY

The heart is a pump that works because of pressure differences inside its cavities. Blood flows to the lungs and the rest of the body because of these pressure differences. If these pressures are altered by structural changes, disease, or infection, heart disease can result, decreasing the ability of the heart to deliver oxygen to the body.

Blood transports nutrients, oxygen, waste, hormones, and enzymes. Blood acts to regulate cell and tissue water content and to monitor body temperature. Blood contains erythrocytes, platelets, and leukocytes. Erythrocytes contain hemoglobin and carry oxygen and carbon dioxide. Platelets are crucial for blood clotting and the control of bleeding. Leukocytes protect the body against the invasion of pathogens, facilitate wound healing, and remove products of cellular destruction. The fluid portion of blood is plasma; plasma contains proteins that are important for blood clotting and immunity.

Circulation is the flow of blood into two circuits, the pulmonary circulation and the systemic circulation. Oxygen and carbon dioxide are exchanged in both systems because of pressure differences; gases always move from a high to a lower pressure. If normal circulatory pressures are changed by a congenital or acquired disorder, the oxygenation of the body is impaired. Inadequate amounts of oxygen lead to hypoxia, the three major types of which are ischemic hypoxia, hypoxic hypoxia, and anemic hypoxia.

Bibliography

Andreoli, K.G., Fowkes, V.H., Zipes, D.P., Wallace, A.G. *Comprehensive Cardiac Care,* ed. 3. St. Louis, C.V. Mosby Co., 1975.

Anthony, C.P., and Kilthoff, N.A. *Textbook of Anatomy and Physiology.* St. Louis, C.V. Mosby Co., 1975.

Cohen, S. Gas and Acid-Base Concepts In Respiratory Care. (Programmed Instruction). *American Journal of Nursing* 76:963, 1976.

Crouch, J.E., and McClintic, J.R. *Human Anatomy and Physiology,* ed. 2. New York, John Wiley & Sons, Inc., 1976.

Frohlich, E.D. (ed.). *Pathophysiology: Altered Regulatory Mechanisms In Disease,* ed. 2. Philadelphia, J.B. Lippincott Co., 1976.

Guyton, A.C. *Basic Human Physiology: Normal Function and Mechanism of Disease,* ed. 2. Philadelphia, W.B. Saunders, Co., 1977.

McIntyre, H.M. (ed.). *Heart Disease: New Dimensions of Nursing Care.* New York, Trainex, 1974.

Price, S.A., and Wilson, L.M. *Pathophysiology: Clinical Concepts of Disease Processes.* New York, McGraw-Hill, 1978.

Vander, A.J., Sherman, J.H., Luciano, D.S. *Human Physiology: The Mechanisms of Body Function,* ed. 2. New York, McGraw-Hill, 1975.

Wade, J.F. *Respiratory Nursing Care: Physiology and Technique,* ed. 2. St. Louis, C.V. Mosby Co., 1977.

CHAPTER **22**

The Child with a Cardiovascular Deviation

BEHAVIORAL OBJECTIVES

After studying this chapter you will be able to:

- Identify factors contributing to congenital cardiac defects.
- Discuss parental reactions to the diagnosis of congenital heart disease in their child.
- Explain common problems and nursing interventions for children with heart disease.
- Discuss complications of congenital and acquired heart disease in the child and how they can be prevented.
- Explain the purpose of diagnostic procedures used to evaluate cardiac involvement.
- Explain treatments used for the child with a cardiac defect; including medical, palliative, and corrective treatment, and nursing implications.
- Discuss the emotional implications of heart disease in the growing child.
- Design a plan of care for the child undergoing corrective cardiac surgery, include both pre- and postoperative care.
- Identify and explain acyanotic and cyanotic heart defects.
- Explain the pathophysiology of rheumatic fever.
- Design a plan of care for the adolescent with moderate carditis.

TERMS AND CONCEPTS

Dyspnea
Tachypnea
Cyanosis
Anoxic spells
Tachycardia
Pulsus alternans
Pulse deficit
Bradycardia
Paroxysmal atrial tachycardia
Valsalva maneuver
Night terrors
Congestive heart failure
Gallop rhythm
Diaphoresis
Pulmonary vascular obstructive disease
Bacterial endocarditis
Cerebral thrombosis
Polycythemia
Murmur
S_1
S_2
Clubbing
Electrocardiogram
Echocardiography
Cardiac catheterization
Angiocardiography
Angiography

Hypothermia
Premature ventricular contractions
Acyanotic defects
Obstructive lesions
Left-to-right shunts
Aortic stenosis
Pulse pressure
Infundibular
Right-to-left shunts
Aschoff body
Carditis
Valvulitis
Myocarditis
Pericarditis
Precordial pain
Mitral regurgitation
Basal pulse rate
Choreiform movements
Pronator sign

INTRODUCTION

Every year, in the United States alone, 30,000 babies are born with a defect of the heart and/or great arteries. This number represents one percent of all live births, or roughly between eight and ten out of every 1,000 live babies. The exact cause of the developmental error that results in congenital heart disease (CHD) is unknown, but there are several contributing factors. An insult to the fetus at five to eight weeks' gestation is responsible for most anomalies. Heredity plays a part, and genetic factors account for five percent of all congenital cardiac defects. Some defects are seen more often in one sex. Between 30 and 40 percent of children with Down's syndrome will have a heart defect. The risk of a parent with a heart defect having a child with a similar anomaly is five percent, and the risk for siblings of a child with a defect is two percent. The exposure of expectant mothers to rubella (German measles) in the first trimester of pregnancy accounts for four percent of all congenital cardiac anomalies. Other viral infections such as mumps, chicken pox, influenza, and rubeola (measles) also contribute to the incidence of CHD, as do radiation, drugs, and vitamin deficiencies. Some anomalies are caused by a persistence of fetal heart structures, such as the ductus arteriosus.

Recent surgical advances coupled with improvements in the management of newborn care now offer a longer life expectancy for the child with a congenital cardiac anomaly. Many defects that were once inoperable can now be corrected by such surgical techniques as optical magnification, microsurgery, and deep hypothermia.

This chapter discusses the problems of the child with a congenital or acquired heart condition. Nursing intervention in the areas of assessment, diagnosis, management, and correction is stressed.

COMMON PROBLEMS AND NURSING INTERVENTIONS

Oxygenation

Anomalies of the heart and/or arteries invariably compromise the child's oxygen usage. Defects of the heart affect oxygenation in a variety of ways. Shunts may carry oxygenated blood to the wrong place, thus depriving the rest of the body of oxygen; they may carry too much blood to the lungs, causing fibrotic changes that lessen the capacity of the lungs. Obstructive lesions prevent the normal flow of blood and cause a backup of blood in the heart, lungs, or venous system. Specific anomalies are presented later in this chapter; first it is necessary to focus on the problems and symptoms caused by oxygen deprivation.

Tissue Hypoxia

Dyspnea

Oxygen deprivation of the tissues is responsible for most of the child's problems and symptoms. *Dyspnea,* labored breathing, is one of the most common signs of congenital heart disease and is more noticeable with the exertion of crying, eating, or defecating (*exertional dyspnea*). Be aware of the normal respiratory rates and patterns for infants and young children so that you can readily recognize a deviation from the norm. The infant with dyspnea frequently uses his accessory muscles of respiration, indicating labored breathing. Watch for signs of impending cardiac failure, such as retractions and flaring nares.

Tachypnea

Tachypnea, an increased respiratory rate, occurring with or without dyspnea, is the most sensitive indicator of CHD in the newborn and the first sign of cardiac failure. It is often overlooked because it is a more subtle sign and is certainly less dramatic than dyspnea. Remove the infant's shirt to expose his chest and neck, then count his respirations for a full minute while he is at rest. The best place to observe respirations in the newborn is the central abdomen just below the xiphoid process. His respirations normally are rapid, shallow, and quiet, but they also can be irregular in rate, depth, and rhythm without being abnormal. The chest and abdomen rise in unison. There should be no sounds, no retractions, and no chin lag.

The infant with respiratory distress may exhibit grunting respirations, retractions, chin lag, and see-saw respirations caused by the involvement of the accessory muscles of respiration in helping to increase oxygenation after the first two hours of life. A respiratory rate in excess of 45 per minute in the full term infant may be indicative of CHD and should be brought to the attention of the physician. Check for other causes of tachypnea, such as a recent feeding, an overheated incubator, crying, or straining to evacuate stool. Record and report your observations. Humidified oxygen is administered (in an isolette, mask, hood, or tent) to help perfuse the child's system and alleviate some of the respiratory distress. Also note the child's response to oxygen therapy. Does he "pink"? (Check the nail beds and mucous membranes of dark-skinned children.) Are his respirations less labored? Does his pulse rate slow? Does he retract less? Is he less restless?

Cyanosis

Cyanosis is a bluish discoloration occurring under the skin and in mucous membranes and is caused by a high level (5 gm/100 ml) of unoxygenated blood in the peripheral circulation. Oxygen exchange in the lungs may not be adequate, thus unoxygenated (rather than oxygenated) blood is returned to the left side of the heart and back out to the body. Or, a defect may exist in the heart or arteries that shunts blood returned to the heart *back* to the body before it is oxygenated by the lungs.

Peripheral cyanosis of the hands and feet is common in newborns for a few hours after birth because blood does not flow freely to the extremities. If cyanosis lasts longer and is present in other than the extremities, CHD can be suspected.

Cyanosis is best seen in the lips, mucous

membranes, and nail beds, especially in dark-skinned persons. Observe the child in a good light, otherwise you may not notice mild cyanosis. Be sure to check his color when he is expending energy, such as during feedings, or when he is crying or defecating. Cyanosis may be present or may increase only during these times. Check the baby's temperature—a subnormal temperature can contribute to cyanosis. Check the hematocrit—anemia may mask cyanosis and an elevated hematocrit may cause cyanosis in the absence of CHD. Respiratory distress syndrome may cause some of the same symptoms as CHD. Table 22–1 offers a quick reference for differentiating between the two problems.

Pallor is seen in some severely ill infants and is caused by anemia, heart failure, or low cardiac output. Cool extremities may indicate shock, severe heart failure, or low cardiac output for any reason.

Oxygen is administered to the cyanotic infant, but if the cyanosis is caused by a heart defect rather than a pulmonary problem, the degree of cyanosis will not change appreciably.

Anoxic spells

When there is an abrupt decrease in pulmonary blood flow the child suffers an anoxic spell. He may suddenly turn cyanotic and become limp. He has cerebral anoxia, which leads to unconsciousness. These episodes are associated with exertion, such as from crying or defecating. Typically, they occur in the morning after awakening. The child becomes irritable (because of a lack of oxygen in the brain), may lose consciousness, and may even die. Anoxic spells are seen primarily in tetralogy of Fallot.

During an anoxic spell, place the infant in the knee-chest position. Turn his head to the side and use a blanket roll to keep his knees tucked under his buttocks, if he is too weak or immature to stay in this position by himself. He may be more comfortable in an infant seat. This position improves venous return to the heart and increases pulmonary blood flow. The older infant or young child will assume the knee-chest position spontaneously by squatting when he is fatigued. Give oxygen to improve saturation of the blood. Morphine is administered

Table 22–1. **Congenital Cardiac Defects *Versus* Respiratory Distress Syndrome**

	Cardiac Defect	*RDS*
Maternal history	Full term pregnancy Normal gestation Normal labor and delivery	Premature delivery Diabetic mother Cesarean section
Cyanosis		
When crying	Worsens (turns bluer)	Less cyanotic (turns to "pink")
After administration of oxygen	Essentially unchanged	Less cyanotic ("pinks")
Liver Palpable	Yes	No

to decrease restlessness and the resulting demand for more oxygen. Handle the child gently to help prevent him from crying.

Tachycardia

The child with CHD will typically have *tachycardia,* an increased heart rate. A normal "fussy" baby may have a rapid heartbeat, but the infant with CHD has a rapid beat—perhaps as high as 160 to 180 beats per minute—*at rest.* Take the pulse apically because some heartbeats may not be strong enough to be palpated at the peripheral pulses. Always count for one full minute. Know the location, character, and quality of the other pulses: radial, carotid, brachial, femoral, and dorsalis pedis (Figure 22–1). Palpate and record them all, especially after cardiac catheterization or heart surgery. If the artery was ligated during cardiac catheterization, the pulse will be absent in the corresponding extremity.

If generalized vasoconstriction is present (due to shock, heart failure, respiratory distress, administration of drugs, or severe acidosis), the pulse will be weak and rapid (See Table 22–2 for pulse variations). A

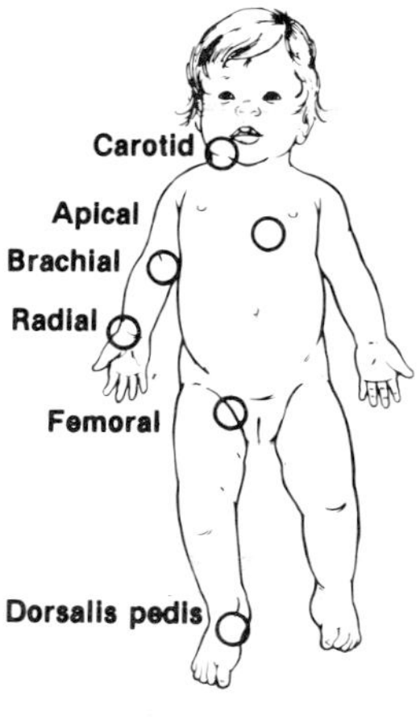

Figure 22–1. *Various pulse locations.*

pulse that is alternately weak and strong, *pulsus alternans,* is an ominous sign indicative of cardiac tamponade, impending failure, or tension pneumothorax. A *pulse deficit* (difference in number of apical beats and peripheral beats) combined with an irregular apical pulse usually means atrial fibrillation and is seen in atrial septal defects and mitral valve disease. A very slow rate, *bradycardia,* is indicative of digitalis overdose or heart block. Loss of consciousness may occur with rates under 50 beats per minute. *Paroxysmal atrial tachycardia* (PAT) occurs when there is a sudden increase in pulse rate exceeding 200 beats per minute. The rate may be as high as 300. Cardiac output is greatly diminished and congestive heart failure may result within 24 to 48 hours. PAT is a medical emergency. There may be a spontaneous return to a normal rate; if not, various maneuvers are tried in an attempt to terminate the episode. Unilateral carotid sinus massage, eyeball pressure, vomiting (induced with syrup of ipecac), or gagging (physically induced) may all be effective. If the child is old enough, deep breathing or the *Valsalva maneuver* (contracting the chest and abdominal muscles as if to defecate) may be used. Digitalis is often administered to the child for a period of time following an episode of PAT.

Observe and record the infant's response to feeding, crying, and defecating. All of the sophisticated equipment used to monitor the infant does not take the place of the nurse at the bedside. Your observations are of upmost importance in the recognition and management of the child with CHD.

When feeding, crying, or defecating does the infant's pulse or respiratory rate increase? Are his respirations more labored? Ask the parents of the older child if he ever

Table 22–2. **Cardiac Causes of Pulse Variations**

Pulse Variation	*Description*	*Probable Causes*
Pulsus alternans	Alternately weak and strong	Cardiac tamponade Impending failure Tension pneumothorax
Pulse deficit (combined with irregular apical pulse)	Difference between number of apical beats and peripheral beats	Atrial fibrillation ASD Mitral valve disease
Bradycardia	Slow pulse	Digitalis overdose Heart block Loss of consciousness
Paroxysmal atrial tachycardia	Sudden increase in pulse rate to over 200	Cardiac output decreased Congestive heart failure
Pulse pressure narrowed	Less margin between systolic and diastolic pressure	Severe aortic stenosis

breathes heavily, gets short of breath, or wheezes upon exertion. Does he have to rest a lot? How far can he walk or climb without tiring? Can he keep up with his peers? Does he have frequent respiratory infections? Does he squat when he is playing hard? Does the infant become more cyanotic? If so, does oxygen relieve the cyanosis? Is the infant's cry weak? A weak cry is indicative of tissue hypoxia because the infant does not have the energy to produce a loud, lusty cry.

These observations and questions will tell you a great deal about how much activity the infant or child can safely tolerate. Plan his care to avoid tiring him and to conserve as much of his energy as possible.

Comfort is a major consideration because even minor discomforts and irritations cause the child to use oxygen he cannot spare. The infant will probably be placed in an isolette to keep him from expending energy to regulate his body temperature. Hypothermia causes vasoconstriction and cyanosis. Poor peripheral circulation (augmented by vasoconstriction) coupled with hypoxia can cause metabolic acidosis. Hyperthermia increases metabolic rate and oxygen needs and can lead to convulsions, shock, and heart arrest. The knee-chest position will lessen the cardiac load by facilitating circulation. If the infant is in an isolette, elevate the mattress and place a blanket roll under his thighs and anchor it to keep him from sliding down. Administer oxygen as ordered to increase the amount available in the lungs for transport. (Remember that making oxygen available to the lungs does not ensure its getting delivered to the body.) Morphine is given to decrease restlessness and the need for more oxygen.

Growth Failure

A lack of oxygen will cause growth failure to some degree. The child with CHD is typically smaller than his peers and lags behind them in developmental milestones. This problem begins in infancy when the infant is using all of his energy to keep his blood oxygenated and has little energy left to eat.

Feeding Difficulties

Poor feeding in the infant is the equivalent of easy fatigability in the adult. The infant tires rapidly during sucking, his major source of active energy expenditure.

The infant is fed on demand. Feed him when he first awakens, before he becomes upset and crys from hunger. Routine nursing care, such as baths and linen changes, are not as important as allowing the child to rest and conserve his energy for feeding. Typically, he will take about 1½ oz, rest for 10 to 15 minutes, then feed again. Do not force him to wake up and eat. Remember that he tires easily and must be allowed to rest and conserve as much energy as possible. It is preferable to hold him in a semi-upright position and offer oxygen with a mask held close to his face. However, if he must be fed in an isolette or oxygen tent, hold him upright to permit him to breathe and swallow better. A soft nipple with a large hole makes it easier for him to suck (try a "premie" nipple). Concentrating the formula will provide more calories in less fluid and helps promote nutrition. Let the infant rest during the feeding and do not let the feeding last too long. Remember that he needs adequate time to rest before the next feeding. Choking spells are common and a suction machine is kept at the bedside in case it is needed. Burp the baby often and place him on his abdomen or right side after feeding. The older child, although he needs independence, may need his mother to help feed him his meals if he tires easily.

Failure-to-Thrive

Failure-to-thrive is common in the child with CHD. Weigh him daily if he can tolerate it. Keeping an accurate record of intake and output will help to determine if weight gain is due to edema or nutrition, or if weight loss is occurring. As mentioned above, the child does not have enough energy to feed properly, and to complicate his nutritional problems, infections, dyspnea, and increased cardiac activity all require additional calories. He has no energy reserves to call on and as a result, anemia and malnutrition are often seen. Feed him as instructed above. Tube feedings are generally contraindicated because they tend to irritate the infant's delicate tissues (see the Skills Manual), and his struggles during the insertion of the tubes use up his precious energy. In addition, the infant derives a lot of pleasure from sucking. However, if he is too weak or too ill to suck, tube feedings may have to be utilized. Hold him while you insert the tube and until he calms down; then proceed with the feeding. Remove the tube between feedings.

Infection

Infection, particularly respiratory tract infection, is a potential threat to the child with CHD, especially if he has congested, edematous lungs. Prevent exposure to communicable diseases by placing the child in a room away from other children with upper respiratory infections. Stress the importance of good handwashing to all personnel, family members, and visitors. Persons with upper respiratory tract infections should avoid contact with the child. An isolette is often used to protect the infant from infection. Reverse isolation is used sparingly because of the psychological problems associated with it.

An elevated temperature is usually indicative of an infection, although the newborn may harbor an infection without a corresponding rise in temperature. A subnormal temperature may indicate sepsis. If the infant is in an isolette, remember to record the isolette temperature as well.

Behavioral Deviations

For centuries, people have thought of the heart as the most important organ in the body. It is thought of as the life-giver, the life-sustainer, and the seat of the emotions. It is indeed a tragic blow to the parents of a newborn to discover that their long-awaited baby will have to start life with an imperfection in such an important organ as the heart. One can live without a palate, without a kidney, without a lung, and without other body parts, but one cannot live without a heart.

Be present when the physician explains the child's defect to the parents. As always, give them some time alone to assimilate the information, then return to answer questions and help clarify their thinking. The infant should be present when the defect is discussed. Recall that bonding (ch. 3) is a necessary part of the healthy parent-infant relationship. If the baby is too ill to go to the mother, take the mother to her baby. If she cannot hold him, let her touch him and look at him. Point out his normal and attractive features in order to promote the bonding process. Also discuss the obvious symptoms of cardiac problems he exhibits, such as difficult respirations and poor color. Involve the parents in the assessment process so that they can better understand the need for further cardiac evaluation and treatment.

The initial reaction of parents is, of course, shock and disbelief, which may change quickly to fear and anxiety. The parents' concern is heightened when the child manifests overt signs of a cardiac defect, such as cyanosis and dyspnea.

If the defect is not corrected in infancy, the child's condition will be chronic, and he will have the same problems as any other child with a chronic illness (ch. 3). Parents find it difficult to punish the child for fear of aggravating the defect. He is overprotected, sheltered, and often forced to be dependent. Some dependency is legitimate (for example, the preschooler who needs help to finish his meals after he tires), but the extreme is to be guarded against.

Overprotection and unnecessary limits on the child's activities may influence his total development. Lack of opportunity to participate with children his own age leads to a lower self-concept and a genuine lack of physical ability. Recall that this child is smaller for his age, and this affects his self-image. Social and perceptual experiences also influence his body image. When asked to draw a picture of himself in a group of peers, the normal child draws himself larger than his peers; the child with heart disease draws himself the same size as his peers. He tends to view himself as dependent, small, and insignificant as an individual.

This child needs support and guidance to see himself as significant. His parents need support and guidance to assist him as necessary and to lessen their protectiveness as the child matures. Encourage them to let him determine his own activity tolerance level. Explain that he will stop when he gets tired.

Gene T., aged four, has tetralogy of Fallot, to be corrected next month. Gene plays well with neighborhood children his own age. His parents have provided him with lightweight, easy-to-manipulate toys to avoid overtaxing him as he plays. Although his mother worries as she watches him running in the yard with his friends, she has learned not to force him to rest. Gene gives up his active play and comes in to watch TV or read when he feels tired. Because his parents have managed to control their anxiety and overprotective tendencies, Gene has become an independent four-year-old who regulates his own activities.

Studies have shown that parents of the child with a cardiac defect seem to live in constant fear of the child dying. This fear derives from their knowledge of a defect, and the child's failure to grow and thrive is a constant reminder of that defect. Their anxiety, of course, is transmitted to the child, who is acutely aware of parental anxiety when he chokes, coughs, and has trouble getting his breath. The parents often put the infant in bed with them at night because they are so afraid that he will die that they cannot bear to let him sleep in his crib alone. This nightly pattern becomes routine and, needless to say, does not permit the parents (or the child) adequate rest. The child will have *night terrors*, which are more frightening than nightmares. He is scared to go to sleep for fear he will die. He awakens in acute anxiety, often screaming and hysterical. It is difficult to calm him and get him to go back to sleep. If the parents complain of these night terrors, ascertain if they have slept with the child since his infancy. If so, do not make them feel guilty, but explain the child's fears to them. Work with them to eliminate the night terrors. Encourage them to reassure the child that they are in the next room. A variety of techniques may be used to help the child express his fears, such as story telling, picture interpretation, or play therapy. It may be necessary to refer the child to a child psychologist.

COMPLICATIONS

Congestive Heart Failure

Congestive heart failure (CHF) occurs when the heart can no longer pump enough blood to meet the energy requirements of the body (Figure 22–2). It occurs in about 7,000 infants born in the United States each year. The symptoms of CHF are a result of the body's attempt to compensate for the heart's inadequacies. According to Strong, the newborn who has cardiac distress in the first week of life has almost a 100 percent chance of dying if his condition is not properly managed. The nurse should be aware of the signs and symptoms of CHD and impending cardiac failure. The nurse in the newborn nursery can observe the infant continuously and is able to detect subtle changes that may be missed by the physician, who sees the child for a limited amount of time.

Signs of CHF are categorized according to cardiac, pulmonary, or gastrointestinal origin, although all are caused primarily by the failure of the heart to pump blood. Cardiac signs include *cardiomegaly* (enlargement of the heart), tachycardia, gallop rhythm, cyanosis, and edema.

Cardiomegaly (together with tachycardia) is the heart's major compensatory mechanism. Within physiological limits, cardiomegaly increases cardiac output, but in CHF, physiological bounds are surpassed and the muscle fibers of the heart cannot contract as well.

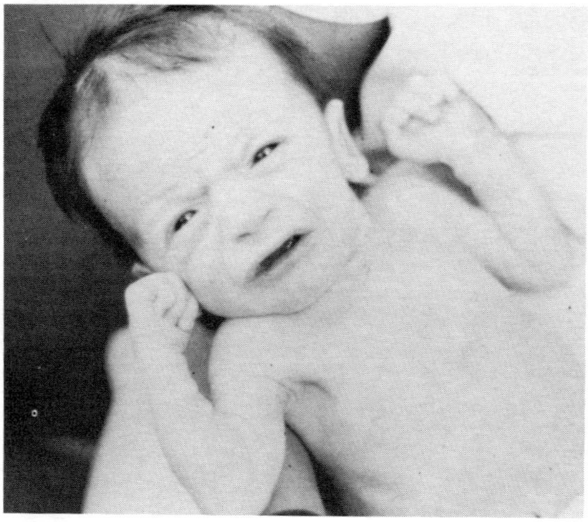

Figure 22–2. *Three-month-old male with a large ventricular septal defect and congestive heart failure; note the irritability and growth failure* (Courtesy, W.B. Strong, M.D., Charbonnier Professor of Pediatrics, Director of Pediatric Cardiology, Medical College of Georgia, Augusta, Ga.)

Tachycardia (a heart rate of over 140 beats per minute) rarely exceeds 180 to 200 beats. *Gallop rhythm* refers to the pronounced third heart sound (S_3) in the presence of tachycardia, and sounds very much like a horse galloping. Cyanosis, already discussed, is seen in CHF. Blood gas analysis is used to document hypoxemia.

Edema is a late sign of heart failure in the neonate and is not as readily apparent as it is in the older child or adult. Check the infant's back and face for edema, depending on whether he has been lying supine or prone.

Respiratory signs of CHF are tachypnea, dyspnea, wheezing, and orthopnea. Tachypnea is an early sign of impending failure in the infant. Respirations may exceed 60 per minute and are exaggerated with feedings. Watch for changes in respiratory rate, especially sustained elevations of 10 breaths per minute in a quiet, sleeping baby. Failure of the left ventricle causes a backup of blood in the lungs resulting in pulmonary engorgement and hypoxia. Together these lead to tachycardia.

Dyspnea indicates respiratory distress. Note retractions of the supraclavicular, subcostal, and intercostal spaces, and flaring nares. Wheezing is caused by edema of the bronchi and bronchioles, which causes expiratory obstruction and, consequently, the wheezing sound heard on expiration. The child may be restless and apprehensive. He is more comfortable and can breathe more easily in a semi-Fowler's position. Propping the infant in an infant seat will achieve the same effect.

Gastrointestinal symptoms include poor feeding, spitting up, and poor weight gain (already discussed), as well as distended neck veins, hepatomegaly (enlargement of the liver), and splenomegaly (enlargement of the spleen). These symptoms are more commonly seen with right ventricular failure, especially the liver enlargement, which is a late sign of CHF. The liver is the most proximal organ to the heart and acts as a reservoir for retained fluids. Both right and left lobes of the liver can be palpated below the costal margin (ribs). In respiratory distress, the left lobe is not palpable (Table 22–1). Hepatomegaly causes an elevation of pressure in the portal vein. Because the splenic vein feeds into the portal vein, portal hypertension can cause splenomegaly and edema of the intestinal mucosa. In turn, edema of the intestinal mucosa may cause malabsorption, anorexia, and spitting up. These factors, together with feeding difficulties, are the major causes of the infant's failure to gain weight and thrive. Remember that excessive energy expended by the heart and lungs also contributes to growth failure.

Diaphoresis, (excessive sweating), especially around the head and neck, is seen frequently in the child with CHF. The exact cause of this sign is unknown. It does act as a safety valve by ridding the body of excess sodium chloride, which causes fluid retention and, therefore, more work for the congested heart.

Treatment for CHF includes reducing energy requirements, improving cardiac efficiency, removing accumulated fluids, and improving oxygenation. Energy requirements are reduced by calming the child and reducing his anxiety with physical contact, TLC, and the administration of a sedative, usually morphine. Help make the child's breathing easier by positioning him in semi-Fowler's position, which relieves pressure on the diaphragm from the abdominal contents and promotes lung expansion. Humidified oxygen is administered to help alleviate the hypoxia caused by pulmonary congestion. Provide rest periods between feedings. Tube feedings may be used, but parenteral fluids are used with caution to avoid further overloading of the circulatory system. Remember to keep the environmental temperature constant to conserve the child's energy.

Cardiac performance is enhanced with the use of digitalis, usually in the form of Lanoxin. Although exact regimens vary, the child may be digitalized by giving one-half of the total digitalizing dose of 0.04 to 0.08 mg/kg of digoxin immediately via an intravenous infusion. One-fourth of the total dose can be given in six-to-eight hours, and prior to the third dose (again, one-fourth of the total), six to twelve hours later, an EKG is obtained to ensure the absence of digitalis toxicity. Intravenous digoxin may be given more rapidly if necessary. The peak action occurs in one to two hours after administration, so a second dose may be given in two hours provided there is no toxicity. Maintenance doses of one-fourth to one-third of the total dose are given in two equally divided doses twelve hours apart. Be alert to manifestations of digitalis toxicity: arrhythmias, anorexia, bradycardia, and nausea. Vomiting is usually a sign of too little digitalis rather than too much.

Digitalis and rest may be adequate to treat mild and moderate CHF, but if signs of CHF persist, diuretic therapy is started. Daily weights are the most accurate monitor of adequate diuresis; measuring urine output is not as reliable because of inadequate collection methods.

Detailed observation and meticulous nursing care are essential if the infant with CHF is to survive. In addition to recording and reporting what may seem to be minor details, the nurse must also keep careful track of the amount of blood withdrawn for laboratory tests. The loss of seemingly small amounts of blood may cause anemia and further compromise the infant's condition because his blood needs maximum oxygen-carrying capacity.

If the infant with cardiac distress is not in a medical center that specializes in the care of infants with CHD, he should be transported as soon as his condition is stable, so that adequate diagnosis and treatment can be initiated.

Pulmonary Vascular Obstructive Disease

Increased blood flow to the lungs, as seen in left-to-right (systemic-to-pulmonary) shunting, causes an increase in the pulmonary artery pressure *(pulmonary hypertension)*. The pulmonary pressure may be twice as high as normal. The increase in pressure, together with polycythemia (an increased number of RBCs with a resultant high hematocrit), leads to fibrotic changes in the lungs. This condition is called *pulmonary vascular obstructive disease* (PVOD). By twelve to eighteen months of age, these lung changes may be irreversible. For this reason, corrective surgery is performed as early as possible. The infant who presents early in CHF may have a *pulmonary artery banding* (PAB) procedure to lessen blood flow to the lungs. This procedure is palliative and requires a second operation for correction. The prognosis is never as good for the child with PVOD as it is for the child with minimal or no lung involvement.

Bacterial Endocarditis

Bacterial invasion of the lining of the heart, *bacterial endocarditis,* usually occurs at the site of a cardiac defect. It is rare in the infant and is more often seen in five-to-fifteen-year-olds; the incidence increases with age. Endocarditis results from streptococcal infections as well as from the introduction of bacteria into the body via catheters, dental work, surgery, or the insertion of instruments for urinary tract observation. Endocarditis may ruin the particular valve, and the child may develop profound heart failure and die. Prevention lies in prophylaxis with penicillin before dental work, surgery, or any invasive procedures, as well as prompt treatment for streptococcal infections.

Peggy G., twelve years old, had a patent ductus arteriosus (PDA). Peggy was asymptomatic, so her cardiologist recommended no treatment. Peggy had dental work done with no prophylaxis three weeks ago, and she developed bacterial endocarditis. She is presently in the ICU of a large medical center, with little chance of surviving heart failure. The ultimate tragedy is that Peggy's endocarditis could have been prevented; also, if Peggy were born today, her PDA would be ligated at an early age, thus eliminating her chances of developing endocarditis.

Cerebral Thrombosis

The child with cyanotic heart disease is at risk for developing *cerebral thrombosis* (cerebral vascular accidents), particularly if he is under the age of two. The greater the degree of the cyanosis, the greater the risk. *Polycythemia,* the body's answer to hypoxia, results from the increased level of desaturated hemoglobin (unoxygenated blood) in the peripheral vessels; the increased number of RBCs carry more oxygen, thus raising the hematocrit and hemoglobin. The circulation becomes sluggish because of the viscous blood, which is more likely to clot. Cerebral vascular accidents (CVAs) may occur spontaneously, but they are more likely to occur if oxygen requirements have been raised by fever, or if blood is made more viscous by dehydration. Fever, vomiting, and diarrhea are treated promptly in the child with cyanotic heart disease in an attempt to prevent cerebral thrombosis.

DIAGNOSTIC STUDIES AND NURSING IMPLICATIONS

Procedures used to evaluate cardiac function often involve complex machinery and equipment that frighten the child. His anxiety, fright, and restlessness may alter the findings. Nursing management during diagnosis includes preparation and reassurance of the child and his parents to decrease their anxiety (See Ch. 2). Explain that most of the tests are painless, and assure the parents that sedation will be used if the test involves prolonged periods of discomfort. The infant may be given a pacifier during testing.

General Assessment

As discussed earlier, the child with CHD will have feeding difficulties. These difficulties may be your first clue that something is amiss. Check the maternal history (See Table 22–1). The child with CHD is usually full-term, whereas the child with respiratory distress syndrome is premature, delivered of a diabetic mother, or via a cesarean section. The newborn with patent ductus arteriosus may be premature or born at high altitudes. The child with CHD is at a 25 percent risk for having other anomalies, so carefully examine him for other defects.

Undress the infant in order to adequately observe him. Observe his overall status, then watch his breathing. Is it symmetrical? Labored? Does he wheeze? Count the rate; is it over 45? Take the pulse; is it regular? Count the femoral and brachial pulses simultaneously; is there a discrepancy? If the femoral pulse is absent, weak, or intermittent, the infant may have coarctation of the aorta. Palpate for a thrill (palpable cardiac murmur). Place your hand on the infant's chest and feel the heartbeat. If a thrill is present, vibration or buzzing is felt. Also, feel the posterior chest wall for a thrill. If you suspect after this examination that the infant has a heart anomaly, notify the physician at once.

Physical Examination

In addition to the clinical manifestations discussed earlier, other physical signs may be found on physical examination. Some of these findings may not be seen in the newborn and are found at the time of a later checkup.

Murmurs

Murmurs are sounds produced by turbulent blood flow through abnormal openings, deformed valves, or roughened vessels. A murmur may be functional (innocent), or it may be organic, i.e., a sign of an abnormal or diseased heart. A general rule for assessing a murmur is to determine if the child's weight and height are normal for his age. If so, the murmur is probably functional, and therefore of no consequence. However, all murmurs should be properly evaluated by a physician.

The first heart sound, S_1, is caused by closing of the mitral and tricuspid valves. It is the atrial impulse and is heard at the beginning of systole. The second heart sound, S_2, marks the beginning of diastole and is caused by closure of the aortic and pulmonic valves. The aortic valve closes slightly ahead of the pulmonic valves. This accounts for the splitting of the S_2 commonly heard during inspiration. Systolic murmurs occur between the "lub" (S_1) and the "dub" (S_2) of the heartbeat, and diastolic murmurs are heard between the "dub" and the "lub."

Clubbing

Clubbing of the fingers and toes occurs in the child with long-standing cyanosis. It usually appears between one and two years of age. The nail bed softens and becomes wider and thicker; the nails have a bulbous appearance (Figure 22–3). The cause is unknown, although a popular theory attributes it to hypoxia.

Blood Studies

A complete blood count can indicate anemia, polycythemia, or infection. Serum electrolyte and blood gas studies will show

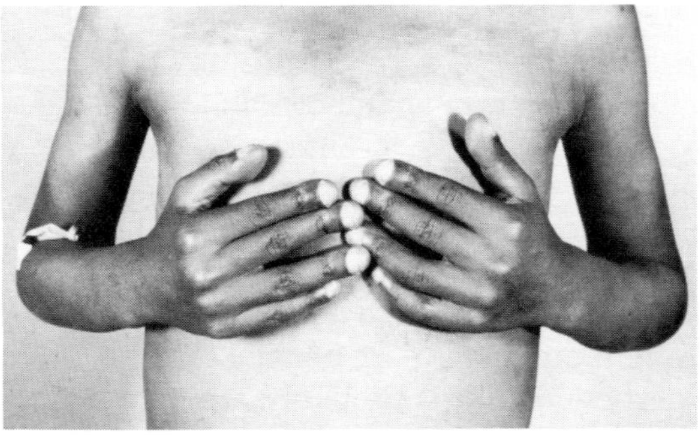

Figure 22–3. *Clubbing in an eight-year-old boy with transposition of the great arteries, ventricular septal defect, and pulmonary stenosis.* (Courtesy, W.B. Strong, M.D., Charbonnier Professor of Pediatrics, Director of Pediatric Cardiology, Medical College of Georgia, Augusta, Ga.)

how well-oxygenated the blood is and will reveal hypoxia and acidosis.

Electrocardiogram

Electrical impulses that stimulate the heart to contract are measured by an *electrocardiogram* (ECG or EKG). The ECG helps the physician to determine which chamber of the heart is involved and to what extent. The, test is painless but requires the child's cooperation because he must remain motionless during the test.

Echocardiography

Ultrasound, the frequency of sound above the range audible to the human ear, is employed in the diagnosis of cardiac anomalies. It orients the physician to cardiac structure and function. The test is painless, and sedation is rarely necessary, but the child's cooperation is important. An ultrasonic transducer is applied to the chest wall, cushioned with water-soluble jelly to form an airtight seal. The child is placed in the supine position and tilted slightly to the left. A beam of sound (ultrasound) is directed toward the heart. The beam is reflected off the tissues (echo), and the amplified output is displayed on an oscilloscope. Polaroid photos can be made of the signal. This procedure is called *echocardiography*.

X-ray Studies

Chest x-ray

The chest x-ray is used to determine the size and shape of the heart and great vessels, and adjacent anatomy. The amount of pulmonary involvement is also demonstrated. The x-ray also differentiates between cardiac and pulmonary involvement.

Angiocardiography

Angiocardiography refers to x-ray studies of the heart and great vessels after injection of a radiopaque dye. It is usually performed during cardiac catheterization. Normal or abnormal blood flow as well as rate of flow is demonstrated. *Angiography*, the x-ray study of an artery, may also be performed during catheterization.

Cardiac Catheterization

Cardiac catheterization involves the insertion of a catheter into the heart, via a vein or artery. X-rays are taken during the catheter insertion. Pressure is measured in the various chambers of the heart, and blood samples are taken from each area. Venous blood (from the venae cavae, right atrium, right ventricle, and pulmonary arteries) is normally 75 percent saturated with oxygen and arterial blood (from the pulmonary veins, left atrium, left ventricle, and aorta) is 98 percent saturated. In cyanotic defects, the oxygen saturation in the left ventricle is decreased. With some acyanotic defects, oxygenation in the right ventricle is higher because of shunting of oxygenated blood from the left ventricle. Systolic pressure is normally higher in the left ventricle and aorta than in the right ventricle and pulmonary artery, but with septal defects, pressure is decreased on the left and increased on the right.

Specific anomalies and their severity are detected during cardiac catheterization. X-rays taken after the introduction of radiopaque dyes (angiocardiography) may be used to further evaluate the child's condition.

The child's cooperation is essential during a cardiac catheterization. He is awake but sedated during the procedure, which is painless except for the injection of local anesthesia at the brachial or femoral catheterization site. In addition to offering routine supportive measures involving touch and a soothing voice, the nurse may read the child a story during the procedure to help decrease his anxiety. This reduction of fear will lessen vascular spasms which cause discomfort. Fear also tends to make the child less cooperative, making the procedure more dangerous, and possibly making it impossible to correctly evaluate critical information.

There is a small risk of fatality in cardiac catheterization, about 0.1 percent, and the parents should be made aware of this. Most of the deaths occur in infants under three months of age with critical disease; a one percent mortality rate exists for these children.

Psychological trauma should not be underestimated, especially if the child is awake during the procedure, as he usually is. (Review Ch. 2 for preparation of the child for procedures.) Apprehension and concern on the part of the parents and child is normal for any surgical or diagnostic procedure, and cardiac catheterization is no exception. There is one major difference between surgery and cardiac catheterization. In surgical procedures, the child is asleep; for a cardiac catheterization, he is awake. He will be aware of strange equipment, strange people, and strange sensations. It is imperative that he be prepared for these things beforehand. The child and his parents should know that the procedure will last from two to four hours, that pain will be minimal, and that medication will be given to ease the pain and make the child sleepy.

The child and his parents may benefit from a tour of the cardiac catheterization room. Explain that this room is *not* an operating room, but a special room where *only* cardiac catheterizations are performed. Have a member of the catheterization team meet you, the child, and his parents, and explain each piece of equipment. Allowing time for questions and touching the equipment is important. The child may like to "try out" the table on which he will lie during the procedure.

After the catheterization, monitor the child's vital signs as well as the color and pulse in the extremity used for the cutdown every hour for six hours. The pulse in that extremity may not be discernible. Fluids are given orally as soon as the child tolerates them. This is especially important for the cyanotic child because of the threat of thrombus formation in the presence of dehydration.

TREATMENT

Palliative Surgery

As recently as the early 1970's, many surgeons favored medical management (see previous section on congestive heart failure) and palliative surgery over corrective surgery. Because the mortality rate for corrective procedures was high (over 15 percent) even with the use of cardiopulmonary bypass, surgery was postponed, if at all possible, until the child was older and better able to tolerate the sometimes complex procedures.

The first palliative surgery for CHD was reported in 1945 by Alfred Blalock and Helen Taussig. Their procedure was a subclavian-to-pulmonary-artery anastomosis. Other procedures followed, including a descending aorta-to-left-pulmonary-artery anastomosis (Potts, 1946) and pulmonary artery banding (Muller and Dammann, 1952).

These and other measures saved the lives of many infants. Unfortunately, many late complications, some of which make corrective surgery impossible, were associated with these procedures. Correction after palliative procedures carries a higher mortality risk than correction without previous palliation. For these reasons, many surgeons prefer to correct all correctable defects in one operation, and to palliate those that are not correctable or are better corrected when the child is older. As mentioned earlier, improved care of the critically ill infant in intensive care units now makes cardiac surgery easier and safer. This policy has several advantages in addition to that of a better prognosis. The child and his family no longer have to live with the psychological threat of a heart defect that is still present and the need for a second operation. The retarded growth and development associated with severe heart disease is avoided or minimized by initial surgical correction. In the event that the lesion is better corrected in an older child, the infant is managed medically with digitalis, diuretics, and support as needed (oxygen, morphine, rest), in addition to palliative surgery if necessary.

Preoperative Care

The child is admitted three to five days before surgery so that final diagnostic procedures can be done. This allows you ample opportunity to work with him in preparation for his surgery. Preparation of the child for cardiac surgery is much the same as for any other procedure with a few exceptions. Never underestimate the emotional impact on the family that accompanies the decision to permit an operation on a child's heart, especially if that surgery involves *opening* the heart. Parents may be hesitant to choose surgery if the child "looks" normal. It is a risk they see no reason to take. Then, too, if the child is sickly and has been hospitalized for a number of times, they may hesitate to consent to surgery for fear of putting the child through still more misery and suffering. They may not feel capable of deciding for the child, who is too young to choose for himself. If the child is old enough, his opinion is usually sought before the final decision is made. Parents need a tremendous amount of support and understanding as they try to make the proper decision, and also *after* they have made their decision.

Pete J., a twelve-year-old boy with a cardiac defect, was scheduled for open heart surgery in four days. The decision was an agonizing one for his parents because Pete did not wish to have the surgery, and he made his decision known to all who would listen. Although he participated in preoperative preparation given by his student nurse and her instructor, he said repeatedly that he did not want the operation. Pete even asked the surgeon to respect his wishes and not operate. After surgery, Pete's heart never resumed pumping on its own, and he died four hours after his chest was closed.

The child undergoing cardiac surgery is usually subjected to more intensive procedures, more complex and frightening machinery, and more psychological trauma than is the child who has another type of surgery.

The child is not prepared for cardiac surgery in one session, as in the case of less complex procedures. Several sessions over a period of two to three days are necessary. Recall that this child and his parents have a high anxiety level, and the child himself is likely to be poorly adjusted. Also, he has usually been hospitalized before and will have a multitude of feelings about the hospital. Extra preparation sessions provide time for you to ascertain his feelings and help him express them. Begin with the least threatening situations in the first session. Give him time to assimilate the information and to ask questions. Save the highly anxiety-provoking situations, such as intrusive and painful procedures, until the last session. Again, permit him to question, to "play back," and to engage in play as necessary. Offer needle play under supervision.

Remember to prepare the child for all things he will be aware of before and after surgery. Do not give details that are not necessary; for example, "then, the doctor will cut open your heart" is *not* necessary—the child will be unconscious when his heart is "being fixed." Telling him he will be asleep is adequate. Resume your narrative when the child awakens in the ICU. He will have an endotracheal tube, or possibly a tracheotomy tube. Prepare him for the endotracheal tube, but do not tell him about the tracheotomy because it is not a usual occurrence. If he awakens with either of these in place, though, he will not be able to speak and will be frightened. Reassure him that the loss of his voice is temporary and is due to the tube in his throat, which is there to help him breathe more easily.

Prepare him for the chest tube(s). Be sure he and his parents know the drainage bottles are to be lower than the level of his chest, and that the tubes themselves will help him breathe more easily by draining air and fluid out of his chest. Tell them the tubes are usually removed in three to four days.

Leads for the cardiac monitor will be attached to the child's chest. Using the analogy of a TV screen is helpful in explaining the monitor. He may be frightened that the leads will electrocute him; reassure him that this is not so. Explain that the leads can feel his heart working and carry these feelings to the TV screen where they make a picture to show the nurses and doctors what a good job his heart is doing.

Offer the child and his parents a tour of the ICU where he will stay immediately postoperatively, but notify the ICU *first.* If conditions are such that they would frighten the child and his parents, another time for a visit will have to be arranged. This visit is important for the child, since he will meet the nurses who will care for him immediately after his surgery. Knowing that *they* know who *he* is is most comforting to the child. The visit gives him a chance to see and feel the strange equipment and to watch "his nurses" at work. He can see them responding to other patients and monitoring the machines.

Preventing hypostatic pneumonia in the child who has had heart surgery is not an easy task because coughing, turning, and deep breathing are painful because of the large incision. Stress that you or another nurse will splint his incision as he tries to cough and breathe deeply. Practice splinting, coughing, and breathing before surgery so that he will know what is expected of him postoperatively. Tell him he will have help in turning, and that pain medication will be given as needed.

An enema is usually given preoperatively to prevent the child from straining to pass a stool in the first few days after surgery. Vital signs are taken preoperatively to serve as a baseline for postoperative comparison. Accurate readings taken when the child is rested are important. Height and weight are used in figuring drug dosages and to help calculate the amount of edema or blood loss after surgery. Heparin is often given preoperatively if a heart-lung bypass is planned. Bleeding and clotting times are determined before heparin is given. The dose will be regulated to prevent both clotting and excessive bleeding. A broad-spectrum antibiotic is usually given as prophylaxis against infection.

Permit the child to take his favorite toy with him to the operating room. Record his choice on the preoperative check sheet so that the toy is not forgotten at the last minute.

Corrective Surgery

Two techniques that have helped make corrective surgery in infants routine are hypothermia and cardiopulmonary bypass. *Cardiopulmonary bypass* refers to the shunting of blood from the venae cavae to the arterial system via a pump or "heart-lung" machine. The result is a bloodless heart on which surgery is more easily performed.

Deep *hypothermia* refers to core, or central, cooling that induces circulatory arrest and permits surgery in a totally motionless, flaccid heart. The infant is surface-cooled with ice packs on the trunk and head (he may also be placed in a tub of ice) until his temperature reaches 25°C (77°F). His chest is then opened and he is connected to the cardiopulmonary bypass with cold (5° to 10°C or 41° to 50°F) perfusate until his temperature reaches 20°C (68°F), thus inducing total circulatory arrest; the tissues will survive under these conditions for 40 to 50 minutes. If the procedure takes longer than this, the child is again perfused (for five minutes) with the cardiopulmonary bypass, and surgery can be continued under total circulatory arrest for another 40 to 50 minutes. After the procedure is completed, the child is warmed with the bypass to a temperature of 33° to 34°C (91.4° to 93.2°F), then warming is continued with the aid of a warming blanket. The heart usually starts beating spontaneously; if not, an electric current is used to begin the heartbeat.

During surgery, Dacron or Teflon patches may be used to close large septal defects; severely damaged valves are replaced with a prosthetic valve. Infection and blood clot formation are hazards when artificial devices are used. Antibiotics are used liberally and anticoagulant therapy is often continued after surgery.

Postoperative Care

The first 48 hours after repair of the heart are critical because the child is most likely to have complications during this time. The child is returned to a pediatric or neonatal intensive care unit where he is cared for by specially trained nurses. The details of care in an intensive care unit are beyond the scope of this book; however, a description of some of the procedures involved follows.

Immediately upon the child's arrival in the unit, check and record his vital signs, color, motion, and level of consciousness every 15 minutes until stable. Start oxygen therapy and connect the cardiac monitor, chest tube, and urinary catheter. Give medications as ordered, and send requisitions for lab work or x-rays to the proper department. Bring the parents to the intensive care unit to see their child. Reassure them about his condition and the strange and frightening equipment. Encourage them to touch the child and talk to him.

Talk to the child as you care for him, even if he seems to be asleep. Recall that if he has a tracheostomy or an endotracheal tube in place he will not be able to talk and will have to communicate with his eyes and facial expressions. When he tries to talk and cannot, he may be frightened; remind him about the tubes, thus reinforcing your preoperative teaching. Tell him you will stay with him and take care of him. The endotracheal tube is usually removed within a few hours postoperatively. Observe the child closely for signs of respiratory distress caused by tracheal edema or inadequate ventilation. The child will receive oxygen via an isolette, hood, or tent (see ch. 23 for care of the child receiving oxygen therapy). Routine respiratory care includes a turning schedule as well as breathing exercises, coughing, and percussion. Deep breathing and coughing may be difficult because of a painful incision, fatigue, fear, or depressant medications. Assist the child by splinting his chest and encouraging his efforts. Let him rest between efforts, but continue until his lungs sound clear. Suctioning may be necessary to stimulate the infant or small child to cough, but it can be dangerous, and must be done with extreme caution. Give the child oxygen to prevent hypoxemia before you begin suctioning. If adequate pulmonary status cannot be maintained, reintubation may be necessary along with mechanical ventilation.

Before the surgical incision is closed, a separate stab wound is made in the chest and a tube inserted into the pleural cavity to drain accumulated blood, fluid, and air. The mechanism of normal respiration is upset when the thoracic cavity is opened during surgery. To ensure effective ventilation, air and fluid are evacuated postoperatively, and negative pressure is maintained by drainage. The most common way of draining the chest is via water seal drainage (Figure 22–4). The system is airtight, thus maintaining negative pressure within

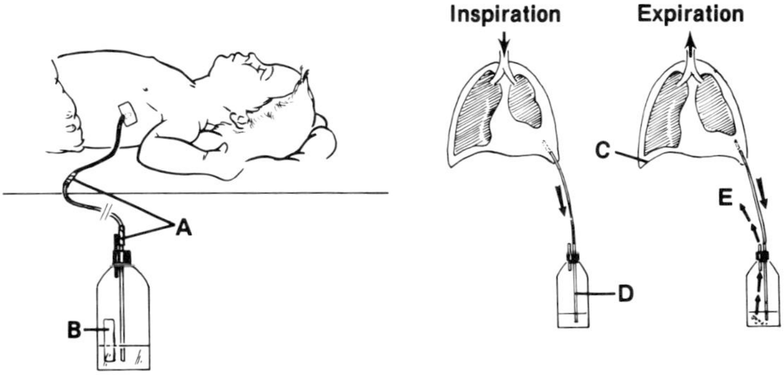

Figure 22–4. *Chest tube to water seal drainage system. A. Adhesive tape to reinforce connection. B. Adhesive tape marker. C. Diaphragm. D. Water level in tube. E. Air escaping from vent.*

the chest cavity. A drainage bottle with a small amount of water in it is secured to the floor under the bed. A long tube inserted through the bottle stopper reaches below the water level and is connected to the chest tube. Place a strip of adhesive on the bottle and mark the amount of water in the bottle initially. Every hour thereafter, mark and record the amount of drainage. If the tube is not draining adequately, gently milk it away from the chest. Do not let the tubing kink. Padded hemostats are kept at the bedside to clamp the tubing should it break or come loose, to prevent air from entering the chest and causing the lungs to collapse. The water level in the tube rises with inspiration and falls with expiration if the chest tube is not obstructed. A short tube placed through the bottle stopper provides an air vent to the outside, or is connected to a suction apparatus in the event additional suction is necessary.

Bubbling is normal when the child coughs; air leaves the pleural cavity and escapes through the water seal to the outside atmosphere. Bubbling at any other time indicates a leak in the system.

Cardiac Status

The child is attached to a cardiac monitor when he returns from the operating room. Conduction paste is used between the skin and the leads to assure proper contact and to prevent skin burns. The child's cardiac status is monitored on a screen at the bedside and/or a central control unit at the nurse's station. The nurse in the pediatric intensive care unit must learn basic electrocardiogram patterns so that she can detect impending problems and notify the physician of any irregularities (Figure 22–5).

Circulatory status can be monitored in part by observing the jugular veins. After blood loss, peripheral veins may collapse and are difficult to palpate. Jugular veins are always visible when the child lies flat and should be barely discernible when he is upright. They should fill on expiration and collapse on inspiration. Distension in the jugulars indicates overtransfusion, cardiac failure, or tamponade (compression of the heart) caused by blood in the pericardial cavity.

Central venous pressure (CVP) monitoring is valuable in determining the adequacy of the heart as a pump as well as the resultant circulatory status. CVP is measured via a catheter threaded into the superior vena cava through the jugular or brachial vein. The normal CVP is 5 to 15 centimeters of water with a mean of 6 to 7 centimeters. Overtransfusion, cardiac failure, or tamponade will produce an elevated reading; hypovolemia will cause a lowered reading.

Fluids and electrolytes are monitored closely. Overtransfusion leads to cerebral edema and forces the heart to work harder. Undertransfusion leads to dehydration and thrombosis (Refer to ch. 29).

Complications of Open-Heart Surgery

Hemorrhage may occur in as many as 50 percent of the children who undergo open-heart surgery. Shock follows rapidly and is fatal if proper treatment is not given. Notify the physician of any of the signs of impending shock: cool, pale skin becoming cold, clammy, and cyanotic; oliguria progressing to anuria; and changes in behavior. The child may be alert and extremely anxious, lethargic, or comatose.

Infection may occur in 25 percent of the children who have undergone open-heart surgery. Vigorous therapy with antibiotics and meticulous nursing care to protect the child from further infection is mandatory.

Arrhythmias are life-threatening and

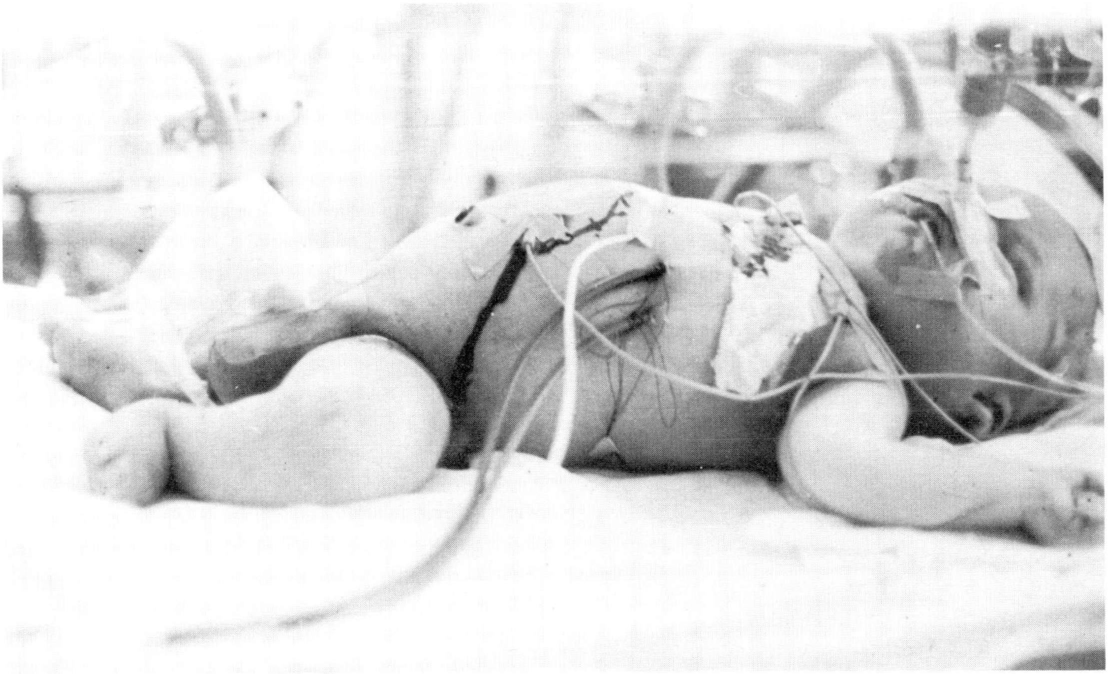

Figure 22–5. *Infant with chronic heart failure with ascites and edema in immediate postoperative period. Note cardiac monitor leads on abdomen and upper chest, chest tubes on left side, temperature probe above stab wound, feeding tube, and nasal oxygen.* (Courtesy, W.B. Strong, M.D., Charbonnier Professor of Pediatrics, Director of Pediatric Cardiology, Medical College of Georgia, Augusta, Ga.)

occur in 10 percent of cases. The first sign of cardiac complication is often *premature ventricular contractions* (PVCs), caused by digitalis intoxication, cardiac hypoxia, or myocardial ischemia. Correction of the arrhythmia may call for the administration of antiarrhythmia drugs, such as quinidine. However, electrical cardioversion (defibrillation) is usually the treatment of choice. A pacemaker may be necessary if damage was incurred by the conduction system of the heart, causing heart block.

Cardiac and respiratory arrest may occur at any time. Be prepared. Know what you will do *before* arrest occurs. Resuscitation equipment is kept at the bedside. Call for help as soon as there is evidence of impending arrest. (See the Skills Manual.)

Emotional Implications

As the child awakens from cardiac surgery, he is frightened and apprehensive, regardless of how well he was prepared preoperatively. Strange equipment, sounds, people, and sensations, coupled with pain and forced dependency, lead to intolerable feelings of helplessness and anxiety. The child regresses and either withdraws or becomes aggressive.

Withdrawal is a way of coping. It "protects" the child and gives him his own refuge from the unfamiliar and from the painful demands on his body. It is a time when he uses his energy for healing. Within limits, this withdrawal is normal and necessary. Dim the lights when possible and respond to the child with a gentle touch and soft voice. Tell him what you are going to do before you do it. Reassure him that his pain is temporary and that you will take care of his needs.

Aggressive or demanding behavior is also normal, but is more difficult for the nurse to deal with. Treat the demanding child as you would the withdrawn child. Meet his needs and be truthful with him. If he wants to talk about his experience or fears, or wants to ask questions, permit him to do so. Encourage this communication, but do not force him.

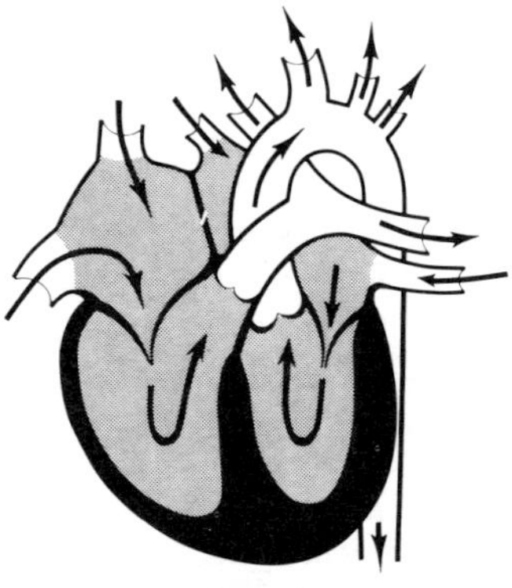

Figure 22–6. *Normal heart.*

After three to five days, the child is returned to his room from the intensive care unit. He gradually becomes involved in his care, thus increasing independence. In many cases, there are no restrictions on the child's activity after complete recovery. For the parents who have overprotected and agonized over this child from birth, "turning him loose" is most difficult. They will need support and encouragement to avoid overprotecting their child. Long-term overprotection is detrimental to the child's emotional well-being.

SPECIFIC CONDITIONS

Congenital Heart Disease

Acyanotic Defects

Figure 22–6 is a diagram of a normal heart, to be compared with diagrams of the defects discussed in this section.

In *acyanotic heart defects,* there is no abnormal mixing of unoxygenated and oxygenated hemoglobin in the systemic circulation, therefore, the child is not cyanotic. Acyanotic defects are classified as either obstructive or left-to-right shunts. Regardless of the classification, the primary characteristic is pulmonary volume overload.

In *obstructive lesions,* abnormal pressure exists across a stenotic area. In *left-to-right shunts,* the oxygenated blood in the left heart (red blood) is shunted to the right heart where it mixes with the unoxygenated (blue) blood. This "purple" blood then goes back to the lungs where it is reoxygenated. It does not go to the systemic circulation, thus the child is not cyanotic.

Severe acyanotic defects may be diagnosed at birth. Otherwise, the child is usually asymptomatic except for frequent respiratory tract infections and mild dyspnea upon exertion.

Obstructive Lesions

Aortic Stenosis

Stenosis of the aortic valve may be congenital or acquired as a result of rheumatic fever. It is an obstructive lesion interfering with left ventricular outflow and may occur at the valve, under it (subaortic stenosis), or above the valve within the aorta itself (supravalvular) (Figure 22–7). Severity depends on the degree of obstruction. Left ventricular pressure increases to push the blood out, thus the left ventricle hypertrophies and may obliterate the orifice of the coronary vessels during systole. This causes a decrease in the amount of blood reaching the heart muscle itself. Angina, ventricular ischemia, and fibrillation may result.

Pulse pressure (the difference between systolic and diastolic pressure) is narrowed in severe cases, which are diagnosed at birth. The infant has symptoms of cardiac failure and shock. In less severe cases, the child may appear normal, and a murmur is discovered at the time of a routine physical examination. This murmur, heard best to the left of the sternum over the base of the heart, is termed a systolic ejection click and is thought to reflect a valvular opening. Often a palpable thrill is present.

Correction is accomplished by a valvotomy to divide the fused cusps (if the defect is at the valvular level). If the lesion is supravalvular or subaortic, the obstructive tissue is excised.

Pulmonary Stenosis

Stenosis of the pulmonary valve may occur as an isolated lesion, but it is frequently seen in association with other defects (Figure 22–8). The valve cusps themselves may be fused, thus narrowing the lumen of the pulmonary artery, or the lesion may be *infundibular,* that is, just beneath the valve in the outflow tract. Rarely, atresia of the valve is present and survival depends on associated defects. Right ventricular hypertrophy occurs because the right ventricle

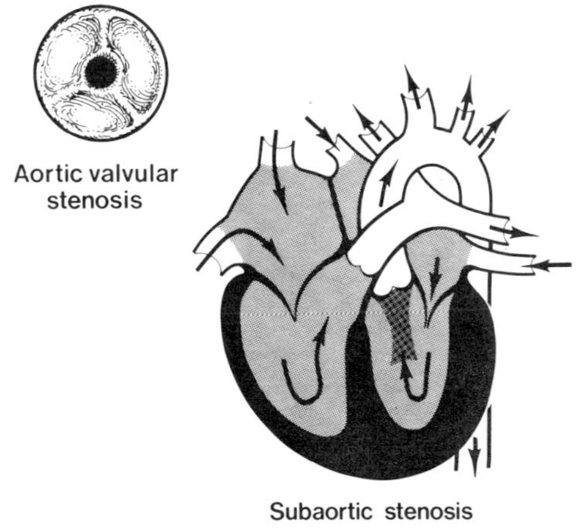

Figure 22–7. *Aortic stenosis.*

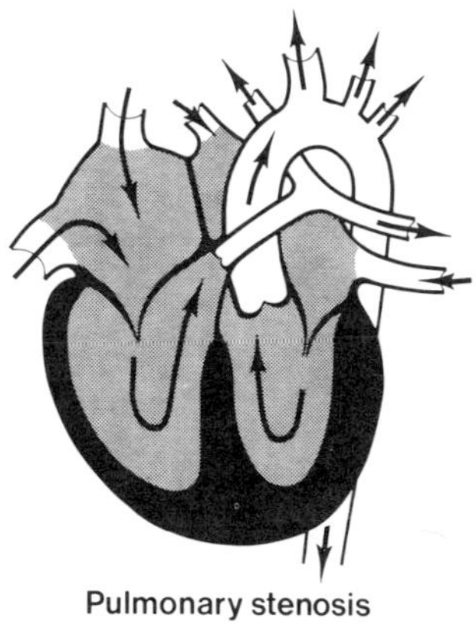

Figure 22–8. *Pulmonary stenosis.*

must work harder to pump blood through the narrowed opening into the pulmonary artery.

If the defect is severe, it is noticed at birth. The infant is in respiratory distress due to lack of oxygenated blood and heart failure. If the foramen ovale is still open, the increase in right atrial pressure produces a right-to-left shunt and the baby will be cyanotic. Usually, though, the child is asymptomatic except for fatigue and dyspnea on exertion.

A harsh systolic ejection murmur may be heard best at the left second intercostal space (ICS) during expiration. A thrill may be palpated, usually over the right third ICS.

Correction involves cutting the fused cusps if the stenosis is valvular, or trimming away excessive tissue if the lesion is infundibular. Atresia of the pulmonic valve does not respond well to surgery, and the prognosis is guarded.

Coarctation of the Aorta

Coarctation refers to narrowing of a lumen. In this case, the aorta is narrowed in the area of the ductus arteriosus just beyond the left subclavian artery (Figure 22–9). Systemic circulation is compromised beyond the defect while circulation proximal to the lesion is increased. This causes high blood pressure and a full, bounding pulse in the upper extremities and a low blood pressure and weak or absent pulse in the lower extremities. Collateral circulation develops, resulting in large intercostal arteries. Congestive heart failure may occur because of the strain on the left ventricle, but if CHF does not occur early, the child is typically asymptomatic and not aware of the defect until it is discovered on routine examination. He may have headaches and

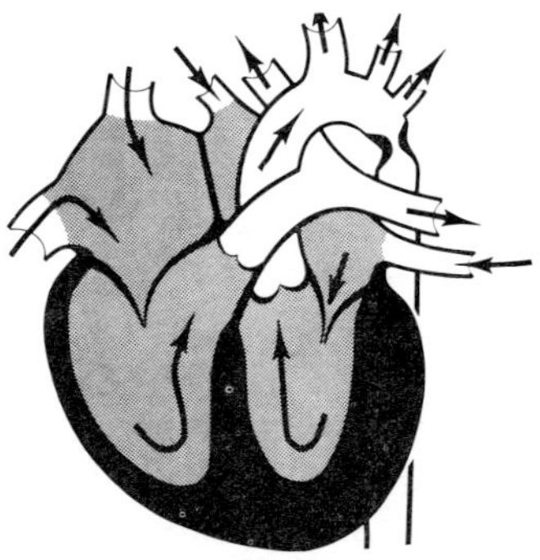

Figure 22–9. *Coarctation of the aorta.*

dizziness caused by the hypertension and cold feet and legs caused by the hypotension. Chest x-ray will show a typical rib notching, which is caused by erosion of the ribs adjacent to the dilated intercostal arteries. If CHF occurs, it is managed medically. Resection of the narrowed aorta is done, if medical management is not effective. The ideal age for correction is between three and ten because the lumen is adequate to support adult life, and fibrotic changes have not yet occurred. End-to-end anastomosis is done if possible, or, if not, a prosthetic graft may be used. The mortality rate is low except when surgery is performed as an emergency measure for heart failure in infancy.

Left-To-Right Shunts

Patent Ductus Arteriosus

The ductus arteriosus is a normal part of the anatomy of the fetal heart. It connects the pulmonary artery at its bifurcation to the aorta. Blood bypasses the lungs and flows into the descending aorta through the open ductus. At birth, pulmonary vascular resistance is decreased as the pulmonary arterioles dilate. The pulmonary blood flow increases and the ductus begins to contract within 24 to 72 hours. Eventually it fibroses, becoming the ligamentum arteriosum.

When the ductus fails to close, it is referred to as a patent ductus arteriosus (PDA) (Figure 22–10). Recall that after birth the systemic pressure (in the left heart) is greater than the pulmonary pressure (in the right heart). This higher pressure causes blood to flow from the systemic to the pulmonary circulation or, in this case, from the aorta, through the ductus, to the pulmonary artery. This is a left-to-right shunt. The blood flow to the lungs is abnormally high, and this in turn increases the return to the left atrium and places a greater work load on the left side of the heart.

Fifteen percent of premature infants have a PDA and in severe cases will develop CHF if the shunt is large. The child is usually asymptomatic, and the defect is detected by the presence of a typical murmur called a "machine-shop" murmur. It is heard best at the second left intercostal space. Mild symptoms are usually seen, such as easy fatigability, frequent respiratory infections, and some physical underdevelopment. Complete repair is done by ligation of the ductus; this is closed-heart surgery (the PDA is outside the heart) and takes only about 15 minutes. The results are excellent. Because of the excellent results and low mortality rate (less than 0.5 percent), this defect should be repaired early, even if the ductus is small. The risk of bacterial endocarditis is significant and can be prevented with early correction. The PDA may be necessary for the survival of the child with a defect involving decreased pulmonary blood flow; in such a case, the ductus must stay patent if the child is to survive. Studies have shown that E-type prostaglandins infused through an umbilical catheter can relax the ductus and delay its closing. Inhibiting prostaglandins by the oral or rectal administration of indomethacin also has been used to close the ductus, thus eliminating the need for surgical correction. Although these agents are not yet available for general use, their potential in the management of PDA is exciting.

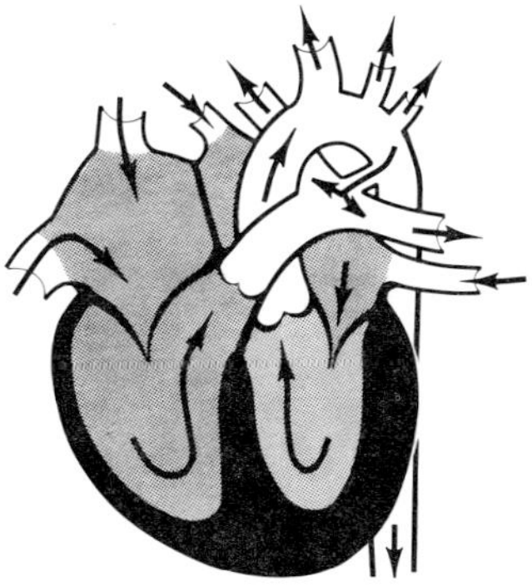

Patent ductus arteriosus

Figure 22–10. *Patent ductus arteriosus.*

Atrial Septal Defects

An atrial septal defect (ASD) is an opening in the septum between the two atria (Figure 22–11). The defect may be high, low, or in the center of the septum. Blood flows from left to right, thus increasing the work load on the right side of the heart and consequently, the pulmonary blood flow.

The severity of symptoms is related to the size of the defect. The child is usually asymptomatic except for respiratory problems and fatigue on exertion. A characteristic pulmonary systolic ejection murmur may be heard at the second and third left

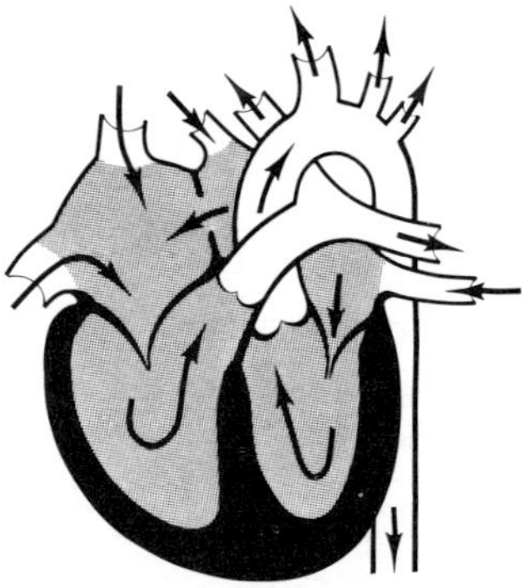

Figure 22–11. *Atrial septal defect.*

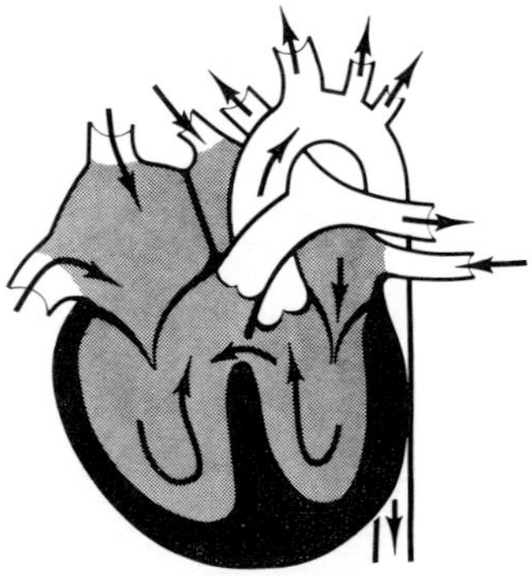

Figure 22–12. *Ventricular septal defect.*

ICS. There is wide splitting of S_2. Surgical correction consists of direct closure, using cardiopulmonary bypass. For large defects, a patch graft is used.

Ventricular Septal Defect

A ventricular septal defect (VSD) is an opening in the septum between the two ventricles (Figure 22–12). It is the most common intracardiac defect and occurs in 3 to 5 out of every 1,000 live births. It accounts for 30 to 50 percent of all congenital heart disease. The defect may be small, or so large that the entire septum is absent. A high defect located just beneath the tricuspid and aortic valves is most common.

Blood flows from left to right, thus the child is acyanotic. Severity of symptoms is related to the size of the defect and the amount of blood shunted to the lungs. Small defects may be asymptomatic, but there is a risk of bacterial endocarditis. A medium-sized VSD is also asymptomatic but the child tires more easily than his peers and has more respiratory infections. With a large VSD, the left ventricle has twice the normal work load, causing congestive failure in infancy. A *pansystolic,* (heard throughout systole) high-pitched, harsh murmur may be heard over the 4 to 6 ICS at the left sternal border. It may be associated with a palpable thrill.

Some physicians treat the child conservatively if the defect is small because spontaneous closure often occurs in the first two years. For CHF, medical management is attempted. If it is not effective, banding of the pulmonary artery may be done to reduce the flow of blood to the lungs. Closure of the VSD is also an option. Some surgeons repair the VSD early even if it is small because of the excellent results (about 100 percent for the infant over three months of age in some hospitals).

Complications of a VSD repair increase if the pulmonary artery pressure is elevated before surgery. The major technical problem in surgery is to suture the defect without injury to the bundle of His. A suture can interrupt the nerve pathway and cause heart block. An artificial pacemaker may be necessary after surgery.

Cyanotic Defects

In cyanotic heart defects, unoxygenated hemoglobin circulates in the peripheral vessels, giving a bluish cast to the skin. All of these defects involve right-to-left shunting. The unoxygenated blood of the pulmonary (right heart) circulation is shunted into the systemic (left heart) circulation where it is pumped back out to the body without being oxygenated by the lungs. (Recall that 5 grams of unsaturated hemoglobin produces noticeable cyanosis.) The determination of the degree of cyanosis in cyanotic heart defects is directly related to the amount of pulmonary blood flow rather than the size of the defect or the amount of blood shunted. Some of these defects cause a massive pulmonary blood flow in the presence of associated anomalies. The child with such a defect may have little cyanosis, yet be seriously ill because of the tremendous blood flow to the lungs, with its consequent heavy load on the left ventricle. On the other hand, some defects produce a marked reduction in flow to the lungs because blood is diverted away from the pulmonary system. Affected infants will be markedly cyanotic. These defects are easily remembered because the more common ones, discussed in this book, begin with the letter *T*.

Tetralogy of Fallot

Tetralogy of Fallot (TF) accounts for 4 to 5 percent of all CHD seen in the first year of life and is the most common cyanotic lesion seen after infancy. Four anomalies occur in TF: 1) pulmonary stenosis, 2) right ventricular hypertrophy, 3) ventricular septal defect, and 4) an overriding aorta, commonly referred to as dextroposition ("to the right,") (See Figure 22–13.) The pulmonary stenosis is typically infundibular but may involve the valve itself. This obstruction forces the right ventricle to work harder; thus, it hypertrophies. The pressure then is increased in the right ventricle, creating a right-to-left shunt that results in cyanosis. Polycythemia and clubbing of the fingers and toes are common, as are anoxic spells resulting in loss of consciousness. The child frequently squats to aid blood flow. A systolic murmur may be heard at the second and third ICS at the left sternal border. S_2 is single.

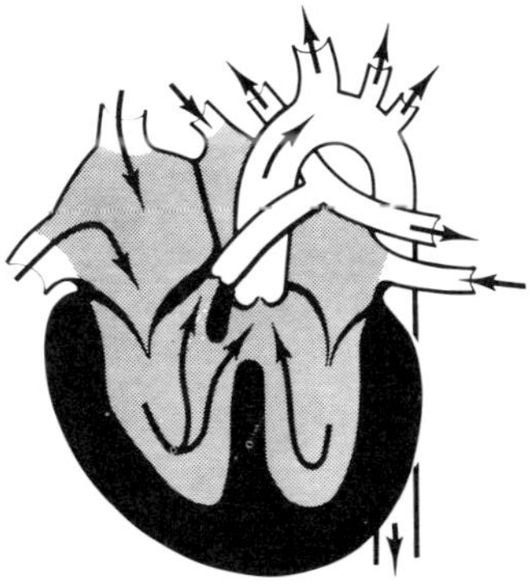

Figure 22–13. *Tetralogy of Fallot.*

If the infant is relatively stable and minimally cyanotic, surgery is postponed; however, the seriously ill infant requires early surgery. Palliative procedures (Blalock-Taussig, Potts, Waterston) may be performed, with total correction postponed until a later date; however, the combined mortality rate for the two-stage repair is from 20 to 50 percent. According to Sade and Castaneda, recent studies have shown that far lower mortality rates result when corrective surgery is done initially. Pericardium is used to enlarge the pulmonary outflow tract, and knitted Dacron is used to patch the VSD.

Transposition of the Great Arteries

Transposition of the great arteries (TGA) is the most common cause of cyanotic congenital heart disease in the infant. It accounts for 5 to 6 percent of all CHD in the first year of life. In TGA, the aorta arises from the right ventricle and the pulmonary artery from the left ventricle (Figure 22–14). Unoxygenated blood is returned to the heart via the venae cavae and is sent directly back to the body through the right ventricle and aorta. Similarly, blood flows from the lungs, to the left heart, and back out the pulmonary artery to the lungs. Two separate circulations exist: the right heart is a systemic circulation; the left heart, a pulmonary circulation. Unless there are other associated defects that permit shunting, death occurs soon after birth. Septal defects and patent ductus arteriosus are commonly associated with TGA.

The affected child is severely cyanotic within the first few days of life. A single intensified heart sound is usually heard in the second left ICS, and a loud systolic murmur is heard if a VSD is present. In cardiac catheterization during the first week of life, a balloon atrioseptostomy (Rashkind procedure) is routinely performed. A balloon catheter is threaded through the foramen ovale, and the balloon is inflated and withdrawn to rupture the atrial septum. This procedure results in improvement of atrial oxygen saturation in most cases. Another procedure (Blalock-Hanlon) involves surgically excising the interatrial septum; however, the mortality rate is 5 to 16 percent. Both of these procedures are palliative and permit mixing of the blood.

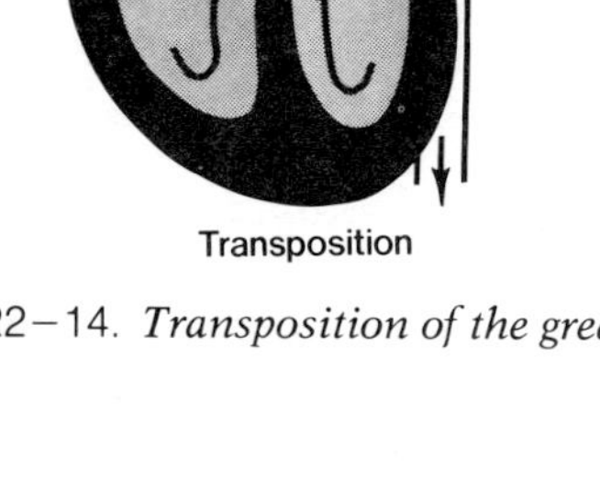

Figure 22–14. *Transposition of the great arteries.*

Corrective surgery consists of a Mustard procedure performed by the age of one year. The mortality rate is less than 10 percent. If the child is doing poorly, the procedure is done at one month or even earlier, although the mortality rate is higher for the younger infant (probably because of his poorer condition). The Mustard procedure involves the use of pericardium to create a new atrial septum, which alters blood flow through the atria. Blood returning to the right atrium from the venae cavae is redirected through the mitral valve into the left ventricle and out the pulmonary artery to the lungs. Blood returning from the lungs to the left atrium is redirected to the tricuspid valve, right ventricle, and out the aorta to the systemic circulation.

Tricuspid Atresia

Tricuspid atresia (TA) accounts for 1 to 2 percent of all CHD in the first year of life. In this defect, there is no opening from the right atrium to the right ventricle. Survival depends on mixing of the blood via associated defects. (Note the ASD, VSD, and smaller-than-normal pulmonary artery in Figure 22–15.) A harsh pansystolic murmur may be heard at the left sternal border (indicative of a left-to-right shunt). A VSD is present. If only a PDA exists, a soft continuous bruit is heard.

Severe anoxic spells in the two- to three-week-old infant signal closure of the patent ductus, frequently the infant's only

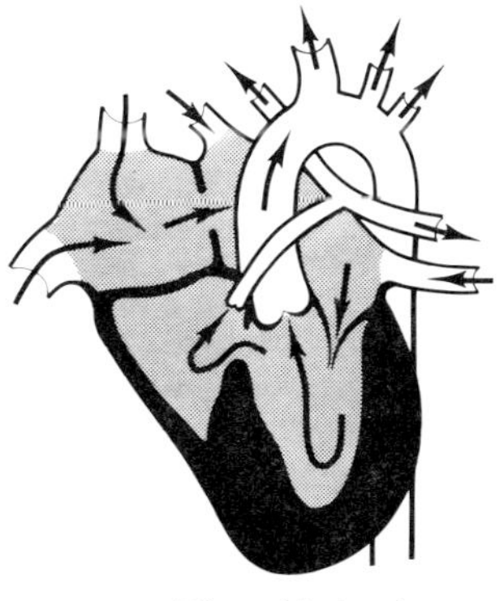

Figure 22–15. *Tricuspid atresia.*

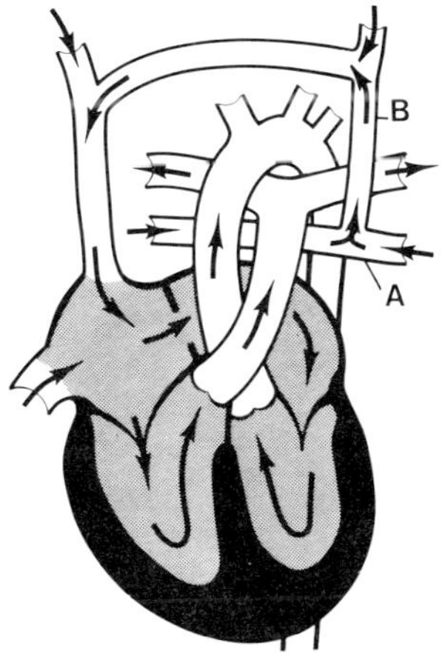

Figure 22–16. *Total anomalous pulmonary venous return, showing A. common vein and B. ascending or descending vein.*

source of pulmonary blood flow. Immediate surgery is indicated. Major or palliative surgery involves shunting of unoxygenated blood to the lungs. Several procedures are in use, but the mortality rate is high. Corrective procedures close the septal defects and divert blood from the right atrium to the pulmonary artery. Intracardiac mixing of blood is prevented. These procedures, too, carry a high mortality rate and are better tolerated in the older child.

Total Anomalous Pulmonary Venous Return

Total anomalous pulmonary venous return (TAPVR) comprises about 2 percent of all congenital heart anomalies seen in the first year of life (Figure 22–16). The pulmonary veins do not return from the lungs to the left atrium. They either return to the right atrium or to other veins feeding the right atrium. In the majority of cases, they form a common vein located behind the left atrium. The affected infant presents early with severe cyanosis, marked respiratory distress, and signs of pulmonary edema caused by obstruction of pulmonary venous drainage. No palliative operation is available, and corrective surgery is undertaken immediately because of the rapid deterioration seen with pulmonary venous obstruction. The ascending or descending vein is ligated, and the common vein is anastomosed to the left atrium. The mortality rate is high—20 to 30 percent.

Truncus arteriosus

Truncus arteriosus (Figure 22–17) is a rare defect characterized by a single arterial trunk arising from the ventricles. A VSD is always present. The pulmonary, systemic, and coronary circulations are all fed from this single trunk. Both ventricles pump into the trunk, thus forcing blood into the lungs at systemic pressure. Because of the high pulmonary blood flow, cyanosis is not marked in the infant. Hemodynamics mimic a large left-to-right shunt: left heart failure, respiratory problems and poor physical development. The S_2 is single be-

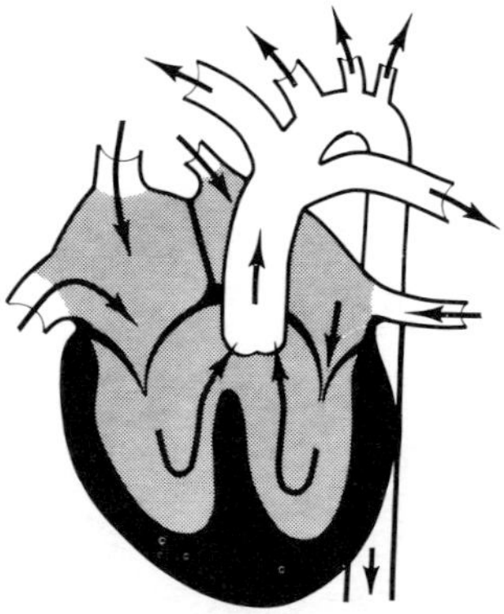

Figure 22–17. *Truncus arteriosus.*

cause of the single set of semilunar valves. A harsh systolic murmur is heard along the left sternal border. Palliative surgery offers poor results and corrective surgery (to separate the pulmonary artery from the aorta) is hazardous.

Acquired Heart Disease: Rheumatic Fever

Acute rheumatic fever (ARF) is an inflammatory disease that affects connective (collagen) tissue in various parts of the body. The heart, joints, central nervous system, and subcutaneous tissue may all be affected.

ARF is seen primarily in the five to fifteen-year-old who lives in a cold, damp climate. It is directly related to low socioeconomic status, poor nutrition, inadequate housing, and crowded conditions. Each year in the United States there are 190,000 new cases. ARF is a major cause of morbidity and mortality in the child and adolescent.

A respiratory infection with group A beta-hemolytic streptococci precedes an attack of ARF. Attacks are more common in the late winter and early spring when respiratory infections are at a peak. There is a seven-day to six-month latent period between the time of streptococcal infection and the onset of symptoms. The length of the latent period varies with the presenting symptom. A hypersensitivity reaction is thought to be responsible for the development of rheumatic fever after a streptococcal infection. Heredity also plays a part because there is a higher incidence among family members.

An *Aschoff body* is an inflammatory lesion unique to rheumatic fever. It results from damage to collagen fibers and is found in the myocardium. Although not all persons with ARF develop *carditis (rheumatic heart disease)*, it is the most outstanding and potentially detrimental symptom, and for this reason rheumatic fever is discussed in conjunction with cardiac disease. Opinions vary as to the percentage of children who develop carditis, but most estimates range from 40 to 60 percent. It is a common mistake to label a person with rheumatic fever as having rheumatic heart disease. Carditis is only one manifestation of ARF.

It is imperative that an accurate diagnosis be made so that recurrence of rheumatic fever can be prevented, and problems associated with a history of ARF are significant. Military service, life insurance, and employment are among the areas that are prejudiced against the ARF victim, even if he never developed carditis. Modified Jones Criteria (Table 22–3) require the presence of two major or one major and two minor manifestations in addition to supportive evidence of a recent streptococcal infection. Fulfillment of these requirements indicates a high probability of rheumatic fever.

Symptoms of ARF are not easily grouped with the common problems of the child who has a congenital heart disease, and

Table 22–3. **Modified Jones Criteria**

Major Manifestations	*Minor Manifestations*	*Supportive Evidence*
Carditis	Clinical	Recent scarlet fever
Murmur	History of previous rheumatic fever	Positive throat culture
Cardiomegaly	Arthralgia	Increased ASO or other streptococcal antibody titers.
Pericarditis	Fever	
Congestive heart failure	Laboratory	
Polyarthritis	Increased ESR	
Chorea	C-reactive protein	
Erythema marginatum	WBC count	
Subcutaneous nodules	Anemia	
	Prolonged P–R interval on EKG	

Adapted from Ammann, A.J. and Wara, D.W. Collagen Vascular Diseases (Rheumatic Diseases), in Rudolph, A.M. (ed). *Pediatrics,* ed. 16. New York, Appleton-Century-Crofts, 1977, p. 385.

they therefore are discussed separately. The major symptoms include migratory polyarthritis, carditis, Sydenham's chorea, subcutaneous nodules, and erythema marginatum. As a general rule, the younger child presents with carditis, and the older child presents with polyarthritis or chorea.

The child has a history of a sore throat or recent scarlet fever (streptococcal infections). One to 3 weeks later (or two to six months later if chorea is the presenting symptom), he presents with symptoms of ARF. These may be mild, such as joint pain, abdominal pain, or fever. Further evaluation may reveal a murmur, reddened throat, or swollen, painful joints. The child should be hospitalized for diagnostic testing.

Major Manifestations

Migratory Polyarthritis

Acute migratory polyarthritis is associated with febrile illness. It is found in 90 percent of the cases of ARF and is more common in the north. In the southern United States, arthralgia, a minor manifestation, is seen more often. The large joints of the extremities (knees and elbows) are most often affected, but the hands, feet, spine, and jaw may also be involved. The joint is red, hot, swollen, and painful to a degree that is disproportionate to physical findings. The joint is affected for about three days, then the symptoms subside and migrate to another joint.

Aspirin should not be given until the diagnosis is certain because its anti-inflammatory properties will mask migration, recognition of which is essential to the diagnosis. Codeine (without aspirin) is given for pain until a positive diagnosis is made.

The involved joint is often so painful that the child cannot even bear to have the bed covers touching him. Use a bed cradle and, if he can tolerate it, place a lightweight blanket over him for a "security blanket." Hot water bottles and heating pads may also add to the child's discomfort even though the warmth is soothing. Try a heat lamp attached to the bed cradle (Remember to use a bulb no stronger than 40 watts). Because migratory polyarthritis leaves no residual effects as does rheumatoid arthritis, the joint may be splinted with sand bags to keep it immobile. Exercise is not necessary, but skin care is important to prevent breakdown. Remember that the child has fever and that he perspires, particularly in skin folds. Gently bathe him with tepid water. He will guard the affected extremity (for example the arm), and the axilla may excoriate. Wash it gently, dry it, and apply talcum powder. Explain the necessity for this thorough bathing to the child and attempt to gain his cooperation. Repeated spraying with deodorant will not help the skin, although it may remove odor for a time. Change damp linens frequently; see that they are wrinkle-free, and check for crumbs, crayons, and other small objects the child tends to drop into his bed. Offer mouth care frequently. If the child is in pain, he is more likely to breathe through his mouth. The mucous membranes will become dry and uncomfortable. Lemon and glycerine swabs actually dry the mouth for the first few days of use, so attempt to get the child to use a toothbrush, toothpaste, and mouthwash rather than relying on swabs.

As long as his joints hurt, the child is content to remain on bed rest. However, when the pain subsides, he is ready for more activity. If the inflammatory process is still active (as evidenced by fever and laboratory tests), bed rest is still necessary. This may present a problem because the child feels good and wants to resume activity. Creativity on your part is mandatory if bed rest is to be enforced. Provide toys, games, and books to interest the child. Place him in a semiprivate room so that he has a roommate. Wheel his bed to the playroom so that he can participate in planned activities. Ask the schoolteacher and "play lady" to visit. Arrange phone calls and letters to friends at home. Basically, any safe activity may be tried in an effort to keep the child from getting bored. He is usually on bed rest for two to three weeks, provided he has no carditis. Restricted activity is ordered for another two to three weeks.

Carditis

Carditis is an inflammatory process involving the endocardium *(valvulitis)*, myocardium *(myocarditis)*, and/or pericardium *(pericarditis)*, The presenting complaint in carditis is often fever with or without arthritis. Chest pain *(precordial pain)* is also a frequent complaint. A pericardial friction rub (scratchy sound) or effusion may be heard. Occasionally, congestive heart failure is the presenting symptom. This is probably a recurrent attack (the first attack having gone unnoticed) because heart damage enough to cause heart failure is uncommon with one attack.

There may be an increase in heart size, appearance of a murmur, or a change in an existing murmur. The most common murmur is that of *mitral regurgitation* (insufficiency). This is a blowing, high-pitched systolic murmur, called a "cooing-dove" murmur. It is heard best at the apex of the heart and occurs more often in females. A gallop rhythm is common, caused by accentuation of the third heart sound, S_3. In severe mitral regurgitation, a Carey-Coombs murmur is heard; this is a low-pitched, mid-diastolic rumble that is transient. It is best heard with the bell of the stethescope rather than the diaphragm. An early diastolic murmur of aortic insufficiency is the second most common murmur and is more common in males.

Tachycardia, with a gallop or "tic-toc" rhythm, is out of proportion to fever. (Recall that the pulse increases 10 beats for every degree of fever.) The pulse is typically over 100 beats per minute with the child at rest. Take the *basal pulse rate* when he is sleeping between 2 P.M. and 4 P.M. Do not awaken him; however, if he does awaken, let him go back to sleep and return in an hour to count his pulse. Record the time you obtained the reading.

Murmurs are graded from I to VI according to severity; grade I is barely audible, and grade VI is very loud and is audible even when the stethoscope is not in direct contact with the chest.

Carditis is considered mild when there is a grade II to VI mitral insufficiency murmur, a Carey-Coombs murmur, and/or second degree heart block, but *no* cardiomegaly. Moderate carditis is characterized by an aortic insufficiency murmur unaccompanied by congestive failure. Carditis is considered severe when cardiomegaly and congestive heart failure are present.

Sydenham's Chorea

Chorea is ultimately self-limiting, but can be disabling during an acute attack. It is a disorder of the central nervous system characterized by *choreiform* (purposeless, writhing) *movements*, weakness, and emotional instability. Chorea is two to three times more common in girls than boys. The movements disappear when the child is asleep. Symptoms may be mild, manifested by facial grimaces and clumsiness, or severe, totally incapacitating the child and requiring bed rest. Typically, the child is of school age. His teacher complains that he has a short attention span, is nervous, and his handwriting is deteriorating. His grades drop. Parents pressure the child to sit still, pay attention, write more carefully, and bring up his grades. This pressure makes matters worse, and a vicious cycle ensues. The child is finally referred to a physician, who checks for the presence of several characteristic signs. When the child is asked to hold his hands up over his head, he exhibits the *pronator* sign—his palms turn outward. When asked to extend his arms, hands, and fingers straight out in front of his body, he hyperextends his fingers and flexes his wrists. He has spasmodic contractions of his hands when he intentionally grasps an object or the examiner's hand. He is unable to hold his tongue still when it is protruded.

Bed rest is necessary if the symptoms are severe. Pad the bed and side rails to prevent the child from hurting himself. Dim the lights to minimize stimulation, which aggravates the choreiform movements. Note his response to his parents when they visit. The movements may worsen during parental visits because of the strain the family and child have been living under prior to the diagnosis. Offer sedation as ordered and be aware of toxic effects of the particular medication. Barbiturates may excite the child.

Subcutaneous Nodules

Subcutaneous nodules are small (1 to 2 centimeters), painless, firm swellings over bony prominences. They are found on the extensor tendons of the hands, feet, elbows, scalp, scapulae, and vertebrae. They tend to occur in crops and persist for days or months. These nodules are not specific to ARF because they also occur in rheumatoid arthritis and systemic lupus erythematosus. Subcutaneous nodules are a late symptom of rheumatic fever, often occurring in the convalescent stage of severe cases.

Erythema Marginatum

Erythema marginatum is a characteristic rash appearing in 5 percent of all cases of rheumatic fever. The rash is found on the trunk and proximal extremities. It is pink with a clear center and serpiginous outline. It tends to be transient, migratory, nonpruritic, and blanches with pressure. Erythema marginatum is also a late sign of rheumatic activity.

Minor Manifestations

Acute Phase Reactants

During an acute attack of rheumatic fever, several laboratory tests are elevated, suggesting the presence of inflammatory activity. An elevated erythrocyte sedimentation rate, the presence of C-reactive protein in the blood, and an elevated white cell count are all indicative of inflammation. These findings are not specific to rheumatic fever.

Changes in the electrocardiogram (prolonged P−R interval), although present in 20 percent of all cases, are also nonspecific.

Supportive Evidence

In addition to major and minor manifestations, the Jones Criteria also require supportive evidence of a recent streptococcal infection. Recent scarlet fever, positive throat culture for group A beta-hemolytic streptococci, and increased antistreptolysin-O titer (ASO titer) or other streptococcal antibody titers are all indicative of a recent streptococcal infection. Throat cultures are positive in 25 percent of the cases. The ASO titer, which shows the presence of streptococcal antibodies in the blood, is elevated in 75 to 85 percent of the cases and one of the streptococcal titers will be elevated 95 percent of the time.

Treatment

Treatment depends on the existence and extent of cardiac involvement and varies with the physician. For this reason, general treatment regimens are discussed herein.

Bed Rest

Bed rest is ordered for a minimum of two weeks to decrease work load on the heart, even if no carditis is evident. If carditis is going to develop, it is usually evident within this period. Some physicians disregard the ESR as a guide to length of bed rest because it tends to stay elevated after all other clinical symptoms of rheumatic activity have ceased. Other physicians do not permit activity until the ESR has returned to normal. Generally, though, bed rest lasts a minimum of two to four weeks if there is minimal or no carditis; then restricted activity is allowed for three months. If moderate carditis is present, bed rest is ordered for one to two months, with restricted activity for six months. With severe carditis, bed rest may last up to six months and activity is gradually increased over the next six months. Remember that these are only guidelines, and specific restrictions depend on the individual child and his physician's preference. Bathroom privileges are allowed if the child can tolerate them.

Medication

In the absence of carditis, aspirin is the drug of choice for the management of polyarthritis. The initial dose is 90 to 120 mg /kg /day divided into four equal doses. This should produce an optimal blood salicylate level of 15 to 25 mg/100 ml. Joint symptoms subside within 12 to 24 hours after initiation of salicylate therapy. After seven to ten days, the dose is reduced to one-half (to avoid rebound symptoms), and continued for another three or four weeks.

In moderate to severe carditis, steroids are administered to suppress the acute inflammatory response. Prednisone is given in a dose of 2.5 mg/kg/day, divided into two doses. Recall that side effects of steroids can be detrimental. For this reason physicians prefer to limit the amount of steroids given. Administration regimens for steroids differ from large doses given for nine days to three months, or until symptoms have ceased. If long-term therapy is required, tapering of the dose is necessary while salicylates are begun. Again, this helps to avoid rebound symptoms.

Chorea requires the administration of a sedative. Phenobarbital has been used with mixed success. Diazepam (Valium), or chlorpromazine may be also used. If chlorpromazine is used, watch for symptoms of toxicity, especially dyskinesia (difficulty in movement).

Prophylaxis

The possibility of heart damage increases with each subsequent attack of ARF. The risk for a second attack is 50 percent after a subsequent streptococcal infection. Benzathine penicillin (Bicillin) is given to eradicate any existing infection at the time of diagnosis. It is then given each month in an IM dose of 1.2 million units as prophylaxis. Sulfadiazine or Erythromycin may be used if the child is allergic to penicillin. Rheumatic fever clinics are set up to meet the continuing needs of the child and his family. His health status can be evaluated and teaching is offered as necessary. The prophylactic penicillin is given at the time of the clinic visit. Oral administration is not successful because the family sees no reason for the child to take pills every day after he is well.

Parent-and-child teaching is most important if the child is to avoid another, more damaging, attack of rheumatic fever. They must understand that the prevention of further episodes is their responsibility. Explain that they should report upper respiratory infections to the physician promptly. Encourage them to keep their clinic appointment so the child can be evaluated and receive his dose of Bicillin.

Prophylaxis with penicillin is necessary for at least five years if the child has no carditis. If he has cardiac involvement, he will likely remain on prophylaxis until the age of 40, or perhaps for the rest of his life.

Complications

Bacterial Endocarditis

Bacterial endocarditis may occur late in the disease process, after valvular disease. Dental prophylaxis, as well as surgical prophylaxis, is necessary. The child tends to have penicillin-resistant viridans streptococci in his dental cavities.

Arrhythmias

First degree heart block is common with carditis. Second degree (or greater) heart block is more serious and requires the use of steroids if the child is not already receiving them. A pacemaker may be required for complete heart block.

Congestive Heart Failure

CHF may occur as a complication of ARF. It is treated with diuretics, digitalis and bed rest, as discussed earlier.

Anxiety

Anxiety is always present in the child and his family. It is usually more evident if the child has chorea or carditis. The child sees the concern of his parents and becomes anxious himself. Parent education is very important. The parents need to learn how they can control their own anxiety, and how to help the child with his anxiety.

Prognosis

Prognosis depends on the extent of cardiac involvement. After one attack most (70 percent) recover, with little or no residual effects. With severe carditis, there may be progressive heart enlargement and severe disability caused by the mitral insufficiency. In 10 percent, mitral stenosis develops over a period of years due to scar tissue formation. Aortic valve involvement has a more guarded prognosis. Surgery may be required to replace damaged valves. Recovery from chorea is usually complete; however many children remain sensitive and unstable throughout life.

SUMMARY

Heart disease may be congenital or acquired. New techniques for surgery and intensive care of the small infant with cardiac defects have improved the prognosis for the child with congenital heart disease. Many defects are correctable, and pallative surgery is possible for others. The implications of cardiac defects often cause the parents to overprotect the child, thus resulting in an insecure, dependent person. The child with acquired heart disease, a result of rheumatic fever, must be maintained on prophylactic penicillin, often for a lifetime, in order to prevent another, more damaging attack with resultant heart damage.

Bibliography

Ammann, A.J. and Ward, D.W. Collagen Vascular Diseases (Rheumatic Diseases), in Rudolph, A.M. (ed.). *Pediatrics,* ed. 16. New York, Appleton-Century-Crofts, 1977, p. 384.

Clark, J. Kelly—An Infant With Heart Defects. *American Journal of Nursing* 77:1823, 1977.

Gildea, J.H., Sacksteder, S., Sutton, P. et al. Congenital Cardiac Defects: Pre- and Postoperative Nursing Care. *American Journal of Nursing* 78:273, 1978.

Hoffman, J.I.E. Circulatory System, in Rudolph, A.M. (ed.). *Pediatrics,* ed. 16. New York, Appleton-Century-Crofts, 1977, p. 1351.

Johnson, A. A Continuing Threat: Rheumatic Fever. *Nursing '74* 4:57, March 1974.

Kaplan, E.L., and Wannamaker, L.W. Rheumatic Fever, in Gellis, S.S. and Kagan, B.M. (eds.). *Current Pediatric Therapy,* ed. 8. Philadelphia, W. B. Saunders Co., 1978, p. 164.

Posey, R.A. Creative Nursing Care of Babies with Heart Disease. *Nursing '74* 4:40, October 1974.

Sacksteder, S., Gildea, J.H., Dassy, C. Common Congenital Cardiac Defects. *American Journal of Nursing* 78:266, 1978.

Sade, R.M. and Castaneda, A.R. Recent Advances in Cardiac Surgery in the Young Infant. *Surgical Clinics of North America* 56:451, 1976.

Shor, V.Z. Congenital Cardiac Defects: Assessment and Case Findings. *American Journal of Nursing* 78:256, 1978.

Strong, W.B. Recognition and Management of Congestive Heart Failure in Infancy, in Green, C.A. and Maragos, G.D. (eds.). *Paediatrician,* 2:296, 1973.

Uzark, K. A Child's Cardiac Catheterization—Avoiding the Potential Risks. *American Journal Maternal-Child Nursing* 3:158, 1978.

Weinberg, A.D., Christiansen, C.H., Wise, D.J. Respiratory Rate: Forgotten Clue in the Early Detection of Congenital Heart Disease. *Pediatric Nursing* 3:38, 1977.

CHAPTER **23**

The Child with a Pulmonary Deviation

BEHAVIORAL OBJECTIVES

After studying this chapter you will be able to:

- Discuss the factors that make respiratory illnesses in the child different from the same illnesses in adults.
- Discuss signs of airway obstruction in the child and the nursing implications for each.
- Write a plan of care for the child with a mild upper respiratory tract infection.
- Discuss parental behaviors seen when the child is having respiratory difficulty; include nursing interventions.
- Explain the complications of respiratory disease, clinical manifestations, and medical management; include nursing implications.
- Identify diagnostic measures for assessment of respiratory involvement, including nursing implications.
- Design a plan of care for a child receiving oxygen therapy via a tent, incubator, or hood; include safety factors.
- Explain the dangers of hyperoxemia and oxygen toxicity.
- Design a plan of care for the child with a tracheostomy.
- Identify and explain common respiratory diseases of the child.

TERMS AND CONCEPTS

PaO_2
Hypoxemia
Hypercarbia
Alveolar hypoventilation
Hyperinflation
Stridor
Wheezing
Expiratory grunt
Coughing
Acute respiratory failure
Atelectasis
Pneumothorax
Mediastinal shift
Respiratory acidosis
$PaCO_2$
Pulmonary edema
Barrel chest
Fremitus
Rhonchi
Rales
Laryngoscopy
Bronchoscopy
Arterial blood gas analysis
Bronchodilators
Hyperoxemia
Oxygen toxicity
Assisted Ventilators
Controlled ventilators
Tracheostomy
Retropharyngeal Abscess
Tonsillitis
Adenoiditis

Acute Epiglottitis
Laryngotracheobronchitis
Bronchiectasis

INTRODUCTION

Respiratory disease is the major cause of death in children under one year of age, accounting for half of all the deaths in this age group (68,000). In 1971, 25,000 deaths were caused by primary respiratory disease; 19,200 of these were caused by idiopathic respiratory distress syndrome of the newborn and another 6,300 caused by influenza and pneumonia. An additional 8,000 to 10,000 deaths were caused by the sudden infant death syndrome (the leading cause of death in infants between one week and one year of age), which is thought to be respiratory in nature. Another 2,000 respiratory-disease-related deaths occur each year in children from one to five years of age.

Over 55 percent of all acute illnesses in the child are respiratory illnesses. Forty-two percent of all childhood hospitalizations are necessitated by respiratory problems, and about 18 percent of all children under seventeen years of age have a chronic respiratory problem, such as chronic bronchitis, asthma, hay fever, hypertrophied tonsils and adenoids, and the like. An average of three school days per schoolchild (or 132 million school days) is lost each year because of respiratory illness.

These statistics indicate that the problem of respiratory disease is of massive proportions. Not all of these conditions are serious, but they may cause discomfort, social deprivation, and the inability to participate in school and recreational activities.

This chapter deals with problems common to the child with respiratory disease. The unique characteristics of respiratory illnesses in the child are presented. Diagnostic and treatment regimens are discussed and nursing interventions are stressed throughout.

COMMON PROBLEMS AND NURSING INTERVENTION

Unique Characteristics of Respiratory Disease in the Child

Airway size

The small size of the airway from the nares to the terminal bronchioles accounts for part of the infant's problem with higher resistance to air flow (15 times that of the adult). The diameter of the tracheal lumen in a one-year-old is smaller than that of a pencil. The airway is further divided into 24 generations, each smaller than the last. Over 85 percent of the child's airway system is less than 1 millimeter in diameter. Therefore, it does not take much mucus or swelling to occlude these tiny airways. An amount of mucus that would be inconsequential in an adult may be deadly to the child.

Muscular Development

The child's lack of muscular development and physical strength causes his cough and respiratory effort to be less effective than the adult's. The child's breathing is faster and more shallow than that of the adult, and his oxygen consumption is twice as high. His body is mostly trunk; therefore, any increase in respirations will tire him more easily because he must move a greater percentage of his body with each breath.

Anatomical Factors

The infant is a nose breather. The small size of the nasal passages causes increased resistance to airflow. The tongue tends to fall back and partially occlude the airway, especially when the infant is supine. Tonsils and adenoids both may hypertrophy and block the airway. The infant's shorter neck poses problems both with respiration and intubation.

There is less room in the baby's chest for expansion and adequate ventilation. His chest wall has little cartilaginous support and is relatively unstable, thus characteristic severe sternal retractions occur (during respiratory distress) which reduce the thoracic content further.

Metabolic Factors

In addition to the higher oxygen consumption already mentioned, the infant's body surface area is greater *in proportion to weight* than is the adult's, and his metabolic rate is twice as high. Therefore, the infant loses more heat from his skin and more water from his increased respiratory rate. He has little muscle glycogen reserve to support this increase in respiration, and acidosis therefore develops rapidly since he is unable to blow off carbon dioxide. The acidosis is complicated by other symptoms of respiratory disease, such as fever, vomiting, and dehydration.

Physiological Factors

In the presence of acidosis, the oxygen-hemoglobin saturation is lower, even with a high PaO_2 (partial pressure of oxygen in the arterial blood). Fever usually accompanies acute respiratory infections in the child and is much higher than fever in adults. The child also has a relative anemia, having about two grams less hemoglobin than an adult. Thus, the oxygen-carrying capacity of his blood is reduced.

Hypoxemia

Obstruction

The end result of respiratory disorders is *alveolar hypoventilation* (a reduction in the amount of air entering the alveoli), leading to a decrease in oxygen *(hypoxemia)* in the arterial blood and an increase in carbon dioxide *(hypercarbia)*. Obstructions may occur in the upper airway, where the *inflow* of air is reduced (although the alveolar exchange of oxygen and carbon dioxide is adequate), or in the lower airway, where the *outflow* of air is impeded, causing air to be trapped distally to the obstruction *(hyperinflation)*. When overinflated, the anteroposterior diameter of the chest increases, and percussion yields a tympanic sound. Alveolar hypoventilation also results from disorders of the terminal airway and the alveoli themselves that hinder the exchange of oxygen and carbon dioxide across the alveolar-capillary membrane. Such conditions include hemorrhage, pulmonary edema, pneumonia, and aspiration.

Restlessness

The hypoxic child will be anxious, restless, and irritable because he cannot breathe with ease. Any restlessness should be noted because it may herald respiratory failure.

Dyspnea

The child with hypoxia has labored breathing (dyspnea). His respirations are rapid and deep; his sternum retracts, as do the suprasternal and intercostal spaces. He uses the accessory muscles of respiration (that is, the neck, pectoral, sternocleidomastoid, and abdominal muscles) in an effort to improve ventilation. The use of the neck muscles pulls the chin down, causing "chin lag," and the nares flare in an attempt to inhale more oxygen. Place the child in a semi-Fowler's position, or strap the infant in an infant seat. This position takes the pressure of the abdominal contents off the diaphragm and permits easier breathing. The prone position is often comfortable for the child, too; it permits better drainage of the airways and puts pressure from the back on the lungs, forcing the air out. The prone position is especially useful for lower airway obstructions. However, if you place an infant with respiratory distress on his abdomen, you must stay with him. The child with dyspnea is seriously ill and demands your close observation; do not disturb him unnecessarily.

Breath Sounds

Audible breath sounds occur with obstruction. *Stridor* is primarily an inspiratory sound. Obstructions of the larynx cause this relatively high-pitched, harsh sound. Stridor may be deceptive; its presence indicates obstruction, therefore, you may tend to think that if the stridor lessens in severity, the child is getting better. This is a dangerous assumption. A sudden lack of inspiratory breath sounds may mean that the child is moving less air, thus, his condition is *worsening.* Lower airway obstructions (in the smaller lumens) tend to cause *wheezing,* which is more high-pitched than stridor and is heard best during expiration. An *expiratory grunt* occurs in an effort to expel all of the air in the alveoli. In moderate respiratory involvement, it can be heard with a stethoscope; in severe distress, grunting is audible to the unaided ear. Careful observation and adequate recording and reporting are imperative in monitoring the child's condition. Note the quality and type as well as the rate of respirations.

Cough

Coughing is an explosive expiration that is triggered when the cough receptors in the trachea and bronchi are irritated by mucus, dust, inflammation, or chemicals. It is a protective response of the body to remove mucus or foreign material before it gets to the lungs. Many cough medicines suppress the cough reflex, thus allowing mucus to accumulate. Rather than suppressing the cough, remove the mucus. Tickling in the throat, caused by irritation, can be soothed with a teaspoon of honey. Soda pop "scratches" the area, and ice cream "freezes" it, thus providing relief.

Paroxysmal coughing is a series of coughs following a deep inspiration. It occurs most often in pertussis. Vigorous coughing may increase pressure in the chest, thus decreasing venous return to the heart. This causes a lowered cardiac output, which may lead to syncope (fainting). Subconjunctival hemorrhage may be seen after prolonged coughing because of the increased pressure in the superior vena cava.

Nighttime coughing is often vigorous because more mucus collects before the cough reflex is elicited. Tell the child's mother to remove the primary cause of the cough by suctioning the mucus from the nose. Apply saline nose drops (one teaspoon salt to one pint of boiled water), and suction again as necessary. Then give one teaspoon of honey to soothe the irritated throat. Cough suppressants should be given only under the direction of a physician, usually to permit rest when the cough is dry, unproductive, and exhausting.

Tachycardia

An increase in the rate and depth of respirations causes an increase in pulse rate, as does an increase in anxiety. Count the pulse apically for a full minute, and note its quality as well as rate.

Cyanosis

Cyanosis is a *late* sign of respiratory distress. It is usually not visible until the PaO_2 falls below 55 mm Hg. It may be masked by the administration of oxygen, or by anemia, acidosis, or shock. *Never* depend on cyanosis as an early and reliable sign of impending respiratory failure.

Pain

The larynx, trachea, and bronchi are especially sensitive to pain. The child may splint his respirations by taking shallow breaths to avoid pain; he is frightened that he cannot get his breath. In the case of obstruction by foreign bodies, the site of obstruction can often be identified by the presence of localized pain.

Secretions

Inflammation of the airway causes an increase in the production of mucus in an effort to clear the airway. Remember that even small amounts of mucus can obstruct the child's airway. Because breathing is impaired in the presence of secretions, the child swallows air and may develop abdominal distention and colicky pain.

Obstruction caused by mucous secretion can be relieved in a number of ways. If the mucus is obstructing the upper airway, try "milking" the nose by placing a warm, moist cloth over the nose to help loosen secretions; then, moisten your forefinger and thumb with warm water and "milk" the infant's nose from bridge to tip. Continue this procedure for several minutes, wetting your finger and thumb as necessary. Copious amounts of mucus may be obtained by this procedure, which may also stimulate crying, which better aerates the lungs.

Another method of clearing mucous obstructions is to use saline nose drops to loosen secretions and an ear syringe to suction them out. Suction excess mucus from the nose with an ear syringe and then instill five to ten drops of normal saline solution in each nostril. Close the opposite nostril while suctioning. Wait five to ten minutes and then suction again. A catheter may also be used to suction nasal secretions as well as the mouth and pharynx. Suctioning is used only when necessary, no more than four or five times a day; before meals and at bedtime is usually sufficient. In the event that blood is suctioned, notify the physician so that the bleeding can be properly evaluated. Nosedrops with vasoconstrictive action should not be used for more than two or three days, since a rebound effect occurs after the initial vasoconstriction; vasodilation and increased mucus secretion makes the obstruction worse. Do not permit nose-blowing because it forces mucus into the ears. The child has a tendency to suck the phlegm back from his nose into his throat and swallows it. Do not discourage this; only after about four years of age will he be able to cough up the phlegm and expectorate it.

Humidification helps to loosen secretions, making them easier to aspirate. Providing adequate hydration also helps to thin the mucus; encourage clear liquids. Milk is considered a food, not a liquid. In the stomach, milk requires the body to give up water, thus it increases dehydration. It also makes the secretions more viscid. The physician will determine the child's fluid requirements. In order to assure that the child is offered adequate fluids, use a fluid plan. One way is to offer a drink of the child's choice every 30 minutes to one hour. (Refer to chapter 18 for tips on encouraging the child to take nourishment.) It may be necessary to give fluids intravenously if the child is not able to take adequate fluids orally. Keep a careful record of all intake and output. Bear in mind that overhydration may result from forcing fluids.

If antihistamines or decongestants are given, offer more fluids. These agents dry out the mucous membranes and cause the secretions to thicken. Dimetapp, Actifed, CoPyrnil, and Novahistamine are examples of antihistamine/decongestants. Some pediatricians prefer to use Sudafed, a pure decongestant, which causes the nose to "run," thus relieving stuffiness by draining, rather than drying, the secretions.

Chest physical therapy, that is, postural drainage with clapping and vibration, may be necessary to help remove secretions from the respiratory tract. The child is placed in a different position for each section of airway to be drained. Know which part of your patient's airway is affected. Clapping and vibration is used in each position, and the child is encouraged to cough up as much sputum as possible. Your hand may be too large to effectively clap and vibrate the small infant's chest. If so, protect the edges of an infant-size oxygen mask or a baby bottle cap with adhesive tape. Use this small "clapper" to percuss the chest. The small infant may not be able to tolerate long periods of postural drainage. Begin with short sessions of five to ten minutes every four hours, and gradually increase the time to twenty minutes per session if the child's tolerance permits this. If therapy tires the child, plan shorter, more frequent sessions. If the child is receiving aerosol therapy to help loosen secretions, this is administered prior to the postural drainage (see the Skills Manual).

Infection

Respiratory tract infections are primarily viral, usually one of the following: respiratory syncytial virus (RSV), parainfluenza virus, adenovirus, or influenza virus. A smaller number of infections (acute epiglottitis, for example) are bacterial. Infection can also be secondary, as when thick mucus traps bacteria in the airways. (Refer to ch. 16.) Problems related to respiratory tract infection include sore throat, anorexia, fever, and lethargy.

Sore Throat and Anorexia

Increased secretions and infection can cause inflammation of the mucous membranes of the throat. Swallowing is painful and may lead to anorexia. Sore throats may be viral or they may be caused by a streptococcal infection, which in turn cause rheumatic fever and kidney inflammation. For this reason, sore throats should be cultured so that if a streptococcal infection is present, proper antibiotics can be administered.

If the child's throat is sore, offer cool, bland liquids. Do not give milk, which thickens secretions, or acid-containing fluids, such as orange juice, for these may be painful. Have the child gargle with a mild saline solution (one teaspoon salt to one pint of water). Provide rest and quiet activities to allow his body time and energy to heal itself. Prevent re-exposure by keeping the child away from other persons with respiratory infections, and dress him appropriately for the weather.

Fever and Lethargy

Between the ages of six months and three years, the child tends to have a high fever—39.4° to 40.5°C (103° to 105°F)—with even minor infections. Watch the young child closely, remembering that he is susceptible to febrile seizures.

The infant with nasal congestion will breath through his mouth. He cannot suck and breathe at the same time, and therefore, he cannot maintain an adequate oral intake. He becomes dehydrated; the fever ◄—► dehydration cycle may then begin. Allow ample time between feedings so that the child can rest between swallows. Aspirin may be given for its anti-inflammatory effects and to help reduce the fever. Provide quiet activity and plenty of rest.

Behavioral Manifestations

The parents of the child with respiratory disease are going to be anxious if the child is having trouble breathing. The child *will* have trouble breathing; therefore, the parents *will be anxious.* Their anxiety is transmitted to the child, and his own anxiety is heightened. As his anxiety level rises, his breathing becomes more difficult and labored, and a vicious circle ensues.

Jamie T., aged eighteen months, was in a mist tent for his croup. He had one episode of breathing difficulty during the afternoon while his mother went home to check on Janie, his twin. He was recovered from the episode and resting quietly when his mother returned. After she learned of his earlier difficulty, she became quite upset and hovered over Jamie's bed, insisting that the nurse suction him again. Jamie then became restless and agitated and his breathing became more difficult. The nurse calmly reassured Mrs. T. that she was watching Jamie carefully and would suction him as necessary. She pointed out how peacefully Jamie was resting after the episode and stressed again the importance of letting Jamie rest. She stayed and continued to reassure them as she let Mrs. T. rock Jamie until they both grew calm.

Because the parents are anxious, you will have to take extra time with them explaining and re-explaining the child's care. Allow them to help plan and participate in the child's care. Praise their efforts and point out improvement in his condition. When the child has an episode of respiratory distress, the parents tend to become very distraught. Your prompt, competent care of their child and your calm reassurance will be most helpful (review ch. 3).

COMMON COMPLICATIONS

Respiratory Failure

The child with a respiratory illness needs close observation because his condition can result in respiratory failure, atelectasis, or pneumothorax, all dangerous complications. The child demands meticulous nursing care.

Acute respiratory failure (acute inability of the lungs to maintain adequate oxygenation of the blood) is a dreaded complication of respiratory illness and a life-threatening medical emergency. There are, unfortunately, no good warning signs of impending failure in the child. He does not have the powers of communication that the adult does. Crying and irritability are seen in a variety of conditions and are often disregarded as a call for help. A scoring system is most helpful in diagnosing acute respiratory failure. Learn the criteria in Table 23–1; clinical observations are crucial to the child's welfare, but the diagnosis of acute respiratory failure depends primarily on repeated arterial blood gas studies.

Table 23–1. Criteria for Diagnosing Respiratory Failure in Infants and Children with Acute Respiratory Disease*

Clinical Signs	*Physiological Signs*
Decreased or absent respiratory breath sounds	$PCO_2 \geq 60-65$mm Hg
Severe inspiratory retractions and use of accessory muscles	$PO_2 < 100$mm Hg in 100% oxygen
Cyanosis in 40% ambient oxygen	
Depressed level of consciousness and response to pain	
Poor skeletal muscle tone	

*Acute respiratory failure should be assumed in the presence of three clinical signs and one physiological sign.

Mechanical ventilation must be started promptly to avoid cardiac arrest.

Atelectasis

Atelectasis (collapse of the lung) secondary to airway occlusion is often seen in respiratory disease, especially with asthma, cystic fibrosis, and aspiration of a foreign body. The air becomes trapped distally to the obstruction; it is absorbed into the bloodstream, and the obstructed portion of the lung collapses. If the obstruction is not complete, it may act as a ball valve and allow air to enter, but not leave, the alveoli. It should be recalled that atmospheric pressure is greater than intrapleural pressure on inspiration, and air therefore rushes into the lungs; on expiration, intrapleural pressure is greater, and air leaves the lungs. However, when the working space of the lungs is lessened by accumulated air or fluid, the lungs cannot push as hard to expel the air. Therefore, air can rush in but cannot be pushed out again. When atelectasis occurs, ventilation in the affected section of the lung is decreased. Furthermore, accumulated secretions provide an ideal breeding ground for bacteria. Symptoms of atelectasis include a decrease in chest expansion and breath sounds as well as a unilateral wheeze. If the well child suddenly exhibits symptoms of respiratory distress, the inhalation of a foreign body should be suspected. Bronchoscopy is performed immediately in order to locate and remove the object.

The child with repeated pulmonary infections does not recover as rapidly. He usually has a long-term history of inability to expel thick secretions. His course of treatment will last longer, and the primary cause of recurrent infections will have to be diagnosed and treated.

Pneumothorax

Pneumothorax (air in the pleural space) causes the lung to collapse. It is usually caused by ruptured alveoli, atelectasis, trauma (as from a puncture wound), or a ruptured lung abscess, as seen in staphylococcal pneumonia. Occasionally, pneumothorax occurs in the newborn as a result of the intense intrathoracic pressure needed to begin respiration.

The child with pneumothorax may have symptoms ranging from tachypnea to severe dyspnea, accompanied by grunting respirations, flaring nares, and cyanosis. Breath sounds are absent or diminished on auscultation, and the lung is hyperresonant on percussion. The heart is displaced toward the affected side (a *mediastinal shift*), and the heart sounds shift from their usual sites. The diaphragm is displaced downward and, with right-sided pneumothorax, the liver is also displaced downward. A chest x-ray will reveal the collapsed lung and displaced heart.

Therapy with 100 percent oxygen is begun promptly. A thoracotomy and water seal drainage is used to suction the accumulated air out of the pleural cavity. If a puncture wound has caused the pneumothorax, the wound must be covered immediately. Use petrolatum gauze if possible, or even your hand. Remember that the child is seriously ill and needs close observation.

Respiratory Acidosis

Respiratory acidosis occurs in severe airway obstruction and is caused by the retention of carbon dioxide. The $PaCO_2$ (partial pressure of carbon dioxide in arterial blood), carbonic acid, and H^+ concentrations rise and the pH falls. (See ch. 29.) The kidneys compensate by reabsorbing bicarbonate (HCO_3) so that the degree of acidosis is lessened. As ventilation improves, more carbon dioxide is blown off, and the $PaCO_2$ level falls. If large amounts of bicarbonate have been given (IV), these factors may combine to produce alkalosis. Blood gas analysis is necessary to monitor the child's status. Fever, vomiting, and decreased oral intake leading to dehydration all contribute to acidosis.

Pulmonary Edema

Pulmonary edema is congestion of the lungs with fluid. Adequate ventilation is impaired. It may occur as a result of heart failure or as a complication of respiratory problems such as pneumonia, trauma, inhalation poisoning, massive atelectasis, and near-drowning. Clinical manifestations of pulmonary edema include tachypnea, retractions, flaring nares, grunting, tachycardia, cyanosis, feeding intolerance, and hepatomegaly. Expiratory wheezing may be heard, and the child may have moist breath sounds and blood-tinged sputum (or frothy saliva in the infant). Diuretics such as Lasix (1.0 mg/kg) are used to draw fluid off the lungs and elminate it via the kidneys. Place the child with his head elevated (infant seat or semi-Fowler's) to pool the blood in the lower part of the body. Mechanical ventilation with positive end-expiratory pressure (PEEP) reduces the venous return by increasing intrathoracic pressure.

COMMON DIAGNOSTIC STUDIES

Assessment

A thorough history and a complete physical examination are necessary in the diagnosis of respiratory disease. One factor in the differential diagnosis of the various conditions is the length of time from the onset of symptoms to the onset of obvious respiratory problems. For example, one form of croup is preceded by a mild upper respiratory tract infection (URI) of several days' duration, while another form of croup has a sudden onset.

Physical assessment begins with observation. Do not touch the child; watch his breathing and count his respirations. Are they labored? Do his nares flare? Is he restless or fighting for breath? Is he cyanotic? Remove his shirt and observe his chest and abdomen and count his respirations. Is he retracting? Is he using his accessory muscles of respiration? Notice the shape of his chest. Trapped air, caused by chronic diseases, such as cystic fibrosis or asthma, leads to an increase in the anteroposterior diameter, or *barrel chest.*

Auscultation and percussion are used to determine the extent to which the lungs are affected. Place your hand on the child's anteroposterior chest walls. You may feel a vibration (caused by air moving past an obstruction) called *fremitus*. Percussion will reveal a tympanic or hyperresonant sound if air is trapped in the alveoli. The sound is dull if the lung is collapsed or filled with fluid.

Listen with your stethoscope for abnormal breath sounds caused by air rushing past an obstruction. Stridor is more evident when the child is supine. Listen for wheezing on expiration. *Rhonchi* are coarse snoring sounds produced by a high obstruction. *Rales* are fine crackling sounds (like the sound made by rubbing hair between two fingers) heard when fluid fills the alveoli. Count the apical pulse for one minute. Tacycardia occurs with tachypnea and anxiety.

X-Ray Studies

Chest x-rays are invaluable as a diagnostic aid. Sites of obstruction as well as the extent of involvement are shown. X-rays are also used during the course of the illness to periodically evaluate the effects of treatment.

Endoscopy

Laryngoscopy is the visual examination of the airway with a laryngoscope. It is useful in diagnosis and is necessary for the removal of foreign objects. *Bronchoscopy*, the visualization of the bronchi through a bronchoscope, is done under general anesthesia. Because this procedure irritates the upper airway, causing increased mucus production and possibly, laryngeal edema, careful observation, suctioning, and postural drainage are necessary afterwards. Preoperatively, atropine is given to decrease bronchial secretion and relax the smooth muscle, thus helping to prevent laryngospasm after the procedure.

Cultures

Cultures of nasopharyngeal mucus, sputum (difficult to obtain in an infant or small child), and blood are obtained to determine the causative agent of the child's illness. Obtaining cultures of the nose and throat is uncomfortable for the child, especially if he has a sore throat. Explain what you must do and what you expect of the child, then do it quickly, but be sure you restrain him adequately first to avoid injury if he should struggle. As you culture the throat, be certain that you touch the exudate, or you will have to do it again; if possible, touch several places. You will have to be quick because holding the child's tongue down will cause him to gag. Send all specimens to the lab promptly; if they dry out, the culture will have to be repeated.

Blood Gases

Blood gases, pH, and electrolytes are monitored routinely in the child with respiratory disease. These studies indicate whether ventilation is adequate, the severity of the illness, and the effectiveness of treatment.

The amount of oxygen administered is determined by the child's PaO_2, (partial pressure of oxygen in the arterial blood). Although the child's clinical signs are of utmost importance, the most reliable indicator of oxygen saturation in the blood is *arterial blood gas analysis*. (Recall that cyanosis is not evident until the PaO_2

reaches a critical level.) This study also reveals the acid-base and electrolyte status of the child.

Specimens may be obtained from the temporal artery in the infant, or the femoral, brachial, or radial artery in the older child. If frequent determinations are needed, an arterial catheter may be inserted to avoid numerous punctures. The specimen is collected in a heparinized syringe, which is placed in a basin of ice and transported immediately to the lab. Apply firm pressure to the puncture site for at least five minutes. Wrap the catheter site with an Ace bandage to prevent the child from pulling on it. Heel or finger sticks may be used if it is impossible to obtain an arterial specimen. Warm the site for 20 minutes in warm water to stimulate local blood flow. The capillary gas levels will then approximate arterial levels.

Pulmonary Function Tests

Pulmonary function tests aid in establishing the diagnosis and in the objective evaluation of therapy. A variety of tests exist, but the physician can determine whether the pulmonary disease is obstructive or restrictive with the use of simple measurements of lung volume and airflow, which can be measured at the bedside. The nostrils are closed with a nose clip or with the fingers. The child breathes through a mouthpiece, and a flowmeter records the amount of lung volume and airflow. Remember to prepare the child and his family for these diagnostic procedures.

COMMON TREATMENTS

Goals of treatment are the removal of obstructions and improvement of ventilation.

Medical Management

The management of secretions, discussed earlier, includes postural drainage, liquifying the secretions, giving expectorants, and managing the effects of cough without repressing the cough reflex.

Medications

Sedatives are given with caution in respiratory illness because most tend to depress respirations, and they may mask restlessness, which is often the first overt indication of respiratory distress. Chloral hydrate is the sedative of choice because it does not depress respirations.

Antibiotics are not given for viral infections. If the causative agent is bacterial, antibiotics are administered in accordance with the culture and sensitivity report. Bacterial infections may occur secondarily to an acute viral infection because thick mucus provides a medium for bacterial growth.

Bronchodilators are given to relax the smooth muscles of the respiratory tract, thus relieving bronchospasms. Epinephrine given subcutaneously relieves bronchospasms in three to five minutes and may be repeated two or three times, every twenty minutes. The inhalation of bronchodilators via aerosol therapy is also effective. Drugs most often used in this manner are epinephrine, racemic epinephrine, isoproterenol, and isoetharine. See chapter 16 for more detailed discussion of bronchodilators.

Oxygen Therapy

Oxygen therapy is indicated for hypoxic conditions. Oxygen is administered to the child via a tent, nasal catheter, mask, incubator, or hood (see the Skills Manual).

The tent is probably the most comfortable because the child can move around in it. However, tents leak, and the oxygen concentration is rarely over 40 percent. (An inspired oxygen level of 30 to 100 percent is necessary for most conditions.) With a flow rate of 4 to 5 liters per minute, a nasal catheter delivers about 50 percent oxygen, and a tight-fitting mask, about 100 percent. Incubators can deliver from 40 to 100 percent oxygen, and a hard plastic hood placed over the infant's head will deliver about 100 percent.

Oxygen is always humidified before it reaches the child; otherwise, it is drying to the tissues. Sterile water is added, along with other agents as necessary (bronchodilators, mucolytic agents, antibiotics, and the like). The fine mist thus produced goes deep into the airways to help loosen secretions.

The care of the child in a tent should be planned to avoid opening the tent excessively. Oxygen and humidity escape every time the tent is opened. The oxygen, which is heavier than air, sinks to the bottom of the tent to provide an oxygen-rich atmosphere, and the warmer carbon dioxide rises to the top and exits. If the tent is not adequately tucked around the bottom, oxygen escapes.

Mist tent therapy is terminated gradually. The tent is left unzipped or open, or the child may be allowed out of the tent for increasing lengths of time (Figure 23–1). Observe his response to this weaning process. Do not hesitate to place him back in a closed tent if he has any signs of respiratory difficulty, and be sure to notify the physician.

Safety rules must be followed when oxygen is in use. Oxygen will not burn, but it *supports combustion*. The more oxygen present, the more readily fires start, and the faster they burn. If a spark ignites in the presence of increased oxygen, an explosive, raging fire can result. In the presence of pure oxygen, fuels can ignite without the aid of a spark. "Use no oil" is a sign posted on all oxygen gauges; this refers to lubricating oil and even oil used on a patient's lips or hair. No volatile chemical should be used on a patient receiving oxygen therapy. Among such chemicals are alcohols, ether, antiseptic tinctures, and oily hair dressings. If a lubricant is needed for the child's lips, use one with a water-soluble base, such as KY Jelly. Electrical equipment, including portable x-ray equipment and electric heating pads, must not be used because of the danger of sparks. Wool and some synthetic fibers also may cause static electricity. The child may want a favorite toy to "live" with him under the tent. If the toy is a stuffed animal that will retain moisture (and therefore bacteria), or an electrical or mechanical toy that may generate sparks, he will have to choose a substitute.

The oxygen hood is a clear plastic dome that fits over the infant's head (Figure 23–2). Different sizes accommodate the in-

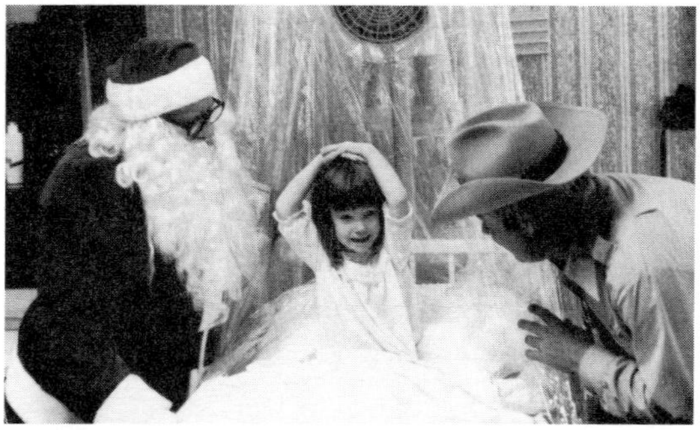

Figure 23–1. *This child can be out of her tent for short periods of time. Special visitors help the day pass more quickly.* (Courtesy, Department of Public Relations, University Hospital, Augusta, Georgia.)

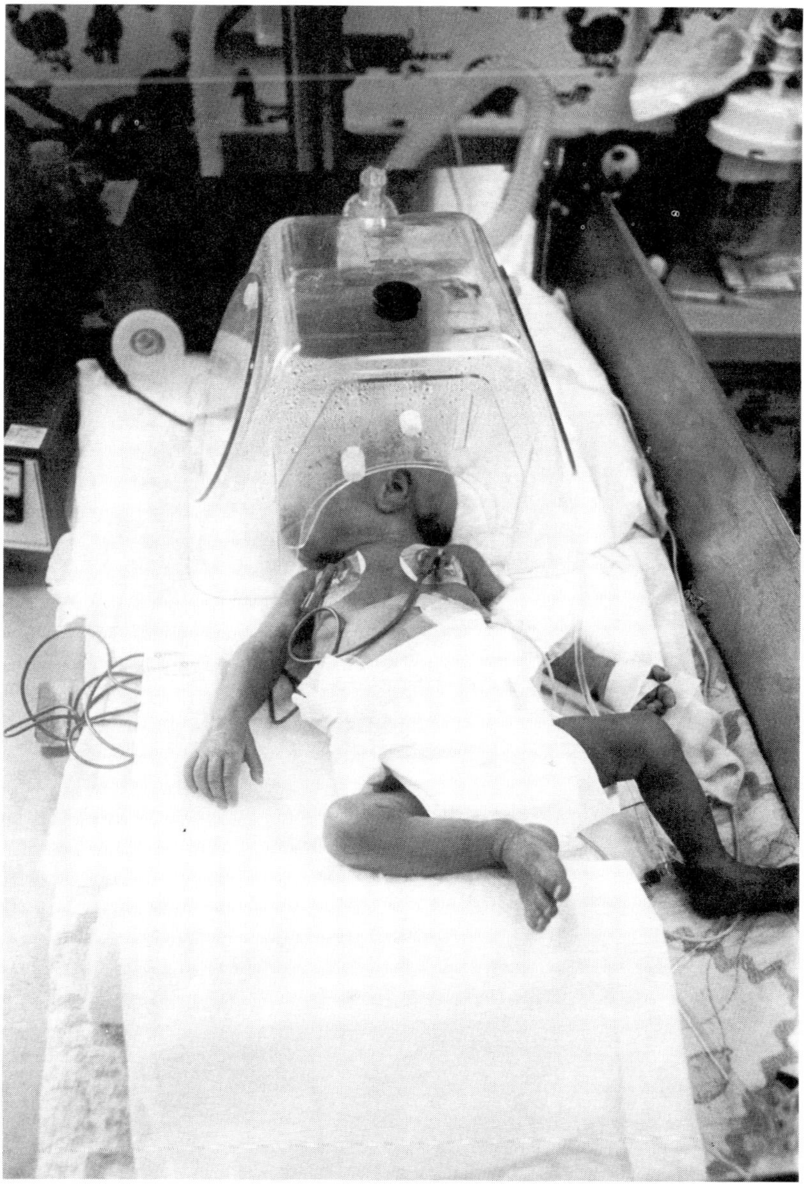

Figure 23–2. *Infant receiving oxygen therapy via Shiley Infant Oxygen Hood.* (Courtesy, Shiley Sales Corporation, 17600 Gilette Avenue, Irvine, California, 92714.)

fant from 1 to 8 kilograms (2 to 18 pounds). The hood can deliver an oxygen concentration of nearly 100 percent. Carbon dioxide dissipates through the neck opening as oxygen enters the hood. When used with a radiant warmer, the hood permits easy access to the child for procedures.

Use an oxygen analyzer every two hours to monitor the concentration within the tent, incubator, or hood. Levels greater than 40 percent are not administered unless ordered by the physician, usually if cyanosis is present.

Hyperoxemia (PaO_2 well above the normal range of 60 to 100 mm Hg) may cause retrolental fibroplasia in the newborn. However, the danger of hyperoxemia is presented by a high *blood level* of oxygen, not the inspired oxygen concentration (FIO_2) which is what the oxygen analyzer measures. The FIO_2 can be 100 percent and the child's PaO_2 may be only 40 percent (for example, in respiratory distress syndrome); in such a case, retrolental fibroplasia would not be a factor.

Oxygen toxicity is a complication of oxygen therapy which must be guarded against. It is suspected when the PaO_2 decreases in an increasing FIO_2. Oxygen toxicity causes damage to the lungs, interfering with the exchange of gases. Secretions build up because of paralysis of the cilia in the respiratory tract, and atelectasis may occur.

Mechanical Ventilation

Mechanical ventilators provide artificial inflation of the lungs. Since ventilators vary in design and usage, be familiar with the equipment used on your patient. Understand how it works, and feel confident in your ability to use it before you enter the child's room. Remember the parental anxiety involved in respiratory disease; if the parents see that you are self-confident and competent, their anxiety may be reduced.

Assisted ventilators detect the start of the child's inspiration and transmit a preset volume or pressure to his airway. *Controlled ventilators* control the volume and depth of the ventilation.

Intubation may also be necessary, especially if ventilations must be assisted for several days. An endotracheal tube is inserted, or a tracheostomy is performed, depending on the child's condition. The tube is then attached to the ventilator, and the prescribed volume or pressure is administered.

The child will be frightened by the ventilator if he is conscious. He may struggle with you or "fight with" the ventilator by breathing against it. Remember the importance of preparing him for procedures in advance if time allows. Be calm and reassuring as you explain the ventilator; your confidence will help to calm the child.

After using the ventilator for a time, the child may resist its discontinuation. He has learned to depend on it to sustain his life and will be afraid to try to breathe on his own again. He will have to be "weaned" gradually. A competent nurse or inhalation therapist must be on hand as the child breathes for short "trial" periods on his own. He needs to know that someone is there, ready to help if he experiences any difficulty. If he is anxious, he will hyperventilate and may grab for the ventilator.

SURGICAL TREATMENT

Endotracheal Intubation

Nasotracheal or oral intubation is performed as an emergency measure to bypass an obstructed upper airway or to provide a direct connection for mechanical ventilators. The child (with the exception of the newborn) is lightly anesthetized for the procedure. These tubes cause local irritation and edema and are not used for more than a week.

Tracheostomy

A *tracheostomy* is an incision into the trachea; the term is also used to mean both the incision and the insertion of an indwelling tube to permit the free passage of air and the removal of secretions. The tracheostomy bypasses obstructions in the upper airway and permits the removal of mucous obstructions in the lower airway.

Endotracheal and tracheostomy tubes interfere with the cleansing action of the mucous lining of the airway and eliminate the warming and filtering of air provided by the nose and pharynx. The child must be suctioned to remove mucus, which he can no longer cough up. Inspired air must be moistened and warmed. Suctioning reduces lung volume and promotes atelectasis because it removes air as well as secretions. The physician may wish you to re-expand the child's lungs with a series of inflations after suctioning him.

The child who must be intubated is frightened, as are his parents. The procedure is usually an emergency, performed when the child suddenly stops breathing, goes limp, and turns cyanotic. If possible, he is carried to the treatment room; otherwise the procedure is done at the bedside. After making an incision into the trachea, the physician inserts an uncuffed tracheostomy tube. Cuffed tubes are not used in the child because of the small size of the trachea. Suction is made available if it is needed to clear blood and mucus.

As the child begins to breathe more easily (and to regain consciousness, if he was unconscious), he tends to fight and thrash out, partly from oxygen hunger and partly from fear. He cries but makes no sound; he becomes terrified, perhaps thinking that his voice box has been "cut out." He needs the reassurance that he will be able to talk once the tube has been removed from his throat. His age and stage of development will determine how and what you tell him. Explain that the tube will help him breathe better. Let his parents hold him, and offer support to them all. Carefully explain why the tracheostomy was necessary and, if it is temporary, emphasize that fact. Explain that the incision was made below the child's vocal cords; therefore, no air passes over the cords when he is breathing through the tube and he cannot make sounds. After the child's anxiety is reduced and his breathing is more stable, show him and his parents that he *can* make sounds when he occludes the tube with his finger. Reducing the parents' anxiety is essential in reducing the child's anxiety. The child may continue to resist the tube and hyperventilate if he senses his parents' fright.

The tracheostomy must be suctioned frequently, sometimes every 15 minutes, sometimes more often. The physician may order you to suction only the tube and not the trachea in order to avoid irritating the mucous membrane and increasing the production of mucus; or, he may order deep suctioning to remove mucus before it forms an obstruction.

Never leave a child with a tracheostomy alone. If he has breathing difficulty he will not be able to call you, or he may panic and will not be able to use the call bell as would an adult. Children have a tendency to pick at the tracheostomy tube and the twill tape holding it in place. Proper restraints are necessary, but remember to release them when the child is being held, fed, or played with (and make it your business to do these things with him). Spend time with him other than for performing painful and intrusive procedures. Cover the tube with a gauze square or bib while the child is eating or drinking; this keeps spilled liquids and crumbs out of the tube. Do not let him play with any objects small enough to go down the tube.

As with the child who has been using a ventilator, weaning from the tracheostomy may frighten the child after he has learned to depend on it. Explain that you or someone else will be with him as the tube is sealed off, and that if he has any difficulty in breathing, you will open the tube. Gradual weaning is necessary. The tube may be partially occluded for a few days and then completely occluded, but not removed, for another day or two. If the child experiences any difficulty or is unduly anxious, the tube can be opened. Leaving the tube in place also provides a means for suctioning should it be necessary (see the Skills Manual).

SPECIFIC CONDITIONS

Respiratory conditions affecting the child can be broadly grouped into four basic categories: respiratory diseases of the newborn, and acute, chronic, and secondary respiratory diseases.

Acute Respiratory Diseases

Retropharyngeal abscess

In the infant, toddler, and preschool child, lymph nodes behind the posterior pharyngeal wall drain the nose and pharynx. These nodes usually disappear by four years of age, but they may become infected when the child has acute nasopharyngitis or pharyngitis, or after a fall in which he sustains a puncture wound to the mouth (for example, when he falls with a stick in his mouth). The causative organism is usually group A beta-hemolytic streptococci or *Staphylococcus aureus*. The child has an abrupt onset of high fever, signs of upper airway obstruction, and difficulty in swallowing that leads to drooling. He tends to hyperextend his head.

Visual examination of the pharynx is done with the child in Trendelenburg position to permit drainage and prevent massive aspiration should the abscess rupture. Restrain the infant with a mummy restraint, and hold his head firmly between your hands during the examination. If the abscess is not yet fluctuant, intravenous antibiotics are the treatment of choice. If the abscess is bulging, it can often be seen on visual examination, and provisions for immediate surgical incision and drainage are made. Lateral neck x-rays will confirm the diagnosis. Surgical incision and drainage require that the child be placed in a Trendelenburg position with suction equipment on hand in case of rupture. If aspiration occurs, immediate bronchoscopy and lavage is performed to remove the purulent material. Postoperatively, keep the foot of the bed elevated to promote drainage and place the child in a semiprone position. Note bleeding as evidenced by swallowing or respiratory distress and give frequent mouth care with warm saline. As soon as the child can swallow, offer warm broths or soups.

Tonsillitis and Adenoiditis

Tonsillitis and *adenoiditis* refer to infection and inflammation of the palatine and pharyngeal tonsils (adenoids), respectively.

Lymphoid tonsillar tissue filters and protects the respiratory and alimentary tracts from invasion by pathogenic organisms. The tonsils tend to atrophy after about five years of age, when the child is no longer as susceptible to respiratory tract invasion. For this reason, and because of the emotional effects of surgery on the young child, surgery is often delayed until after five years of age. In spite of this, the tonsillectomy with adenoidectomy (T&A) is the most common surgical procedure performed on the child in the United States today.

Symptoms of acute tonsillitis resemble those of severe pharyngitis, with the throat being so painful that the child tends to drool rather than swallow his saliva. High fever accompanies tonsillitis, and pus can be seen on the bright red edematous tonsils. Chronic tonsillitis is diagnosed when the child is sickly, has recurrent sore throats with bouts of low-grade fever, enlarged anterior cervical lymph nodes, and pus on the tonsils.

Adenoiditis produces symptoms *in addition to* those of acute tonsillitis: mouth breathing, nasal quality of speech, offensive breath, and impairment of hearing, taste, and smell. The child may acquire the typical facies of adenoiditis, which includes droopy eyes and open mouth, as well as noisy respirations during sleep. Hypertrophied adenoids can obstruct the nose and the eustachian tube, contributing to chronic otitis media. If recurrent or chronic otitis occurs without enlarged adenoids, polyethylene tubes are inserted into the eardrums to promote drainage of the middle ear.

Although common, T&A is a major surgical procedure that still has a significant mortality rate. The tonsils are scraped during surgery and are not sutured; the risk of hemorrhage and respiratory complications is therefore great.

History of bleeding tendencies and bleeding and clotting times are obtained before surgery, often on an outpatient basis. A complete blood count and urinalysis is also indicated. If any infection is present, surgery is postponed. Surgery is never done on the child with infected tonsils because the spread of pathogens can cause septicemia. Check the child's mouth for loose teeth or chewing gum, both of which can be aspirated during surgery. A barbiturate and atropine are given preoperatively.

Postoperatively, place the child in a semi-prone position with a pillow under his chest; with his head lower than his chest, the risk of aspiration is lessened. Watch for any signs of bleeding, such as frequent swallowing, or bright red vomitus. (Dark blood is old blood from the surgery and does not indicate fresh bleeding.) Vital signs are also a clue to hemorrhage. Watch for a rapid, thready pulse (over 120 beats at rest) and pallor. The child's face will normally be flushed because of the preoperative atropine combined with dehydration.

As soon as the child is alert enough to take fluids orally, offer clear liquids, shaved ice, popsicles, or Jello. Swallowing stimulates blood flow to the throat, which enhances healing. An ice collar and aspirin are used for pain. If there are no complications, the child may be discharged the afternoon of surgery, or the next morning. Caution his parents to observe him carefully for signs of bleeding, which is most common during the first 24 hours after surgery (while clots are forming) and five to seven days later when the clots slough off. Tell them to restrict the child's activity for a week and to gradually add soft foods to his diet after a few days. Before the child is discharged, offer him ice cream. He was probably promised it before surgery, although he may not care for it because it tends to make secretions more viscid as does milk.

Croup-type Syndromes

Acute epiglottitis, laryngotracheobronchitis (LTB), and acute spasmodic laryngitis are the most common of the croup-type syndromes. LTB is commonly referred to as "croup" and is often thought of as including the "allergic" or "spasmodic" form of laryngitis. These syndromes produce marked dyspnea with abnormal inspiratory sounds, such as stridor, wheezing, whistling, and snoring. The croup-type syndromes cause airway obstruction in the area of the larynx. The critical point is above the vocal cords (supraglottic) in epiglottitis and below them in croup (subglottic). Differential diagnosis is imperative because croup, although serious, is usually self-limiting, but epiglottitis is life-threatening and may cause rapid death if untreated.

Acute epiglottitis is a fulminating, inflammatory edema of the epiglottis caused by bacterial invasion, most often with Hemophilus influenzae type b. Affected children are usually over the age of three. A prodromal URI of less than 24 hours' duration is usually seen, after which a fever over 38.9°C (102°F) develops rapidly. The child has a sore throat and dysphagia which progresses to drooling before or at the onset of respiratory distress. His tongue protrudes to make room for his edematous epiglottis, and he bends forward to keep the floppy epiglottis from obstructing his airway.

Diagnosis involves three procedures: inspection of the epiglottis, lateral neck x-ray, and laryngoscopy. Inspection is simple yet dangerous because the use of a tongue blade will induce the gag reflex, which may cause acute airway obstruction and death. If epiglottitis is suspected, the throat is never examined unless emergency equipment is on hand. If the cherry red, edematous epiglottis is seen, the diagnosis of epiglottitis is established. If the epiglottis is *not* edematous, LTB is diagnosed. X-rays will show an enlarged epiglottis; the physician accompanies the child to x-ray and stays with him during the study and its immediate interpretation. If the diagnosis is positive, the child is taken directly to the operating room or intensive care unit where a laryngoscopy and intubation are performed. There must be no delay in establishing an artificial airway. Complete obstruction and death is certain if adequate treatment is not instituted early; the mortality rate is 100 percent in untreated cases. Intravenous antibiotic therapy is begun at once until blood culture sensitivities are reported.

Laryngotracheobronchitis, or croup, is mucosal edema in the larynx, trachea, and bronchi (beneath the vocal cords or subglottic area). It is almost always caused by a viral infection. The affected child is under three years of age and has a mild URI for over 24 hours before the appearance of symptoms of respiratory obstruction. Attacks usually occur at night and are accompanied by fever, hoarseness, croupy cough, inspiratory stridor, and respiratory distress, which is usually mild but may be life-threatening. the epiglottis, although inflamed in some cases, is never edematous.

Diagnosis is made from the history and physical examination, although in some cases, direct laryngoscopy is done to rule out epiglottitis. Treatment usually does not include antibiotics because LTB is viral; death, when it occurs, is caused by obstruction and rarely by bacterial complications.

Humidification of inspired air reduces symptoms and is the cornerstone of croup therapy. Cool humidity is usually administered. Oxygen is given if the child is hypoxic, and he requires close observation to detect impending respiratory obstruction. Racemic epinephrine (RE) may be used to treat croup. It is inhaled in aerosol form, usually via IPPB or mask, and should not be given at intervals of less than one hour. The relief may be transitory, so you must watch the child closely for rebound (return of symptoms). Occasionally the child's condition deteriorates and respiratory failure ensues, necessitating the creation of an artificial airway. Tracheostomy is the procedure of choice because the tube enters the airway below the obstruction; nasotracheal intubation tends to cause tracheal necrosis because the tube traverses the obstructed area.

Acute nasopharyngitis, pharyngitis, sinusitis, and acute spasmodic laryngitis, or "allergic" croup, are discussed in chapter 16.

Lower Respiratory Tract Infections

In *bronchitis* and *bronchiolitis,* mucus and edema in the airway cause air to become trapped in the lungs, resulting in overinflation (which can lead to atelectasis). The form of *pneumonia* that most often affects the infant and small child is bronchopneumonia, in which infiltration is scattered over a large portion of the lung. The older child and adult tend to have lobar pneumonia, in which one or more lobes is affected.

Aspiration of Foreign Bodies

The older infant and toddler are particularly prone to aspiration of foreign bodies because they are constantly exploring. Objects most frequently aspirated are bones, hardware, coins, nuts, and safety pins. Because the right bronchus is straighter and wider than the left, objects pass into it more easily and tend to lodge in the right lung. If complete obstruction occurs, atelectasis results. If partial obstruction occurs, the object acts as a ball valve, and permits air to enter but not leave the lung, causing hyperinflation.

The child coughs violently, and if the airway is lacerated by the object or if infection is present, hemoptysis, purulent sputum, fever, and leucocytosis develop. X-ray reveals radiopaque objects, but other objects cannot be visualized. Vegetable products, such as peanuts, popcorn, and pumpkin seeds, are coated in oil and will swell in the respiratory tract, thus causing obstruction or even lipid pneumonia. Bronchoscopy is performed to remove the object.

The child is seen in the emergency room in respiratory distress. He and his parents are frightened and anxious. The parents feel guilty for "letting" the child get hold of the object he swallowed. They need reassurance and support.

Chronic Respiratory Diseases

Asthma

Asthma is an allergic disease and as such it is discussed in chapter 16. The earlier sections of this chapter on dyspnea, wheezing, and secretions apply to asthma.

Bronchiectasis

Bronchiectasis is a chronic inflammatory disease of the bronchi. It appears gradually after repeated pulmonary infections such as cystic fibrosis. The child has symptoms of chronic lung disease including a barrel chest and retarded growth. He fatigues easily and has clubbing of the fingers and toes. Treatment includes bronchodilation, postural drainage, administration of antibiotics and, sometimes, surgical removal of the affected lobe of the lung.

Cystic Fibrosis

Respiratory involvement in CF children results from blockage of the bronchioles and then the bronchi by thick secretions. The alveoli overinflate in an attempt to compensate, and emphysema results, evidenced by a barrel chest. Clubbing of the fingers and toes may occur. Eventually, right-sided heart failure *(cor pulmonale)* occurs. The child is particularly susceptible to pulmonary infections, which compromise his condition further.

Treatment for pulmonary involvement consists of the prevention of infection and the control of disease. Antibiotics are given as indicated by deep throat culture. Intermittent aerosol therapy is used to deliver small amounts of medication or water (to liquefy secretions) to the lower respiratory tract. Among the medications used are decongestants, bronchodilators, antibiotics, and mucolytic and/or anti-inflammatory agents. Drugs that suppress the cough reflex are never given to the CF child. Aerosol therapy is followed by postural drainage in twelve positions. Clapping for one to two minutes in each position is followed by vibrating during five exhalations (see the Skills Manual). Encourage coughing after each segment, and if the cough is productive, repeat the therapy for that segment. Regular exercise and deep breathing are encouraged to aid in the expectoration of mucus and to maintain muscle mass. The child usually sleeps in a mist tent to aid in liquefying the abnormally thick secretions.

SUMMARY

Respiratory disease in the child is potentially more serious than in the adult due to the physical differences in the two and to the fact that the child cannot verbalize his distress as readily. The child is frightened because he cannot get his breath easily. His fright is compounded by the use of frightening equipment and procedures, such as the oxygen tent and tracheostomy. Respiratory diseases in the child range in duration and severity. The medical and nursing management depends primarily on the clinical manifestations. Careful observation and competent nursing care of the child are essential.

CLINICAL APPLICATION

Lyman, aged two, is admitted at 3 AM in obvious respiratory distress. He is sitting upright, retracting with an inspiratory stridor, using his accessory muscles of respiration, and is cyanotic; he appears anxious. The diagnosis is laryngotracheobronchitis. He is placed in an oxygen tent with humidified oxygen at 10 liters per minute.

1. Explain how Lyman's illness differs from acute spasmodic croup.
2. What is stridor? What might it mean if Lyman's stridor diminishes?
3. How can you tell that Lyman is cyanotic?
4. Why was he placed in an oxygen tent?
5. Explain your nursing responsibilities while Lyman is in the tent.
6. How will you know if the tent is helping Lyman?

   Lyman becomes more restless. He hyperextends his neck and crawls up on two pillows to elevate his chest. His pulse rate has increased from 110 to 140 beats. His retractions are more severe. You notify the physician, and he elects to perform a tracheostomy on Lyman.

7. After Lyman returns from the operating room his cyanosis has disappeared, he seems less anxious, and he is not retracting. Why?
8. What do you think the tracheostomy means to Lyman?
9. How will your nursing responsibilities change now that Lyman has a tracheostomy?
10. Given that Lyman has a tracheostomy and is in an oxygen tent, what toys will be suitable for him? Unsuitable?

Bibliography

Burnette, B.A. Family Adjustment to Cystic Fibrosis. *American Journal of Nursing* 75:1986, 1975.

Cohen, S. Blood-gas and Acid-Base Concepts in Respiratory Care: Programmed Instructions. *American Journal of Nursing* 76:P.I. 1, 1976.

Holsclaw, D.S. Early Recognition of Acute Respiratory Failure in Children. *Pediatric Annals* 6:467, 1977.

———. Recognition and Management of Patients with Cystic Fibrosis. *Pediatric Annals* 7:9, 1978.

———. Pediatric Pulmonary Disease: An Overview. *Pediatric Annals* 6:438, 1977.

Lockhart, C.H. and Battaglia, J.D. Croup (Laryngotracheal Bronchitis) and Epiglottitis. *Pediatric Annals* 6:262, 1977.

Nalepka, C.D. The Oxygen Hood for Newborns in Respiratory Distress. *American Journal of Nursing* 75:2185, 1975.

Rapkin, R.H. Acute Infectious Laryngitis in Children. *Resident and Staff Physician* 24:86, 1978.

Shaw, L.L. and Mansmann, H.C. Decisions in the Evaluation and Treatment of Acute Viral Croup. *Pediatric Annals* 6:476, 1977.

Tooley, W.H. and Lipow, H.W. Respiratory Function and Pulmonary Disease in Older Infants and Children, in Rudolph, A.M. (ed). *Pediatrics*, ed. 16, New York, Appleton-Century-Crofts, 1977, p. 1544.

CHAPTER **24**

The Child with Anemia

BEHAVIORAL OBJECTIVES

After studying this chapter you will be able to:

- Discuss the cardiac and respiratory changes produced by anemic hypoxia.
- Explain why fatigue and infection are problems associated with anemia.
- Compare the studies of hemoglobin, hematocrit, red cell indices, and hemoglobin electrophoresis, explaining the purpose of each test and the information yielded.
- Prepare a nutritional replacement menu for a child deficient in Vitamin B_{12}, folic acid, and iron.
- Explain the different uses for transfusion therapy and categorize the types of transfusion reactions.
- Discuss the function of the spleen and the purpose of a splenectomy.
- Design a teaching plan for explaining anemia and hypoxia to the parents of a child newly diagnosed with an inherited, chronic, hemolytic anemia.

TERMS AND CONCEPTS

Anemia
Anemic hypoxia
Red cell indices
Hemoglobin electrophoresis
Hemolytic anemia
Transfusion reactions
  Hemolytic reactions
  Pyrogenic reactions
  Allergic reactions
  Hypothermic reactions
Hemolysis
Splenomegaly
Splenectomy

The child with anemia is deficient in the *quantity* or *quality* of his red blood cells. Either the *total number of erythrocytes* or the *concentration of hemoglobin* packed inside each red blood cell is reduced. One or both of these problems result in anemia. The specific type of anemia, named according to the characteristics of the erythrocyte or the cause of the anemia (see Figure 24–1), determines treatment and nursing care. Frequently anemia does not occur alone but rather as a result of other conditions, such as undernutrition, cancer, or congenital anomalies.

Anemia is a deficiency in the oxygen-carrying ability of erythrocytes. The body immediately tries to compensate for this deficiency in two ways: the heart rate and force of contractions increase, resulting in tachycardia; the forces controlling respirations increase, resulting in dyspnea. Despite these compensatory mechanisms, *anemic hypoxia*, or a deficiency in the

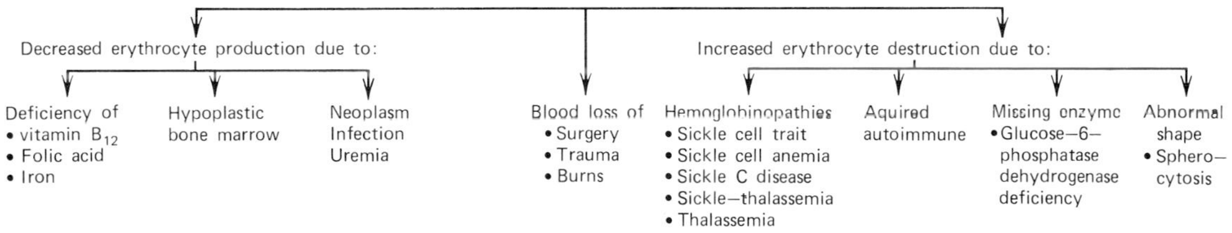

Figure 24–1. *Causes of anemia.*

amount of oxygen delivered to the body's tissues, occurs. Since tissues in the myocardium, brain, and muscle are most dependent on adequate oxygen delivery, they are the most vulnerable to a reduction in oxygen availability. In addition to signs of tachycardia and dyspnea, the child with anemia shows such effects of tissue hypoxia as fatigue, infection, and decompensation of functions in major organs, for example, the heart and spleen.

This chapter discusses anemia and the effects produced by an alteration in normal erythrocyte production, destruction, or hereditary coding. Common diagnostic methods and treatments as well as the nursing interventions are discussed. Table 24–1 presents descriptions of specific anemias, their treatment and nursing care.

COMMON PROBLEMS AND NURSING INTERVENTIONS

Compensatory Changes

Increased Circulatory Output

The heart increases its pumping action in an effort to deliver more oxygen-saturated blood to waiting tissue. Cardiac hyperactivity causes tachycardia, which is measured as an increased pulse rate, and felt as palpitations. The normal myocardium can tolerate sustained hyperactivity for prolonged periods. However, if the anemia is extreme and chronic, the continual, accelerated rate and force of the heart's contractions may lead to heart enlargement, and eventually to congestive heart failure.

Increased Pulmonary Function

To enhance alveolar ventilation, respirations increase. Consequently, following exertion, the child may experience dyspnea and *orthopnea*, a condition in which breathing is possible only in a sitting or standing position. These are signs of increased pulmonary function and the compensatory effort to deliver adequate amounts of oxygen to waiting cells. If increased pulmonary function continues, decompensatory changes, such as pulmonary congestion, ascites, and edema, may result. Despite compensatory changes, tissues are deprived of oxygen, and anemic hypoxia results.

Anemic Hypoxia

Fatigue

Muscle cells deprived of oxygen have less power to contract, fatigue easily, and are unable to persist at tasks. Even after rest, these hypoxic cells fail to regain their energy. Insufficient oxygenation of body tissue results in feelings of fatigue, weakness, and lightheadedness. Observe the

Table 24–1. **Anemias**

Name	*Definition*	*Treatment*	*Special Nursing Considerations*
	Anemias Due To Impaired Erythrocyte Production		
Folic acid deficiency	Deficiency or inability to use folic acid. Low serum and red blood cell (rbc) folic acid levels confirm the deficiency.	Oral 1-mg tablets. Injections given deep subcutaneously, or intramuscularly, if malabsorption is suspected.	Body reserves of folic acid are normally small; dietary deficits develop quickly with symptoms. Folic acid deficiencies occur when foods are cooked for long periods. Obtain information about food preparation and dietary intake. Children at risk for the deficiency are: young infants on cow's milk diet not receiving vegetables, meats and eggs; premature infants with already small folic acid reserves; children with hemolytic anemia and increased folic acid needs due to acute or chronic overactivity of the bone marrow.
Iron deficiency anemia	Deficiency or inability to use iron. Hemoglobin, hematocrit, serum iron, and iron binding studies confirm the deficiency.	Give oral iron on an empty stomach with orange juice. When given parenterally, Z-track the injection.	Administer with a dropper or straw, since iron may stain teeth. Stools may be dark green or black. Continue therapy until iron stores are replenished, possibly six to twelve months *after* hemoglobin and hematocrit return to normal. Teach proper infant feeding, using iron-supplemented formulas, iron-fortified cereals, and limited amounts of whole milk. Be aware of iron intoxication and hemosiderosis.

Pernicious anemia	Deficiency or inability to use Vitamin B_{12}. Diagnosis confirmed by Shilling Test (the ingestion of radioactive tagged B_{12}) and B_{12} serum assay test. For B_{12} to be absorbed from the intestine, an intrinsic factor (IF) must be present in gastric mucosa. IF is usually absent in pernicious anemia.	Lifelong injections of Vitamin B_{12} (cyanocobalamin). Transfusions for low hemoglobin.	Vitamin B_{12} deficits cause central nervous system disturbances such as alterations in gait, bladder and bowel control, irritability, poor memory, and depression. Advise family of importance of continued therapy to avoid neurologic complications.
Hypoplastic anemia (Aplastic anemia)	Failure of the bone marrow to deliver blood cells into the circulation; can occur following excessive exposure to radiation or exposure to certain drugs or chemicals. Child is deficient in red blood cells, platelets, and leukocytes.	Use of steroids and androgens. Transfusions with packed red blood cells, platelets, and leukocyte concentrates. Splenectomy. Bone marrow transplant.	Side effects of steroids include Cushingoid appearance, hypertension, and extreme weight gain. Androgens, when used for long periods, produce masculine effects, i.e., facial and body hair, acne and voice changes. Complications of infection and/or bleeding cause morbidity and mortality. Offer care measures to minimize infection and bleeding (see Ch. 20).
Sickle cell trait (SCT)	A benign condition with no physical abnormalities occurring in 1 in 10 black births. The child inherited *one* allele for sickle hemoglobin that is confirmed by hemoglobin electrophoresis.	Family education about the SCT and the difference between SCT and SCA (see below). Offer genetic education. If both mates have SCT, *each* conception has a one in four chance of having SCA, a serious chronic disease.	The child with SCT is not anemic; hemoglobin and hematocrit values are normal. If available oxygen is reduced, e.g., higher altitudes, scuba diving or in unpressurized aircraft, he could experience intravascular sickling, vaso-occulsions, and infarctions. For the same reason, medical personnel need to be aware of SCT in the case of accident, shock, or anesthesia. A hemoglobin electrophoresis should be done on each black child admitted to a health care facility.

(continued)

Table 24–1. *(Continued)*

Name	*Definition*	*Treatment*	*Special Nursing Considerations*
Sickle cell anemia (SCA)	An autosomal recessive condition occurring in 1 in 400 black births, causing a severe hemolytic anemia and ill episodes called crises. Four types of crises occur: *pain or vaso-occulsive, acute sequestration, aplastic,* and *hyperhemolytic.* The child inherited *two* alleles for sickle hemoglobin confirmed by hemoglobin electrophoresis.	Supportive and symptomatic care for crises: *Pain/vaso-occulsive* (due to intravascular sickling): provide increased oral hydration and monitor intravenous therapy if indicated. Record intake and output. Offer analgesics, e.g., Tylenol or aspirin. Guard against high dosages of drugs that make child drowsy, sleepy, and unable to consume fluids. Take temperature before administering any analgesic. Be alert to early signs of infection during and after the crisis.*Acute Sequestration* (due to massive entrapment of sickled cells in the spleen): the child is in hypovolemic shock. Death occurs if oxygen and blood transfusions are not given quickly. Splenectomy if child survives the crisis. *Aplastic* (a decreased production of erythrocytes by the bone marrow): usually occurs in wake of infection, e.g., flu, otitis media, gastroenteritis. Transfusions. *Hyperhemolytic* (due to increased destruction of red blood cells): jaundice and dark urine. Offer added hydration.	Prophylactic and health maintenance care: Monthly or bimonthly hematology evaluations for children under two; for older children, every three to six months. Good basic nutrition; advise family that no special foods or diet will correct anemia. All routine immunizations must be given. No activity restriction. Allow child to set his own limits. Children with SCA die more often from infection than any other single cause. Be alert to early signs of infection, e.g., fever, malaise, and anorexia. Offer preventive care and teach family early recognition of infection. Teach family to assess early signs of increasing anemia, e.g., pallor and lethargy. Chronic complications involve major organs that become congested with sickle cells, producing *cardiomegaly, hepatomegaly,* and *splenomegaly.* Hemoglobin values range from 5.5-9.5 gm/100 ml.

Sickle-C disease	A chronic hemolytic anemia occurring in 1 in 800 black births, resulting from inheritance of *one* allele for sickle hemoglobin and *one* allele for hemoglobin C.	Same as SCA.	Onset and severity of crises and chronic care problems are usually later in life and milder than SCA. Cardiomegaly is an occasional occurrence in contrast to frequent cardiac changes in SCA. Same prophylactic and health maintenance care. Hemoglobin values range from 8-10 gm/100 ml.
Sickle thalassemia	A chronic hemolytic anemia occurring in 1 in 1,600 black births. The child inherited *one* allele for thalassemia and *one* allele for sickle hemoglobin. Diagnosis is confirmed by hemoglobin electrophoresis.	Same as SCA.	Thalassemia is a decreased production of hemoglobin. Thalassemia combined with sickle hemoglobin results in crises that may be mild or severe. Prophylactic, acute, and chronic care needs are the same as for SCA. Hemoglobin values range from 6-13 gm/100 ml.
Thalassemia Thalassemia minor Thalassemia major	A decreased production of a specific hemoglobin chain, i.e., beta thalassemia is a reduction of beta hemoglobin. If the child receives *one* allele for thalassemia, he has *thalassemia minor*, a mild condition; if *two* alleles for thalassemia are inherited, the child has *thalassemia major*, a serious, life-threatening disorder.	Thalassemia minor usually requires no treatment. Thalassemia major requires routine transfusions to maintain hemoglobin at 10 gm. Splenectomy for hypersplenism.	Growth retardation throughout life. Hemosiderosis, especially cardiac. Frequent infections; minimize with prophylactic care.

(continued)

Table 24–1. *(Continued)*

Name	*Definition*	*Treatment*	*Special Nursing Considerations*
	Anemias Due To Increased Erythrocyte Destruction		
Glucose-6-phosphatase dehydrogenase deficiency (G6-P-D)	A sex-linked disorder occurring in 13 percent of all black males and 3 percent of black females. A deficit of the enzyme G6-P-D, resulting in a hemolytic anemia only after exposure to *certain* drugs or chemicals (see Table 24–2). Screening and diagnosis confirmed with a blood assay test.	Avoid all drugs and chemicals listed in Table 24–2. If compounds ingested, the child experiences seven to twelve days of acute hemolysis, followed by an increase in hemoglobin and reticulocytes.	Hemolytic anemia with symptoms of shortness of breath, fatigue, jaundice, and dark urine following ingestion of compounds listed in Table 24–2. Provide families with a list of drugs and chemicals to be avoided. Offer instructions on how to read drug labels because many of the offending agents are included in nonprescription medicines. Advise that drug lists be left with pharmacist, health department, physician, and each person who may prescribe or monitor drugs for the child. Advise against any medication given to the child by a person not knowledgable about the G6-P-D deficiency.
Hereditary spherocytosis (HS)	An autosomal dominant condition occurring in 1 in 4,500 births. Abnormally shaped erythrocytes are produced that are prematurely destroyed in the spleen; a mild hemolytic anemia results. Diagnosis confirmed with an abnormal osmotic fragility study and presence of disease in another family member.	Splenectomy after ages three to four and before ages eight to ten. Splenectomy delayed because of increased incidence of pneumococcal meningitis after splenectomy.	Before splenectomy, the child has chronic jaundice and splenomegaly. Following splenectomy, the erythrocytes have a normal life span but their shape remains abnormal. After splenectomy, prophylactic penicillin is usually recommended.

Acquired immunohemolytic anemia (AHA)	An abnormal immune system response caused by mechanisms *outside* the erythrocyte, such as antibody-antigen reactions that begin within the child but are not intrinsic to the erythrocyte. The reason for the abnormal immune response is not known. Diagnostic tests are the direct and indirect Coombs test. The direct Coombs detects the presence of antibodies in the red blood cell. The indirect Coombs detects red blood cell antibodies in the serum.	Based on results of the Coombs test. Frequently corticosteroids, e.g., prednisone, are given. If corticosteroids are ineffective, a splenectomy may be necessary. Transfusions are avoided, since they accelerate hemolysis; however, they are used as life saving measures.	Systemic lupus erythematosus, ulcerative colitis, rheumatic fever, and viral diseases such as infectious mononucleosis are associated with symptoms of AHA. The child has a low-grade fever, anorexia, lethargy, pallor, and jaundice from hemolysis. AHA is often acute and may be severe but is usually self-limiting. If prednisone is given, be alert to side effects, e.g., fluid retention, potassium loss, muscle wasting, hypertension, gastrointestinal irritation, increased appetite and weight gain. Prednisone is immunosuppressive; use measures to minimize infection.

child's body following exertion, noting changes in skin color, breathing, and posture. One indicator of tolerance for activity is cardiac pulse rate. Although tachycardia is a compensatory change, activities that cause the pulse rate to increase greatly are probably too strenuous and need to be reconsidered or replanned.

Each child's energy level is different, depending on his personality, development age, and abilities. If an anemic condition develops in an already inactive, quiet, solitary child it may go unnoticed. Anemia frequently develops slowly, especially when it is caused by nutritional deficiencies. If the anemic symptoms of fatigue and weakness also develop slowly, they may be ignored or attributed to the child's personality, and needed treatment may be delayed or not sought. When assessing tissue hypoxia and its effect on present activity level, consider the child's past and present personality, the duration of the anemia, and present blood values. Each of these factors influences his energy level and the degree of fatigue following exertion. The child with a chronic anemia frequently adapts to his low hemoglobin level, so that the amount of energy he has differs little from that of the child with normal blood values.

A child with chronic, noncorrectable, anemia is encouraged to establish his tolerance level for all activities, exerting himself according to his individual ability. Activity restrictions should not be imposed, and rest periods should be enforced only as needed. Competitive and contact sports, however, should be avoided because team goals usually take precedence over the individual child's tolerance level during these activities. Allow each child to set his own pace. He will stop and rest when he is fatigued. Self-pacing gives the child a sense of control over his body and promotes a positive self-concept and body image. If the child's energy must be conserved, refer to chapter 22 for nursing interventions. Prolonged fatigue may precipitate appetite and weight loss. Dietary measures discussed in chapter 18 for anorexia are equally applicable to the anorexic child with anemia.

Infection

Hypoxic tissues are more susceptible to infection than are adequately oxygenated tissues. Thus, the anemic child needs protection from organisms that cause infection. Advise parents to minimize the child's contact with others who have a known infection. They should avoid crowded places when possible, especially during the winter months when respiratory infections are prevalent. Preventive measures include keeping immunizations up-to-date, prompt cleansing of cuts, bites, and other easy portals of infection, regular dental checkups, and adequate clothing for damp or cold weather. During hospitalization, the child must be protected from other children with coughs, draining wounds, respiratory infections, or other obvious infectious conditions. Emphasize the importance of thorough handwashing, offering role modeling to help the child and his parents remember this simple but important measure. Since hypoxia hinders healing of traumatized tissue, protect the skin from trauma by maintaining skin integrity. Dry skin benefits from emollients and humidity. If the child is bedridden, change his position frequently to alleviate pressure and aid circulation.

In addition to being susceptible to fatigue and infection, the anemic child may experience nocturnal muscle cramps (muscular hypoxia) or headache, dizziness and irritability (cerebral hypoxia). For the child with ischemic hypoxia (see ch. 22), carefully observe and record the color and integrity of his skin, lips, nail beds, and mucous membranes. Energy level, mood, and tolerance for activity are additional information that can be reassessed after treatment.

COMMON DIAGNOSTIC TESTS AND NURSING CONSIDERATIONS

Erythrocyte Studies

To identify the specific type of anemia, it is necessary to look closely at the size, shape, and color of the red blood cells. A small amount of peripheral blood is extracted during a finger or heel stick, or venipuncture. It is then treated in a special manner and viewed under a microscope. Morphological classification of erythrocytes is based on laboratory findings. If an anemia is suspected, frequently ordered blood tests are a total red blood cell count, hemoglobin concentration, hematocrit level, and red blood cell indices.

Red blood cell indices are corpuscular values of erythrocytes which are determined by specific mathematical computations, using the child's predetermined red blood cell count, hemoglobin, and hematocrit. There are three indices: the *MCV*, or *mean corpuscular volume*, the *volume* of the average erythrocyte; the *MCH*, *mean corpuscular hemoglobin*, the *amount* of hemoglobin in the average erythrocyte; and the *MCHC, mean corpuscular hemoglobin concentration*, the *concentration* of hemoglobin in the average erythrocyte. The child's red blood cell indices, like the hemoglobin and hematocrit, are compared with normal blood values (see Tables 21–2 and 21–3).

Be aware of how often and exactly how much blood the child is losing from repeated venipunctures. Record the exact number of milliliters of blood extracted daily. This record will be used to assess blood loss, a serious threat to children needing repeated venipunctures. The blood plasma rapidly replaces itself, but the erythrocytes may not be replaced completely, especially if the bone marrow is depressed (e.g., during myelosuppression of a neoplasm or anticancer chemotherapy). Extensive blood studies can result in appreciable blood loss or an exacerbation of the anemia. Explain the venipuncture procedure to the child, applying a restraint if necessary (see the Skills Manual).

Bone Marrow Aspiration

A sample of bone marrow is used for close study of the erythropoietic tissue, which makes erythrocytes. Refer to chapter 20 for a description of a bone marrow aspiration and nursing considerations.

Hemoglobin Electrophoresis

Over 200 different kinds of hemoglobin exist. Each one can be identified by its electrical property. *Hemoglobin electrophoresis* is a sophisticated laboratory test that separates hemoglobins according to their electrical properties. This makes exact identification of different hemoglobins, and diagnosis of abnormal hemoglobins possible. New, inexpensive, electrophoretic methods use small amounts of capillary blood. The results are dependable and offer screening and diagnostic possibilities at local community health facilities. However, careful transport of the blood sample to a properly equipped laboratory is essential for reliable results. Hemoglobin electrophoresis can quickly diagnose abnormal hemoglobins, or *hemoglobinopathies*.

Most of the over 200 hemoglobinopathies *do not* cause clinical symptoms, but the presence of sickle hemoglobin can cause an increased rate of erythrocyte destruction, or *hemolytic anemia* (Figures 24–2 and 24–3). If a hemoglobinopathy is suspected, it is important that a hemoglobin electrophoresis be done immediately to differentiate between sickle cell trait, a totally benign hemoglobinopathy, and sickle cell anemia, a chronic debilitating hemoglobinopathy (see Table 24–1).

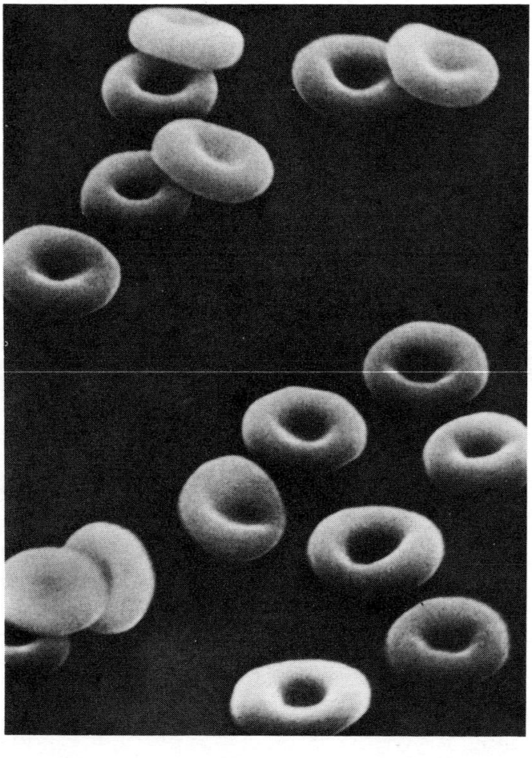

Figure 24–2. *Normal red blood cells as they appear under a scanning electron microscope. The disk shape allows the RBCs to move easily through blood vessels.* (From Barnhart, M.I., Henry, R.L., Lusher, J.M. Sickel Cell, A Scope Monograph, The Upjohn Company Kalamazoo, Mich., 1974.)

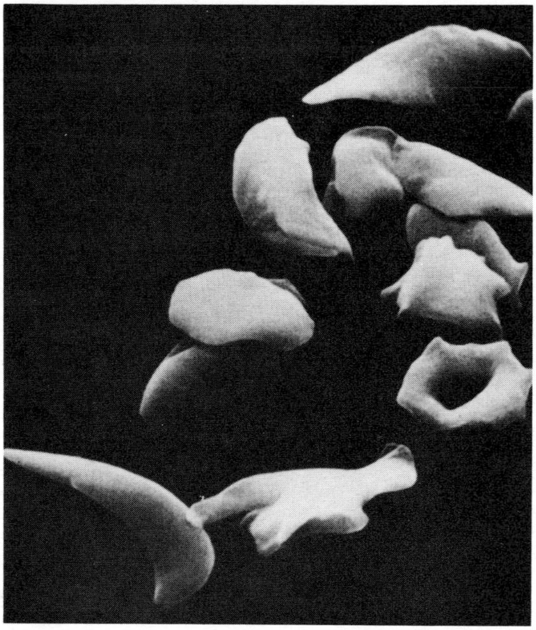

Figure 24 –3. *Sickled red blood cells. The crescent shape can easily cause jamming in blood vessels and lead to a vaso-occlusive crisis.* (From Barnhart, M.I., Henry, R.L., Lusher, J.M. Sickle Cell, A Scope Monograph, The Upjohn Company, Kalamazoo, Mich., 1974.)

A complete hemoglobin study is essential for an assessment of the child's hemoglobin and for planning his care. The optimal time for hemoglobin testing and/or screening of well children is debatable. Infant hemoglobin testing is usually *not* done until after the age of six months because of the presence of fetal hemoglobin, and the consequent difficulty in reading capillary blood samples. However, some hospitals test umbilical cord blood in order to identify newborns with a sickle hemoglobinopathy. Early identification, education, and medical follow-up of infants with a sickle hemoglobinopathy disease can alert the family and medical staff to special care needs long before symptoms indicate a diagnosis. Figures 24–4, 24–5, 24–6, and 24–7 illustrate how several common sickle hemoglobinopathies are inherited.

Physical Appearance

The appearance and behavior of the child, as well as lab values and vital signs, provide diagnostic information and considerations for care. Closely observe the child's skin, sclera, and mucous membranes for color changes. The anemic child may be pallid. As the anemia increases, so does the pallor. If his anemia is due to increased de-

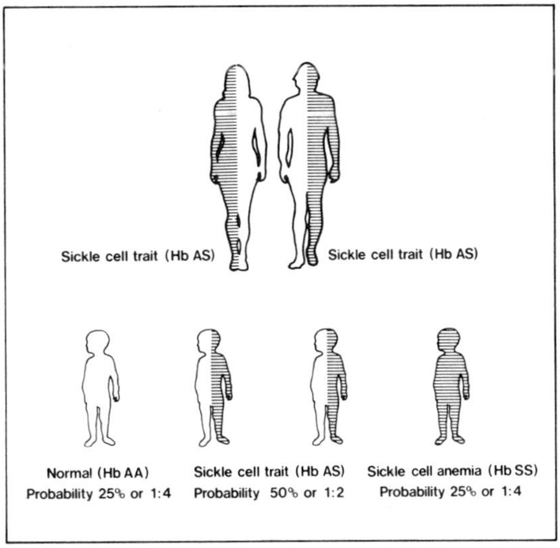

Figure 24–5. *How sickle cell anemia is inherited. Each child receives one hemoglobin gene from each parent at conception. The probability of occurrence is the same in each pregnancy.*

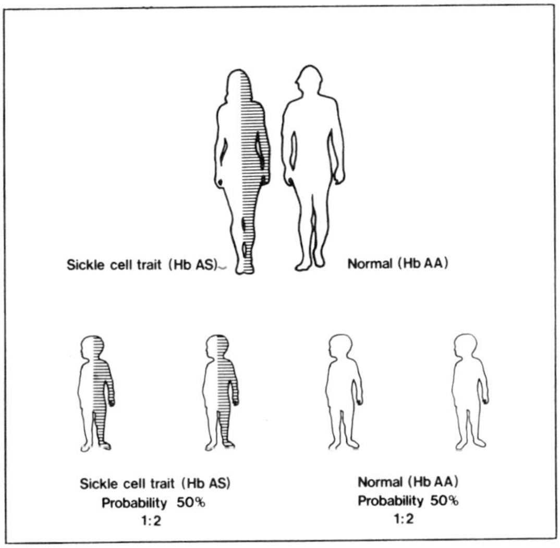

Figure 24–4. *How sickle cell trait is inherited. Each child receives one hemoglobin gene from each parent at conception. The probability of occurrence for each of the possible hemoglobin combinations is the same in each pregnancy.*

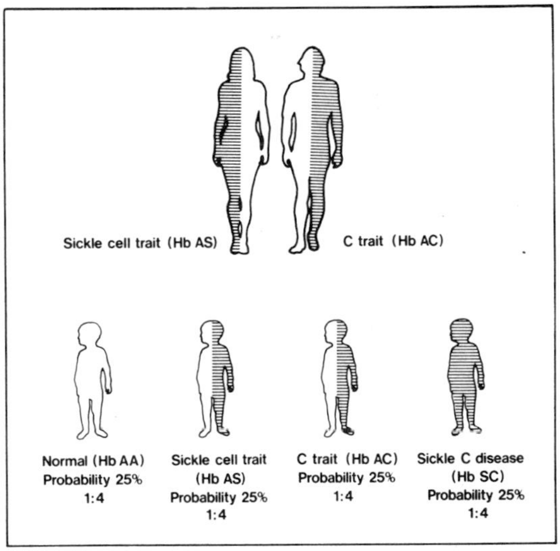

Figure 24–6. *How sickle C disease is inherited. Each child receives one hemoglobin gene from each parent at conception. The probability of occurrence is the same in each pregnancy.*

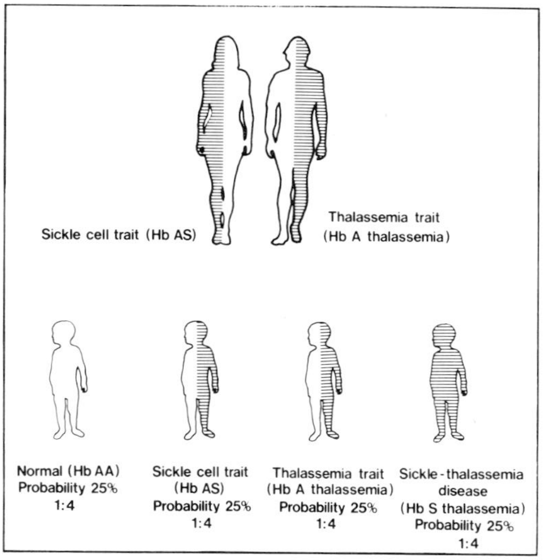

Figure 24–7. *How sickle-thalassemia disease is inherited. Each child receives one hemoglobin gene from each parent at conception. The probability of occurrence of each of the possible hemoglobin combinations is the same in each pregnancy.*

struction of erythrocytes, jaundice also may be present. If the jaundice increases, medical attention is needed. Teach the family normal skin, sclera, and mucous membrane coloring for their anemic child. Do this by studying the child's palms, sclera, conjunctiva, and tongue, since each site can be easily observed for color and any color changes. Advise the family to report increased pallor and/or jaundice. Increased pallor can be life-threatening and requires immediate care. Increased jaundice is not as serious but needs attention. Inform the family that with increased jaundice, the urine becomes a dark amber color.

An anemic child may be active and alert even though his erythrocyte values are very low. The extent of his symptoms is not necessarily related to the severity of the anemia. For example, children whose anemia has developed over many months, or years, will probably experience minimal or mild physical symptoms. These children have adapted slowly to lower hemoglobin levels and appear rather healthy. In contrast, children whose anemia is due to a sudden blood loss have acute symptoms, such as weakness, fatigue, shortness of breath, and irritability. They have not had time to adapt to their lower hemoglobin levels. When planning care, consider the laboratory test and the duration of the anemia and its cause.

COMMON TREATMENTS AND NURSING CONSIDERATIONS

Nutritional Replacement

Certain nutrients are crucial to the process of *erythropoiesis*, or erythrocyte formation. If one or more of these compounds are lacking, anemia can result. For example, deficiency anemias result from a lack of Vitamin B_{12}, *iron*, and *folic acid*. Dietary treatment for these anemias is the daily inclusion of foods high in the lacking nutrients. For example, Vitamin B_{12} is important for erythrocyte maturation, and the best sources of Vitamin B_{12} are organ and muscle meats. Since plant foods are very poor sources, children who eat primarily vegetables may develop Vitamin B_{12} deficiency anemia. Folic acid, also needed for erythrocyte maturation, is contained in green, leafy vegetables, such as broccoli, spinach, lettuce, and asparagus. Organ meats, whole grains, lemons, and bananas are additional sources of folic acid. Iron is essential for making hemoglobin and is found in liver, muscle meats, egg yolks, shellfish, dried fruits, and green leafy vegetables. Since only 11 to 14 percent of ingested iron is absorbed, intake must be high. Vitamin B_6 is also important for hemoglobin synthesis and is contained in meats, wheat germ, and whole grain cereals. Vitamin C is essential for the use of folic acid and aids in the absorption of iron. Citrus fruits and green, leafy vegetables contain Vitamin C.

All of these important nutrients for erythropoiesis are found in the more expensive food groups. This added economic burden creates a problem for families with limited financial resources and several children to feed. This, coupled with the frequent anorexia and irritability caused by anemia, taxes anyone's patience. Adding the needed nutrients to already preferred foods may be a possible solution for the family who cannot afford the costly diet. For example, a beaten egg, ground liver, or wheat germ can be added to a hamburger *without* a change in taste, but with a tremendous increase in iron and folic acid (see ch. 18).

Dietary management alone will rarely correct a deficiency anemia but it can be helpful in preventing an anemia or controlling an already existing anemia. The importance of adequate intake of nutrients essential for the production of erythrocytes should be emphasized during the growth periods of early childhood and adolescence, and during periods of illness or emotional stress.

Drug Therapy

The medicines used most commonly in the treatment of anemia are vitamins and minerals, especially iron, folic acid, and Vitamin B_{12}.

Iron

Intramuscular injections of iron are used only if adequate oral iron absorption is impossible, or if a rapid production of hemoglobin is sought. If intramuscular iron is given, use a Z–track injection technique (see the Skills Manual). Even when the Z–track technique is used, intramuscular iron may cause local skin discoloration and discomfort.

Oral iron is the safest, cheapest, and most readily accepted form of iron. Adequate iron absorption requires an acid environment, and iron should be given *between* meals when the absorbing surface of the duodenum is likely to be in an acid state. Since Vitamin C (ascorbic acid) aids iron absorption, iron administered with orange juice, makes the iron more acceptable to taste and more readily absorbed. Mild gastrointestinal complaints of constipation or loose stools may occur after oral iron therapy. If the child develops nausea, heartburn, abdominal distension, or cramping following oral iron, give the iron with food, and gradually wean him to taking it on an empty stomach.

Iron dosage is dependent on the child's blood values and the type of iron given. The child's response to iron is evaluated with reticulocyte counts and hemoglobin concentration. In iron deficiency anemia, a reticulocyte rise should occur within three days after starting iron therapy. It should continue to rise for eight to ten days. Hemoglobin levels rise about 1.5 grams every ten days in the early phase of treatment. The rate of increase decreases as normal levels are attained. It is important to continue iron therapy until body iron stores are replaced. This replenishing may take six months to one year.

In mild anemia, hemoglobin and hematocrit values will not change for ten to fourteen days after the beginning of treatment. After two weeks, the anemia is corrected quickly. Hemoglobin should be halfway back to normal in four to five weeks, and normal in two months. The hemoglobin *is* normal but body stores are *not* replenished. Iron must be continued for some children for six to twelve months. The need for replacing depleted iron and the reason for continual treatment must be stressed to the family. Explanations help to maintain the motivation needed for continuing therapy.

Because of the large number of iron-deficient persons, the wide use of therapy, and the easy accessibility of over-the-counter iron preparations for self-treatment, acute iron poisoning due to iron ingestion by children has become a national health problem. Ingestion of six ferrous sulfate tablets by a child can cause serious iron poisoning. The child ingesting excessive iron usually vomits within an hour after ingestion. The vomiting is followed by hypotension, tachypnea, cyanosis, coma, and death in a few hours. The first step in treating a child with suspected iron ingestion is to evacuate the stomach contents rapidly. Use syrup of ipecac, a nonprescription emetic, to induce vomiting, or place your finger in the back of the child's throat to stimulate vomiting. Another way to induce vomiting is an oral, tepid solution of baking soda and water. The bicarbonate ion in the baking soda helps to retard the iron absorption. Children who survive three to four days usually recover.

Vitamin B_{12} and Folic Acid

Deficiencies of folic acid or Vitamin B_{12} can impair the synthesis of DNA, resulting in the production of large, abnormal erythrocytes called *megaloblasts*. When the body lacks Vitamin B_{12} or folic acid, fewer red blood cells are produced, and the concentration of hemoglobin inside each megaloblast is less than normal. Since large reserves of Vitamin B_{12} exist in the body, several years pass before a deficiency develops, and Vitamin B_{12} deficiency in children is rare. Folic acid deficiency is far more common. Unlike Vitamin B_{12}, body reserves of folic acid are normally small, and dietary deficits quickly cause deficiency. A folic acid deficiency may result from inadequate intake, faulty absorption, or impaired utilization caused by the action of certain drugs that are folic acid antagonists, for example, methotrexate and Dilantin. Oral folic acid is given with favorable results.

Transfusions

Transfusions are given to restore blood volume and treat shock after acute sudden blood loss or to provide needed blood products, such as platelets or erythrocytes.

Blood Loss

When 15 to 20 percent of the circulating blood volume is suddenly lost (for example, following trauma, burns, or surgery), tachycardia, hypotension, and shock may develop, accompanied by weakness and restlessness. Whole-blood transfusions are given to restore blood volume and treat shock, usually at the rate of 20 milliliters for each kilogram of body weight. Plasma or plasma expanders may be used to sustain the child in shock until blood is available.

Slow, continual blood loss, which can occur with bleeding ulcers, ulcerative colitis, and certain neoplasms, causes anemia. Whole blood, plasma, or packed red blood cells are given.

Transfusions for Chronic Anemias

Transfusions are given to children with chronic anemias during an exacerbation, such as a low hemoglobin, an infection, or congestive heart failure (CHF). If CHF exists, or if the child receiving a transfusion is an infant, an exchange transfusion may be done. During this process, equal amounts of the child's blood are removed as transfused blood is added. To minimize heart stress due to the extra blood volume that must be circulated, packed red blood cells (prepared by removing most of the plasma from whole blood) are transfused. The amount and flow rate of packed cell transfusion depend on the child's condition and the reason for the infusion. A safe guideline for amount and flow rate is 15 milliliters of packed erythrocytes for each kilogram of body weight, at a flow rate of 10 to 15 drops a minute. It is best for blood to infuse over a three- to four-hour period. Be sure to check the infusion set for information on drops per milliliter because manufacturing companies differ, and there is no standard.

Nursing the Child During a Transfusion

Nursing responsibilities during a transfusion focus on the child's *safety* and *comfort*. A transfusion tends to be lengthy and tiring to child, family, and staff. Although blood transfusions are not reserved solely for emergency or life-sustaining care, they are used with discretion and administered with great care. Not only is a transfusion reaction a possibility during each transfusion, but the child with chronic anemia frequently has an overworked heart. This stressed heart may have difficulty coping with the added blood volume infused during the transfusion. For this reason, all transfusions are given slowly over a three- to four-hour period, and close observations are made on vital signs and general behavior.

Hospital policy should be followed during a transfusion. The following are guidelines:

1. Check and double check the donor's blood, making sure the ABO and Rh type are the same as the receiving child's. Verify all identifying information with another nurse. Make sure that the blood has not passed its expiration date.
2. Explain the procedure to the child and his family, allowing him to touch the tubing, tourniquet, and blood container.
3. Select a comfortable position (usually semi-Fowler's), and use a vein in the left arm if the child is right-handed, or vice versa. A large-gauge IV insert (19- or 21-gauge) facilitates blood flow. If restraints are necessary, refer to the Skills Manual.
4. Use a Y-tube infusion set, hanging a small bottle of normal saline. If the transfusion needs to be stopped permanently or temporarily, the patency of the vein can be maintained by fusing the saline. If the infusing cells are viscous and not infusing well, flush the IV line with the normal saline through the Y-connector.
5. Record the baseline temperature, pulse, respiration, and blood pressure *before* starting the infusion.
6. Note the exact time the infusion begins.
7. Since most transfusion reactions occur during the absorption of the first 50 cc of blood, stay with the child until 50 cc are infused. This may take thirty minutes or longer for a small child, and twenty to thirty minutes for a large, older child. Use this time to involve the child with coloring, painting, or other quiet activities, such as TV, games, or reading. This is a good time to re-explain the

purpose of the transfusion and the reason for frequent checking of vital signs. Tell both the parents and the child to report quickly unusual feelings, such as irritability, restlessness, pain, or discomfort (particularly back pain), rashes or changes in skin color, and chills.

8. Record vital signs every thirty minutes, noting any changes. Question the child and observe him for chills, fever, headache, dyspnea, and back pain. Check the infusion site for edema, pain, or redness of infiltration. Mix the blood gently two or three times during the transfusion to prevent packed cells from entering the blood stream first.
9. Do not add medications to a blood transfusion.
10. Observe and record the amount of intake and output.
11. Note the exact time the blood is completely infused. Flush the tubing with saline so that all blood enters the bloodstream. Tubing may hold as much as 20 milliliters of blood.

Transfusion Reactions

Adverse reactions occur in 2 to 5 percent of all transfusions, usually as a result of clerical or technical error, or limitations in the cross-matching procedure in the laboratory. The following steps should be taken immediately for a suspected transfusion reaction: 1) *stop the transfusion* (infuse the saline to keep the vein patent); 2) *obtain blood and urine samples;* 3) *notify the physician in charge.*

Hemolytic Reaction

A *hemolytic* reaction is caused by donor-recipient ABO incompatibility and is the *most dangerous* type of transfusion reaction. If incompatible blood mixes, antigens and antibodies combine, causing lysis of the red blood cells (see ch. 21). When the erythrocytes are destroyed, free hemoglobin is released and enters the kidneys, causing severe renal damage. The hemolytic reaction occurs quickly, usually within the first five or ten minutes of the transfusion. The signs of a hemolytic reaction are chills, headache, fever, tachycardia, chest pain, dyspnea, nausea, vomiting, facial flushing, apprehension, and backache.

Pyrogenic Reaction

The pyrogenic, or febrile, reaction is the *most common* type of transfusion reaction. It occurs when the donor's leukocytes are transfused into a child with antibodies directed against leukocytes. The antigen-antibody reaction releases pyrogens that produce fever and chills, usually starting about an hour after the infusion begins. These symptoms are indistinguishable from the serious hemolytic reaction. Antipyretics are given to treat this type of reaction. Later transfusions with leukocyte-pool red blood cells or frozen-washed red blood cells may prevent a recurrence of the pyrogenic reaction.

Allergic Reaction

The *allergic reaction* is common and usually does not progress to a lethal state. An allergic transfusion reaction can be caused by an antigen-antibody reaction in the child to allergens in the donor's blood. Assessment signs are itching, hives, edema, chills and wheezing, headache, a drop in blood pressure, and a weak thready pulse. If the reaction is severe, dyspnea and bronchospasms occur. Antihistamines are given for mild reactions, and epinephrine with or without cortisone is used for severe reactions.

Hypothermia Reaction

When chilled or cold blood is infused, a *hypothermic* reaction can occur. A hypothermic reaction can be avoided by using a warming coil for a rapid infusion, and by covering the child.

Latent complications of a blood transfusion include the transmission of an infection present in the donor's blood, such as serum hepatitis or syphilis. Each donor needs careful cross-matching and screening for allergy or infection to help prevent transfusion reactions.

Hemosiderosis

Repeated transfusions can lead to *hemosiderosis* or increased iron storages in the body. The child receiving frequent transfusions (some children with chronic hemolytic anemia receive a transfusion every three to four weeks) has added deposits of iron following the breakdown of transfused erythrocytes. The extra iron accumulates in the liver, pancreas, myocardium, and skin, causing heart failure, liver disease, and diabetes. Hemosiderosis is a problem associated with continual transfusions and may accompany *excessive* therapeutic iron dosages.

Platelet Transfusions

When red blood cells are removed from whole blood, the remaining plasma can be divided into platelets, clotting factors such as Factors VIII and IX (which will be discussed fully in chapter 25), immunoglobulins, and albumin. Platelet transfusions are given to children with low platelet counts (less than 10,000/cu mm) or for a child with active bleeding who has a dangerously low platelet count (less than 20,000/cu mm). The guidelines for administration of platelets are the same as those for a safe transfusion. Platelets are transfused rapidly and survive only a few days in the circulation, and their transfusion may have to be repeated frequently.

Occasionally, leukocyte concentrates are transfused, usually because of bone marrow suppression or failure. A special process termed pheresis was described in chapter 20. Pheresis extracts only the needed blood product from a donor, returning all remaining blood.

Functions of the Spleen

The spleen engulfs microorganisms, as well as imperfect or worn-out erythrocytes and platelets. The spleen then separates the hemoglobin from the fragmented erythrocyte, collecting the iron and globin for circulation back to the bone marrow and liver for future use. This efficient cleaning system of the spleen can promote a hemolytic anemia. Hemolysis is the premature destruction of erythrocytes. It can be caused by forces that enter the body such as toxins, certain chemicals or medicines, an incompatible blood transfusion, or an infection. Hemolysis also occurs when abnormal changes in the erythrocyte cause a shape or function change, making passage through the spleen difficult. If hemolysis continues, the erythrocyte population decreases, causing a hemolytic anemia. Hemolysis is frequently used to explain anemia. Always ask what is causing the hemolysis, and what type of hemolytic anemia exists. The answers will determine the nursing care.

Much of hemolysis occurs in the reticuloendothelial lining of the spleen. Since erythrocytes must be smooth and malleable to pass through the spleen, imperfectly shaped erythrocytes are caught and hemolyzed. If the spleen continually

Table 24–2. **Agents Associated with Hemolysis in G6-P-D Deficient Children**

Agent	*Examples*
Headache and cold medicines	APC tablets Super Anahist Empirin Bromo-Seltzer Stanback 4-Way Cold Tablets Anacin Aspirin (use an acetominophen preparation instead)
Constipation remedies	Black Drought
Prescription drugs	All sulfa drugs Furadantin, Furoxone, Furacin, Alta-fur Para-aminosalicylic acid (PAS) Vitamin K (water-soluble analogues)
Other chemicals	Naphthalene mothballs Chloramphenicol Quinine

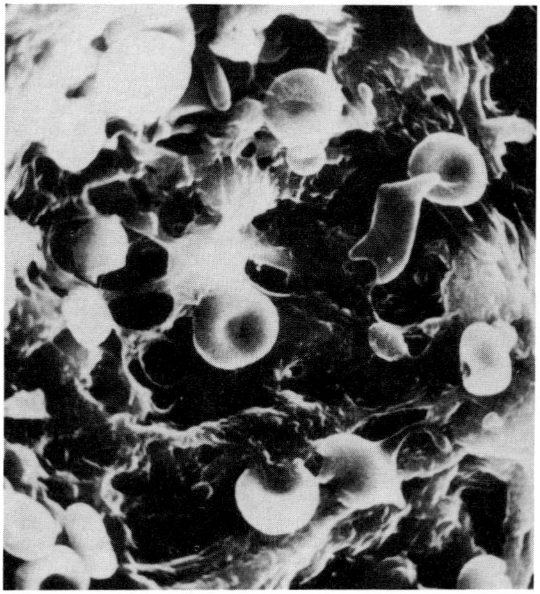

Figure 24–8. *Sickled red blood cells and normal red blood cells in the pulp of the spleen. The normal RBCs easily pass through the small openings in the spleen and return to the venous circulation, but the sickled RBCs are likely to be trapped in the spleen and will plung exit paths.* (From Barnhart, M.I., Henry, R.L., Lusher, J.M., Sickle Cell, A Scope Monograph, The Upjohn Company Kalamazoo, Mich., 1974.)

hemolyzes erythrocytes, it becomes congested with them and enlarges. This condition is called *splenomegaly*.

In sickle cell anemia, a chronic inherited hemolytic anemia (see Table 24–1), the spleen becomes plugged with abnormally shaped sickled erythrocytes. The small lumens of the spleen infarct, scar, and atrophy, resulting in functional asplenia. The reticuloendothelial elements of the spleen are bypassed, since they are plugged with sickled cells, and the child is liable to overwhelming infection (Figure 24–8).

The spleen may also suddenly pluck large numbers of sickled red blood cells from the circulation, resulting in hypovolemic shock. If this condition is not corrected quickly with transfusions, death results.

Splenectomy

A *splenectomy,* or surgical removal of the spleen, may be necessary for many reasons, including a rupture, tumor, or infection of the spleen. Certain chronic conditions, such as thrombocytopenia (ch. 25), improve after a splenectomy. Complications of several anemias are also treated with a splenectomy.

When preparing a child for a splenectomy, review chapter 2 and the general nursing considerations for preoperative and postoperative procedures. Blood transfusions may be administered if the spleen has ruptured and blood values need stabilization. The insertion of a gastric tube before surgery helps to keep the stomach deflated during the splenectomy.

Following a splenectomy, splenic defense action of bacterial phagocytosis is eliminated as it is during "functional asplenism." Bacteria previously removed are now free to multiply and cause infection. Since there is an increased susceptibility to pneumococcus meningitis after a splenectomy, particularly in young children, prophylactic penicillin is frequently given to reduce the incidence of bacterial infection.

Teach the family the early signs of infection and the measures necessary to minimize exposure to infectious microorganisms. Every child who has had a splenectomy should be routinely assessed for infection.

EXPLAINING ANEMIA

Anemia is a common word echoed daily in the newspaper, television, and radio. The word evokes little emotional impact; no tears are shed, pity felt, or doom predicted. The child with anemia looks very much like any other child; external body changes are minimal. Since most anemias develop slowly, the family adjusts to the child's fatigue, shortness of breath, and lethargy. Parents suddenly informed that their seemingly normal child has a health problem, and, if the anemia is inherited, that the disorder will be present for a lifetime, often feel confused, angry, and helpless. How could this have happened without someone knowing? What caused the anemia? Is there a cure? Will the child grow up, go to school, get married? Parents ponder many such questions when the diagnosis of anemia is explained. For most chronic, hemolytic anemias, there are no cures or medicines to increase blood counts or reverse symptoms. Care is specific to symptoms and supportive, with emphasis on prophylaxis and health maintenance. The child will always need hematologic evaluations, daily assessment of increasing anemia or infection, and special care during exacerbations. Families with anemic children are families in stress.

During health agency visits, it is commonly assumed that since the chronically anemic child is continually exposed to medical care, the family understands all aspects of the child's care. This is a dangerous assumption. Continually review the meaning of the child's anemia with the family. Discuss the disease, re-explaining its physiology and accompanying symptoms. Pamphlets, audiovisual aids, and group discussions are meaningful, supportive ways to evaluate the family's understanding and to tailor teaching information (see Figures 24–9A through D). Be knowledgeable, interested, and available to consult with the family about daily care needs and first aid for illness.

Parents of a child with an inherited anemia frequently agonize over whether or not to have more children. Awareness that one can pass a chronic, life-threatening disease to an offspring is frightening and guilt-producing. Both parents require support to make a decision about having more children. Offer support by allowing and providing an opportunity for parents to

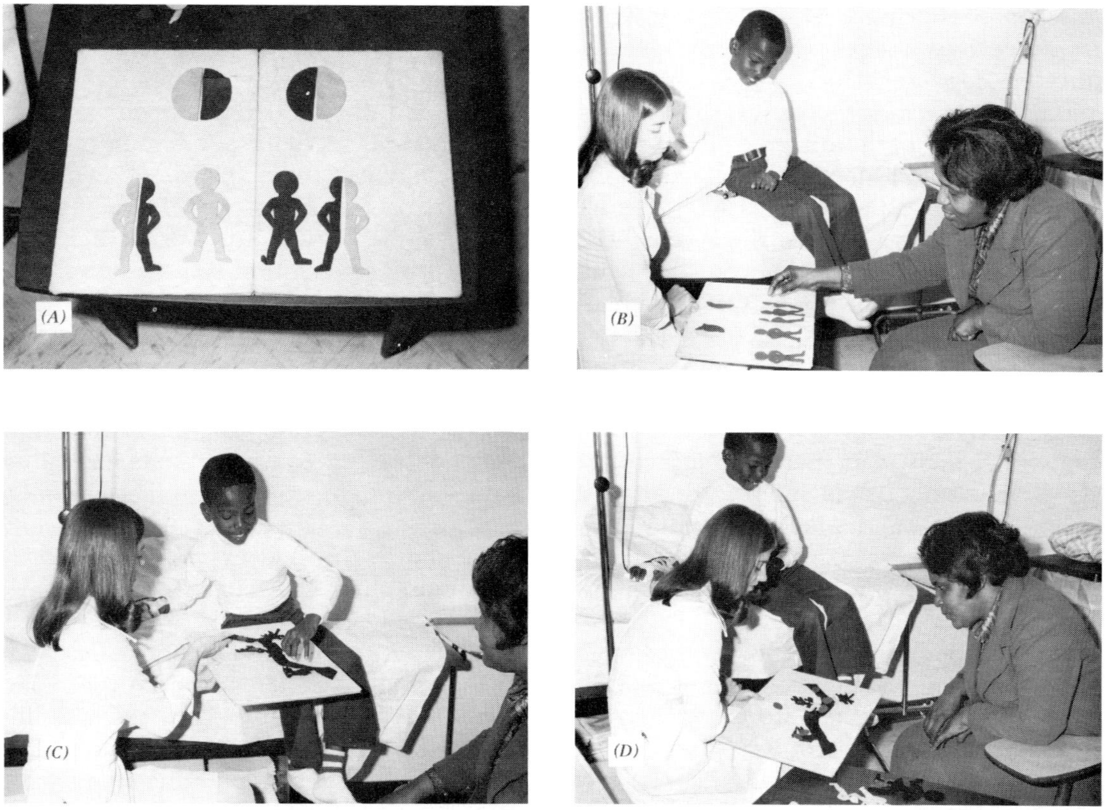

Figure 24–9. *(A) Use two plywood pieces attached with a hinge and covered with flannel to show how sickle cell anemia is inherited. The dark semicircles represent sickle hemoglobin, the light semicircles, normal hemoglobin. The circles represent persons with sickle cell trait, and the cut-out figures represent the possible hemoglobin types of each child conceived. (B) Change the semicircles to represent a person with normal hemoglobin mating with a person who has sickle cell trait; rearrange the cut-out figures to show the possible hemoglobin types of each pregnancy. (C) Felt is cut in the shape of a blood vessel; crescents represent sickled red blood cells that may jam and cause a sickle cell pain crisis. (D) Discussing pain crises leads to a discussion of how to manage crises.*

discuss their concerns and fears. Group parent meetings are one therapeutic means of offering information on how others have coped with family planning decisions. Providing information on various effective methods of contraception is another intervention that offers parents time to make a decision about having more children. Hematologic testing of infants born to parents with a known hereditary condition can be offered to aid in reducing anxiety.

When planning continual care for the child with a chronic anemia, include other nonmedical community professionals. For example, a conference with the parents, child, nurse, and teacher early in the school year can result in an understanding of the child's exercise needs and abilities, and the fact that anemia *does not* affect intelligence can be emphasized.

Children with chronic anemias frequently receive care in ambulatory health care facilities; the principles of continuity of care are important for optimal care, and are best expressed by using written and verbal correspondence between the acute care facility and community personnel.

SUMMARY

Oxygen, essential for respiration, is bound to hemoglobin within each erythrocyte and transported to every niche in the body. When normal erythrocyte production, destruction, and hereditary coding are changed, anemia can result. Anemias that are due to inherited abnormalities are congenital and lifelong; no cure exists. Deficiency anemias are not present at birth but are acquired due to inadequate intake of certain important compounds. Acquired immune anemias result from unexplained events which promote the body's destruction of its own cells.

Regardless of the cause, each anemic child lacks sufficient oxygen. When tissues are hypoxic, cardiac and respiratory rates change, muscles fatigue, and skin color changes. Anemia is diagnosed by studying the shape, size, color, volume, and total number of erythrocytes. The type and amount of hemoglobin and iron contained within each erythrocyte is classified by hemoglobin electrophoresis and assay test.

Some anemias can be treated with vitamins and minerals, food supplements, transfusions, or a splenectomy. Other inherited chronic anemias defy cures, and the care for these anemias is directed at symptoms, with emphasis on prevention of complications and health promotion. The anemic child is in stress and needs continual education and support to cope with his disease.

CLINICAL APPLICATION

During the past two years, Marie has intermittently complained of pain in her stomach, arms, legs, and back. The pain episodes have lasted several days, and then disappeared. However, this time the pain has not been relieved by rest, aspirin, or a heating pad. Yesterday, Marie refused to drink or eat, and today she was admitted for intravenous hydration and tests to determine the cause of her pain.

Although small for her age, Marie is an active three-year-old and her parents attribute the pain episodes to "growing pains." Admission hemoglobin and hematocrit levels are very low. When Marie's mother, Mrs. S., was told that Marie had anemia, and that additional blood tests and a hemoglobin electrophoresis are being done to help determine the cause of the anemia, she became extremely upset, voicing a fear that Marie has leukemia.

> Explain to Mrs. S. what a hemoglobin electrophoresis is, and the difference between anemia and leukemia. Reviewing the common problems of anemia, what specific questions will you ask Mrs. S. about Marie?

The electrophoresis result is hemoglobin SS. Mrs. S. is told that Marie has sickle cell anemia (SCA), an inherited chronic anemia due to abnormal hemoglobin. Presently, no cure exists and the anemia will always exist. After twenty-four hours of IV hydration, Marie is sitting up in bed, playing. When you ask Mrs. S. what she understands about SCA, she responds that a mistake must have been made about the SCA being inherited, since no one else in the family has SCA.

> Remembering that SCA is an autosomal recessive condition, explain to Mrs. S. why it is possible that no other family members have SCA. Also offer an explanation about sickle cell trait (SCT) to Mrs. S.

You explain to Mrs. S. that a cure or special medicines do not exist for SCA because the abnormal hemoglobin is inherited and present in every erythrocyte. When the red blood cells give up oxygen (air), their shape changes from a round flexible donut to a stiff curved sickle shape. The sickled red blood cells frequently become clumped together, blocking the passageway of tiny blood vessels. These masses of sickled cells stop blood from reaching cells that need oxygen. The sickled occlusions cause pain and discomfort and can happen anywhere in the body. These pain periods are common in persons with SCA. When Marie has a pain period, extra fluids, rest, and aspirin or acetaminophen are important treatments. Extra fluids help to prevent dehydration and further sickling and promote circulation through all vessels. If the pain is severe, or if Marie begins to vomit or refuses fluids, IV hydration is advisable. Although Marie's pain periods, or crises, are uncomfortable, they will subside in five to seven days. Each pain period is different. A severe pain crisis does not mean the next one will be equally severe.

It is important to be alert to pain episodes, especially following the stress of an illness. Pain crises may or may not be associated with fever. However, if Marie has a low grade fever (38°C) for more than two days or suddenly develops a high fever (39°–40°C), she should see a physician. Pain crises are not associated with increased anemia, are usually not serious, and frequently can be cared for at home.

Although not as common as pain crises, there are three other types of crises that a child with SCA may experience.

> Describe to Mrs. S. the needed medical care for an aplastic crisis, an acute sequestration crisis, and a hyperhemolytic crisis (see Table 24–1). Offer specific information on how she can distinguish these crises from a pain episode.

Mrs. S. asks about adding spinach, liver, and peanut butter to Marie's meals to build up Marie's hemoglobin, and extra naps to save her energy. She also inquires if Marie should be excused from outside play at school.

> Explain about activity for the anemic child. Discuss what is meant by a hemolytic anemia, and why extra protein and iron will not raise Marie's hemoglobin level.

Knowing that children with SCA are more prone to infection, offer measures to minimize infection and promote health.

Mrs. S. asks if Marie will be able to have children, and if they will all have SCA.

> Explain that women with SCA have conceived and delivered children, but that a pregnant woman with SCA is likely to have many problems, needing transfusions and medical attention.

Explain to Mrs. S. what the chances are of Marie's children having SCA or SCT.

Mrs. S. asks if SCA kills children. You explain that some children with SCA die because of complications, but many others live, grow up, and become active, working adults, some with families. Today, more information is known about SCA and the accompanying problems than ever before. It is important for Mrs. S. to plan a future for Marie, thinking about her individual needs for love and growth. Marie has a lifelong health problem that she can fully understand and care for with time. Her SCA will be a major consideration in her life, but equally important is how Marie feels about herself and her need for developing a healthy self-concept.

Review chapter 9, offering Mrs. S. suggestions on how to reinforce a positive body image and self-concept for Marie.

Bibliography

Barber, J.M., Stokes, L.G., Billings, D.M. *Adult and Child Care: A Client Approach to Nursing,* ed.2. St. Louis, C.V. Mosby Co., 1977.

Beck, W.S. (ed). *Hematology*. Cambridge, Mass., MIT Press, 1973.

Buickus, B. Administering Blood Components. *American Journal of Nursing* 79:937, 1979.

Cullins, L.C. Preventing and Treating Transfusion Reactions. *American Journal of Nursing* 79:935, 1979.

Gorst, D.W. Sickle Cell Disease. *Nursing Times* 72:1436, 1976.

Griesemer, D.A., Winkelstein, J.A., Luddy, R. Pneumococcal Meningitis in Patients with a Major Sickle Hemoglobinopathy. *Journal of Pediatrics* 92:82, 1978.

Kazak, A. Processing Blood for Transfusion. *American Journal of Nursing* 79:931, 1979.

McFarlane, J.M. Sickle Cell Diseases. *American Journal of Nursing* 77:1948, 1977.

———, Disturbances in the Oxygen Carrying Mechanisms, in Jones, D., Dunbar, C., Jirovec, M. (eds). *Medical Surgical Nursing.* New York, McGraw-Hill, 1978.

Powers, D., Schroeder, W.A., Vavaseur, J. et al. On the Birth of an Infant with Sickle Cell Anemia. *Hemoglobin* 1:409, 1977.

Rossman, M., Slavin, R., Taft, E. Pheresis Therapy: Patient Care. *American Journal of Nursing* 77:1135, 1977.

Scarlato, M. Blood Transfusion: What You Should Know and Do. *Nursing '78* 8:68, 1978.

Thomas, S. Transfusing Granulocytes. *American Journal of Nursing* 79:442, 1979.

Vaughan, V.C. and McKay, R.J. *Nelson's Textbook of Pediatrics,* ed. 10. Philadelphia, W.B. Saunders Co., 1975.

CHAPTER **25**

The Child with a Bleeding Disorder

BEHAVIORAL OBJECTIVES

After studying this chapter you will be able to:

- Contrast spontaneous and traumatic bleeding and discuss the differences in cause, appearance, and care.
- Design nursing care interventions that can prevent or minimize trauma and bleeding.
- Manage a bleeding episode.
- Identify different types of shock.
- Recognize early signs of shock, and begin appropriate nursing care.
- Explain common diagnostic tests that evaluate platelet and coagulation function.
- Discuss the uses, benefits, and problems of plasma concentrates.

TERMS AND CONCEPTS

Spontaneous bleeding
Traumatic bleeding
Thrombocytopenia
Hemorrhage
Hypovolemic shock
Cardiogenic shock
Distributive shock
Obstructive shock

When a finger is cut, vessels are torn; platelets are mobilized and cluster at the site of the wound. Plasma proteins quickly arrive and interact with factor compounds in a rapid series of events called coagulation. A sticky cot of fibrin is formed and healing begins. This is a normal process.

The child with a bleeding problem cannot respond to trauma quickly and efficiently. Because of a defect in the number or quality of platelets or a deficiency in one of the many crucial ingredients of coagulation, bleeding does not stop but continues, and blood may accumulate in joints and tissue. Bruises dot the child's body, and he experiences pain and fear. This chapter discusses the different types of bleeding, care intervention, special diagnostic tests, and treatment plans.

COMMON PROBLEMS AND NURSING INTERVENTIONS

Bleeding

Bleeding is termed *spontaneous* or *traumatic*. Spontaneous, or *purpuric* bleeding occurs in the microcirculation and involves the mucous membranes. Bleeding gums (gingival bleeding), nosebleeds (epistaxis), and gastrointestinal hemorrhages are examples of purpuric bleeding. Purpuric bleeding is usually caused by platelets that are not functioning normally, and may appear as small purplish, hemorrhagic spots (*petechiae*) dotting the child's body or as large hemorrhagic areas (*ecchymoses*). Purpuric bleeding is profuse but can be stopped permanently with pressure.

In contrast, *traumatic bleeding* (e.g., bleeding into joints (hemarthosis), hematuria, or deep intramuscular bleeding) results from injury to arterioles and small arteries. Massive subcutaneous bruises are common, and large hematomas follow injury. The bleeding may be delayed, not beginning until one to two hours after the initial trauma was experienced. Traumatic bleeding is difficult to stop and may begin again even after pressure has been applied. Defects in coagulation, such as hemophilia, are common causes of traumatic bleeding.

The type of bleeding is very important. If the bleeding is spontaneous, the child may have a disorder in the quantity or quality of his platelets. If bleeding is traumatic, however, the cause is usually a defect in the coagulation process. (Remember from chapter 21 that platelets are only one of the ingredients needed for coagulation.) Numerous crucial plasma factors are needed to make thrombin, a vital precursor of fibrin, the central component of the clot. A deficiency of just *one* plasma factor can cause traumatic bleeding; this is exactly what occurs in hemophilia (see Table 25–1).

Thrombocytopenia

Purpura is a group of disorders characterized by hemorrhagic rash, usually caused by a reduction in the number of platelets, a state called *thrombocytopenia*. Thrombocytopenia has many causes. It can be inherited, or it can be acquired following neonatal rubella or the antepartal ingestion of a thiazide diuretic. Acquired factors already discussed in previous chapters, such as aplastic anemia, bone marrow infiltration by a neoplasm, leukemia, and irradiation, and myelosuppressive drugs, such as methotrexate, can also decrease platelet production and result in thrombocytopenia and spontaneous purpuric bleeding. Nutritional deficiencies, such as those of folic acid or B_{12}, can also cause a reduction in platelet number. Cyclic thrombocytopenia occurs in normal women, causing platelet-count decreases of up to 20 percent during the last two weeks before menstruation. Each of these conditions causes a decreased production of platelets. Platelets, like erythrocytes, also may be destroyed at an increased rate as a result of certain bacterial, viral, and rickettsial infections. The accelerated platelet destruction results in thrombocytopenia.

A Bleeding History is Important

A bleeding history, noting the site and duration of bleeding, and preceding activity is essential for the diagnosis of any bleeding disorder. Do other family members have a similar problem? Has the child had a recent infection, has he received medications, or does he seem undernourished? Ask about blood in stools or urine; black, tarry stools indicate blood loss, as do nosebleeds. Record the size, location, and color of hemorrhagic lesions, asking when the lesions were first noticed. Although nursing care focuses on the specific type of bleeding problem (see Table 25–1), there are several measures to minimize bleeding that are applicable to all children with bleeding disorders.

The use of side rails for children of all ages guards against a fall from bed and possible injury, and their use is extremely im-

Table 25–1. **Common Bleeding and Coagulation Disorders in Children**

Name	*Description*	*Treatment*	*Special Nursing Considerations*
Acute idiopathic thrombocytopenia purpura (ITP)	An autoimmune response that frequently follows a mild respiratory or measles infection. The child, usually aged two to six, has petechial hemorrhages, purpura, and bleeding from the gums and gastrointestinal and urinary tracts. The platelet count is low, usually less than 100,000/ml, and platelet life is short, due to destruction of platelets in the spleen.	Eighty percent of affected children have spontaneous, permanent remissions within one to four months regardless of the treatment plan. If the child does not recover in six months, corticosteroids and/or splenectomy are used. Following a splenectomy, platelet counts increase greatly. Children with florid purpura are hospitalized and carefully observed. Platelet transfusions may be given but are of limited value because of the very short platelet life span.	Following diagnosis, most children are managed at home. During the severe thrombocytopenia stage (usually immediately after diagnosis), offer the parents instructions on ways to minimize bleeding. For example, restrict the young infant's activity to a crib or playbed lined with bumpers. The older crawling infant and toddler need extra padding at the knees, ankles, and other pressure areas. Sewing extra fabric on to clothing at these sites affords sufficient protection. Have child wear socks and long pants regardless of the weather. Temporarily stop tree climbing, bike riding, or other possibly abrasive play. Instruct parents to report black tarry stools, hematuria, or nosebleeds to the physician. Weekly platelet counts are necessary until the counts return to normal.
Hemophilia	A hereditary sex-linked recessive coagulation disorder caused by a functional deficiency of a certain plasma clotting factor. Bleeding is prolonged, but is no faster than in a normal child. Hemophilia is passed from an unaffected carrier	Depends on site of bleeding: For *minor* lacerations, apply firm manual pressure or a pressure dressing to the cut or abrasion. Apply ice bags to stimulate vasoconstriction. Immobilize the affected area to prevent clot dislodgement. If the above	Five to 20 percent of children develop an inhibitor (antibody) to the needed factor and their bodies therefore destroy infused factors; special management therapy is needed for these children. Allergic reactions can occur during factor

mother to her male affected offspring (see Figure 3–4). Hemophilia occurs in 1 of every 10,000 births. There are two main types of hemophilia: *Classical hemophilia, or hemophilia A* (Factor VIII deficiency), and *Christmas disease, or hemophilia B* (Factor IX deficiency). Hemophilia is classified as *mild, moderate,* or *severe* according to the amount of Factor VIII or IX present: the child with *severe* hemophilia has *less than 1 percent* of the deficient factor; the child with *moderate* hemophilia has *5 percent or more* of the deficient factor; the child with *mild* hemophilia has *25 to 50 percent* of the deficient factor. (Normal values for Factor VIII are 60 to 120 percent; normal values for Factor IX are 60 to 130 percent.)

measures do not stop the bleeding in 15 minutes, administration of factor concentrate is necessary. For *severe* bleeding (e.g., joint bleeding, hemarthrosis), infuse the deficient clotting factor (several clotting factor concentrates are available for hemophilia A and hemophilia B; cryoprecipitate is *one*). Prophylactic infusions are given to some children to prevent hemorrhage or to decrease existing problems. For all bleeding: the earlier the treatment, the better. If treatment is given *before* swelling and limitation of joint mobility, the amount of pain and injury is decreased.

concentrate infusion. Observe for wheezing, pruritus, flushing, or urticaria. Benadryl or epinephrine is used to treat allergic reactions. Avoid drugs that increase bleeding tendencies or prolong bleeding time, e.g., aspirin, glyceryl guaiacolate (contained in many cough syrups), phenacetin, phenothiazines, and Indocin. Teach parents and child to identify early signs of *serious bleeding,* which are severe pain and swelling of muscles or joints that limit movement; a serious or hard blow to the head; swelling in the tissues of the neck and/or floor of the mouth; severe abdominal pains; hematuria; and melena. Superficial bruises and cuts *rarely* result in serious bleeding and need mild laceration treatment only. Life-threatening complications do occur. The most common are airway obstruction caused by hemorrhage into neck or pharynx; intestinal obstruction caused by bleeding into intestinal walls; nerve compression with paralysis caused by hemorrhage into deep tissue; intracranial bleeding with seizures. Hemophilia is a frightening condition; both parents and child need continual support and help. Offer referral to the local chapter of the national Hemophilia Foundation.

(continued)

Table 25–1. *(Continued)*

Name	*Description*	*Treatment*	*Special Nursing Considerations*
Diffuse intravascular coagulation (DIC), or consumption coagulation	An acute bleeding syndrome occurring when certain illnesses introduce substances into the circulation that begin or speed up the intravascular use of clotting factors and platelets. This rapid consumption leads to hemorrhage and widespread deposits of fibrin thrombi in small blood vessels as coagulation factors are depleted. Serious bacterial and viral infections, neoplasms, tissue damage caused by burns or trauma, hemolytic transfusion reaction, and snakebites can introduce substances capable of beginning DIC. The DIC causes bleeding and/or hemorrhage; blockage of capillary flow in an organ, causing tissue ischemia necrosis; damage to erythrocytes, causing hemolytic anemia.	Identify and control the mechanisms (e.g., infection or burns) that triggered the DIC. Administer heparin to stop clotting although it may worsen bleeding. Replace depleted factors (e.g., fibrinogen, platelets, etc.); however, replaced factors offer fresh ingredients for new fibrin formation. Provide supportive care. Provide oxygenation. Restore blood volume. Monitor vital signs with special attention to urinary output.	Any severely ill child may develop DIC. Any of the following may indicate DIC: a bleeding tendency (e.g., purpura, or oozing from puncture sites); pallor or jaundice caused by an acute hemolytic anemia; shock; evidence of thrombi and emboli in major organs (e.g., respiratory distress, hematuria and renal shutdown, coma, convulsions, gastrointestinal distension, and ileus).

portant to children with bleeding problems. Avoid intramuscular injections when possible. When these children need injections, select the needle of the smallest gauge possible and apply firm pressure for five minutes following the injection. When restraining the child for procedures, support the extremities to avoid trauma. Use a soft-bristled brush for oral hygiene in order to preserve delicate tissue. (Chapter 20 describes additional preventative measures for the child with thrombocytopenia.)

Bleeding Episodes

When external bleeding occurs, first assure the child and family that it can be controlled. Apply firm, steady pressure to the bleeding area. Elevate the bleeding area so that it is higher than the heart in order to decrease blood pressure in the vessels and to allow for vasoconstriction. Ice also speeds up vasoconstriction and should be applied. Carefully immobilize the bleeding area to prevent clot dislodgement. If the bleeding site is a puncture wound, apply a pressure bandage. When giving analgesics for pain caused by bleeding remember that aspirin affects normal platelet function and prolongs bleeding time. A nonaspirin analgesic, such as an acetaminophen preparation, is preferable. Keep the traumatized area clean because blood is an excellent medium for bacterial growth. If these first aid measures do not stop the bleeding within 15 minutes, consult a physician. Do not persist unassisted.

Hemorrhage

A *hemorrhage* is a large blood loss from a blood vessel. The blood loss may be *internal* or *external*. As was discussed in chapter 21, blood is the body's transportation system, responsible for delivering nutrients, chemicals, and oxygen to cells and for picking up cellular waste products. Without this pick-up and delivery system, life is halted. The heart, brain, and kidneys are especially sensitive to oxygen loss and may be permanently damaged following three to five minutes of hypoxia. When blood is lost, oxygen delivery is decreased. If the blood loss is from arterial vessels, the blood is bright red and spurts out; if the hemorrhage is from a vein, the blood is dark and flows slowly from the bleeding site. If the hemorrhage is internal, signs and symptoms are related to fluid and oxygen loss; the child is apprehensive, restless, thirsty and pale; respiration and pulse rates are rapid; and the skin is cold and moist. Internal bleeding can be stopped only by surgical intervention.

Bleeding from external or peripheral vessels is stopped by elevation and the application of pressure and cold. Elevation of the bleeding site decreases the flow of blood in the area. Pressure closes the bleeding vessel sources. Apply pressure with an open hand or sterile dressing. The application of a tourniquet is a last resort since it may cause ischemia and even the loss of a limb. If a tourniquet must be applied, place it as close to the wound as possible and secure it tightly. Note the exact time the tourniquet was applied, and leave it in place until additional medical help arrives. Place the child who is bleeding in a supine position to provide as much circulation as possible to brain cells. Some authorities recommend a Trendelenburg position, in which the head is lower than the legs, to increase blood supply to the head and trunk. However, this position may increase respiratory effort, and the heart will be forced to exert more force to pump blood against gravity into the kidneys. Venous return from the head is also stifled. Therefore, place the child in a modified Trendelenburg with only the legs elevated; this reduces some of the problems of a Trendelenburg position while taking advantage of gravity to enhance arterial blood flow to the brain and the return of venous blood from the trunk and lower limbs. Keep the child warm by covering him with blankets. A blood transfusion is usually given; however, until the blood is ready for transfusion, plasma or other fluids may be given to expand blood volume and raise blood pressure.

Shock

When the circulation of blood is inadequate to meet the metabolic demands of tissue, the child goes into physiologic shock. Shock is usually caused by a *decrease in blood volume* or a *redistribution of the blood within the body*. There are several types and many classification systems of shock. Characteristically, shock is categorized according to the cause rather than to the underlying problem. In recent years, however, shock has been classified in four categories, each representing a different circulatory problem.

Hypovolemic Shock

Hypovolemic shock occurs when the blood volume is too low to perfuse the body with oxygen. Hemorrhage, plasma loss due to burns or inflammation, and electrolyte losses arising from diarrhea and dehydration are common causes of hypovolemic shock.

Cardiogenic Shock

Cardiogenic shock is pump failure; the heart cannot circulate the needed volume of intravascular fluid. Its causes include severe heart failure from any cause, and cardiac arrhythmias.

Distributive Shock

Distributive shock is an abnormality in the distribution of blood and may be caused by bacterial toxins (*endotoxins*), barbiturate overdose, or a central nervous system (CNS) injury. A barbiturate overdosage can depress the CNS, causing loss of vessel tone. As a result, vessels may dilate, and hypotension ensues, resulting in a decrease of tissue perfusion. Endotoxins circulating in the blood can cause small vessels to dilate, causing pooling of blood into capillary beds. Less blood is returned to the heart for processing, and the child is hypotensive; survival depends on proper antibiotic therapy for the primary infection.

Obstructive Shock

Obstructive shock is any condition that interferes with blood flow (e.g., pulmonary embolus and vena cava compression).

Signs and symptoms of shock are evident when blood losses approach 20 to 40 percent of total volume. Regardless of the type of shock or cause, the effects of decreased blood volume are uniform. The child in shock has a reduction in venous blood return, a decreased cardiac output, and reduced arterial pressure. The child responds to shock by using all available resources to restore adequate circulation. The adrenal medulla secretes epinephrine and norepinephrine that cause vasoconstriction and an increase in cardiac output. In addition, peripheral veins constrict emptying their blood into the circulation. To save body fluids, increased amounts of antidiuretic hormone (ADH) and aldosterone are secreted. Coronary and cerebral vessels dilate so that blood flow to the brain is improved. Fluids shift from interstitial to capillary spaces to increase plasma volume and help maintain an adequate blood pressure, venous return, and cardiac output. These forms of adaptation enable the cells to extract more oxygen from blood and maximize its use. Simultaneously, the heart and respiratory rates increase to aid oxygenation. These are some of the forces that work to reverse shock. This massive effort by the body to adapt and to respond to shock and to conserve vital organs with compensatory mechanisms, characterizes *reversible shock*, that is, any kind of shock producing changes that are not fatal and that can be corrected by treatment.

Complications of Shock

If shock continues, the reduced blood volume causes cells to be deprived of oxygen and nutrients. With oxygen in short supply, cells are forced to use chemical reactions for energy that do not require oxygen, a process called *anaerobic metabolism*. However, anaerobic metabolism leads to metabolic acidosis. The child with metabolic acidosis has an imbalance in the body's crucial acid-base balance. Prolonged acidosis leads to coma and death.

Lack of oxygen to the brain causes lethargy, restlessness, anxiety, and personality changes. The child's level of consciousness varies. The sluggish blood flow to vital brain centers may cause changes in perception and coordination with possible paralysis and *aphasia* (inability to speak).

Vasoconstriction in the systemic circulation blocks blood flow to the intestines, depriving the bowel cells of oxygen and leading to necrosis of the tissue. Prolonged vasoconstriction of the large vessels to the liver, for example, impair the liver's ability to to detoxify substances. In addition, the kidneys cannot adequately filter out waste substances, a state that further adds to the amount of toxic products in the body.

Lack of oxygen and nutrients, combined with the accumulation of toxic substances, severely impairs vital organ functions. If compensatory mechanisms fail, the reduced blood flow leads to heart failure, which in turn leads to less cardiac output and a further decrease in blood pressure. If not corrected quickly, the decreased cardiac output, arterial pressure, and tissue perfusion lead to death.

Immediate care for shock lies in the early recognition of its initial signs and symptoms. Signs of cerebral anoxia (e.g., restlessness, anxiety, and personality changes) appear long before a change in vital signs. A decrease in blood pressure and heart rate is a sign of *advanced* shock.

The child in shock will have physical characteristics that correspond to the cause of the shock. For example, the child in distributive shock caused by bacterial toxins will be febrile and flushed. The child with hypovolemic shock is often pale or ashen and may be shivering because of peripheral vasoconstriction.

Carefully note the vital signs. The apical pulse will be rapid initially but will become slower as shock progresses. The respirations will be rapid and shallow because of accumulations of carbon dioxide, which stimulate respiration rate. If heart failure is occurring, the child may have a cough, and fluid may be heard in the lungs. Hypotension is not usually noted until 15 to 20 percent of the blood volume is lost. When changes occur in blood pressure, both the systolic and diastolic pressures decrease.

The treatment for shock is directed to:

1. Maintaining arterial blood pressure;
2. Supplementing blood volume;
3. Ensuring blood flow;
4. Increasing oxygen consumption;

5. Providing calories and nutrients for cellular metabolism.

Oxygen and intravenous fluids and drugs are begun with close attention to vital signs and urinary output. Urine output for infants and children should be 10 to 20 milliliters an hour.

Since the skin may be cold and moist because of peripheral vasoconstriction, use blankets to keep the child warm but not so warm that he will perspire and lose fluids. If the child can drink, offer warm fluids to help elevate his body temperature. Both elevated temperature and chills increase metabolism and the need for oxygen. Each degree of fever increases the child's respiratory rate by about four breaths a minute. Intake, output, and vital signs are crucial and must be monitored on a regular basis.

COMMON DIAGNOSTIC TESTS AND NURSING IMPLICATIONS

A normal platelet count is 150,000 to 300,000 platelets/cu mm of blood. Platelet counts of less than 50,000/cu mm may be associated with hemorrhagic phenomena. Counts of less than 10,000/cu mm may be life-threatening. When a platelet bleeding problem is suspected, platelets are counted and studied. A bone marrow aspiration is done to determine the quantity of platelet production. A bleeding time (BT) is a simple technique used to evaluate qualitative platelet disorders. Bleeding time is determined by placing a puncture wound 2.5 millimeters deep on the inner surface of the forearm after a blood pressure cuff has been placed on the arm and the pressure maintained at 40 mm Hg. The blood is blotted at 30-second intervals until the flow ceases; a normal bleeding time is three to six minutes. If the platelet count is normal, prolongation of the BT indicates that platelet function is abnormal because of congenital or acquired abnormalities.

When a defect in coagulation (e.g., hemophilia) is suspected, standard coagulation tests are done to determine the specific disorder. The results of tests that measure platelet numbers and function, such as a platelet count, bleeding time, platelet adhesiveness, prothrombin time, and fibrinogen concentration, are all *normal* for the child with hemophilia. This is to be expected, since the hemophiliac child's platelets are normal in quantity and function, but he lacks a factor necessary for coagulation. As will be recalled from chapter 21, several factors must be present to form a clot. The whole blood clotting time is greatly prolonged in severe hemophilia but is *normal* in mild hemophilia. The test most sensitive for identifying low levels of factor VIII is the partial thromboplastin time (PTT). This simple test can detect levels of factor VIII below 30 percent of normal. Additional factor assays may also be done.

Extensive data is collected about the family history, the child's medical history, the mother's prenatal history, and the daily functioning of the child. The entire diagnostic process is stressful for child and family; repeated venipunctures are traumatizing and contribute to blood loss. When a diagnosis of a bleeding problem is explained to the family, intense emotions usually result. Seek to minimize trauma and maximize comfort during the entire diagnostic ordeal.

COMMON TREATMENTS AND NURSING IMPLICATIONS

Platelet Transfusion

Because of their very short life span (eight to ten days), platelets are not routinely given for bleeding disorders although they are used as emergency treatment for severe purpura or for life-sustaining measures.

Plasma Concentrates

The necessary factors for coagulation are contained in the plasma. If the child has a deficiency of a certain factor, such as in hemophilia, treatment consists of replacing the deficient factor.

From 1950 to 1965, fresh frozen plasma was the primary treatment for persons with hemophilia. Because of the low concentration of clotting factors in plasma, large volumes of it had to be given to control bleeding. This practice was dangerous since the large volumes of plasma caused an excessive volume of circulating blood, a condition that can lead to congestive heart failure. In 1966, a plasma concentrate, *cryoprecipitate*, was introduced and began to be used to replace fresh frozen plasma. By 1970, high potency plasma concentrates became available. Since only very small amounts of the high potency concentrates are needed, they are given by syringe. The cost of these concentrates is extremely high, however. It is not unusual for a child with hemophilia to need thousands of dollars worth of plasma concentrates in one year. Such large sums represent a financial burden to the family, the institution, and the community.

For some children with extensive muscle or joint degeneration, or children whose bleeding cycle is very frequent, prophylactic concentrates are given on a fixed schedule of two or three times a week. This represents an added financial problem. In order to help defray this added expense, to decrease the use of medical facilities, to improve school attendance, and to decrease the chronic problems associated with frequent bleeding, a large number of children with hemophilia are receiving their clotting factors at home, with assistance from a family member. Families with an interest in home therapy need a thorough evaluation by the health team, with all positive and negative aspects of home care presented. Possible dangers of home transfusions include poor long-term care, improper handling of materials and possible sepsis, wrong dosage, damage to veins, serious transfusion reaction, and delay or omission of therapy. If a decision is made by staff and family for home care, make sure that trained personnel will be available for technical assistance as well as for continued emotional support.

Summary

Bleeding may be spontaneous or traumatic. Spontaneous, or purpuric, bleeding is frequently caused by a lack of platelets (thrombocytopenia). Spontaneous bleeding occurs as nose or gum bleeds and is usually profuse but can be stopped with pressure. Traumatic bleeding produces large bruises, frequently involving joints or muscles, and is difficult to stop; the cause is usually a deficiency of a coagulation factor. Diagnostic tests determine whether the bleeding is caused by a platelet or by coagulation problem.

When large amounts of blood are lost, the child hemorrhages. The hemorrhage may be external or internal and must be managed quickly. External hemorrhage is treated with pressure, elevation, and cold. If the circulatory flow of blood is inadequate to perfuse oxygen and meet metabolic needs, shock occurs. There are several types of shock, each caused by a reduction in the volume of circulating fluids or a redistribution of circulating fluids within the body.

Bleeding, hemorrhage, and shock are potential problems of the child with a bleeding disorder. Care must center on minimizing trauma and on quick intervention when bleeding occurs.

Bibliography

Barber, J.M., Stokes, L.G., Billings, D.M. *Adult and Child Care*, ed. 2. St. Louis, C.V. Mosby Co., 1977.

Boutaugh, M. and Patterson P.C.: Summer Camp for Hemophiliacs. *American Journal of Nursing* 77:1288, 1977.

Boutaugh, M. and Patterson, P.C. Hemophilia: The Disease. *American Journal of Nursing* 77:1289, 1977.

Inwood, M. Aids for Hemophilia Children on a Self Infusion Program. *Journal of Pediatrics* 92:78, 1978.

Roberts, F.B. *Review of Pediatric Nursing*, ed. 2. St. Louis, C.V. Mosby Co., 1978.

Reardon, N. Idiopathic Thrombocytopenic Purpura. *Nursing Times* 72:980, 1976.

Sergis, E. and Hilgartner, M. Hemophilia, in O'Connor, A.B. (ed). *Nursing of Children and Adolescents*. New York, American Journal of Nursing Company, 1975.

Williams, W.J., Beutler, E., Ersler, A.J., Rundles, R.W. *Hematology*. New York, McGraw-Hill, 1972.

Wintrobe, M. *Clinical Hematology*. Philadelphia, Lea and Febiger, 1975.

SECTION FIVE

Mobility

CHAPTER **26**

Mobility

BEHAVIORAL OBJECTIVES

After studying this chapter you will be able to:

- Identify and discuss the basic parts and functions of the nervous system.
- Identify and discuss the basic parts and functions of the musculoskeletal system.
- Explain how the musculoskeletal system and the nervous system act to produce purposeful movements.

TERMS AND CONCEPTS

Mobility
Muscle contraction
Purposeful movement
Central nervous system
Cerebrum
Cerebellum
Brain stem
Spinal cord
Meninges
Dura mater
Pia mater
Arachnoid membrane
Cerebrospinal fluid
Epiphyseal plate
Skeletal muscle
Cardiac muscle
Visceral muscle
Ligaments
Tendons
Cartilage
Joints
Epiphyses
Voluntary muscles
Involuntary muscles

Jim, aged three, stoops over, grasps a red block, and gingerly places it atop his tower. To accomplish this seemingly simple task, Jim must *extend* (straighten) his fingers, then *flex* (bend) them. The degree of finger extension depends on the size of the block and the force of flexion on the weight and consistency of the block. At the same time, Jim's waist, elbow, and shoulder extend, and his trunk inclines forward. His shoulder must remain stabilized to support the weight on his aim and of the block. Jim manages all these motions while maintaining an upright posture. Jim's exact movements depend on information received from his senses about the distanct of the block from him and the direction in which it lies. However, none of these considerations concerns Jim, who has been thinking and talking about the kind of sandwich he wants for lunch during the entire operation.

An intact musculoskeletal system and nervous system are needed for *purposeful movement.* This chapter discusses the main parts and functions of the musculoskeletal and nervous systems, and alterations in normal *mobility*.

THE NERVOUS SYSTEM

The *nervous system* is composed of the *central nervous system* (CNS) and the *peripheral nervous system.* The CNS includes the *brain, spinal cord,* and surrounding *membranes.* The peripheral nervous system consists of nerves that connect the CNS with the rest of the body. Included in the peripheral nervous system are 12 pairs of *cranial nerves,* 31 pairs of *spinal nerves,* and *autonomic nerves.* Nerve tissue is made of *neurons* (nerve cells), which can be stimulated to conduct impulses to body cells. To produce movement, motor neurons are stimulated to conduct impulses to muscle cells.

The brain has three sections: the *cerebrum,* the *cerebellum,* and the *brain stem* (Figure 26–1). The cerebrum is the largest part of the brain and is divided into right and left *hemispheres* (halves). Each hemisphere is further divided into four *lobes: frontal, parietal, temporal,* and *occipital.* The cerebrum can interpret sensations, coordinate voluntary actions, and exert control over many reflex actions. In addition, the cerebrum can retain, modify, and reuse information. The cerebrum is the physical locus of memory and knowledge. The cerebellum, located between the cerebrum and brain stem, coordinates muscle activity and is responsible for balance and posture.

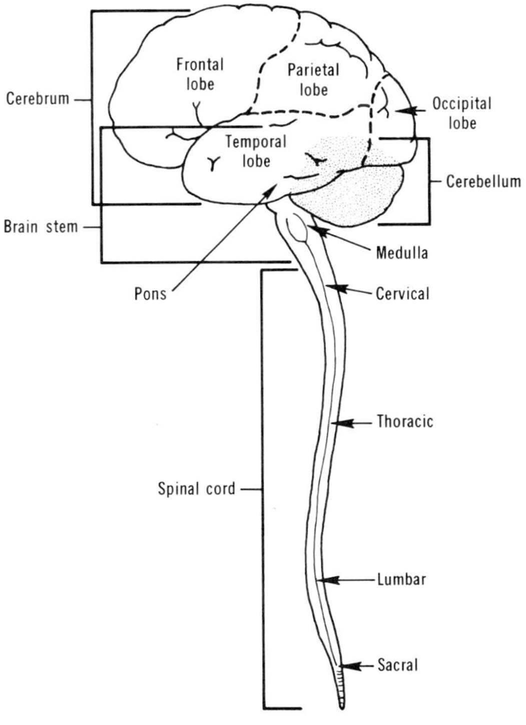

Figure 26–1. *A lateral view of the central nervous system.* (Adapted from L.L. Langley et al., Dynamic Anatomy and Physiology, 4th ed., McGraw-Hill Book Company, New York, 1974.)

The *brain stem,* or medulla oblongata, is a continuation of the spinal cord and contains vital centers for the regulation of respirations, heartbeat, and vasomotor activity. Reflexes such as coughing, vomiting, sneezing, and yawning are controlled by the brain stem. The *pons,* the superior portion of the brain stem, connects the two halves of the cerebellum and contains conduction pathways between the brain stem and cerebrum.

The spinal cord, located in the cerebral canal, is the site at which 31 pairs of spinal nerves originate. The spinal cord is protected by the bony vertebral column and by *meninges* (coverings). Special tracts in the spinal cord carry sensory impulses to the brain; other tracts in the cord transmit motor impulses from the brain. Most of the functions of locomotion are provided by the spinal cord and brain stem; the cerebrum controls these functions according to the desires of the person. In other words, to return to the example of Jim at play, he uses his cerebrum to decide which block to pick up next, which direction to move in, when to stop moving, and where to place the block. As the rote actions of muscle bending and straightening are accomplished by messages sent from the spinal cord and brain stem to muscle cells, the cerebrum is free for thinking.

Three coverings surround the brain: the *dura mater,* the *arachnoid membrane,* and the *pia mater.* Each of these coverings are continuous with the meningeal coverings of the spinal cord. The spaces between the coverings are called the *subdural space* and the *subarachnoid space. Cerebrospinal fluid* (CSF) is in the subarachnoid space and is produced in the two lateral ventricles. It functions as a fluid cushion for the brain and spinal cord against possible trauma. The fluid is under pressure and is constantly being produced and circulated. The path of the CSF is shown in Figure 26–2. Cerebrospinal fluid flows from the lateral ventricles through the foramen of Monro into the third ventricle, through a narrow canal called the aqueduct of Sylvius, to the fourth ventricle. Leaving the fourth ventricle, the CSF flows into the subarachnoid space via the foramens of Magendie and Luschka. In addition to providing protection, CSF continually bathes the brain and spinal cord with nutrients, and carries off waste products from nerve cells.

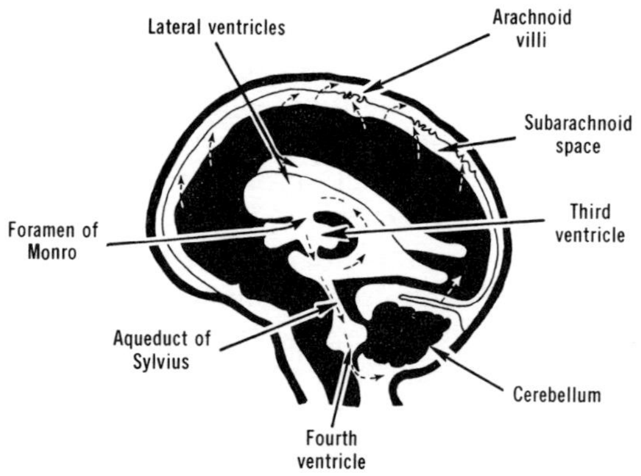

Figure 26–2. *The normal circulatory path of cerebrospinal fluid.*

THE MUSCULOSKELETAL SYSTEM

The *skeletal system* consists of *bones* and *joints* that together form the *skeleton,* which supports and protects body parts. Bones provide rigid support for the body frame. They serve as storage sites of minerals, such as calcium, phosphorus, and magnesium, and produce blood cells. Bones consist of a *diaphysis,* or shaft, and an *epiphysis,* or end (see Figure 26–3). Epiphysal cells are subject to growth hormone regulation by the anterior pituitary. Bone growth occurs at the *epiphyseal plate*. Bones can grow while continuing their other functions.

Ligaments and *tendons* connect bones to contiguous structures. Ligaments attach bones to one another, and tendons attach muscle to bone. Both ligaments and tendons are made of very strong fibrous strands of tissue termed *fibrous connective* tissue. This same tissue covers muscles. At the end of each bone is *cartilage,* an opaque

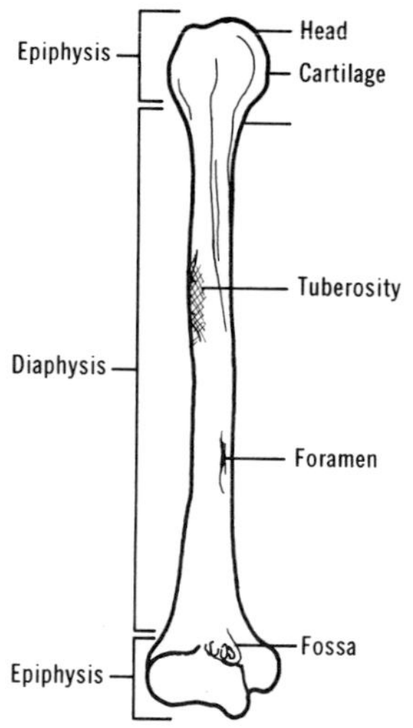

Figure 26–3. *A typical long bone.*

white tissue that is made of a firm rubbery material called *matrix*. Cartilage cushions bony prominences and offers protection against stress. For this reason, cartilage is ideally suited for its placement between the spinal vertebra. Except for the bones of the skull and face, most bone is cartilage that has been hardened by the deposits of calcium in the matrix.

Two very important substances regulate the formation of bone—Vitamin D and parathyroid hormone. Vitamin D aids the absorption of calcium and phosphate from the digestive tract, and parathyroid hormone regulates the concentration of calcium in body fluids. Calcium phosphate is the primary determinant of proper bone density.

Mechanical stress aids bone formation; inactivity favors bone dissolution. For this reason, children with fractures of the weight-bearing bones are usually put in traction. Traction supplies the mechanical stress that facilitates bone healing while the child is inactive. Of course, traction also helps to keep bone fragments in proper alignment.

The *marrow* inside all bones is called *reticuloendothelial tissue*. Marrow is red or yellow. Red marrow forms erythrocytes, granular leukocytes, and platelets. In addition, it destroys worn out erythrocytes and some foreign materials. Yellow marrow contains fat and is used for fat storage.

The 206 bones of the body are classified into four groups according to their shape. *Long bones* are found in the extremities. Most bone problems in children involve the long bones. If the growth area (i.e., the epiphyseal plate) is injured, growth may stop, be stimulated, or become irregular. *Short bones* are located in the ankle and wrist. *Flat bones* are found in the skull, ribs, scapula, and sternum. *Irregular bones* are in the vertebra and face. Special terms are used to refer to markings found on the surfaces of bones. For example, *foramen* means "hole"; *fossa*, a depression; *meatus*, a tube-shaped opening; and *sinus*, a cavity or space.

A *joint* is the point at which bones come together. Joints are classified according to the degree and variety of movement they permit. Joints accomplish several types of movement, including *flexion* and *extension*, which decrease and increase the angles between bones. Joints *abduct* (draw a body part *away from* the midline), *adduct* (move a part toward the midline), and *rotate* (turn a part on an axis). Figure 26–4 illustrates each of these movements.

Muscle

Muscle is made of tissue and has the special ability to contract. By contracting, muscle can provide external movement of body parts for locomotion, and internal movement for the functioning of body organs.

There are three types of muscle tissue: *skeletal muscle, visceral muscle,* and *cardiac muscle.* Skeletal muscles, attached to the skeleton, receive their nerve stimuli from cerebrospinal nerves and are voluntarily controlled. They are referred to as *voluntary muscles*. Skeletal muscles contract only in response to stimulation. In the event that nerves to the skeletal muscles become diseased or injured so that impulses cannot reach the muscles, the muscles cannot contract and are paralysed. Visceral muscle is found in walls of intestines, blood vessels and other internal structures. Cardiac muscle is found in the heart. Both visceral and cardiac muscle are *involuntary* and have the inherent ability to contract rhythmically.

When a muscle contracts, its cells become shorter and thicker. Muscle contrac-

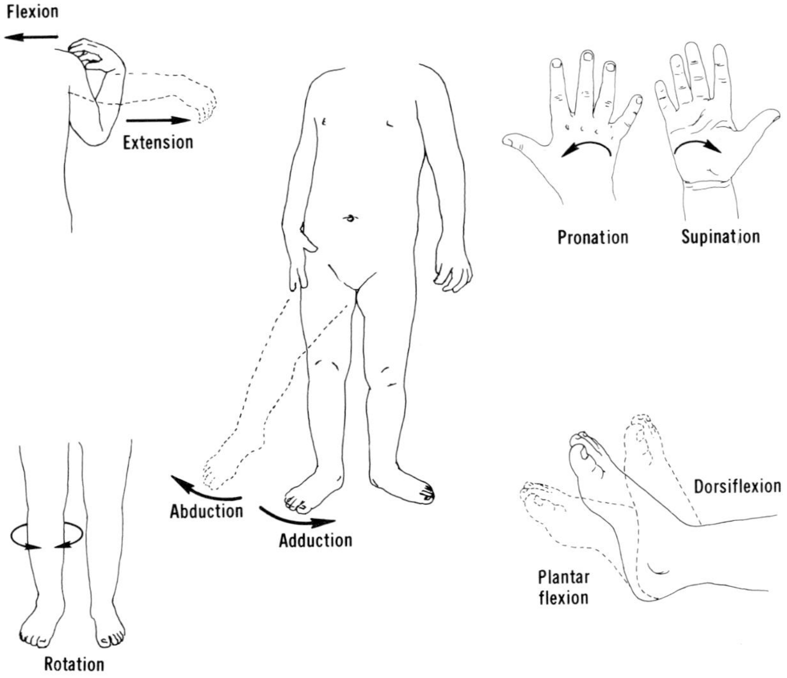

Figure 26–4. *Terms used to describe movements.*

tion causes the body part to move. The chemical reaction of contraction produces heat, which helps to maintain normal body temperature. All healthy muscle tissue is continually in a state of partial contraction. Muscle tone is lowest when a person is sleeping or when nerve supply is interrupted, such as following trauma. Muscles become fatigued after excessive and continuous contraction. Complete fatigue occurs when a muscle is unable to contract. Disuse of a muscle causes *atrophy,* or wasting.

Muscles move the parts of the body as strings operate a puppet. Shortening of the puppet's leg string causes the limb to move. Similarly, when a muscle contracts, it shortens and causes the bone to which it is attached to move. When a muscle contracts, one bone must remain stationary to act as an anchor for the muscle to pull against as it draws the other bone toward it. Muscles act in groups, not individually. For any given movement, several muscles act in a coordinated process; while some muscles contract, others relax. The type of movement produced depends on the place the muscle is attached to the bone and the type of joint involved. In movement, bones work as levers, and the joints are pivots for the levers.

The orchestration of the complex patterns of voluntary muscle activity is accomplished by the central nervous system. Muscles are made to shorten or lengthen according to messages transmitted by nerves from the brain and/or spinal cord to the muscles. To return once more to the example of Jim, in order to voluntarily pick up the red block, he had to have conscious control of his arm and hand movements. His arm straightened as he reached for the block, and muscles of the shoulder provided stability while his arm moved at the same time, muscles in his trunk and limb enabled him to keep his balance. But in order for Jim's CNS to control his movements, information must be received from receptors in muscles, ligaments, joints, and skin, about body position (erect, prone, or tilted) and consistency of the block (hard, spongy, or rough). All voluntary movement occurs in response to a constant flow of information. The information must be transmitted on intact pathways to be received in the CNS, interpreted, and retransmitted to stimulate muscles for movement. If pathways to or from the CNS become diseased, traumatized, degenerate, or are nonexistent, the child cannot perform willful movements. Similarly, if changes occur inside the brain or spinal cord and arriving information cannot be adequately processed, movement is affected.

ALTERATION IN MOBILITY

Mobility can be temporarily or permanently interrupted by prolonged bed rest, or the use of mechanical devices such as splints or braces. Sometimes mobility is voluntarily curtailed to conserve energy and maintain equilibrium. Usually, however, alterations in mobility are caused by disease or trauma.

Trauma is the most common cause of mobility problems in children. Birth injuries, falls, and automobile accidents frequently necessitate immobilization with casts or traction. A head injury caused by trauma is one of the most common causes of direct injury to the brain. *Fractures,* a break in any bone of the body, and *dislocation,* the disjoining of bones from their sockets, are common injuries that alter normal movement.

Illnesses that alter mobility include *congenital disorders, inflammation and infection,* and *structural or degenerative changes* within the body.

John was born yesterday with a large bulging sac on his lower back. He does not move either leg and his feet are clubbed. Faulty development allowed meninges and spinal cord elements to protrude through the vertebral column in a sac. John has a *meningomyelocele,* a *congenital interference* with mobility.

Congenital interferences with activity frequently prevent normal growth and development. They may be caused by errors of embryonic development, genetic defects, or birth injuries. Although many congenital defects of the musculoskeletal system and central nervous system are minor and can be corrected, some are especially serious because they affect not only the child's appearance, but his intelligence.

Inflammation and/or infection can affect muscles, bones, and joints, making them painful and limiting movement. An infection can lodge inside the bone marrow after a fracture, open wound, or surgery. The microorganisms may then be carried in the bloodstream and cause a systemic infection. Microorganisms may invade the nervous system, causing temporary or permanent limitation of movement. Inflammation of brain tissue is very critical and may be fatal.

Structural changes in the skeleton, muscles, or nervous system may be slow and insidious or rapid and acute. Some diseases of the nervous system cause progressive functional incapacities and a loss of effective nervous tissue. As a result, the child's muscles may become weak and atrophy.

Motor development is retarded and may eventually cease.

Jennie, aged fourteen, can never get her dresses and skirts to hang evenly and lately it has been impossible to buy jeans that fit. Jennie has *scoliosis*, a lateral curve of her spine. In addition, several vertebrae are damaged. The structural change in Jennie's skeleton will require braces and, perhaps, surgical correction.

John's problem began in the nervous system; Jennie's originated in the musculoskeletal system; both children have an interference in normal mobility. In addition to mobility, growth, development, and emotional integrity are affected. The development of every child is accomplished by sensory and motor interactions with his world. If normal activity is impeded, the quantity and quality of available sensory information is reduced, as is the ability of the child to respond and incorporate stimuli. Similarly, if nervous pathways are diseased, traumatized or nonexistent, the child cannot take in, use, and respond to stimuli; development is stifled.

Bibliography

Anthony, C. and Kilthoff, N. *Anatomy and Physiology*, ed. 9. St. Louis, C.V. Mosby Co., 1975.

Barber, J., Stokes, L. Billings, D. *Adult and Child Care: A Client Approach to Nursing*, ed. 2. St. Louis, C.V. Mosby Co., 1977.

Burke, S.R. *Human Biology in Health and Disease*. New York, John Wiley & Sons, Inc., 1975.

Conway, B. *Pediatric Neurologic Nursing*. St. Louis, C.V. Mosby Co., 1977.

Elhart, D., Firsich, S., Gragg, S., Rees, G. *Scientific Principles in Nursing*, ed. 8. St. Louis, C.V. Mosby Co., 1978.

Hamilton, M. *Basic Pediatrics*, ed. 3. St. Louis, C.V. Mosby Co., 1978.

Hirschberg, G., Lewis, L., Vaughan, P. Promoting Patient Mobility. *Nursing '77* 7:42, 1977.

Larson, C. and Gould, M. *Orthopedic Nursing*, ed. 9. St. Louis, C.V. Mosby Co., 1978.

Mitchell, P.H. *Concepts Basic to Nursing*, ed. 2. New York, McGraw-Hill, 1978.

O'Neil, S. Mobility, in Burgess, A. (ed). *Nursing: Levels of Health Intervention*. Englewood Cliffs, N.J., Prentice-Hall, 1978.

Parry, S. and Eales, C. The Neurophysiology of Normal Movement. *Nursing Times* 72:1590, 1976.

Vander, A., Sherman, J., Luciano, D. *Human Physiology: The Mechanisms of Body Function*, ed. 2. New York, McGraw-Hill, 1975.

CHAPTER **27**

The Child with a Neurological Deviation

BEHAVIORAL OBJECTIVES

After studying this chapter, you will be able to:

- Identify the signs of increased intracranial pressure and the nursing implications for each.
- Design a plan of care, for a child with seizures, including parental teaching.
- State how you would manage the physical care of a paraplegic child.
- Discuss the emotional ramifications of a coma as it affects the child, the parents, and you as the nurse.
- Design a plan of care for the child who is comatose, including an assessment of his neurological status.
- Discuss the problems of establishing or reestablishing a positive body image in the child with a neurological dysfunction.
- Explain the diagnostic procedures used to evaluate neurological status.
- Discuss the treatment regimens for the child with a neurological disorder.

TERMS AND CONCEPTS

Increased intracranial pressure
Ataxia
Cerebral ischemia
Herniation
Seizure
Convulsion
Aura
Epileptic cry
Status epilepticus
Neurogenic bladder
Neurogenic bowel
Coma
Neurological danger orders
Meningitis
Nuchal rigidity
Opisthotonos
Kernig's sign
Brudzinski's sign
Hyperpyrexia
Hypocalcemia
Computerized axial tomography
Ventriculography
Pneumoencephalography
Cerebral arteriography
Echoencephalogram
Subdural puncture
Brain scan
Hypercarbia
Credé's maneuver
Nonsterile intermittent catheterization
External collecting devices
Ventriculoperitoneal shunt
Ventriculoatrial shunt
Ventriculoureterostomy

INTRODUCTION

Neurological deviations in the child pose a myriad of problems, not only for the child and his family, but for you, his nurse. The family must cope with such questions as "Why did this happen to me?"; "Will my child have brain damage?"; "Will he ever regain consciousness?"; "Will he ever walk?". They may feel resentment towards him for needing such time-consuming care, and then feel guilty about their anger. Whether the child's problem is congenital or acquired, the parents will have to go through the grief process (as will the child, if his dysfunction is acquired).

This chapter discusses problems common to the child with neurological deviations. Nursing care during the diagnosis, treatment, and acute illness is stressed. (See Table 27–4, at the end of this chapter, for specific conditions.)

COMMON PROBLEMS AND NURSING INTERVENTIONS

Increased Intracranial Pressure

The cranial contents (the brain, nervous tissue, cerebrospinal fluid, and blood) are located within the skull, a protective, unyielding case (except in the infant, whose cranial sutures have not fused, and in the young child, whose sutures may widen in the presence of increased intracranial pressure). An increase in the size or volume of any of the cranial contents (e.g., as a result of edema, a tumor, or hemorrhage) increases the pressure within the skull.

Symptoms and signs of *increased intracranial pressure* may be associated with focal neurological symptoms that vary with the portion of the brain affected. Early symptoms are often vague, and may not seem like cause for alarm. The child may have personality changes. He may become irritable and lethargic, or begin losing his vision, speech, strength, sensation, and memory. These changes are often subtle enough to go unnoticed by the child and his parents. More frightening symptoms, such as hallucinations and convulsions, may also be seen. The classic symptoms of increased intracranial pressure are headache, vomiting, and diplopia. These early signs are often seen after the more subtle personality changes.

Headache

Unlike stomachaches, headaches are not a common complaint of children. And if a child complains of a headache, it is important to note the location, duration, and intensity. Headaches due to increased intracranial pressure often occur in the morning, or after the child has been recumbent for a time. They may or may not be associated with vomiting. If they are, the vomiting often relieves the headache. These headaches tend to occur with increasing frequency, and are aggravated by coughing or straining at stool. The child may tilt his head to lessen the pain, and will not change this position voluntarily. The infant cannot tell you his head hurts, but he may be irritable or restless; he may cry, pull away from you, bang his head, or rub it on the bed. Nursing care for headaches caused by increased intracranial pressure is specific to symptoms because, as long as the intracranial pressure is elevated, the child is likely to have a headache. Rock and comfort the child as necessary and give medications in accordance with the physician's orders.

Vomiting

Vomiting is frequently an early sign of increased intracranial pressure, or it may be an early sign of a brain tumor caused by a local irritation that precedes the onset of increased pressure. Vomiting tends to occur after arising in the morning, or right after breakfast, and may or may not be associated with nausea and headaches. As with headaches, *recurrent* vomiting may indicate intracranial causes.

The child may also be anorectic, a condition that causes nutritional problems. The anorexia is complicated by his irritability and lethargy. In addition to the general nursing implications regarding anorexia (see ch. 18), arrange the child's meals to prevent vomiting and to encourage his appetite. Time the feedings or meals so that treatments are given at least 30 minutes before meals. This will allow the child time to rest and calm down before eating. Do not give any treatments within an hour after meals; permit the child to rest during this period. This may require coordinating efforts with the other members of the health team, such as the laboratory technician who comes to draw blood midway through a meal. Hold the infant for feedings, unless this is contraindicated (e.g., if he has a newly repaired spinal defect). Make the child comfortable in bed, or if possible, let him eat in the playroom with other children. If the playroom activity is too strenuous for him, he may fare better in a quiet environment in his own room. If he wants to eat in his room, but not in bed, get a child-sized chair and table from the playroom, and let him have his own "picnic" or party. Do not hurry meal/feeding times. Allow the infant to rest during his feedings. Bubble him frequently, and after he eats, place him on his abdomen or right side.

Diplopia

Diplopia (double vision) will develop if extraocular muscle function is impaired by the involvement of cranial nerves II, IV, or VI, such that the visual axes are not parallel (disconjugate gaze). Diplopia is difficult to assess in the infant and young child. Even the school-age child with long-term diplopia may not realize he has a problem. He may think everybody sees two of everything. However, if he only recently developed double vision, he will be able to describe it. The younger child may tilt his head to one side in an effort to avoid double vision. Voluntary closure of one eye, another attempt to avoid double images, may also occur, but is often erroneously attributed to ptosis (drooping eyelid) rather than to compensation for diplopia.

If the child has trouble with his vision, chart your observations accurately in order to help the physician determine the cause of the problem. Be as specific as possible; a statement such as "child does not see well" is not as helpful as "child sees double."

Papilledema

Papilledema is a swelling of the optic nerve head, seen on funduscopic examination with the opthalmoscope. It can be an early sign of increased pressure, often occuring before the headache, vomiting, and diplopia. However, this sign is not always present in infants and young children because of the capacity of the skull to expand.

Enlarged Head

Head enlargement is often the only sign of increased intracranial pressure in the infant. If increasing head size is suspected, measure the circumference of the head daily or every other day (see the Skills Manual). Growth will be more than the normal half inch a month. Palpate the fontanelles to see if they are bulging or tense and the sutures to determine if they are widening. Observe the infant's eyes. Are they looking downward? Can you see the sclera above the iris? This "setting sun" appearance of the eye is due to pressure on the roof of the orbit.

The enlarged head is heavy, and the infant is not able to lift and turn it as does a normal infant. You will have to pick his head up and reposition it at regular intervals to prevent or minimize pressure sores. The enlarged head places an increased strain on the neck, so handle it carefully. Gentle massaging around pressure areas will increase blood supply to the area and help prevent decubitus ulcers. Daily hygienic care is important. A thin rubber pillow or sheepskin may be used to cushion the head.

Feeding the infant with an enlarged head is time-consuming. Pick him up, unless contraindicated. You, the mother, or the father should be comfortable before the feeding is begun. Use a chair with armrests, and pad the armrest with a pillow to support the arm that cradles the infant's head. As you and the parents discover ways to help the infant with feedings, share this information with other members of the health team and make notations on the care plan.

Ataxia

Ataxia, muscular incoordination or an unsteady gait, may occur as a result of increased intracranial pressure, or if a tumor mass involves cerebellar pathways. Other causes of ataxia are infection and degenerative processes.

The child may appear unsteady, and walk with a broad-based gait or waddle. Safety measures for this child include using side rails on his bed and walking with him to ensure that he does not lose his balance and injure himself.

Late Signs

In addition to the nursing implications for the early symptoms of increased intracranial pressure, carefully observe the child for any signs of *increasing* pressure. The nurse is the child's first line of defense against intracranial pressure. Because many of the obvious signs of increased intracranial pressure are late signs, subtle changes in the child's personality must be monitored constantly. Irritability, lethargy, picking at his bed linens or pajamas, and restlessness are some frequently occurring changes. Remember to heed the parent's comments that he is "just not himself." A change in the level of consciousness is the most important criterion in evaluating the child's condition, but subtle changes often precede a decrease in the level of consciousness, except in acute head trauma, when loss of consciousness may be immediate.

Increasing intracranial pressure may result in *cerebral ischemia* because the blood cannot adequately perfuse the brain in the presence of this pressure. The systolic blood pressure rises in a compensatory attempt to supply the brain with blood, and the pulse rate falls (bradycardia) in response to arterial hypertension. The combination of increased intracranial pressure, arterial hypertension, and bradycardia is known as *Cushing's triad.* If these signs are not recognized and treated promptly, decompensation occurs; blood pressure falls and the pulse rises to minimize shock. Death soon follows. A problem in recognizing these danger signs is that they tend to occur intermittently, during peaks of high intracranial pressure. By the time the physician is notified and gets to the bedside, the signs have subsided, only to recur later. This transient worsening of the neurological status is significant. It indicates that pressure within the cranium is already high, and the small increases are causing pressure peaks, with the resultant vital sign changes. When the signs are progressive and continuous, they may indicate impending herniation, or compression, of the brain.

Herniation occurs when the pressure in the cranium is so great that the brain has no place to escape, and it shifts within the skull (Figure 27–1). The vital centers are damaged or destroyed by compression of brain structures. In the final stages, hyperthermia and respiratory changes, such as central neurogenic hyperventilation, occur. Pupillary changes may be an ominous sign of brain herniation. The type of pupil reaction reflects the area of the brain involved. Check the pupils in a darkened room. Note any difference in size, measuring the pupils with a millimeter rule. Shine a penlight at one pupil from an angle. Does the pupil constrict? Is it a rapid or a sluggish reaction? Check the other eye. Does it react similarly? Record and report any abnormal dilation or constriction. Drugs such as atropine and scopolamine may cause pupil dilation, and opiates such as morphine cause pupil constriction. A metabolically caused coma does not affect the pupils until very late in the course. If both pupils are dilated and do not react to light, brain damage may be irreversible.

If the medulla herniates, acute apnea occurs, and death follows rapidly if immediate intervention with life support systems is not begun. If the medulla herniates, or drops, through the foramen magnum (Figure 27–2), death is almost instantaneous.

Altered Motor-Sensory Functioning

Seizures

Generalized, psychomotor, and focal motor, or sensory, seizures may be the initial symptom of a lesion in the brain. A *seizure* is a transitory change in behavior reflecting a disturbance in brain functioning caused by uncontrolled electrical impulses in the brain. The disturbance may be in the child's consciousness, or in his motor, sensory, or autonomic functioning. The terms *seizure disorder,* and *epilepsy* are used

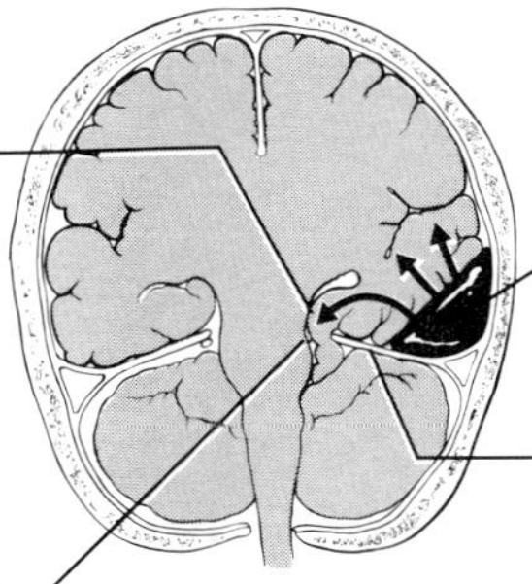

Figure 27–1. *Brain herniation through the tentorium. Note compression of third cranial nerve.*

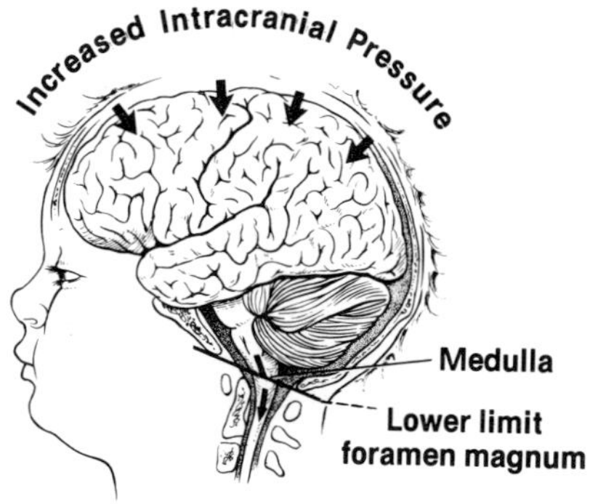

Figure 27–2. *If the medulla herniates, or drops, through the foramen magnum (e.g., in cases of increased intracranial pressure), death is almost instantaneous.*

synonymously; both terms imply a chronic state with recurrent seizures. A *convulsion* is a seizure manifested by jerking movements of the entire body. Seizures may be a symptom of tumors, infections, trauma, and drug toxicity or withdrawal. If no cause is found, the condition is called idiopathic epilepsy. This condition will be discussed at the end of this chapter.

A generalized seizure begins in the central brain, causing an immediate loss of consciousness. A focal seizure is restricted to one part of the cortex, causing symptoms characteristic of that area of the brain. A third type of seizure begins in an area of the cortex and spreads to the midbrain. This type of seizure may include an *aura,* which was formerly thought to be a warning sign of a seizure. The aura is actually a part of the seizure, occurring in the early focal stage before the generalized or central brain seizure occurs. Figure 27–3 illustrates the three types of seizures; Table 27–1 explains each type, including the cause, treatment and nursing interventions for each.

The patient who experiences an aura as a part of his seizure will often lie down immediately on the bed or the floor to prevent himself from falling when he loses consciousness. A signal to an impending seizure is the *epileptic cry* at the beginning of the generalized seizure. This cry may last a few seconds and is heard when the abdominal muscles contract and force air across the tightly closed vocal cords.

Stay with the child and remain calm. Your attitude will be conveyed to the child and his family. If you are calm, they will be reassured. Help the child to the floor if he is not there when you arrive (if he is in bed, be sure the side rails are up). If he has generalized convulsions, his side rails

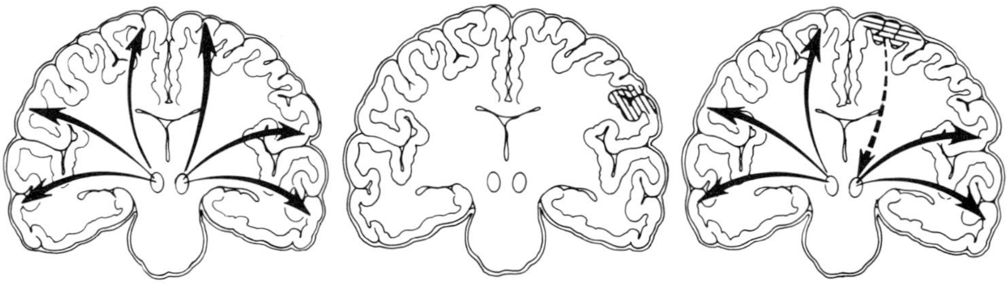

Figure 27–3. *Three types of seizures.* (Adapted with permission from Neil O. Hardy).

should be padded. If his teeth are already clenched, do not try to pry them open to insert a padded tongue blade or rolled washcloth. Any damage to the tongue will have already occurred, and you may break his teeth or injure his gums if you try to forcibly insert anything into his mouth. However, if you are with him before he clenches his teeth, pad them to prevent tongue injury.

If the child is on the floor, use a pillow or blanket to pad his head, and place it on your lap to keep it from banging on the floor. Move objects that he might strike during the convulsion away from him. *Do not attempt to restrain the child in any way.* You may cause his arm or leg to break if you hold it, since the jerking movements are so violent. Loosen any tight clothing, and try to hyperextend his head to help clear his airway. As soon as the seizure is over, turn him on his side, and suction him if necessary.

While doing your best to keep the child safe, you must also carefully observe what is happening. This is not an easy task, but your observations are important in helping the physician diagnose the type of seizure and its cause. Note the seizure's duration (remember to glance at your watch as soon as you are aware that the child is having a seizure). Note where and how the seizure starts. Is there an immediate loss of consciousness? Does the child seem to hallucinate? Did movement start on one side of the face, or with one hand or foot? How did it progress? Was the entire body stiff or jerking? If you can see the pupils, note any reaction to light. In a generalized seizure, the pupils are often dilated and do not react to light; in a focal seizure, they may deviate away from the lesion. Does the child urinate or pass a stool during the seizure? (Incontinence occurs in 50 percent of generalized seizures.) Check the plantar reflex after the seizure (Figure 27–4) by firmly stroking the sole of the foot with a pointed object, such as a key, from the heel to the ball, and then across the middle of the foot. A normal response, after twelve to eighteen months of age, is plantar flexion of the toes. An abnormal response is fanning and dorsiflexion of the toes; this is termed a *positive Babinski response* and indicates a neurological dysfunction. Occasionally, the child will have another seizure before regaining consciousness. This may be the onset of *status epilepticus*, a medical emergency. After the seizure, the child may fall into a deep sleep. Be sure that the side rails of the bed are up, and that the lights are dim. Record and report the episode in as much detail as possible.

Paralysis

Depending on their site and severity, spinal cord lesions can cause motor and sensory dysfunction in varying degrees. Paralysis often occurs in muscles served by the portion of the spinal cord caudal to the lesion. Flaccid muscles are typical early in the course during the period of spinal shock.

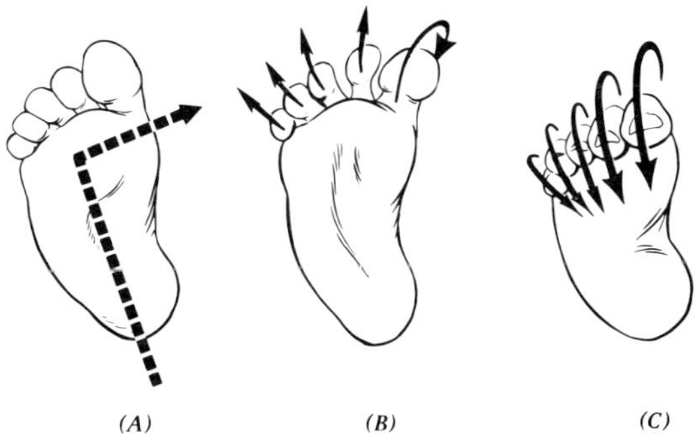

Figure 27–4. *Babinski response. (A) Direction of stimulus. (B) Babinski response (extensor plantar response). (C) Negative Babinski (flexor plantar response).*

Table 27–1. **Types of Seizures**

Type	*Cause*	*Course*
Miscellaneous: Febrile	Acute febrile illness in a susceptible person.	Occurs with high temperature. Resembles grand mal. Lasts about five minutes.
Generalized: Grand mal seizures (Major motor)	Abnormal electrical discharges overwhelm central brain.	Immediate loss of consciousness; if standing, falls to floor. Tonic phase lasts 10 to 20 seconds. Symmetrical involvement of all skeletal muscles. Body stiffens, arms flex; legs, head, neck extend; jaws clamp shut; epileptic cry. Becomes cyanotic because breathing ceases during tonic phase; increased secretions. Clonic phase lasts 30 seconds. Violent jerking of entire body; foams at mouth as he breathes through accumulated secretions. Bladder and bowel sphincters relax, causing incontinence. After seizure, may sleep several hours. On awakening, has headache, sore muscles, and cannot remember the seizure.

Table 27–1. **Types of Seizures** *(continued)*

Age	*Predisposing Factors*	*Treatment*	*Management/Parent Teaching*
Six months to three years, but may occur up to eight years. More common in boys than girls. Outgrows febrile seizures as CNS matures.	Family history of seizures.	IV Diazepam (Valium) for uncontrolled seizure (status epilepticus); IM phenobarb to control seizures. Maintenance, phenobarbitol p.o. for two to four years. Sponge to reduce fever.	Prevent subsequent seizures by keeping temperature down. Review temperature taking. Be sure they can read thermometer and recognize signs that accompany fever: irritability, behavioral changes, anorexia, vomiting, diarrhea, sore throat, cough, pulling at ears. Sponging (see Skills Manual). Teach side effects of medications.
Childhood, usually before the age of twenty.	Petit mal seizures.	Phenytoin (Dilantin) Phenobarbital (Luminal) Primidone (Mysoline)	*Must* take medicine as prescribed. Precipitating factors: emotional or physical stress, excessive fluid retention (premenstrual edema), flashing lights, direct sunlight, alcohol. If an aura occurs, child should lie down and have someone call for help. If seizure does not stop, may have status epilepticus. Call physician immediately. Provide a schedule of sleep, activity, recreation. Keep stress at a minimum without overprotecting child. Encourage activity: swimming or biking only with companion, field sports; no high risk sports, such as skin diving, mountain climbing. Wear Medic Alert bracelet.

Table 27–1. Types of Seizures *(continued)*

Type	*Cause*	*Course*
Petit mal (Absence attacks)		Momentary loss of consciousness, appears to be staring or daydreaming; activity stops or becomes automatic in character. Can occur 50 to 100 times a day. Returns to normal activity, sometimes without being aware of seizure.
Myoclonic (Minor motor)		Sudden brief muscle contractions; may or may not be symmetrical. Arms jerk together and upward; trunk flexes. Movement may be severe enough to throw child to ground. Myoclonus is a normal part of the sleep cycle and occurs as one falls asleep.
Akinetic		Sudden loss of muscle tone and postural control; may fall and injure head. Does not bite tongue or become incontinent. No aura, may have to wear football helmet to avoid head trauma.
Partial/Focal		
Partial/Focal Seizures Motor/Sensory	Abnormal electrical discharges in localized area of cortex; occur secondarily to underlying condition that damages brain tissue, such as birth trauma, congenital anomalies, and brain trauma or tumors.	Symptoms related to site. Motor: hand and face most commonly affected. Movements last 20 to 30 seconds with no loss of consciousness. Sensory: numbness and tingling in affected part of body. Auditory, vestibular, and visual seizures also seen.

Table 27–1. **Types of Seizures** *(continued)*

Age	*Predisposing Factors*	*Treatment*	*Management/Parent Teaching*
Early childhood; sometimes stops at puberty.	Family history.	Ethosuximide (Zarontin) Clonazepam Valproic acid (VPA). Ketogenic diet (increased fats and decreased carbohydrates)	
Childhood and adolescence.	Hereditary; appears before age of fifteen.	Methsuximide (Celontin) Clonazepam Ketogenic diet	
Any age.		Phenobarbital Carbamazepine (Tegretol) Primidone (Mysoline)	

Table 27–1. Types of Seizures *(continued)*

Type	*Cause*	*Course*
Psychomotor/Temporal Lobe (complex partial seizures)	Involves higher level cerebral functioning: affects memory, cognition. Temporal lobe most common site. Behavioral manifestations plus motor movements yield the term "psychomotor."	Ranges from brief loss of consciousness to longer periods of purposeless activity (e.g., walking up and down stairs repeatedly). Inappropriate activity may be mistaken for psychotic behavior. At onset, may have strange feeling in pit of stomach, which rises to throat. May smell an unpleasant odor, and hear strange noises. Memory disturbances, distorted perception of time and self, and strong emotions such as fear and anxiety are common. Seizures last four to five minutes. Afterwards, confusion and amnesia exist.
Secondary generalization	Spread of focal seizure. Abnormal impulses begin at localized site in cortex and spread to the central brain, then generalized convulsive seizures occur.	Symptoms of focal seizure (motor, sensory, psychic) may precede a general seizure. This *aura* is not a symptom or warning sign, but a part of the seizure, occurring in the early stage.
Jacksonian march		Localized clonic movements which spread or "march" to other parts on the same side of the body. Rare.
Infantile spasms	Associated with major cerebral anomalies.	Brief spasms; child may have up to 200 per day. May include jerking of head and clonic movements of extremities. Child may laugh or cry during spasms. Seizures may be mistaken for colic. Child is likely

Table 27–1. Types of Seizures *(continued)*

Age	*Predisposing Factors*	*Treatment*	*Management/Parent Teaching*
More common in adults but may begin at any age.			
Begin during first year of life; usually disappear spontaneously by age three or four but are replaced by major motor seizures in most cases.			

Table 27–1. **Types of Seizures** *(continued)*

Type	*Cause*	*Course*
		to have other developmental disabilities such as severe retardation or cerebral palsy. Ninety percent of affected children are mentally retarded.
Status epilepticus	Failure to take prescribed medication.	Series of any type seizure in rapid succession. In grand mal, the child does not regain consciousness between attacks.

Table 27–1. **Types of Seizures** *(continued)*

Age	*Predisposing Factors*	*Treatment*	*Management/Parent Teaching*
		Oral airway suctioning; tracheostomy if necessary. Drugs—Diazepam (Valium) IV, then Phenytoin (Dilantin). If no results, general anesthesia and curare. Death or permanent brain damage may occur from hyperpyrexia and hypoxia. Treatment may cause cardiac or respiratory arrest.	

Because the child cannot feel or move his own legs, you must move them for him. At least every two hours, change his position and inspect his legs and feet, particularly the buttocks, knees, ankles, and toes, for proper alignment and the presence of pressure areas. Include a quick inspection when you approach the bedside for any reason. Because the child cannot feel his legs, he is vulnerable to injury. He cannot tell if his ankle is being irritated by his other leg. He cannot tell if the gooseneck lamp you are using for his diaper rash is burning him. Special care must be taken with his legs because he cannot feel or control them. If he is old enough to play on the floor, pad his legs and feet with long pants and socks.

As the child grows older, he will be given increased responsibility to see that his legs are straight and protected from injury. He will learn to use a mirror to inspect his buttocks and thighs for pressure areas, and to avoid environmental hazards, such as floor furnaces, radiators, and sharp objects, such as abrasive cement.

Passive range of motion exercises are given to minimize muscle atrophy and contracture. Even if your institution has a physical therapy department, include a range of motion movements during daily care. Bath time is usually an excellent time to exercise the muscles and joints.

Braces may be used to help the child attain an upright posture. Together with crutches, they make it possible for him to have some mobility. A crutchless walker and parapodium are devices which permit an upright position and some mobility, yet leave the arms and hands free to touch and explore the environment (e.g., petting a dog, picking a flower, or opening a door). After spinal cord injury, the older child or adolescent may be determined to walk, even though he is paralyzed from the waist down. Much time and effort are spent in conquering this psychological challenge. A tremendous effort, coupled with strength, is required for walking without the use of one's legs. Typically, after the child learns to walk with the aid of braces and crutches, he puts them aside and returns to his wheelchair, which is more manageable and maneuverable, and provides greater mobility.

Bladder and Bowel Dysfunctions

The terms *neurogenic bladder* and *neurogenic bowel* refer to bladder and bowel dysfunctions in which incontinence is caused by a lack of innervation. Constant dribbling of urine and feces is irritating to the skin, and predisposes the child to diaper rash. Change diapers frequently, gently cleansing the skin and patting it dry with each change. Cloth diapers do not soak up the urine as readily as do disposable diapers. Thus, you will be more likely to notice that the baby is wet if he is wearing a cloth diaper. However, the disposable diaper may be preferred because it tends to keep the infant drier. Remember to check for wetness and soiling more often if you use a disposable diaper. (See chapter 18 for more details of care of diaper rash.)

Be especially careful not to let stool or urine contaminate a spinal defect. It may help to position a plastic drape between the spinal lesion, or incision, and the buttocks. The infant may be placed on a Bradford frame so that urine and feces drain away from the lesion and into a bed pan. Use of the frame also eliminates frequent linen changes. In addition to the Bradford frame, a standard incubator or crib can be modified somewhat to accommodate the infant with a spinal defect (Figures 27–5). Note the slight Trendelenburg slope, which helps to reduce pressure in the lesion and keeps

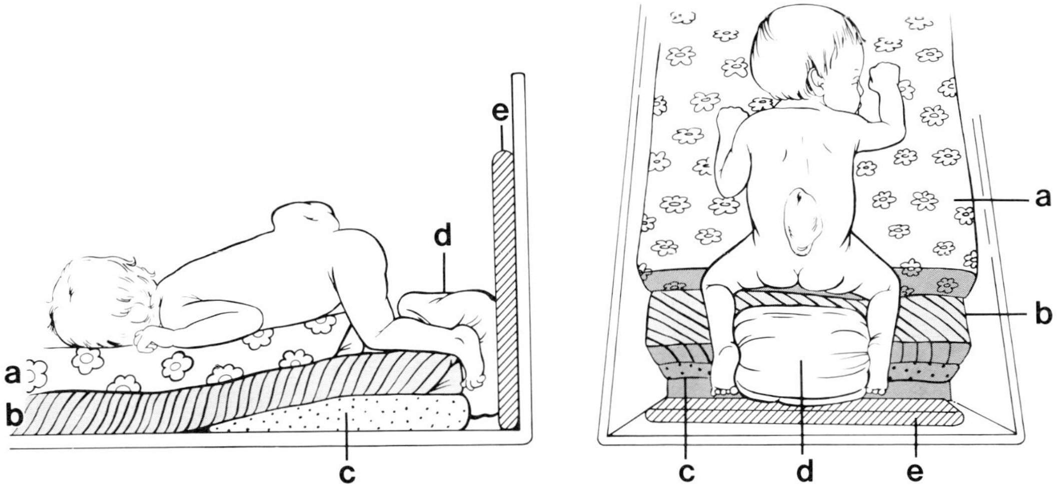

Figure 27–5. *Crib modified for infant with spinal defect:* (a) *short mattress or pad used to keep hips flexed;* (b) *crib mattress;* (c) *extra pad to keep infant from sliding to foot of bed;* (d) *pad placed between legs to keep them in position of abduction;* (e) *covered pad to keep infant from touching foot of crib.*

the infant from sliding to the foot of the bed. The hips are slightly flexed so that pressure over the lesion is not increased. As with the Bradford frame, the urine and feces drain down away from the spinal lesion. A pad is placed between the legs to keep the hips abducted, helping to prevent or minimize subluxation (a dislocated hip). The feet hang freely to prevent worsening of foot deformities. Although lower than the body, the legs and feet usually are high enough to prevent edema.

Varying degrees of neurogenic bladder and bowel dysfunction are seen. After medical and surgical intervention have stabilized the major defects or injury, management of the neurogenic bladder and bowel becomes the most distressing problem for the child and his family. Bladder and bowel management should be started in infancy or soon after the accident, depending on the cause of the paralysis. Early management is necessary to preserve renal function and to manage the incontinence. The biggest hurdle to beginning and maintaining such a program is the parents themselves, or the child if he is older. Parents have difficulty realizing the impact of their child's incontinence until he reaches the age of toilet training and cannot be trained. The older child or adolescent, paralyzed in an accident, may have trouble realizing that his paralysis and incontinence are permanent. Bladder and bowel training programs are discussed under common treatments and nursing implications.

Coma

As pressure within the cranium builds, the child's level of consciousness may change, progressing to a coma. A *coma* is a state in which there is no verbalization, no eye contact, and no responses, except for basic reflexive ones.

Management of the comatose child is a tremendous responsibility. His care requires skillful observation, assessment, and planning. The actual implementation of the plan is taxing and time-consuming. Rewards in terms of feedback from the child may not be forthcoming. A coma may last for weeks, months, or years. Of course, the child may recover from coma with little or no residual damage, but if the coma lasts for more than two weeks, the chances for a complete recovery with normal functioning are lessened.

Emotional Impact of Coma

The parents will experience grief as the coma continues, and the child they knew and nurtured seems less and less accessible. They mourn the loss of the child they love. At the same time, they tend to deny the reality of the situation, and hope for total recovery. The parents' grief reaction means that they will be angry at the situation and may transfer their anger to the nurse, the outsider closest to the situation. Refer to Chapter 3 for a complete discussion of the process of grief, the parent's reactions, and your reactions. Recall that understanding your own feelings and responses will help you in dealing with this child and his family.

As you are exposed to illness, suffering, and death, you become more aware of your own vulnerability. How you deal with this awareness will affect you in other areas of your life, not just in your professional life. You may think about this comatose child after hours, and even dream about him. You ask the same questions the parents ask, "Why this child?", and search for answers that may not be forthcoming. It is difficult to remain unaffected by the sight of a previously healthy, whole child who has become helpless and nonfunctional. A normal reaction is to feel angry with the child for needing such intensive nursing care, and then to feel guilty for feeling angry. This cycle may continue if you then become angry with the child for making you feel guilty. Guilt is often intensified when unspoken thoughts run through your head, such as "This child would be better off dead." Professional frustration builds if you cannot see any positive changes in the child's condition. Nursing is a helping profession, and if you do not feel that you are helping you probably will become frustrated.

Parents usually want you to know the child as he was before the coma. They may bring in pictures of him as a happy, active child. They may bring his favorite toy, or record if he is an older child. You begin to imagine him as he was, to see him as a functioning member of that family, and to become more fully appreciative of their loss. This step also draws you further into the grief process. You may begin to experience anxiety as you wait in a state of limbo with the family to see if there is any improvement.

Every trauma care unit, intensive care unit, and general nursing unit that cares for seriously ill patients should have a support group for the health personnel involved in the care of critically ill patients. This group can act as an outlet for feelings of frustration, anxiety, hope, fear and depression. If your institution or unit does not have such a support group, or a "screaming room," talk with your instructor, peers, supervisor, or a friend about your feelings concerning this patient. Recognize your feelings, and deal with them, because if you suppress them, they will surface later.

Physical Care During Coma

Physical care of the comatose child is geared towards maintaining optimal physical condition, and preventing complications caused by his immobility and impaired neurological status.

Respiratory Status

Respiratory failure is the leading cause of death in the comatose child. It is usually the result of an airway blockage caused by a mucus plug, or aspiration of food or a foreign object. Minimize this risk by elevating the head of the bed at least 30°. Elevate the head by putting shock blocks under it. Cranking up the head of the bed puts an excessive amount of pressure on the child's buttocks. Initially, the physician may wish the child to remain flat. If so, place him in a semiprone position on his side; do not place him flat on his back.

Aspiration occurs most often during tube feedings, when the child's stomach becomes distended. To minimize this risk, measure (but do not remove) residual stomach contents before each feeding and subtract this volume from the next feeding. This prevents stomach distention. Remember to elevate the head of the bed during and after feeding to help prevent aspiration. (Refer to chapter 18 and the Skills Manual for a more detailed discussion of tube feedings.)

Monitoring the stomach residual also aids in evaluating GI tract status. A consistently large or increasing residual may indicate ileus. Listen with your stethescope for bowel sounds. If they are diminished or absent, notify the physician.

The child may retain secretions and require suctioning to prevent aspiration and infection. (Secretions are an ideal medium for bacterial growth). Frequent, deep, tracheal suctioning, along with mechanical ventilation, postural drainage, percussion, and turning are necessary. Profound hypoxia is most likely to occur during suctioning. Therefore, hyperventilate the child with 100 percent oxygen before and after you suction him. (Of course, the use of 100 percent oxygen requires a physician's order.) A humidifier at the bedside will help to liquify secretions. If respiratory difficulty persists, a tracheostomy may be necessary. Be sure that the tracheostomy tube does not get occluded by bed linens or other items. Watch for signs of airway obstruction. (Refer to chapter 23 and the Skills Manual for tracheostomy care.)

Clean the nares with a saline-soaked, cotton-tipped applicator; then moisten them with another applicator dipped in mineral oil. If the child has a brain injury or a craniotomy, check with the physician before inserting anything into his nose or ears. Note and report immediately any bleeding or drainage from the nose or ears. Bloody cerebrospinal fluid drainage will not clot and leaves a telltale water ring on the linens; the outer circle will be lighter because cerebrospinal fluid (CSF) is less dense and spreads further than the inner circle of blood. Test the drainage for glucose; a positive test indicates CSF. In the case of CSF drainage, do not pack the nose or ears; tape a gauze pad loosely over the ear or under the nostrils. Packing may suppress drainage and lead to a retrograde infection.

Skin and Muscle Integrity

Immobility leads to skin breakdown, muscle atrophy, and contractures of the extremities into nonfunctional positions (e.g., foot drop). An air mattress is helpful in preventing skin breakdown, but it should be used without linen savers or drawsheets because these increase pressure on the skin, negating the effects of the air mattress. Use pillows and blanket rolls to position the child. Lightweight plastic splints may be used to maintain the arms and legs in functional positions. Remove them every four hours, inspect the underlying skin, and offer skin care and range of motion exercises. Make a turning plan that designates specific positions, and post it in the child's room. Each time the child is turned, check off that position so that the next person caring for him can immediately tell which position to use.

Corneal Care

If the eyes do not close completely, the cornea will dry out, resulting in damage and possible blindness. Every four hours, remove dried sections from the canthi and lids of the eyes with saline-moistened cotton balls, and instill artificial tears (methylcellulose eyedrops). It may be necessary to keep the eyelids closed with Steristrips, which are changed when eye care is given.

Oral Hygiene

Proper oral care involves much more than swabbing the teeth, gums, and tongue with lemon-glycerin swabs. Turn the child on his side and brush his teeth with a soft brush. Have someone else suction if necessary. If brushing the teeth is not possible (e.g., if the child's mouth is clamped shut), try irrigating his mouth with mouthwash and hydrogen peroxide in a 3 to 1 concentration. Use a 20-cc syringe with a two-inch plastic tube attached. Again, have someone suction while you irrigate. Lubricate the lips with mineral oil at intervals throughout the day. If the child clenches his jaws and grinds his teeth, an oral surgeon may provide a bite block to protect the teeth and tongue.

Bladder and Bowel Function

Urinary output should be measured carefully. A large increase in volume may indicate diabetes insipidus. a decrease in volume may mean dehydration, a state that is sometimes medically induced to relieve increased intracranial pressure.

A Foley catheter is used to collect and measure urine output. A "wee-bag" or external collecting device may be used on the infant. (Refer to chapter 30 for care of the child who requires urinary tract monitoring.)

Although the child is also incontinent of feces, he may also suffer from fecal impactions, or inadequate emptying of the bowel. He should have a daily rectal exam, with manual removal of retained stools. If the stools are hard, a liquid stool softener or glycerin suppository should be used. If diarrhea is present, the child may not be adequately absorbing his feeding. Diarrhea can also indicate fecal impaction. Check all stools for occult blood, a possible sign of stress ulcers.

Assessing Neurological Status

Rehabilitation is a primary goal for the comatose child. Assessing his neurological status provides clues to his condition. If it improves or deteriorates, appropriate changes in his treatment and nursing management should be instituted.

Neurological status checks, referred to as "neurological danger orders" or "neurosurgical danger orders" in different institutions, are a set protocol for assessing the patient's condition. These protocols vary according to the institution, and even within some institutions. The protocol used should be clearly stated so that each person using it knows what it means. Protocols using the terms comatose, confused, or delirious, and the like are often confusing. Table 27–2 offers an example of a workable protocol.

The terms *confusion* and *delirium* describe a state of consciousness at about the same level as *obtunded,* but they imply thought and behavior impairments caused by a cortical dysfunction. Confusion means the child appears dazed and disoriented.

Decorticate rigidity is seen when the child flexes his arms, wrists, and fingers, hugging them to his body. The thumb is folded into the palm with the fingers closed over it. The legs are extended, plantar flexed, and internally rotated. In *decerebrate rigidity,* the child is opisthotonoid, his teeth clenched, arms adducted and hyperpronated, and his legs stiffly extended. He may shiver and breathe rapidly; this is an ominous sign.

To test muscular strength, ask the child to squeeze your hand, or lift his legs. Test each limb separately in order to compare strength and function. Questions such as "Can you pretend you are riding a bike?" or "Can you squeeze the ball," may elicit a response from a young child. Pick up both of his legs or arms, and allow them to fall back to the bed. If one side is affected, that limb drops more quickly.

Test his cough, swallow, and gag reflexes by inserting an airway and suctioning, or by using a similar maneuver. If these reflexes are absent, establish and maintain a parent airway. Check pupillary response to light by shining a penlight into the pupil at a slight angle (Figure 27–6). Note whether the response is equal and reactive (in which case both eyes react equally to light) or sluggish, brisk, and so on. Measure the reaction and record it (see the Skills Manual).

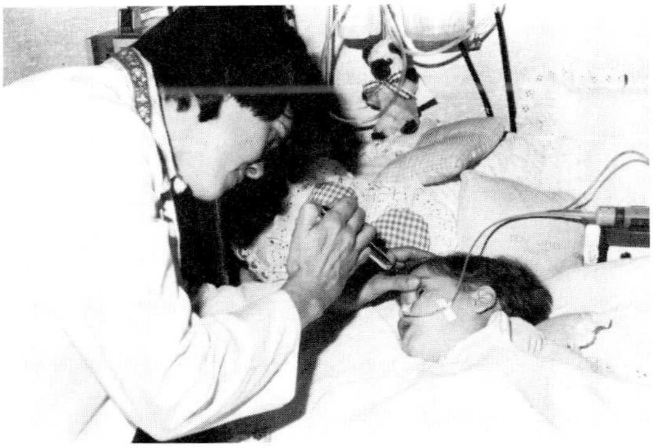

Figure 27–6. *Nurse checking pupillary response of comatose child.*

Test for the blink reflex by touching a corner of the cornea with a wisp of cotton. If this reflex is absent, protect the eye with artificial tears. Try to elicit the Babinski reflex; record the child's response.

Psychosocial Needs

Because the physical care of the comatose child is so demanding, it is easy to forget to provide emotional care. Since the patient cannot overtly respond, we tend to think that he cannot comprehend. Although communication with the child and his family is often the least considered part of care, it is not the least important. The uncertainty of the prognosis contributes to the lack of communication. Explain to the parents the necessity of each procedure, and let them help if they are able to. The high quality of care the child receives is a great comfort to the family even if he doesn't recover. Never assume the child is oblivious to his environment. Talk to him and explain what

Table 27–2 Neurological Checklist*

Date	*Time*	*B/P*	*T*	*P*	*R*	*Patent Airway*	*Level of Consciousness*	*Pupil Reaction and Eye Movement*	*Reaction to Verbal Stimuli*	*Reaction to Painful Stimuli*	*Muscular Response Strength*	*Reflexes*	*Signature*
	7												
	8												
	9												
	10												
	11												
	12												
	1												
	2												
	3												
	4												
	5												
	6												
	7												

Note: Patient NPO unless othersie ordered.
Check every hour unless otherwise ordered.
See next page for code.
Notify physician if any of the following occur:
Pulse changes:

Full-term newborn	↓ 90 or ↑ 190
Infant	↓ 75 or ↑ 175
1–6 years	↓ 70 or ↑ 140
6–12 years	↓ 65 or ↑ 125
12–18 years	↓ 60 or ↑ 110

Respirations: any irregular pattern
Blood pressure: any rise over child's base line
Temperature: 38.8° (102°F)

*The checklist that appears here is adapted from a form in use in many clinical settings. The code that appears on page 635 is usually printed on the reverse of the checklist.

Neurological Checklist Code

Level of Consciousness

1. **Alert.** Fully aware of surroundings; oriented to time, place, person. Appropriate response to auditory, visual, motor, and sensory stimuli. (For a child, you must know his normal responses. Play "peek-a-boo" or "patty cake" with him. If he is afraid, let his mother interact with him.)
2. **Obtunded.** Responds slowly or incompletely when stimulated, otherwise appears drowsy, indifferent, confused, dazed, disoriented, delirious, uncooperative, easily agitated.
3. **Stuporous.** Responds after repeated vigorous stimuli. When aroused, is not oriented to time, place, and person.
4. **Coma.** Responds to painful stimuli with decorticate posturing (arms, wrists, and fingers flexed and clutched to body; legs extended, plantor flexed, and internally rotated) or decerebrate posturing (opisthotonoid, clenched teeth; arms adducted and hyperpronated; legs stiffly extended).
5. **Deep coma.** No response to painful stimuli. No deep tendon, corneal, cough, or gag reflexes.

Pupillary Response

E/R = Equal and react to light; otherwise, measure reaction and use descriptive terms, such as pinpoint, dilated, sluggish, brisk, and so on.
L = Left
R = Right

Eye Movement

Light coma. Doll's eye sign—when head is turned briskly, eyes roll in opposite direction.
Deep coma. Motionless, slightly divergent (in position of rest).

Muscular Strength

Test each extremity for paralysis, strength, and equal movement.
LA = left arm
RA = right arm
LL = left leg
RL = right leg

Reflexes

Test cough, swallow, and gas reflexes.
Babinski response: Stroke sole of foot with pointed object from heel to ball then across foot medially. Babinski response consists of fanning and dorsiflexion of toes in patients over 12 to 18 months of age.

The following are signs of meningeal irritation:

Brudzinski's sign. With child supine, passively flex his neck; if Brudzinski's sign is present, he will involuntarily flex his kees.
Kernig's sign. Flex child's hip by raising his leg, then attempt to straighten the knee. If Kernig's sign is present, knee will not straighten and child will experience pain and muscle spasm.
Nuchal rigidity. Stiff neck.

you are doing just as you would for an alert child. Tell him nursery rhymes while you provide his care, or sing his favorite songs. If his condition is stable, he can usually be held. Encourage his family to hold, cuddle, rock, and talk to him. Ask them to bring his favorite storybooks and let them read to him.

Jeff, aged five, had been comatose for six weeks when Ms. Bell was assigned to care for him. He required gastrostomy feedings every two hours. His abdomen was constantly rigid, which made the feedings more time-consuming. Ms. Bell asked Jeff's mother to read his favorite story during the feeding. During the third and subsequent feeding-story times, Jeff's abdomen visibly became more relaxed.

Often the child who awakens from a coma will recognize his nurses' voices.

Belinda, aged seven, awakened after a three week coma following a head injury. She had a big smile for her favorite nurse and said, "You're the one that sang the song about the frog."

Because the comatose child may be able to hear, do not discuss his condition in his presence. It may be necessary to remind parents, visitors, and even physicians that the child may be able to hear their conversations.

Infection

Meningitis, or infection of the meninges, may be a primary cause of, or a complication of a neurological dysfunction. Wound infection or contamination during surgery is a common cause of meningitis. The child will have headaches, fever, hyperirritability, *nuchal rigidity* (a stiff neck), *opisthotonos* (extreme arching of the back with retraction of the head), and perhaps seizures. Positive *Kernig's and Brudzinski's* signs can be elicited. To elicit either sign, place the child in a supine position. For Kernig's sign, flex the hip by raising the leg; then attempt to straighten the knee. If Kernig's sign is present, the knee will not straighten, and the child will experience pain and muscle spasm. Brudzinski's sign is positive if the child flexes his knees involuntarily when you passively flex his neck. Improperly treated meningitis can lead to brain damage, coma, and death.

Status Epilepticus

Status epilepticus is a state of continuous seizures in which the child does not recover consciousness between attacks. This condition is a life-threatening emergency which may lead to brain damage or death due to *hyperpyrexia* (fever) and hypoxia. The usual cause of status epilepticus is failure to take prescribed medications. Establishing an airway takes first priority and is followed by suctioning to prevent aspiration and pulmonary involvement. A tracheostomy may be necessary.

Drug therapy to control the seizures includes diazepam (Valium) given IV push, followed by phenobarbital and phenytoin (Dilantin) for maintenance therapy. If these methods fail, general anesthesia and curare are used.

Orthopedic Anomalies

Congenital dislocation of the hips and clubbed feet often occur in conjunction with spinal defects. These conditions are discussed in chapter 28.

Body Image Disturbances

The child with a neurological deficit often suffers from a chronic condition. All of the problems presented in the chronic illness section of chapter 3 pertain to this child. Encourage the parents to let the child do what he can. He needs emotional support and carefully planned habilitation or rehabilitation. Physical therapy may be necessary. Encourage interaction with the peer group (Figure 27–7) and participation in school activities. Tutoring should be made available when the child cannot get to school.

The adolescent is particularly vulnerable to changes in body image. If he has a spinal cord injury, for example, he must modify concepts of himself and his relationships to people. He also may have to alter career and personal decisions, and he must be helped to rebuild a body image consistent with a useful life.

DIAGNOSTIC PROCEDURES AND NURSING IMPLICATIONS

History

A complete and accurate history is mandatory for assessing neurological problems. The past medical history must include information about the prenatal period, labor and delivery, and the postnatal period as well as accidents and illnesses. Ask the mother when she first noticed something was amiss. With a child with cerebral palsy, for example, she probably will have noticed very early that the child was not progressing normally. Determine if the child has ever had any lapses of consciousness, seizures, or problems with balance, and if the older child or adolescent has used alcohol or drugs. Recall that the family may not understand medical language. You may have to ask if the child has "fits" or "spells," or if he "drinks," "does drugs," or is "into dope." If seizures have occurred, ask the parent or other witness to describe exactly what happened. Ask the child what he remembers. Refer to the section on common problems and nursing interventions for other questions regarding the seizure. Frequently, a parent will say, "He is just not himself. I can't put my finger on it, but he just doesn't act right." Pay attention to remarks such as this. *Subtle changes are often the first sign of a tumor or increased pressure in the cranium.*

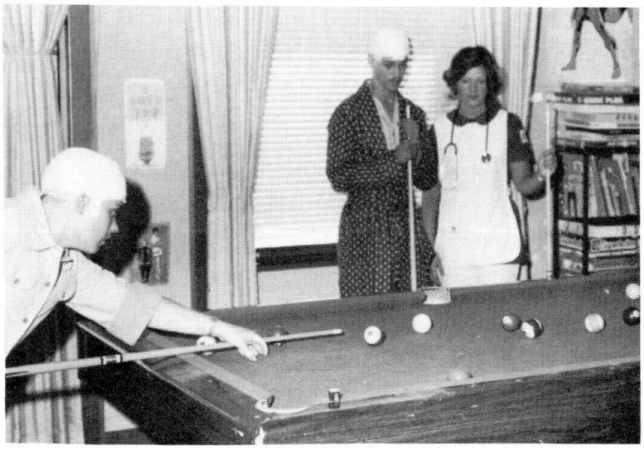

Figure 27–7. *These two adolescents play pool with a student nurse while recovering from brain surgery.*

Assessment

The neurological assessment, a detailed evaluation of neurological functioning is not within the scope of this text. However, some general guidelines will help you in evaluating your patient's neurological status.

Cerebellar Functioning (Balance and Coordination)

If the child can walk, watch him. Does he stagger or drag one leg? Do his legs scissor (cross) when he walks? Do his toes drop? Does he waddle? You must be aware of the developmental changes in the child's gait in order to detect abnormalities. For example, the toddler has a wide-based gait, or waddle, but a wide-based gait in an older child may indicate muscular dystrophy. Can he stand on one foot? (By the age of four, he should be able to do so for about five seconds). Have him close his eyes and touch his nose with his index finger, alternating hands. For the infant, note his coordination in sucking, swallowing, kicking, reaching, and grasping.

Motor Function

Note the size, tone, strength, and abnormal movement of muscles. If you suspect hypertrophy or atrophy, measure the muscles for comparison. Assessment of muscle tone is particularly important in the infant. Lay him on his back, grasp his hands, and slowly pull him to sitting. Does his head lag? A full term newborn should be able to hold his head fairly straight until he is upright. Then he will balance it a second or two, and let it fall forward. Are his arms and legs floppy? Turn him over and hold him with your hand under his chest. Does his head hang more than 45° from the horizontal? If so, he may not have good muscle tone.

One of the earliest signs of cerebral palsy (CP) is spasticity and can be observed after the age of two months when the infant begins to use his extensor muscles. Check for spasticity by pushing the baby's head forward. The child with cerebral palsy will resist and push against your hand. Flex his legs onto his abdomen and quickly release them; if he has spasticity, the legs spring back into extension and then adduction, perhaps scissoring, or crossing. With the infant prone in his crib, lift his head. If he fails to extend his arms in an effort to protect himself, this may be a sign of cerebral palsy.

Check the child's muscle strength by having him hold his arms straight out in front of him. Ask him to resist while you try to push them apart. Try to straighten his fingers while he attempts to keep them bent. Muscle strength in the infant and toddler can be checked by noting the suck reflex and the development of motor skills. Also note any irregular movements, such as twitching, jerking, and slow, irregular, wormlike movements, which are seen with athetoid cerebral palsy after eighteen months of age.

Laboratory Studies

A complete blood count is done to assess the oxygen-carrying capacity of the blood, to check for anemia or a blood loss, and to look for indications of infection. Blood gas analysis will determine if there are respiratory and/or metabolic imbalances and may help pinpoint the cause of the child's signs and symptoms (e.g., respiratory acidosis). Recall that respiratory changes may be caused by metabolic processes, as well as by neurological disturbances.

Serum electrolytes will be ordered to help the physician determine if the dysfunction is caused by hypoglycemia, *hypocalcemia* (low calcium level), drug overdose, renal failure, electrolytic abnormalities, or hypoxia. If the blood glucose is below 40 mg/100 ml, or the calcium below 7 to 7.5 mg/100 ml, coma and convulsions may occur. A blood urea nitrogen (BUN) will be necessary if dehydrating measures are used to treat the child. A urinalysis will monitor hydration and renal status. Hypertensive encephalopathy is the likely diagnosis if hematuria and proteinuria are present along with hypertension.

Radiographic Studies

Skull films are used to diagnose fractures and suture separation (indicative of increased intracranial pressure, or of a space-occupying lesion) and to help identify child abuse. However, they are of limited value in assessing the degree of intracranial damage. X-rays of the spine are used in the diagnosis of spinal tumors and congenital abnormalities.

Computerized axial tomography, or CAT scan, is a noninvasive, radiologocal technique for scanning the patient's head (Figure 27–8). It is often the procedure of choice for evaluating intracranial pathology. The scan is then analyzed by computer, and pictures of the skull and its contents are obtained. Tumors, a hemorrhage, ventricular shape and size, and shifts of brain tissue are revealed. Sedation or general anesthesia may be necessary because the child must be absolutely still during the procedure. *Contrast studies* are invasive radiographic procedures performed only for specific indications. They have largely been replaced by the CAT scan. *Ventriculography* is the direct introduction of air into the ventricles. *Pneumoencephalography,* in which air is introduced into the lumbar subarachnoid space, is more commonly used. X-rays are taken during and after each procedure. *Cerebral arteriography* requires injection of a radiopaque substance into a major artery in order to visualize the vessels of the brain. General anesthesia is used in each of these contrast studies.

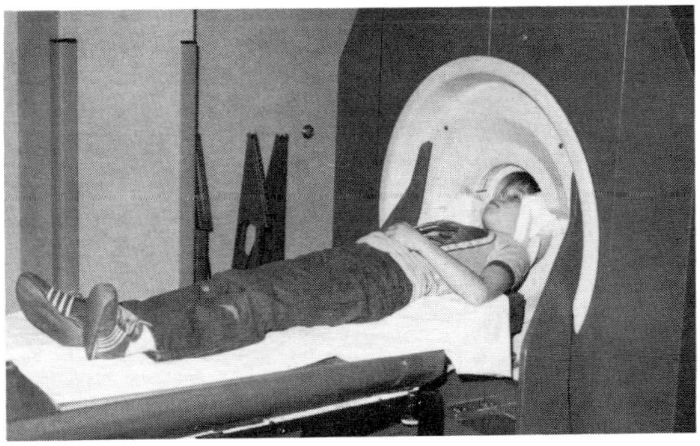

Figure 27–8. *Child having CAT scan to check for possible recurrence of brain tumor.*

After the test, keep the child flat and at rest. Check his neurological signs every half hour for two hours, then every two hours. A severe headache is common after the ventriculogram and pneumoencephalogram. Other signs, such as vomiting, fever, irritability, and meningeal irritation may also be seen. Encourage the child to drink fluids to replenish the CSF. If arteriography is done, observe him for seizures, a transient loss of vision, a thrombus or hemorrhage at the injection site, and an altered level of consciousness. See chapter 2 for preparation of the child and his family for procedures and therapeutic play afterwards.

An *echoencephalogram* is a high-frequency sound recording used to evaluate displacement of brain structures from the midline, which may occur in cases of subdural hematoma or brain tumor.

A lumbar puncture is mandatory when infection of the central nervous system (CNS) is suspected. However, it is usually contraindicated in the presence of increased intracranial pressure (ICP) if there is no infection. If the pressure is high, the sudden outlet of pressure in the lumbar area may cause the medulla to herniate into the foramen magnum, resulting in death. Lumbar punctures (spinal taps) are less frequently necessary for the diagnosis of brain abnormalities because of the newer techniques available. Normally, the CSF is clear and colorless. Hemorrhagic fluid may indicate a traumatic puncture or hemorrhage in the CNS (Figure 27–9). (See the Skills Manual.)

A *subdural puncture* is done on the child suspected of having a subdural hematoma or an effusion. This procedure is diagnostic as well as therapeutic. It determines if an

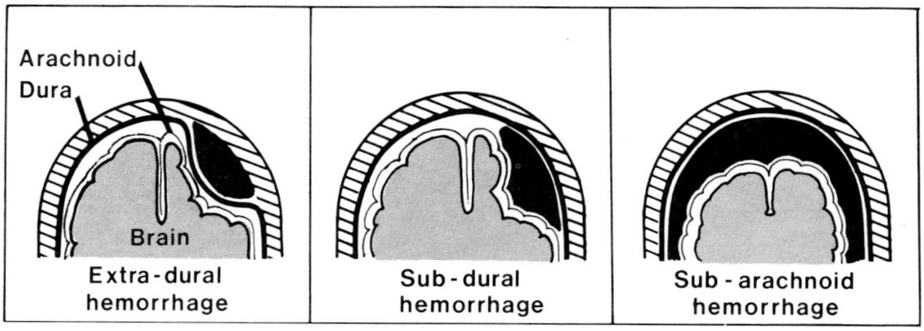

Figure 27–9. *Extradural, subdural, and subarachnoid hemorrhages.*

infection is present, and enables medicine to be instilled, or fluid to be aspirated to relieve pressure. A ventricular tap may also be done. Both of these procedures are demonstrated in the Skills Manual, and both require that an area of the child's head be shaved.

A *radioisotope brain scan* is useful for identifying brain tumors and vascular lesions. Scanning of the head is done after a radioisotope is given IV. The child may be sedated.

The *electroencephalogram* (EEG) is used to identify seizure disorders and space-occupying lesions and to monitor the progress of encephalitis and head injury.

COMMON TREATMENTS AND NURSING IMPLICATIONS

Medical Management of Increased Intracranial Pressure

Controlled Dehydration

Controlled dehydration is often used in the management of increased intracranial pressure. The pressure may be reduced temporarily by using osmotic diuretics, such as mannitol or urea, given intravenously. These agents rapidly remove water from the cells, inducing dehydration and reducing cerebral edema. However, a rebound effect may occur after the diuretic is excreted by the kidneys. For this reason, osmotic diuretics are useful only in the initial phase. Steroids then may be given to further reduce the edema.

Since mannitol may contain crystals, warm the container in water to dissolve any crystals, and use an infusion set with a filter. Monitor the child carefully during hyperosmotic therapy to prevent hypovolemic shock from fluid loss. In the case of kidney failure, the child may not be able to excrete the increased volume; thus, his edema may increase. Care must be taken not to administer hypotonic solutions by mistake, since they will further increase the cerebral edema.

During controlled dehydration, the physician may restrict the child's fluid intake. If so, make a fluid plan, dividing the permissible amount of fluid into the three shifts on a two-fifths, two-fifths, one-fifth basis.

Hypothermia

Fever may accompany increased intracranial pressure. The fever can increase the pressure further by causing cerebral vasodilation. Hypothermic measures may be employed. Hypothermia induces vasoconstriction, which helps to decrease the cerebral pressure. It also lowers the cerebral oxygen and glucose requirements. A cooling blanket or pad is used, and the core temperature is monitored every 30 minutes. A rectal probe is used for the comatose child.

Antipyretics, such as Tylenol, may also be used to combat elevated temperature. Aspirin is used with caution because it prolongs the clotting time and may cause gastric disturbances.

Hyperventilation

Hypercarbia (an excess of carbon dioxide in the blood) causes cerebral vasodilation, which increases intracranial pressure by increasing intracranial blood volume. Hyperventilation is artificially induced to lower the pressure by inducing respiratory alkalosis. This lowers the arterial carbon dioxide levels, helping to reduce intracranial pressure.

Seizures

Seizures are controlled with the use of anticonvulsant drugs (see Table 27–3 for drugs of choice). Treatment is begun as soon as the type of seizure is identified, because there is some evidence that the longer epilepsy remains untreated, the more difficult it is to control. During early treatment, while various drugs, dosages, and combinations are being tried, the child and his parents may become disappointed and frustrated. The medication may make him sleepy, or even stuporous or it may not completely control the seizures. Offer support and encouragement to the family at this time. Explain the necessity for trying different drugs, and insist that they comply with the treatment regimen.

The best drug schedule is one which controls the seizures, yet permits normal functioning. The school child may need to have his dosage adjusted so that he does not have to take medication at school, where he is often teased into not taking the medicine.

Liquid medication must be shaken enough to avoid undermedication from the top of the bottle and overmedication from the bottom of the bottle. Liquids may be lost if the child drools or spits when taking his medicine. A discrepancy in spoon sizes may also cause inaccurate dosages, resulting in under- or overmedication. Capsules or tablets are more accurate, and can be crushed and mixed with syrup or honey, if necessary.

Recall that the most frequent cause of seizures is failure to take medication regularly. This is usually caused by a lack of understanding about the illness itself, and about the necessity for carefully following the medication regimen. This noncompliance may be a form of denial. Your responsibility includes properly educating the child and his family about his illness and drugs.

Explain that taking the drugs as prescribed can allow the child to lead a relatively normal life. Not taking them will result in recurrent seizures. Warn them against overconfidence; when the seizures are completely controlled, they may feel that the child is cured and discontinue the medication. Tell them this will only lead to more seizures. Explain the side effects of the drugs so that their occurence will not cause undue alarm.

Many of the drugs may cause blood dyscrasias. Therefore, the physician may request white blood cell and hemoglobin counts periodically. Visual and motor dis-

Table 27–3. **Anticonvulsant Drugs of Choice**

Drug	*Dose*	*Indications*	*Side Effects*	*Toxic Effects*
Phenobarbital (Luminal)	5–10 mg/kg/day given in one dose	Grand mal Focal seizures Psychomotor seizures	Drowsiness Megaloblastic anemia	Nystagmus Ataxia
Phenytoin sodium (Dilantin)	5–10 mg/kg/day given in one dose	Grand mal Focal seizures	Gum hyperplasia Megaloblastic anemia	Nystagmus Ataxia Lethargy
Primidone (Mysoline)	10–20 mg/kg/day given in three or four doses	Grand mal Focal seizures Psychomotor seizures	Drowsiness Nausea and vomiting	Ataxia Nystagmus Lethargy
Ethosuximide (Zarontin)	250 mg bid. given in three or four doses	Petit mal	Rash Leukopenia	Dizziness Nausea and vomiting
Diazepam (Valium)	2–5 mg IV push q 30 minutes until seizures subside	Status Epilepticus	Rash	Lethargy Respiratory depression Ataxia

turbances should be reported promptly. Gum hyperplasia may be lessened by good tooth brushing to remove food particles and prevent infection and by frequent massaging of the gums. Oral surgery is necessary in some cases to remove excess gingiva.

If nausea and vomiting are a problem, have the child take his medication with meals. If side effects are troublesome, the physician may change medications. Encourage the parents to return to the physician or clinic for the scheduled followup visits, and always allow the child and his parents adequate time to absorb the information and to ask questions.

Headaches

Analgesics may be necessary to ease headache pain. Aspirin or codeine are the drugs of choice. Caution must be taken not to sedate the child with a head injury, especially with opiates, barbiturates, or Valium. Sedation interferes with accurate assessment of the level of consciousness and may depress the respirations, resulting in an accumulation of carbon dioxide. Recall that carbon dioxide is a vasodilator which can increase cerebral edema and intracranial pressure.

Vomiting and Straining at Stool

Antiemetics are ordered to reduce vomiting, and stool softeners are given to prevent straining at stool, both of which increase intracranial pressure.

Infection

Antibiotics are given to prevent and combat infections, especially meningitis.

Tumors

Radiotherapy with or without surgery is often used in the treatment of cerebral tumors. It is begun as soon as the surgical incision heals. The entire tumor area and a generous portion of normal tissue are included in the radiation therapy field. In tumors that tend to involve the spinal cord, such as medulloblastoma and ependymoma, spinal irradiation is also done.

Chemotherapy is useful for some tumors, especially medulloblastomas and astrocytomas. (Refer to chapter 20 for nursing care of the child undergoing radiation therapy or chemotherapy.)

Bladder Management

Early assessment and continued urinary monitoring at regular intervals are a necessary part of bladder management. The objective is to identify recurrent infections and to detect any changes which could lead to progressive obstruction.

Urinary stasis resulting in infection can be prevented partially by a good urinary flow and complete emptying of the bladder. An adequate urinary flow for a child requires a minimum fluid intake of 125 ml/kg/day. Encourage the parents to offer fluids frequently, and teach them to calculate the necessary amount. Unless they understand the importance of maintaining a good urinary flow, they may restrict the child's intake to help control incontinence.

Bacteria thrives more easily in an alkaline environment. Therefore, keeping the urine acidic helps to control infection, as well as salt and stone formation. Foods high in acid are meats, eggs, cheese, starches, corn, lentils, cranberries, plums, and prunes. Alkaline foods are milk products and all other fruits and vegetables. Ascorbic or mandelic acid may be given to lower the urine pH.

Parents must be taught to recognize urinary tract infections because the child with a neurogenic bladder will not experience the usual signs of infection, such as burning and frequency. Teach them to look for unexplained fever, decreased appetite, vomiting, lethargy, and foul smelling urine.

Several methods are available for reducing the amount of residual urine and preventing obstruction of the urinary tract. Manual bladder expression, or the *Credé maneuver* is easily learned by the child and his parents. The parents are taught to manually express the urine from the bladder with each diaper change. With the fingers a firm but gentle pressure is applied on or above the dome of the bladder, and the whole hand is used to gently press downward. When the child is old enough to sit on the toilet, he can be taught to strain in an effort to empty his bladder. Afterwards, he can use the Credé maneuver to express the residual urine. This method is contraindicated if the child has vesicourethral reflux (see ch. 30).

Nonsterile intermittent catheterization is becoming more popular, but nurses and parents alike may resist introducing a nonsterile catheter into the child's bladder. The crucial factor of the success of this method is not the sterility of the catheter but the frequency and thoroughness of emptying the bladder. Overdistension leads to decreased blood supply which in turn results in an increased susceptibility to infection. Intermittent self-catheterization, three to four times a day, helps to keep the bladder small and undistended and prevents the stasis of residual urine. The child over the age of five with good hand coordination can learn to catheterize himself. Parents should be taught to catheterize the younger or less able child.

The parents and child should be taught such basic information as the location of the external anatomy of the urinary and reproductive tracts, and should be able to identify the external urethral meatus.

Have the child or parents wash their hands and then the perineal area with warm water. The child doing self-catheterization will sit on the toilet. If the parent is catheterizing the child, suggest that the child be kept in the recumbent position. Have a container available to catch the urine. Hold the catheter near the tip, and lubricate it with a water-soluble lubricant. For girls, separate the labia with one hand, identify the meatus, and insert the catheter about 1 inch to 1½ inches. For boys, insert the catheter 1 inch to 1½ inches, plus the length of the penis. Allow the bladder to drain completely. (If you insert the catheter into the vagina, rinse the catheter under warm water, and try again). Wash the catheter in mild soapy water, rinse it well, allow it to air dry, and store it in a clean container. Boil the catheter for a few minutes each week.

External collecting devices, such as padded panties for girls and penile sheaths for boys, are commonly used to control urinary incontinence. Odor and skin breakdown are associated with the use of external devices. If penile ulceration and skin irritation develops, instruct the parents to discontinue use of the device until healing occurs. A collection bag is attached to the leg if a penile sheath is used. The bag is emptied every two to three hours. If no reflux occurs, straining and the Credé maneuver may be used when the bag is emptied.

Bowel Management

Management of the neurogenic bowel involves two objectives: managing constipation and incontinence, and preventing complications. Retained stool may cause obstruction of the bladder neck (resulting in urinary tract infections), rectal prolapse, hemorrhoids, high fecal impactions, anal fissures caused by passing hard stools, and skin breakdown caused by constant soiling. Controlling constipation is the key to preventing all of these complications, and managing incontinence.

When the child is in the newborn period, parents are taught to watch for signs of constipation, and to prevent it. Dietary management is started early. Teach the parents to avoid constipating foods, such as rice cereal, applesauce, bananas, and desserts. As age and nutrition permit, the intake of milk and milk products should be limited. Encourage foods which decrease constipation, such as barley, bran, whole grain cereals and breads, fruits, fruit juices, and vegetables. Teach the parents to place the child on a potty-chair as soon as he can sit and maintain an adequate attention span. This position increases intraabdominal pressure, and helps to evacuate the bowel. Explain that activity also helps to decrease constipation.

Stool softeners and/or stimulants may be given daily to aid in defecation. Careful explanation of the reasons for these medications is necessary if the parents are to comply on a long-term basis. It is difficult to understand why a young child needs a laxative and a stool softener, especially when advertisements warn that these agents may be habit-forming. Reinforce your previous teaching about the child's lack of innervation to the bowel. Explain again why it is important to avoid the complications of constipation.

A mild stimulant, such as standardized senna (Senokot) is safe, inexpensive, and is available without a prescription. Senokot-S is a combination stool softener/stimulant. An initial dose of a half to one teaspoon is given daily for three days to empty the colon. A maintenance dose of one quarter to one half teaspoon is then given daily, as needed, to keep the stools soft.

Bowel training is begun when the child is able to sit on the potty-chair. Place him on the potty-chair after each meal for three to five minutes, gradually increasing the time to 15 to 20 minutes as his tolerance builds. If the child has already established a pattern of stool elimination, place him on the potty-chair at these times, too. Initially, reinforce him only for sitting on the potty-chair; do not worry if he does not have a bowel movement. This scheduled toileting increases the chances of a successful stool evacuation because the gastrocolic reflex (a general increase in bowel tone after eating) is employed, and the intraabdominal pressure is increased with the sitting position. The child may be encouraged to strain in order to further increase the intraabdominal pressure.

If an additional stimulant is needed for stool evacuation, glycerin suppositories may be used in conjunction with the Senokot. Give the Senokot at supper or bedtime if you want the bowel movement to occur in the morning. After breakfast, insert the suppository, and let it dissolve for 15 to 20 minutes. Then place the child on the potty-chair and ask him to push or grunt. This schedule takes advantage of the morning gastrocolic reflex. The schedule may be varied according to the family's routines and needs.

Habilitation and Rehabilitation

Depending on whether the child's condition is present from birth or occurred as the result of an accident or infection, he will need to be habilitated or rehabilitated. He may need to spend some time in a rehabilitation center to learn to live and function within the limits of his disability. In some areas, special arrangements may be made to accommodate the child in a normal school setting, depending on the degree and extent of his handicap. Special schooling or home-bound teachers are other options.

SURGICAL MANAGEMENT

Cerebrospinal Fluid Drainage

Management of increased intracranial pressure often involves the draining of excess cerebrospinal fluid from the cranium. In the child under the age of two, subdural or ventricular taps are performed via the anterior fontanel to remove acute accumulations of fluid. A burr hole will be necessary for the older child or adult. The child is sedated and restrained in a mummy restraint (see the Skills Manual). An area around the anterior fontanel of his head is then shaved and scrubbed with an antiseptic solution. The physician inserts an appropriately sized needle, measures the initial pressure, and withdraws excess fluid. Dye may be instilled for further studies. Aftercare includes observation for any untoward effects of the sedative or the procedure. Note the child's color, vital signs, and any leakage of CSF from the puncture site. After he has recovered from the sedation, a normal diet and routine are resumed, although some physicians may wish to keep the child flat in bed, or at least quiet, for four to six hours.

Internal drainage of CSF involves the use of a permanent shunt. This type of shunt is used primarily with the child who has hydrocephalus, an abnormal amount of CSF under increased pressure within the cranium. Occasionally, a shunt is employed during surgery for removal of a brain tumor.

Physicians differ about the type of shunt to be used. With each type, cerebrospinal fluid is shunted from a lateral ventricle into a portion of the body where it is absorbed. A *ventriculoperitoneal shunt* runs from the ventricle to the peritoneal cavity. This is currently the most popular site for drainage. A *ventriculoatrial shunt* runs through the jugular vein to the right atrium (Figure 27–10). The *ventriculoureterostomy* connects the ventricle with a ureter. This shunt requires the removal of a kidney, and because CSF is excreted rather than absorbed, the child must have an increase in fluids and salt to compensate for the electrolytic imbalance.

After a shunting procedure, daily head circumference measurements are necessary to determine if the shunt is working properly. Improvement in the child's general condition will be seen within a few hours. He will be less irritable, and the anterior

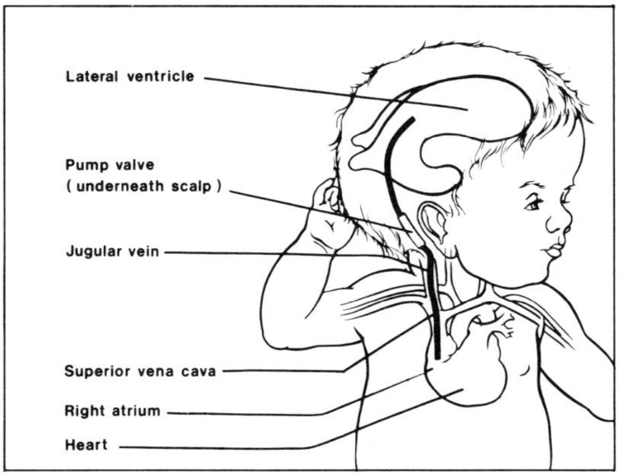

Figure 27–10. *Ventriculoatrial shunt running from ventricle through the jugular vein to the right atrium.*

fontanelle will no longer be tense and bulging, but may actually be depressed. The venous engorgement and sunset eyes will improve in about 12 hours.

Most shunts will have to be replaced as growth occurs, and a number will need replacement because of infection. The objective of early shunting is to prevent brain compression and damage during the period of rapid brain growth in the first years of life. If the brain can be protected in this fashion until the hydrocephalus is arrested, the child has a 70-percent chance of achieving normal growth and intellectual development. Less than 10 percent of these children are grossly retarded.

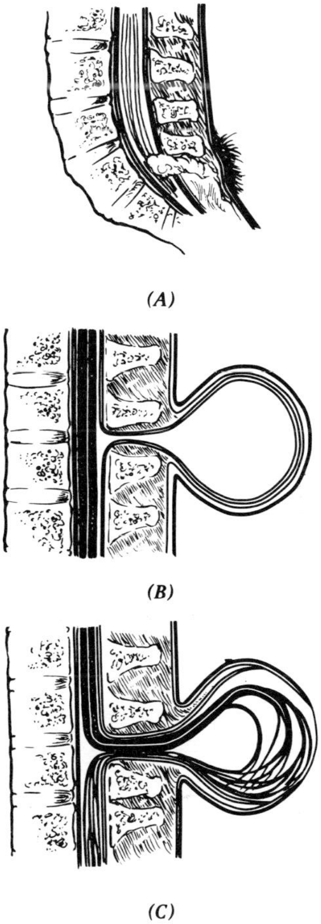

Figure 27–11. *Spinal cord anomalies. (A) Spina bifida—failure of bony arch of vertebrae to fuse and cover spinal cord; note dimple and tuft of hair. (B) Meningocele—sac forms through defect in neural arch of vertebrae; meninges protrude into sac, which is filled with CSF. (C) Meningomyelocele—in addition to CSF and meninges, sac contains spinal cord and/or nerve roots.*

Cosmetic Surgery

Closure of a spinal defect does not improve the child's functional level, but it does help to prevent meningitis, and enhances daily care. Once the spinal cord itself is injured or stretched, as in meningomyelocele (Figure 27–11), the damage is irreversible. Repair will not return sphincter control to the bladder or bowel, nor will it enable paralyzed legs to move and feel. Surgery can prevent or forestall meningitis by closing the often delicate sac, thus making it more resistant to infection. Without the fluctuant sac on the child's back, daily care is easier and less time-consuming. After the wound has healed, the child can lay on his back and be held in a normal fashion.

Immediately after surgery, keep the infant prone for two to ten days, or until primary healing takes place. During this time, he usually cannot be picked up. This prone position complicates not only physical care, but psychological care, as well. Touch and stroke the infant often and speak soothingly to him.

Keep the wound clean from urine and feces. Note any CSF drainage from the incision. Pay special attention to paralyzed extremities, giving meticulous skin care and passive range of motion exercises, according to physicians orders. Palpate the bladder every hour to be sure it is emptying, using the Credé maneuver to fully express the urine. Note the number and consistency of stools; constipation may be a problem. Mild laxatives and stool softeners will be ordered if necessary. Hydrocephalus is a complication after repair of a spinal defect, so measure the head circumference daily to detect any increase in size.

Craniotomy

An incision into the cranium is made to partially or completely remove brain tumors, debris, such as bone fragments and foreign bodies after head injuries, or to control a hemorrhage.

Brain surgery is a frightening treatment, both for the child and his family. It is natural for them to fear disability and/or death. They will need reassurance and support throughout the child's illness and hospitalization. If the child was injured in an accident, the surgery will probably be of an emergency nature with little or no time for emotional and psychological preparation. The parents may be in a state of shock, not knowing if their child will live or die. (Refer to chapter 3 for a discussion of acute illness and grief.)

If the child is suspected of having a brain tumor, the family probably has feared this diagnosis for some time. With television and other media carrying stories about leukemia, brain tumors, and the like, many parents are aware of signs and symptoms of such illnesses and immediately suspect the worst with the onset of the first symptoms.

Establish a trusting relationship with the family on admission. Such a relationship will enable you to work effectively with them and to support them during subsequent admissions. They very much need an ally whom they can trust throughout the often long and involved course of the disease.

The child's head is shaved preoperatively, and the hair given to his parents. This is always traumatic, and especially so if the child has not been adequately prepared, and if the person shaving him is not gentle and understanding. (Refer to chapter 2 for preparation of the child.) Explain to the parents that after surgery, the child may have facial edema, black eyes, a massive dressing, and may even be in a coma. Tell them these are usually transient effects caused by a disturbance of the cranial contents during surgery, and that they will subside.

Postoperatively, the child will go to the pediatric intensive care unit, if one is available. Monitor his vital signs and neurological changes every 15 minutes until he is stable, then every two hours for 24 hours. Position him on the unaffected side and change his position often. If the incision was in the occipital region, you may have to "logroll" the child to keep his neck and head in perfect alignment.

Monitor intravenous fluids and urine output carefully to avoid circulatory overload and the resultant cerebral edema. Prevent vomiting and straining at stool by limiting oral intake until bowel sounds are heard, and by giving stool softeners and laxatives as ordered. Raising the head of the bed about 30° will help to reduce intracranial pressure and facial edema. (Refer to common problems and nursing interventions for other nursing care measures.)

If the child does have facial edema, black eyes, or is in a coma, remind the parents of this before they are allowed to see him. Remind them also that these are transitory effects.

Check the dressing frequently for drainage. Note the amount and color of the drainage, and reinforce the dressing as necessary with sterile sponges or a sterile towel. Record and report your findings.

Restraints may be needed, particularly if the child is not fully conscious, to keep the child from pulling at his IV or his dressing, or from injuring himself. As discussed earlier, if the child resists or struggles against the restraints, do not use them because the resistance will increase his intracranial pressure.

Complications of brain surgery include hyperthermia, shock, meningitis, wound infection, headache, vomiting, swallowing difficulties, and respiratory involvement.

SUMMARY

Neurological deficits may be caused by a variety of conditions. Many of these conditions are life-threatening; all are frightening.

Nursing care of the child with neurological deficits is often complex, demanding, and emotionally draining. You will need to muster all of your skills, knowledge, and compassion to work with him and his family. Unfortunately, the child who is not able to function at what society deems a "normal" level is often thought of as a second-class citizen rather than as a person who happens to have a problem. As his nurse, you can help him to build or rebuild a positive self-image, which is so necessary to his continued well-being and adjustment.

CLINICAL APPLICATION

Peggy T., two days old, is admitted to the pediatric unit with a diagnosis of meningomyelocele. She has a large sac on the lumbosacral portion of her back. Reflexes below the sac are absent, and her legs are flaccid. They do not respond to pin prick. Peggy's head is larger than her chest by four centimeters. She is admitted for a workup, pending parental consent for surgery.

1. Define hydrocephalus, distinguishing between communicating and noncommunicating types.
2. Identify the physical manifestations of hydrocephalus and explain why each occurs.
3. Explain how increased intracranial pressure differs between an infant and an older child.
4. Contrast meningocele and meningomyelocele; include complications most often seen.
5. State how you will manage Peggy's neurogenic bladder and bowel.

Peggy's parents give permission for surgery, which is performed when she is five days old. She has a ventroperitoneal shunt and closure of the meningomyelocele. After surgery, Peggy's father asks, "When will she be able to walk?"

6. What do you say? On what information do you base your answer?
7. Peggy is to remain prone for 48 hours after surgery. How will this affect your nursing care plan?
8. List at least three nursing goals for Peggy that you expect to meet while she is hospitalized. Explain how you intend to meet these goals.
9. Design a teaching plan for helping Mr. and Mrs. T. to manage Peggy's neurogenic bowel and bladder.

Table 27–4. Specific Neurological Conditions

Condition	*Description*	*Treatment*	*Special Nursing Considerations*
Head Injury			
Skull Fractures			
Linear	Simple break in the continuity of the bone, but no alteration of the relationship of the parts.	Symptomatic treatment on basis of degree of brain injury. Simple fractures require minimum care.	
Comminuted	Splintered bone caused by multiple linear fractures.		
Depressed	Broken skull pushed inward, may impinge on local area of the brain, causing seizures or focal neurological signs.	Surgical correction as soon as the child's condition permits.	
Compound	Any fracture complicated by an external wound.		
Basal	At the base of the skull; more serious because torn meninges permit leakage of CSF from ears and nose. Characteristic water-ring stain on linens points to basilar skull fracture. The danger is not leakage of CSF, but entrance of bacteria into the subarachnoid space, resulting in meningitis.	Bedrest until drainage subsides; cool soaks for orbital edema and ecchymosis.	Special attention to drainage from ears and nose. Protect the eyes with an ophthalmic ointment.
Cerebral Trauma			
Concussion	Minor head injury characterized by brief loss of consciousness and spontaneous recovery.		Careful observation including neurological check; notify physician of any change.
Contracoup concussion	The brain bounces against the skull opposite the site of impact/injury.		

Contusion	Brain is actually bruised; consciousness lost for longer period of time. Neurological dysfunction likely. Memory loss at time of the injury is characteristic.	See section on coma care.	
Laceration	Tearing of the pia mater, resulting in hemorrhages on the convolutions of the brain.		
Hemorrhage			
Subdural	Acute or insidious collection of blood and fluid below the dura mater, compressing brain.	Removal of fluid and blood via subdural tap. Surgery may be necessary if taps do not decrease the amount of fluid significantly. Prognosis depends on amount of brain damage incurred before treatment.	Observe and report changes in neurological status.
Extradural	Tear in middle meningeal artery (lying just inside the skull), usually due to skull fracture. Rapid bleeding which must be treated promptly. Classic picture is initial loss of consciousness followed by arousal (lucid interval), then rapidly progressing neurological changes.	Immediate surgery	
Subarachnoid	A bleed between arachnoid and pia mater from a vessel on surface of brain. Signs of meningitis (headache and stiff neck) occur within 24 to 48 hours after injury.	Rest and/or surgical intervention.	

(Continued)

Table 27–4. *(Continued)*

Condition	*Description*	*Treatment*	*Special Nursing Considerations*
Spinal Cord Anomalies/Injuries			
Spina bifida occulta	Failure of bony arch of vertebrae to fuse and cover spinal cord; usually in lumbosacral area. May have dimple or tuft of hair over the site. No symptoms; defect seen on Xray.	No treatment necessary.	
Spina bifida cystica	A cyst or sac forms through the defect in the neural arch of the vertebrae.		
Meningocele	Meninges protrude into sac, which is filled with CSF. No nerves protrude, thus there is no sensory loss.	Surgical repair to remove the sac.	Keep incision site free from urine and feces.
Meningomyelocele	In addition to CSF and meninges, the sac also contains spinal cord and/or nerve roots. Residual defects range from muscle imbalance with orthopedic anomalies (dislocated hips and clubfoot) to full paralysis of the legs and incontinence of urine and feces. Seventy percent develop hydrocephalus.	Option of the parents with guidance from the neurosurgeon. May elect not to operate. If treatment is to be pursued, the sac, which may be thin and transparent, or covered with normal skin, is excised to facilitate care and cosmetic appearance. Nerve roots are placed back into the spinal canal. If surgery is postponed, the infant must not lay on his back.	See section on paralysis in altered motor-sensory functioning. Position patient on side or abdomen.
Spinal cord injury			
contusion	Bruise of spinal cord; gradual return of function over several weeks. Initial paralysis and loss of sphincter control.	Immediate medical attention to prevent further injury.	Protect from further neurological injury, pressure points on skin, urinary infections.

Laceration	Loss of inervation below the level of injury.	Immediate life-saving measures and usually surgery to stabilize the spine and prevent further neurological damage. Rehabilitation.
*Brain Tumors**		
Infratentorial tumors	Account for 50 percent of childhood tumors; located below the tentorium in the cerebellum or posterior fossa.	
Cerebellar Medulloblastoma	Most common malignant tumor of childhood; 20 percent of intracranial tumors. Twice as common in boys than girls; peak incidence between ages three and eight. Tumor originates in cerebellum, grows rapidly. Grade IV malignancy.	Surgery, irradiation, chemotherapy. Tumors usually reoccur. Average survival time is eight to twenty-four months.
Spongioblastoma (Cerebellar astrocytoma)	Peak incidence between ages seven and nine; more common in girls. Accounts for over 15 percent of all childhood tumors. Slow growing, noninvasive. Grade I malignancy; most benign childhood tumor.	Excision; if totally removed, does not metastasize or recur. Radiation, if complete removal is not possible.
Ependymoma	No sex or age predilection. Occurs most often in fourth ventricle. Cauliflower-like growth. Seeding (spread) throughout the CNS is spontaneous or surgically induced. Grade I malignancy.	Excision; if totally removed, does not recur, but the tumor usually is inaccessible. Surgery and radiation combined extend life three to ten years.

(continued)

Table 27–4. *(Continued)*

Condition	*Description*	*Treatment*	*Special Nursing Considerations*
Brain Stem Tumor	Peak age seven. No sex dominance. Accounts for over 10 percent of infratentorial tumors. Brain stem, pons, and medulla oblongata may be involved. Astrocytoma of the brain stem is most common.	Surgical removal is not possible. Radiation extends survival time.	
Supratentorial tumors	Occur above the tentorium. Symptoms and diagnosis occur late, after tumor is large.		
Cerebral Ependymoma	Most common in males two to five years of age. Primary site is frontal or parietal lobe; may also originate in temporal lobe. Cauliflower-like mass which may expand to fill entire hemispheric spaces. Grade II malignancy.	Surgery, but recurrence is common. Most are sensitive to irradiation.	
Astrocytoma	Incidence higher after age thirteen. Does not metastasize, but may change into malignant glioblastoma. Frontal, temporal, and centroparietal regions are primary sites. May be semibenign or malignant.	Surgery and radiation prolongs life, but the prognosis is generally poor.	
Spongioblastoma	Astrocytoma of juvenile type. Located near ventricles. Longer survival than in cases of astrocytomas. Slow-growing; do not metastasize or seed into CSF.	Surgery, irradiation. Poor prognosis associated with incomplete removal.	

Glioblastoma	Located primarily in cerebrum, but also in brain stem. Rapid growth. Extensive brain edema is common. Death occurs within 12 to 15 months even after extensive treatment. Grade IV malignancy.	Surgery to excise tumor, followed by irradiation.	
Craniopharyngioma	Accounts for about 20 percent of supratentorial tumors. Originates prenatally; peak ages five to fifteen; twice as often in males. Located near pituitary; may cause hormonal disturbances, such as delayed puberty, diabetes insipidus, myxedema, and visual disturbances.	Surgery. These tumors are radioresistant.	
Optic Nerve Glioma	Exopthalmos is often the first symptom. Recall that young children generally do not complain of visual disturbances.	Surgery with complete or partial removal, followed by irradiation.	
Hydrocephalus	Abnormal accumulation of CSF in the brain. *Obstructive or noncommunicating:* tumor, hemorrhage, or congenital defects obstruct the free flow of CSF; fluid accumulates in the ventricles, pushing the brain against the skull. The fontanels bulge and the head enlarges. *Communicating:* CSF is not absorbed after it reaches the subarachnoid space because of hemorrhage, scar tissue, or congenital anomalies. Fluid accumulates outside the brain. Head enlargement is not as great as with obstructive hydrocephalus.	Shunting procedure.	See the section on cerebrospinal fluid drainage with surgical management.

(continued)

Table 27–4. *(Continued)*

Condition	*Description*	*Treatment*	*Special Nursing Considerations*
Encephalocele	Incomplete closure of bones of the skull in utero; meninges and brain protrude. Most common site is occipital region.	Surgical excision of sac and repair of bony defect. No treatment when there is gross evidence of brain damage.	See hydrocephalus.
Craniosynostosis	Premature closure of the sutures, leads to brain damage, mental retardation, convulsions.	Surgical opening of sutures.	See brain tumors.
Epilepsy	Seizure activity caused by abnormal impulses in the brain.	Refer to Table 27–1	
Idiopathic	No known cause; onset prior to puberty, some family tendency.		
Acute	Related to metabolic disorders, such as hypoglycemia, hypocalcemia, or drug withdrawal.		
Chronic	Recurrent seizures; no external cause. The term "epilepsy" is generally used in this context.		
Cerebral Palsy	An aggregate of handicaps: emotional, neuromuscular, and sensory; caused by fixed (nonprogressive) brain damage. Usually due to anoxia prenatally or perinatally. The infant at risk is "small for date", weighs less than 2000 gm, has poor socioeconomic status, and complications at birth. (Refer to section on diagnostic procedures.)	Treatment is long-term and requires a team approach, including the neurologist, pediatrician, nurse, physical therapist, and social worker.	Encourage the family to accept the child and his disability (see bonding, ch. 3). Precautions to prevent painful muscle spasms are necessary.

Spastic (50–60%)	Increased muscle tone; exaggerated deep tendon reflexes; abnormal continuation of neonatal reflexes; typical posture include scissoring, whereby the tight abductor muscles pull his legs together so that they cross. Toe-walking is also common due to tightening of the heel cord. Spasticity may involve all extremities, the legs, or one side of the body. Speech and swallowing may be impaired, particularly if all extremities are involved. The child will drool constantly and is more likely to be mentally retarded.	Many communities have clinics and rehabilitation centers which treat the child, guide and support the family, and provide financial assistance. Preventing contractures is a major goal of therapy. Exercises and braces are utilized. Special feeding techniques may be necessary, such as suction cups to keep dishes stable, weighted cups, and special silverware designed to strap on to the child's hand.	Bathe in warm water (cold or hot will trigger spasms). Spastic thighs and buttocks make bowel movements difficult. Gently separate the buttocks to facilitate bowel movements; release if spasms occur. Allowing ample time for relaxation of tight muscles before beginning exercises helps to prevent spasms.
Dyskinesia (20 to 25 percent) A thetosis (most common type of dyskinesia)	Slow, writhing, worm-like movements which increase under pressure or stress, and decrease during sleep. Movements usually include all extremities as well as the head and neck. Drooling may be excessive.		
Ataxia (1 to 10 percent)	Incoordination due to disturbance in sense of balance, posture, kinesthetic feedback.		
Mixed (15 to 40 percent)	Most common combinations of the above are spasticity with athetosis, and ataxia with athetosis.		

*Central nervous system tumors are second only to leukemia as the leading group of neoplasms in the child. These tumors arise from the brain tissue itself, not as a result of metastasis from other organs.

Bibliography

Adams NR. Prolonged Coma: Your Care Makes All the Difference. *Nursing '77* 7:21, August, 1977.

Alexander, M.M. and Brown, M.S.: Physical Examination: Part 18, Performing the Neurologic Examination. *Nursing '76* 6:50, July, 1976.

Bindler, R.M. and Lowry, L.B. Nursing Care of Children With Febrile Seizures. *American Journal of Maternal-Child Nursing* 3:270, 1978.

Bruya, M.A. and Bohn, R.H. Epilepsy: A Controllable Disease. *American Journal of Nursing* 76:388, 1976.

Conway, B.L. *Carini and Owens' Neurological and Neurosurgical Nursing,* ed. 7. St. Louis, C.V. Mosby Co., 1978.

Conway, B.L. *Pediatric Neurological Nursing.* St. Louis, C.V. Mosby Co., 1977.

Cooper, C.R. Anticonvulsant Drugs and the Epileptics Dilemma. *Nursing '76* 6:44, January, 1976.

Cruickshank, W.M. *Cerebral Palsy: A Developmental Disability,* ed. 3. New York, Syracuse University Press, 1976.

Ertel, I.J. and Boesel, C. Brain Tumors. *Pediatric Annals* 7:560, 1978.

Fochtman, D., Raimondi, A.J., Gutierrez, F.A. Nursing Care of the Pediatric Neurosurgery Patient, in Fochtman, D. and Raffensperger, J.G. (eds). *Principles of Nursing Care for the Pediatric Surgery Patient,* ed. 2. Boston, Little, Brown & Co., 1976, p. 189.

Geddes, N. Intermittent Catheterization for Patients with Spina Bifida. *The Canadian Nurse* 74:34, 1978.

Hawley, D. and Reiser, D.W. Reducing Muscle Spasms in a Child with Cerebral Palsy. *American Journal of Nursing* 78:1214, 1978.

Henderson, M.L. and Synhorst, D.M. Bladder and Bowel Management in the Child with Myelomeningocele. *Pediatric Nursing* 3:24, 1977.

Hendry, J. and Geddes, N. Living with a Congenital Anomaly: How Nurses Can Help the Parents of Children Born with Spina Bifida to Develop Lasting Patterns of Creative Caring. *The Canadian Nurse* 74:29, 1978.

McLaurine, R.L. et al. Nervous System, in Gellis, S.S. and Kagan, B.M. (eds). *Current Pediatric Therapy.* Philadelphia, W.B. Saunders Co., 1978.

Meyd, C.J. Acute Brain Trauma, *American Journal of Nursing,* 78:40, 1978.

Mitchell, P.H. and Mauss, N. Intracranial Pressure: Fact and Fancy. *Nursing '76* 6:53, June, 1976.

Muehl, J.N. Seizure Disorders in Children: Prevention and Care. *American Journal Maternal-Child Nursing* 4:154, 1979.

Nursing Grand Rounds: Family-Centered Conferences for Better Trauma Care. *Nursing '78* 8:70, October, 1978.

Passo, S.D. Positioning Infants with Myelomeningocele. *American Journal of Nursing* 74:1658, 1974.

Rudy, E. Early Omens of Cerebral Disaster. *Nursing '77* 7:59, February, 1977.

Shearer, J.D. The Adolescent Wheelchair Athlete. *Pediatric Nursing* 3:20, 1977.

Spitz, P.S. and Sweetwood, H. Kids in Crisis Part I: Bedside Assessment—Special Considerations. *Nursing '78* 8:70, March, 1978.

Surveyer, J.A. The Emotional Toll on Nurses Who Care for Comatose Children. *American Journal Maternal-Child Nursing* 1:243, 1976.

Swift, N. Helping Patients Live with Seizures. *Nursing '78* 8:25, June, 1978.

Wahl, S. Only a Concussion. *Nursing '76* 6:44, August, 1976.

RESOURCES

Epilepsy

Americal Epilepsy Society
Stanford University Medical Center
Stanford, California 94305

Epilepsy Foundation of America
1828 L Street, N.W.
Washington, D.C. 20036

National Epilepsy League
116 S. Michigan Avenue
Chicago, Illinois 60603

Spinal Cord Trauma

Sister Kenny Institute
1800 Chicago Avenue
Minneapolis, Minnesota 55405

CHAPTER **28**

The Child with a Musculoskeletal Disorder

BEHAVIORAL OBJECTIVES

After studying this chapter you will be able to:

- Assess the physical and emotional effects of immobility on the child.
- Explain diagnostic procedures to the child and his family.
- Discuss the various modes of treatment for the child with a musculoskeletal deviation.
- Design a plan of care for the child immobilized by a cast or traction.
- Describe specific musculoskeletal conditions common to the child.

TERMS AND CONCEPTS

Ortolani's sign
Trendelenburg's sign
Electromyogram
Cast petaling
Window edema
Cast syndrome
Traction (skeletal and skin)
Restraints (sling, jacket, frame, and diaper)
Osteomyelitis
Bradford frame
Halo-femoral traction
Halo-pelvic traction
Risser cast

IMMOBILITY

Musculoskeletal anomalies in children are many and varied. This chapter focuses on those conditions that are rarely or never seen in adults (except in instances in which the condition was present since birth or childhood and allowed to go without proper treatment). Common problems and diagnostic and treatment regimens are discussed, along with the nursing interventions for each condition. Nursing responsibilities for the child in a cast or traction are covered in depth.

COMMON PROBLEMS AND NURSING INTERVENTIONS

Immobility

Immobility affects the child both physically and emotionally. Physical effects are varied and often complex. Some emotional response to immobility is to be expected; the child should be *encouraged* to react to his immobility in whatever way is natural for him.

The normal child's life centers around his mobility; he learns about himself and his world through movement. He reaches out to touch a flower or a rock. He rolls in the green grass, smelling and feeling it as he rolls. He stands tiptoe to reach the countertop. The young child hops, skips, and jumps his way through the world. He uses fine muscles to build with blocks and scribble a picture. Through each of these activities he is learning and *moving.* The school child catches the bus to ride to school; he climbs on the monkey bars at recess, and pushes his way to the front of the lunch line. His fine muscle movement is refined as he writes his lessons or learns to play the piano. He is *constantly* interacting and *moving.* The adolescent depends on his mobility to engage in sports, to dance, and to walk hand-in-hand with his new "love." Interaction with his peers and establishing his self-identity depend to a large extent on his ability to be mobile.

Mobility is important not only to the child's normal growth and development but also for the release of energy and aggression. He releases his frustration through activity. If the child is immobile (because of traction, a cast, or bed rest for another reason) he is denied this normal release. If provisions are not made for the expression of his frustration, his anxiety level rises. Every immobilized child should be permitted some form of activity. Provide a punching bag for the release of aggression; use a large balloon or rubber ball attached to traction bars or an IV pole. For the young child, try using a peg-board he can hammer. Modeling clay to pound, squash, and manipulate is excellent for the older child.

Not only does the child need play to release his frustration, he needs it to alleviate the boredom of restricted activity. If possible, move the child (bed and all if he's in traction) to the playroom or recreation area. He can participate in music, art, and games offered by the "play lady." If these facilities are not available, move him into the hall or near the nurse's station. He should be in the center of activity, his condition permitting. Perhaps he can help cut out holiday decorations for the unit.

Television can be useful as a diversion, especially if educational programs (or cartoons for the young child) are available. Do not depend on the television to entertain the child all day, or to take the place of meaningful interaction and activity, however. It is far better to schedule TV watching than to turn it on and leave it on. Special tutoring, or "school" if your institution has a school teacher, will enable the child to continue to learn and to keep up with his grade while he is hospitalized.

If the child is going to be immobile for a long time, he should not have a private room. Place him in a room with a child near his own age who has a similar condition. They will be able to share experiences and feelings. Explain to the parents why it is important for the child to have a roommate, because they may prefer a private room for a number of reasons.

Circulatory Status

Immobility causes a decrease in cardiac output. Circulation is slowed because of inactivity, and if the child is in a cast or traction, circulation to the affected area of the body may be even more sluggish. The nurse can stimulate the circulation through passive exercise and by letting the child move as much as possible. He may be able to help turn, bathe, dress, or feed himself; move around in bed; or engage in fine motor activities such as handicrafts, writing letters, and so on, depending on his age and disability. *Let the child do what he can.* This self-help attitude promotes independence and helps restore (or build) self-confidence.

Digestive Status

Immobility leads to sluggish digestion in several ways. The circulation to the gastrointestinal tract is decreased; the child's appetite is decreased because of his lack of activity; and his anorexia leads to inadequate intake, which contributes to constipation. Check the child's menu after he selects his food. Is he choosing bland foods with little roughage? (Roughage is found in fruits and vegetables, whole-grain breads, cereals, and fruit juices.) Explain to the child and his family why he is having bowel problems and what can be done to correct them. Encourage a well-balanced diet that includes roughage. Remember that allowing the child a choice will gain his cooperation more quickly than will choosing for him. You can encourage a proper diet *and* permit him to choose by saying, "Bill, tomorrow's dinner menu includes potatoes, carrots, and rice. The potatoes and carrots are roughage; the rice is not. Since you need roughage, which would you like, potatotes or carrots? Of course, you can have the rice, too."

Check the child's fluid intake. Is it adequate? (See Table 29–1 for water needs at various ages.) If not, encourage increased fluid intake to help prevent constipation. Laxatives and enemas are given as necessary.

Kidney Function

Sluggish kidney function is always a problem during periods of immobilization, and renal calculi (stones) are more likely to form because calcium is pulled from the bones and is deposited in the kidneys. The nursing goal is to improve renal function and to prevent the formation of calculi. Encourage an intake of at least twice the normal daily fluid requirements. Make a chart or "progress poster" to help the child keep up with his fluid intake; everytime he drinks a glass of liquid, allow him to put a star or other decoration on his chart. Be sure to offer fluids the child prefers. Milk consumption should be limited to a glass with each meal since an increased calcium intake will increase the likelihood of renal deposits. Keeping the urine acidic will help to prevent the formation of calculi and urinary tract infections, both of which occur more readily in an alkaline urine. Offer acid-ash foods and cranberry juice daily to prevent the formation of alkaline urine.

Skin Integrity

Pressure areas tend to develop when a child must be immobilized. Skin care and a change of position every four hours will help to prevent the formation of decubitus ulcers. If the child has a past history of pressure problems, or a meningomyelocele, turn him and give skin care at least every two hours.

Musculoskeletal Integrity

Disuse of muscles leads to atrophy; the muscles decrease in size and become flabby. Calcium loss in the bones causes *osteoporosis* (loss of bone density). The bones become softer and may fracture easily. The nurse's responsibilities begin with the prevention of musculoskeletal disuse problems. Passive and active exercises help prevent these complications. Often the physical and/or occupational therapist will design a plan of activity and exercise for the child. All extremities not in a cast or traction are exercised in an attempt to maintain muscle strength and function. Self-help activities, such as bathing, eating, and turning, are an important part of therapy for the immobilized child.

Body Image

The child who is handicapped is exposed to the trauma of the treatment regimen and also to emotional trauma. He is often ridiculed by his peers. He is subjected to jokes about his condition and is frequently rejected. His family may overprotect and pity him. He often has guilt feelings about his condition, thinking he is a burden. If his problem is the result of an accident, he will feel guilty for having "caused" the accident. Perhaps he was told not to ride his bike in the street; he did and was struck by a car. As a result, he feels that he was "bad" because he didn't obey, and he sees his injury as punishment for his wrongdoing.

If the child was born with his handicap, he and his family usually accept it better because he has known no other way of living. If his injury was caused by an accident, he and his family will have a more difficult time adjusting. He will have to grieve for the loss of his healthy body before he can cope with his new handicapped body.

Pain

Pain is common with musculoskeletal disorders. After surgery on bone, the pain is more severe than when soft tissue alone is cut or manipulated. Saws, chisels, and hammers are all used in bone surgery, and the aftermath will certainly be painful. Anxiety may increase pain, as do muscle spasms. The child may refuse to change position, turn, or even cough or breathe deeply because he is in pain. He will need pain medication, and it should be offered, especially after surgery or manipulation of a fracture. Assure the child that he can have pain medication as needed, and be sure to get it for him.

Handle the painful body part gently but firmly. Never let it slip out of your hands because this can cause extreme pain and may alter the proper alignment. Reassure the child that you will be as gentle as possible.

COMMON DIAGNOSTIC STUDIES

Physical Examination

A number of musculoskeletal disorders (e.g., some fractures, and curvature of the spine) are readily observable. Knowing what to look for is imperative if these problems are to be detected on physical examination.

Screening for scoliosis is a simple procedure used in many schools and health clinics. The child's back must be exposed if the spine is to be properly visualized. Girls may prefer to wear a halter or bathing suit top. Stand behind the child and ask him to stand erect but relaxed (Figure 28–1). Does his head line up directly over the crease in his buttocks? Is one shoulder or scapula (usually the right) higher than the other? Is there a difference in the neck-to-shoulder angle on either side? Is one scapula or hip (usually the left) more prominent than the other? Is there a deeper crease on one side of the waist or a difference in the size of the space between arms and trunk? Does the spine appear to curve? Ask the child to bend forward, letting his arms hang freely (Figure 28–2). His knees should be unbent and his back parallel to the floor. Look from both the front and back, inspecting for any curvature of the spine or a visible hump (prominence) on one side of the back. Hold your index and middle fingers together and gently palpate the spine. Can you feel any curvature? If the answer to any of these questions is "Yes," refer the child to a physician for further diagnostic studies, such as x-rays.

To check for congenital dislocated hips, place the infant flat on his back or stomach and extend his legs (Figures 28–3 and 28–4). Does he have extra gluteal folds on one thigh? Is one leg shorter than the other? Can you see a prominent trochanter? With

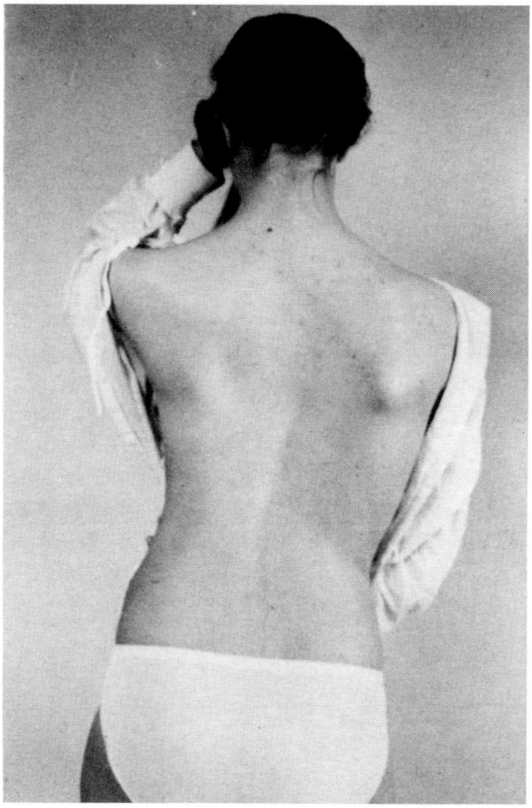

Figure 28–1. *Scoliosis, erect. Note prominent right scapula and left hip.* (Courtesy, E.A. Saunders, M.D., Professor of Surgery; Chief, Section of Orthopedics, Medical College of Georgia, Augusta, Ga.)

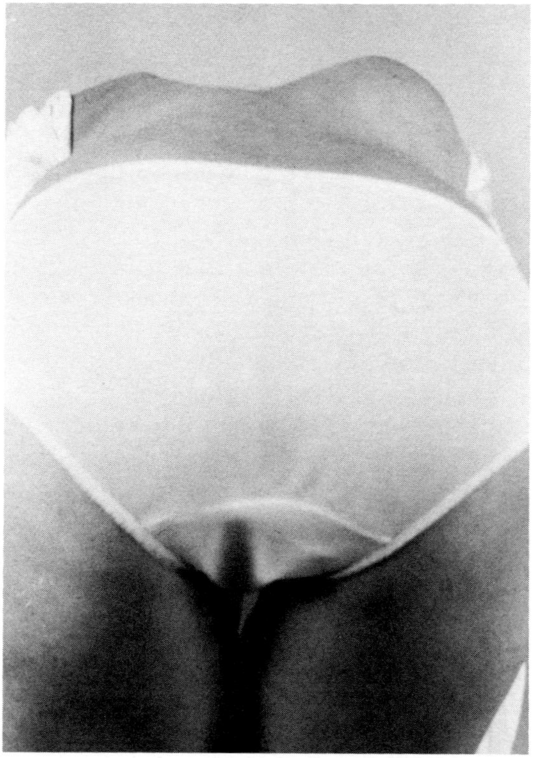

Figure 28–2. *Scoliosis, bending forward. Note rib hump on right.* (Courtesy, E.A. Saunders, M.D., Professor of Surgery; Chief, Section of Orthopedics, Medical College of Georgia, Augusta, Ga.)

the infant on his back, flex the knees and hold them at a right angle to the body; does one leg appear shorter? If so, this is a positive Allis's sign and indicates dislocation of the hip (Figure 28–5). Place your third finger on the trochanter and gently abduct one leg. Does it have limited abduction? (If the infant is under one month old, a telltale click, *Ortolani's sign,* is heard as the trochanter slides out of the acetabulum. If he is older than one month, the affected leg will not abduct). Repeat for the other leg.

In the older child with dislocated hip, *Trendelenburg's sign,* or a "duck-waddle" gait, may be observed. To check for Trendelenburg's sign, have the child stand on one foot with his back to you. If the opposite pelvis dips, the sign is positive (Figure 28–6). A duck-waddle gait is seen in cases of bilateral dislocation.

Talipes (clubfoot) is an obvious deformity diagnosed in the newborn. It may be structural (true clubfoot) or positional. Positional clubfoot is a result of intrauterine

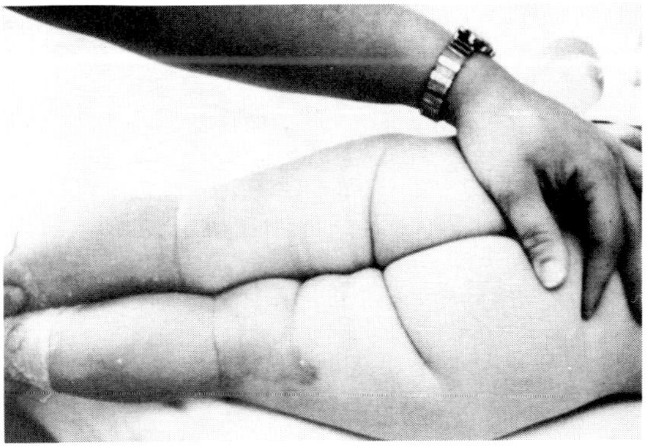

Figure 28–3. *Congenital dislocated hip in infant Note extra skin folds and prominent trochanter on right side.* (Courtesy, E.W. Berg, M.D., Associate Professor of Surgery, Section of Orthopedics, Medical College of Georgia, Augusta, Ga.)

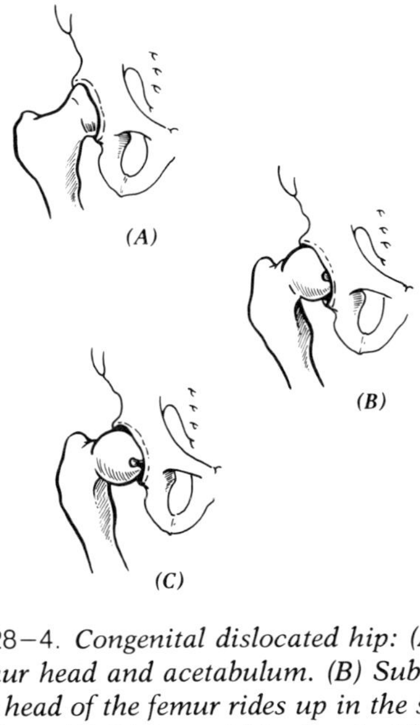

Figure 28–4. *Congenital dislocated hip: (A) Normal femur head and acetabulum. (B) Subluxated hip; the head of the femur rides up in the shallow acetabulum. (C) Dislocated hip; head of femur is not in acetabulum.*

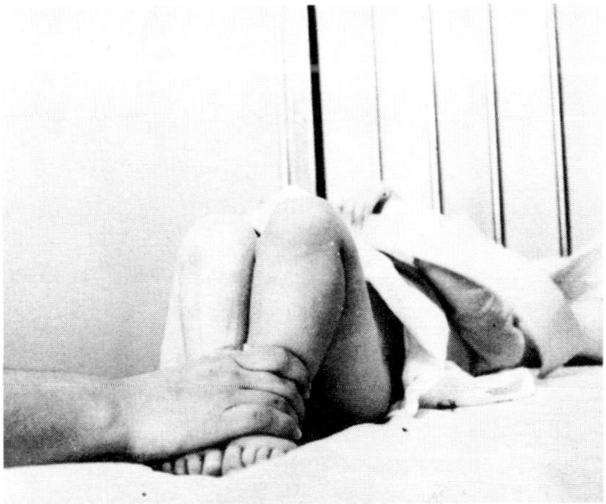

Figure 28–5. *Allis's sign for dislocated hip. Right knee is lower than left, indicating dislocation of right hip.* (Courtesy, E.W. Berg, M.D., Associate Professor of Surgery, Section of Orthopedics, Medical College of Georgia, Augusta, Ga.)

positioning and can be passively corrected. Attempt to gently correct the clubfoot. If it can be easily moved, it is positional; if the foot cannot be easily manipulated, the child has true clubfoot (Figure 28–7).

Other Studies

Suspicion of musculoskeletal disorders warrants x-ray examination to confirm or deny the diagnosis and to determine the severity of positive cases.

Routine blood studies may reveal anemia, leukocytosis, and altered serum electrolytes. In muscular dystrophy, for example, the creatine phosphokinase (CPK) level is elevated, as is the erythrocyte sedimentation rate (ESR) in juvenile rheumatoid arthritis. The nurse's responsibility includes preparing the child for venipuncture, assisting with the procedure, offering comfort and support to the child, and providing needle play afterward.

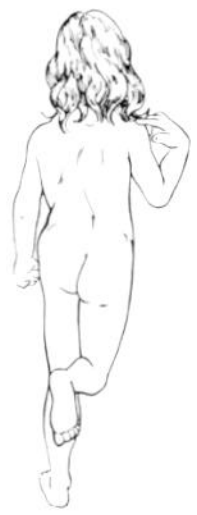

Figure 28–6. *Positive Trendelenburg's sign. Note prominent trochanter on left side.*

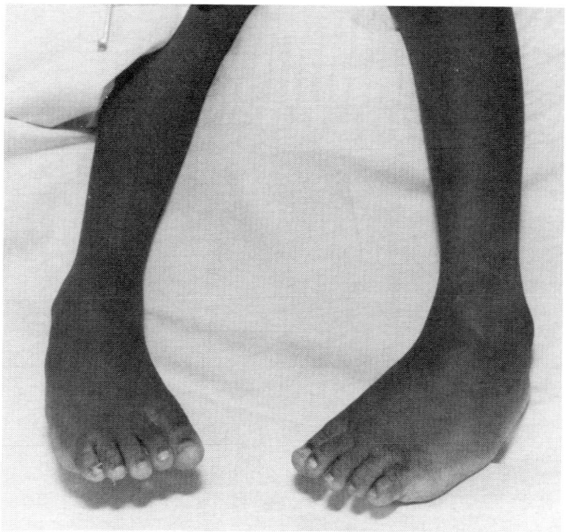

Figure 28–7. *Bilateral clubfoot in five-year-old girl after one attempt at surgical correction.*

An *electromyogram* (EMG) is a necessary part of the dianostic process for muscular dystrophy. Its purpose is to determine if muscle weakness is due to abnormal nerves or muscles. Thin, wirelike needles are inserted into the child's muscles, and a recording of muscular contractions is made on a screen. This is a frightening and painful test that requires much support for the child. Carefully explain the procedure to both the child and his parents, provide needle play beforehand, and stay with the child during the test.

Muscle biopsy is also necessary when muscular dystrophy is suspected. This is a surgical procedure in which the child will be anesthetized, Explain that only a small sample of the muscle mass will be removed.

COMMON TREATMENTS

The treatment of musculoskeletal disorders often involves the use of a variety of devices to correct and maintain proper alignment and to immobilize the body part until healing has taken place or to prevent further deterioration of the child's condition.

Casts

Plaster casts are a commonly used method of immobilizing a body part. Casting is frightening to the child. Offer the infant a bottle, or let the young child take his teddy bear or doll to the cast room. Sedation may be necessary if the child is in pain, and anesthesia may be administered if manipulation of his body or extremity is required during the casting procedure. If there is time before cast application to explain the procedure to the child, do so. (If he suffers a fracture as a result of an accident, for example, there may be no time for an adequate explanation.) Let him apply a cast to a doll or teddy bear so that he can become familiar with the feel of the plaster and the procedure. Explain that the cast will feel warm while it is drying, but that it will not burn him and will cool as the cast dries.

Before the cast is applied, a stockinette is fitted over the part to be casted to protect the skin from irritation. Cotton padding is wrapped over the stockinette with special attention to bony prominences. Plaster of paris bandage rolls are immersed in water, wrapped around the extremity and/or body in the desired position, and then allowed to dry and harden.

Handle a wet cast with the palm of your hand to avoid finger indentations which create pressure areas. Allow the cast to dry on pillows to avoid mashing the soft plaster. Turn the child every two hours until the cast dries, which takes 48 to 72 hours. It is usually necessary to elevate the extremity and apply ice bags to reduce edema. Do not place full ice bags on top of the cast because the weight of the ice will flatten the cast, causing a pressure area to develop. Fill ice bags one-third to one-half full and prop them on the side of the cast. Refill them every three hours, checking to make sure they are not indenting the plaster.

As soon as the cast is properly positioned on pillows to dry, remove excess plaster from the child with a warm wet washcloth. He will likely have plaster from head to toe and will feel more comfortable when it is removed. Carefully remove plaster crumbs from under the edge of the cast. If a stockinette is used to pad the cast, the ends will likely be pulled down over the cast's edges and secured with a light coating of plaster. This makes a smooth edge that decreases skin irritation. Check the edges to see if there are any thin spots where the stockinette is not adequately padded. If there are, cut the stockinette where it is attached on the outside of the cast, lift it up and pad the area, then tape the stockinette back in place to form a smooth edge. If a stockinette is not used, *petal* the cast with strips of tape beginning under the cast and folding the tape over to the outside. (See the Skills Manual.)

Neurovascular Assessment

Neurovascular assessments are an important part of cast care. Neurovascular impairment is relatively common after casting and may be caused by the cast application and molding, edema, or the constrictive force of the cast. It is imperative that the child receive meticulous nursing care after casting. With conscientious care, there is no reason for the child to suffer complications of cast treatment. Check the child's neurovascular status every hour for the first 24 hours after casting, or until his normal status has returned; then check him every four hours until the cast is removed. Assess each extremity encased or affected by the cast. If the trunk is also enclosed in the cast, assess all four extremities.

To evaluate the circulatory status, check the color, temperature, extent of edema, and capillary filling of the toes or fingers, in adequate light. Using inadequate lighting causes nursing errors. Assess neurological status by checking the child's reaction to a pinch or pinprick. If he cries, moves, or wiggles his toes or fingers, sensation is intact. To check for motion, ask the child to wiggle his toes. Remember that the child cannot be depended on to verbalize symptoms, so be sure to obtain objective proof of neurovascular status on the child under ten years of age.

Record your observation in easily understood terms; do not use ambiguous terms such as "good" or "poor." Record the actual results of your assessment, such as "fingers pink and warm to touch, capillary filling rapid, no edema, responds to pinprick, moves fingers on command, denies numbness and tingling." The use of an orthopedic neurovascular assessment sheet facilitates the continuous documentation of the child's status.

Skin Care

Skin care is another important aspect of cast care. Skin around the cast edges readily becomes irritated because of friction produced as the child moves around. Toughen the skin around the cast edges and over bony prominences and pressure areas by rubbing it with 70 percent isopropyl alcohol every four hours as long as the cast is in place (Figure 28–8). If a reddened area is noted, increase the alcohol application to every hour, and relieve pressure on the area. Do not use powders, oils, or lotions on the skin; powders tend to cake, causing further irritation, and oils and lotions soften the skin, increasing its vulnerability to breakdown.

Reposition or turn the child every two hours to help prevent pressure sores from developing. If he has a problem with sensation (e.g., with a meningolyelocele), reposition him every two hours. If he is on a Bradford frame, he can turn from front to back only. Most other casts permit sidelying also. (See the Skills Manual.)

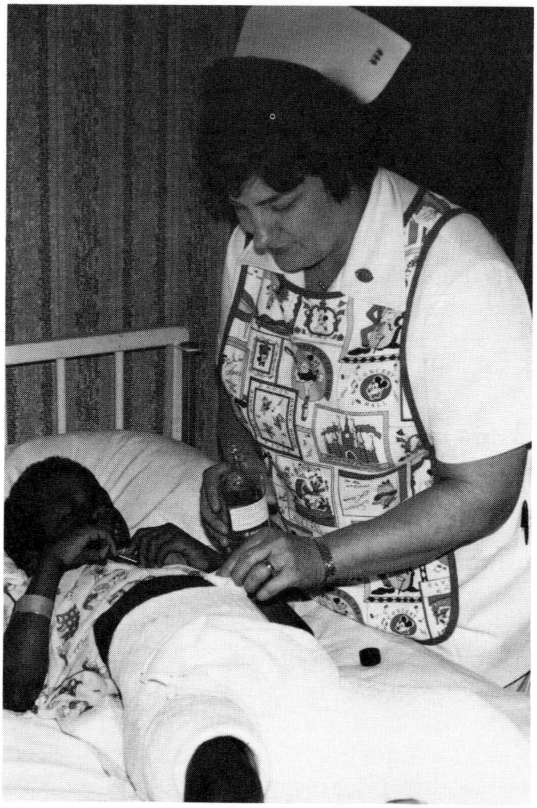

Figure 28–8. *To toughen skin, nurse applies alcohol to skin around cast edges; note waist of cast petaled with adhesive tape.*

Skin Care Under the Cast

In addition to the problems just discussed, the child himself may contribute to skin breakdown if he drops articles into his cast. Food crumbs and small toys are the most likely culprits. Do not permit the child to play with small toys or other objects that may drop into the cast (coins, paper clips, buttons, etc.). Cover the cast with a towel when the child eats so that crumbs do not fall into the cast. If the child complains of itching, he or his parents may introduce a coat-hanger, pencil, back scratcher, ruler, or other object into the cast in an effort to scratch; this is dangerous because it may harm the skin or may be inadvertently dropped into the cast. Planning ahead to place a gauze "scratcher" under the cast before application will allevaite much of the child's discomfort (see the Skills Manual). When it needs to be changed, attach a new piece to one end and pull it through.

Smell under the cast at close range each day, and inspect the skin under the cast with a flashlight several times a day. If the older child consistently complains of pain under the cast, or if the young child cries or is fussy or irritable after the initial period of adjustment, assume that there is a pressure area under the cast. Such symptoms as elevated temperature or an unfamiliar odor from the cast indicate an open sore or skin sloughing and should be reported immediately. The physician may bivalve the cast (i.e., cut it in two lengthwise), or he may prefer to cut a window over the suspicious area to observe the skin. A bivalved cast is strapped back in place after the skin is treated, and a cast window is replaced with padding and tape. The replaced window must exert the same pressure as the rest of the cast or window edema will occur at the site.

Keeping the Cast Clean and Dry

Perhaps the most difficult aspect of caring for the child in a cast is keeping the cast clean and dry. Soiled casts soften, often compromising the desired position of alignment. If the padding becomes wet from urine or feces it will not dry, thus predisposing the child to urine dermatitis or skin infections. The odor is most unpleasant and cannot be eliminated. It is embarrassing and emotionally traumatic to the child, who must wear the soiled and offensive smelling cast. Such soiling of the cast can be prevented with consistent nursing care and parent teaching. The perineal area of the cast must be protected with plastic. For the young child, tuck plastic wrap inside the cast in the perineal area, front and back, bringing the plastic out to cover a portion of the cast. Fold a cloth diaper to cover the genital area, or use a sanitary pad or disposable diaper to absorb wastes. Change the plastic as necessary. (See the Skills Manual.) If the child is on a Bradford frame, funnel the plastic into a bedpan at all times. For the older child, apply the plastic when he needs to void or defecate, then remove it.

Body casts pose a particular problem, that of *cast syndrome;* the child experiences gastric disturbances such as nausea, vomiting, and severe pain. The physician will cut a "belly hole" in the cast to relieve the constriction.

Parent teaching is vital to the child's continued healthy status when he goes home in a cast. Permit the parents to participate in their child's care as soon as he returns to the room after casting. Explain each step in the process of cast care. If they are allowed and encouraged to care for the child with your guidance while he is hospitalized, the transition to home will not be as frightening to them. Provide them with written instructions for care and a number to call if they have questions or need additional support.

Removal of a cast is usually more frightening than is its application. The plaster saw makes a terrifying noise, and the child may be afraid that the saw will cut him. Reassure him that it will *not* cut him, but tell him that he may feel some vibration and heat. As with cast application, it may help to offer the infant a bottle.

Braces

Braces are tailor-made to fit the child (Figure 28–9). They are used to correct a deformity, to prevent weightbearing, to immobilize a paralyzed limb in the position of function, or to stabilize a joint. For example, if the foot drags, a short leg brace attached to the shoe will permit a normal gait.

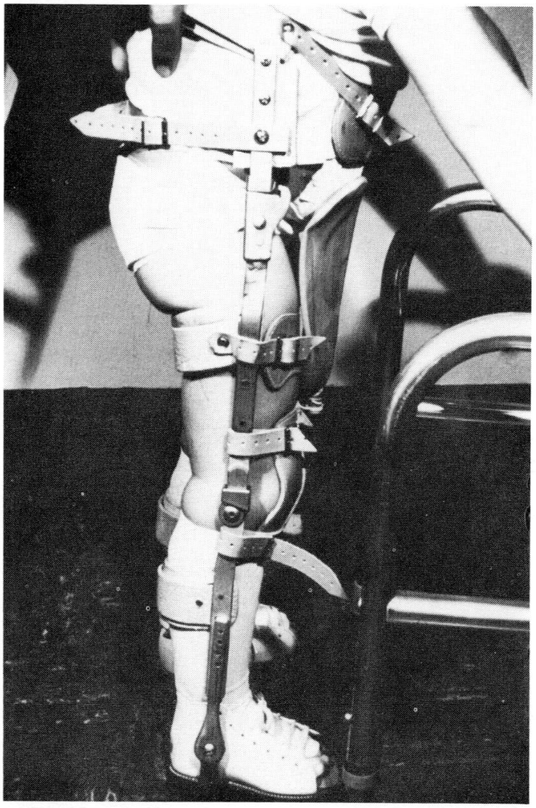

Figure 28–9. *Long leg braces on a child with meningomyelocele. Note ileostomy bag in place.* (Courtesy of E.A. Saunders, M.D., Professor of Surgery; Chief, Section of Orthopedics, Medical College of Georgia, Augusta, Ga.)

Inspect the skin around all pressure areas, and use alcohol to toughen it as is done for cast care. Check all straps, shoe laces, buckles, and joints for wear, and be sure they are in proper working condition. The child will outgrow the brace; check frequently to see that it is not too tight or too short. Remind the parents to have the brace checked at regular intervals.

Except for extremity braces, the most common brace used for pediatric musculoskeletal disorders is the Milwaukee brace, used for treatment of scoliosis (S-shaped curvature of the spine). The brace is worn 23 hours a day. The one hour without the brace is used to bathe and rub the skin with alcohol, to do rigorous exercises as a part of the therapy, and to clean the brace. The brace is commonly used for the adolescent with a mild curve (20 to 40 percent); it may improve the curve up to 50 percent. However, it is also used in the younger child with a severe curve (up to 60 percent) to prevent progression of the defect until surgery can be performed.

Scoliosis affects girls six times more often than boys. The girl will have trouble adjusting to the brace and will need reassurance and support. Being an adolescent is trying in its own right without the added burden of having to wear a visible and awkward brace. Teach the child and her family the following aids for living with a brace. Daub moist tea bags on pressure areas; the tannic acid will toughen the skin. Tincture of benzoin may also be used. Wear a T-shirt under the brace to protect the skin. Be sure the shirt is not wrinkled. (A bra may be worn under the T-shirt.) Wear underpants on top of the brace, otherwise the elastic band and wrinkles may cause pressure areas. If a chin bar is part of the traction, the child should visit the orthodontist regularly so that he can prevent jaw deformities caused by the pressure. Many new braces use a throat mold rather than the chin bar, thus eliminating this problem. Activity generally is not restricted except for contact sports.

Traction

Traction provides a mechanical pull on a part or parts of the body. *Skeletal traction* utilizes a pin or wire that has been surgically inserted into bone (Figure 28–10 and 28–11). *Skin traction* involves the application to the extremity of straps that are attached via a spreader or footplate to weights, providing pull. Adhesive straps, such as moleskin, are used when continuous traction is necessary, as it is with a fracture. Nonadhesive straps, made with foam-backed material, are used when the traction need not be continuous. This is the only type of traction that the nurse can apply or release; in fact, the nonadhesive straps are designed to be released at regular intervals.

The objective of traction therapy is to achieve maximum benefit in the shortest amount of time. To meet this goal, the child must be kept in good body alignment and must be immobilized properly. Unless otherwise ordered, the supine position is used. The Bradford frame is used for some types of traction, according to the age of the child. In addition, restraints are necessary to keep the child immobile and in proper alignment. Properly used, the restraints need not be traumatic to the child. The

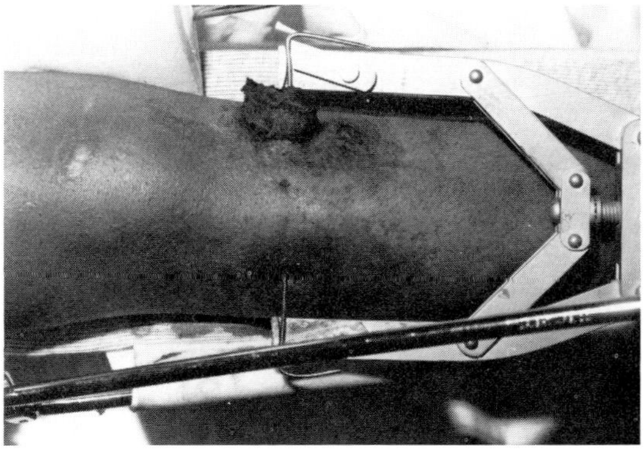

Figure 28–10. *Skeletal traction pin in place. Betadine-soaked gauze has been removed from lower insertion site to permit visualization of pin.*

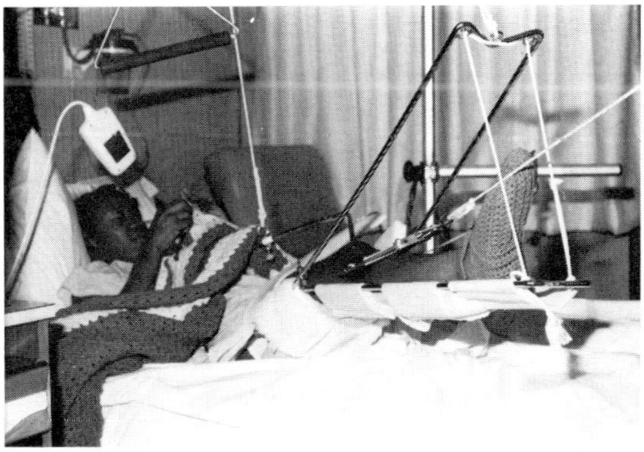

Figure 28–11. *Skeletal traction for fractured femur in seventeen-year-old girl. Note call bell within easy reach.*

major period of adjustment to traction is the first few days. If you place the child in the proper restraint from the outset and see that each staff member is consistent in its use, the child will accept it as part of the treatment and readily adjust to it. Adding the restraint after the child has been in traction will cause him to view it as punishment. Use bright colors and patterns to make the restraints, as these are more easily accepted than drab, patternless materials. Explain to the parents, and to the child if he is old enough, why the restraints are necessary. Be sure not to restrain the child any more than is necessary to accomplish the goals of treatment. Check the restraints often to be sure they fit properly.

Types of restraints used for the child in traction are the *sling, jacket, frame,* and *diaper* restraint. The diaper restraint is used *only* when routine countertraction (such as elevating the head of the bed or using other restraints) has not been successful. It is not routinely used because of the complications associated with its use, notably urinary tract infections, skin irritations on the thighs, and diaper rash. When this restraint is used, check the diaper at least every half hour and change it as necessary. (These restraints, as well as types of traction, are illustrated, and their use explained, in the Skills Manual.)

The type of traction used varies with the child's condition and the physician's preference. The basic nursing care of the child is not altered by the type of traction used. Know the type of traction, whether skeletal or skin, adhesive or nonadhesive. Maintain good body alignment and immobility to obtain maximum benefit from the therapy. Check the equipment frequently. See that the ropes are in the center track of the pulleys and that they are not frayed. Weights must hang free. If they are resting on or against the bed, their actual pull will be decreased. Know the amount of weights that the child should have. Record it on the Kardex and in the nursing notes. If in doubt about any aspect of the child's traction therapy, ask the physician.

Care of the child in traction follows the same guidelines as those for the child in a cast. Neurovascular checks are necessary every hour for the first 24 hours after the application of skeletal or adhesive skin traction. Nonadhesive skin traction is checked 30 minutes after application. If impairment is noted, the traction is probably wrapped too tightly. Rewrap the traction and check neurovascular status again in 30 minutes. If all is well, recheck every four hours, and a half hour after each rewrapping. Continue to check all extremities involved in traction every four hours until the traction is discontinued.

Skin care with alcohol is imperative. Remember to use no powders, oil, or lotion. If adhesive skin traction is used, observe for an allergic reaction to the adhesive. If the child complains of severe itching under the straps, the physician probably will remove the straps and apply benzoin or Ace adherent, and then stockinette to the extremity before reapplying the adhesive. The nursing history may reveal previous tape allergy.

If skeletal traction is used, it is best to get a written order for pin or wire care. The physician may want nothing done outside of frequent inspection, or he may order antibiotic sprays or ointments, or antiseptic solutions to cleanse the area. In any case, inspect the areas for signs of infection, such as redness, heat, and drainage. Report these signs promptly because the physician will probably want to remove the pins or wires to avoid *osteomyelitis* (inflammation of the bone). Because the pins and wires can slip or break, look for any irregularity in pin or wire placement. If there is a difference in length on either side, the pin may have slipped; if both ends appear unstable, it may be broken. Report your suspicions to the physician immediately.

Bradford Frame

The Bradford frame is an important tool of orthopedic nursing. The frame may be solid or split. The split frame is used for the child in a hip spica cast (which encases part or all of the trunk and one or more extremities; see Figure 28–12) to help keep the cast dry and prevent soiling. The solid frame is used to help immobilize the child in traction, to promote body alignment, and to provide countertraction if needed. The sole criterion for the use of the split frame is incontinence; the child who is continent need not be placed on the frame. The criteria for using the solid frame are age, hyperactivity, and retardation. The child under the age of five who is put in traction should also be

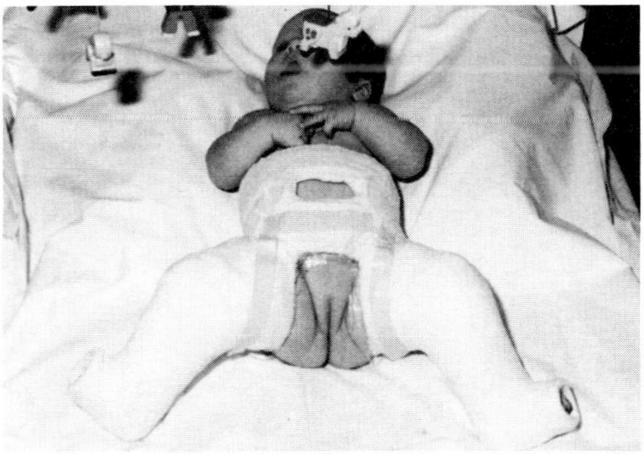

Figure 28–12. *Hip spica cast for treatment of dislocated hips. Note baby is elevated on pillows, window in cast, adhesive tape petaling, and plastic wrap for protection of perineum. Diaper removed for visualization.*

placed on a solid Bradford frame. If he is hyperactive or retarded, he is placed on the frame, regardless of his age. However, if he violently resists the frame, do not use it. The principle behind the use of the frame is that it is much easier to properly immobilize the child on a small area (frame) than on a large area (bed).

SURGERY

Surgical procedures are sometimes necessary in the management of musculoskeletal dysfunctions. Anesthesia may be required for manipulation of a fracture (closed reduction). Open reduction, involving an incision, may be needed to properly align the bone. Pins and wires may be inserted as a prelude to skeletal traction.

The child with severe scoliosis may require spinal fusion to stabilize the spine. Preoperatively, the child is placed in traction, either *halo-femoral* or *halo-pelvic* (Figure 28–13). The *halo* is a circular bar attached to the skull by four pins. If halo-femoral traction is used, traction pins are placed through the distal femur, and the weights pull against both the halo and the femoral pins; this stretching of the spine may take up to three weeks. Halo-pelvic traction requires the insertion of two pins into the iliac crests. A pelvic hoop surrounds the pelvis and is attached to the pins. Traction is exerted by turning the four connecting rods which run from halo to hoop.

Before insertion of the halo pins, the hair in the pin area is removed. Reassure the child that his head will not be shaved. Tell him that after the pins are removed, the scars will be very tiny and will be covered by his hair.

After surgery for spinal fusion, logroll the child every two hours, turning the head, spine, and legs as one unit. Pay special attention to pulmonary status because the prolonged immobility and the crowding of

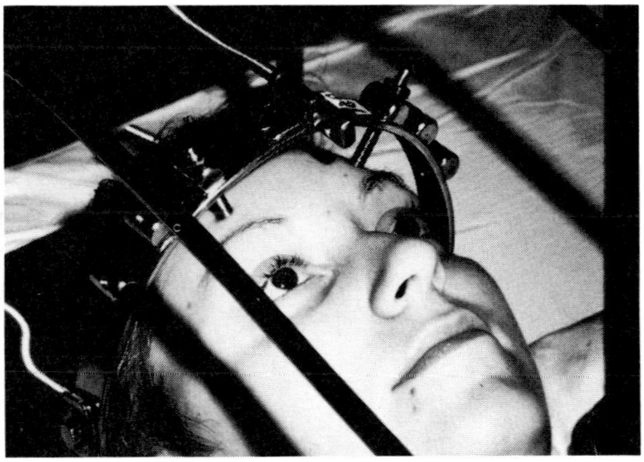

Figure 28–13. *Halo traction attached to skull with screws.* (Courtesy, E.W. Berg, M.D., Associate Professor of Surgery, Section of Orthopedics, Medical College of Georgia, Augusta, Ga.)

Table 28–1. **Specific Musculoskeletal Conditions**

Name	*Definition*	*Treatment*	*Special Nursing Considerations*
Congenital anomalies			
Talipes (clubfoot)	Ranges from minor forefoot adduction ("toeing in") to severe deformities that prevent walking. Four primary deformities are: *Talipes varus:* heel inverted; forefoot adducted and inverted. *Talipes valgus:* heel everted; forefoot abducted and everted. *Talipes equinus:* plantar flexion of foot with toes lower than heel. *Talipes calcaneus:* dorsiflexion of foot with heel lower than toes. Four combinations of deformities may occur: equinovarus, equinovalgus, calcaneovarus, and calcaneovalgus. Talipes equinovarus is the most common, occurring about once in every 1,000 live births. Anatomical changes involve bone, muscle, ligament, and tendons; may be unilateral or bilateral.	Beginning in the first few days of life, weekly applications of plaster casts after gentle and progressive correction. This step takes about ten weeks. Maintenance of correction with Denis Browne splint worn day and night (removed for bathing) for three months. Gradually worn for shorter periods during the day, but worn all night for another year or more. Orthopedic shoes until three years of age. Followed by physician until end of growth. Sixty percent respond to this nonoperative therapy. The other 40 percent who resist correction undergo heelcord lengthening at three months of age and then follow the above therapy.	Neurovascular assessment after manipulation and casting. Emphasize to the parents the importance of adhering to the prescribed therapy, especially if they are required to exercise the foot.
Dislocation of the hips	Incidence: from 1:600 to 1:1,000 live births. Acetabulum fails to develop normally; it is too shallow to hold the head of the	Optimally, diagnosis made at birth. Birth to three months: gentle reduction followed by maintenance in position of	Careful assessment of hips during newborn exam in nursery. Refer to physician as necessary.

femur. The femur slides out of the acetabulum and lies above it. Failure to correct at an early age leads to crippling degenerative arthritis in adulthood. Four times more common in girls than in boys.

flexion and passive abduction (the "human" position). The "frog leg" position, which places the hip in extreme abduction, can cause a vascular necrosis of the head of the femur. A Frejka pillow splint is used for the infant. Occasionally a plaster cast is necessary to hold the hip in the desired position. Three to eighteen months: shortening of the hip adductor muscles is marked by this age. Muscles must be lengthened by skin or skeletal traction for a few weeks, followed by gentle closed reduction under anesthesia. An adductor tenotomy may be necessary. A hip spica cast is used postoperatively to maintain the correction. Immobilization may be required for as many months as the hip was left untreated. Eighteen months to five years: skeletal traction and open reduction, followed by casting. Results are much less satisfactory than with early diagnosis and treatment. Over five years of age: complicated, extensive surgical procedures necessary, with little hope for success. After six or seven years, reduction is not usually attempted.

(continued)

Table 28–1. *(Continued)*

Name	*Definition*	*Treatment*	*Special Nursing considerations*
Torticollis (wryneck)	Shortened sternocleidomastoid muscle on one side of the neck causes the head to tilt to that side; the face is turned toward the unaffected side. Asymmetry of face, eyes, ears, and skull often present, as well as other anomalies such as clubfoot and dislocated hip. May be congenital, in which case a mass is usually felt in the muscle. Mass subsides in three to six months. Torticollis also is seen in other conditions (not congenital), especially following infections and trauma.	Stretching exercises done four to six times a day. Use of sandbags or towels to position the head during sleep; 90 percent cure rate with this conservative treatment. Surgical intervention necessary if response is inadequate by six to nine months. Postoperative head halter traction seven to ten days, then brace three to six months.	usu. effective
Birth injuries			
Brachial plexus injury (Erb's palsy)	Most common cause is injury to brachial plexus during delivery. Arm is extended and internally rotated.	Full range of passive motion. Judicious use of bracing with physical therapy. Less than 20 percent obtain full neurological function. Reconstructive procedures attempted when the child is older and can cooperate.	Explain to parents the importance of maintaining normal joint motion.
Cerebral palsy	(See ch. 27 for a discussion of cerebral palsy.)		
Fractures	Accidents are the most frequent cause of fractures. More severe trauma is necessary to produce a complete fracture in the child than in the adult; the child's bones can tolerate a greater degree of deformity. Pain,	Immobilize the part until x-rays can be taken. The fracture is usually set under general anesthesia. The child will be in a cast or traction according to age and severity of fracture. Majority of fractures treated	Check neurovascular status before the part is corrected.

	swelling, and deformity occur with a fracture. The child may refuse to move the part because of muscle spasms and severe pain. In the case of trauma, assume multiple injuries have been sustained until the contrary is proven.	on outpatient basis with closed reduction and plaster casts. Fractures of the femur and supracondylar area of the humerus are treated in the hospital.	
		Multiple system injuries are treated in this order (the "Six B's"): breathing, bleeding, brain, bowel, bladder, bone.	Maintain patent airway, stop bleeding, start IV fluids, assess neurological status. Support the child and his family.
Hereditary Anomalies			
Osteogenesis imperfecta	"Brittle bones" that fracture with minimal trauma. Autosomal dominant trait; may be congenital, with fractures at birth, or may occur later in childhood. Dwarfism and restricted activity common due to recurring deforming fractures. Fractures are less common after puberty.	Good orthopedic management, otherwise no effective therapy.	Handle gently to avoid additional fractures.
Duchenne's muscular dystrophy	Most common muscular dystrophy in the child; a crippling disease caused by muscular weakness and atrophy. Presents by three or four years of age and progressively worsens. Victim rarely lives past second decade. Sex-linked recessive trait.	Keep child as mobile and independent as possible. Long leg bracing extends walking one or two years. Tendon lengthening, transfer, and release usually necessary. Physical therapy helps keep the child active and modifies development of contractures. Nonambulatory stage represents 30 to 50 percent of the child's life; the problem is to prevent progressive spinal deformities. Back braces and surgery may be used. Maintenance of respiratory function necessary.	Familial support, understanding and encouragement during time of diagnosis.

(continued)

Table 28–1. *(Continued)*

Name	*Definition*	*Treatment*	*Special Nursing considerations*
Musculoskeletal infections	Results from introduction or "seeding" of bacteria into the bones or joints, following a blood-bone infection or trauma. Initial manifestations are those of an acute inflammatory process (tenderness, swelling, and fever).	Culture specimen of fluid obtained from the affected area via needle biopsy. Appropriate antibiotic given in accordance with culture report. Analgesics and splinting of the extremity help alleviate pain. Surgery with postoperative drainage is often necessary.	Provide rest and adequate splinting as needed. Offer analgesics if prescribed. Monitor drainage and infusion of fluids.
Septive arthritis	Affects large joints, such as hip, knee, shoulder, ankle. Symptoms of pain and swelling in the joint, plus fever.	Daily aspiration of synovial fluid. If amount of fluid does not decrease, open surgical incision and drainage is done; the joint space is cleansed with saline irrigations during surgery.	
Osteomyelitis	Inflammation of bone, usually caused by Staphylococcus aureus.	Penicillin G IV is drug of choice, unless the organism is penicillin resistant. Carbenicillin or other drugs may also be used. IV therapy is continued for *at least* three weeks. If the erythrocyte sedimentation rate (ESR) is still elevated after three weeks, treatment is continued. If pus is obtained by diagnostic needle aspiration, surgery is performed to drain the bone. Early ambulation with moderate weight-bearing is indicated once the local pain has disappeared.	Place extremity in functional position with splints or sandbags; a plaster cast may be used after surgery.

Torsional Deformities	Caused by heredity or intrauterine positioning.		
External femoral torsion (Toeing-out)	Both knees and feet turn outward; due to intrauterine positioning.	Usually corrects itself; if not, a Denis Browne splint may be used at night.	
Internal tibial torsion (Toeing-in)	Most common cause of toeing-in in the preschool child. Knee faces forward, toes turned inward. Secondary to cross-legged position in utero.	Corrects spontaneously unless the child habitually sits or sleeps with knees flexed and feet turned in, in which case the internal torsion may worse. Treatment aimed at training the child to avoid harmful sitting and sleeping positions. Denis Browne splint may be required at night for the child over two or three years of age.	
Internal femoral torsion (Toeing-in)	Common cause of toeing-in in the older child and adolescent. Develops by five years of age due to habit of sitting on floor in "television" position, with the femora internally rotated and the feet out to the side.	Teach the child to avoid the "television" position, replacing it with the cross-legged or "Indian" style position. A night splint may be necessary for the child over age eight.	
Curvature of the spine			
Kyphosis	Increase in dorsal prominence of thoracic spine ("roundback"). Caused by bad posture in 95 percent of cases, especially in adolescent girl; caused by rounding of back to hide breast development.	Exercise program with instructions on proper posture.	Requires understanding of the emotional problems of "growing up." Suggest exercises such as swimming and dancing for girls and weightlifting or track for boys. These activities seem less like "posture exercises" and are well-tolerated.

(continued)

Table 28–1. *(Continued)*

Name	*Definition*	*Treatment*	*Special Nursing Considerations*
Juvenile kyphosis (Scheuermann's disease)	Anterior wedging of the thoracic vertebrae secondary to osteochondrosis of spine (disorder of bony epiphysis caused by interference with blood supply).	Milwaukee brace; occasionally casting is necessary prior to bracing.	Lordosis = lumbar curvature
Scoliosis	S-shaped curvature of spine. Idiopathic; thought to be genetically transmitted as an x-linked trait. Usually, the younger the child at time of diagnosis, the more serious the prognosis, because the curve tends to progress with growth.	Exercise program in combination with more definite treatment, such as Milwaukee brace, halo traction, spinal fusion, or body casting, depending on severity of defect. (Exercise alone will *not* correct the deformity).	
Infantile	Occurs between birth and three years of age. Left thoracic curve. More common in males; due to intrauterine positioning. Usually resolves spontaneously. May be associated with congenital dislocation of the hips.		
Juvenile	Occurs between ages of four and ten. Usually seen after six years; right thoracic curve; both sexes affected equally.	Milwaukee brace or modified Milwaukee brace. Risser localizer cast, Cotrel traction or surgery to stabilize the spine.	strengthen muscle of torso longitudinal tx & latitudinal pressure - wear @ all x's

Adolescent	Occurs between age of ten and skeletal maturity. Most curves are to the right; 80 percent occur in girls.		
Slipped capital femoral epiphysis	Epiphysis of head of femur slips downward and backward on the neck. Acetabulum is normal. Leg is adducted and externally rotated. Child has a limp and pain in hip or knee. Boys between ages of ten and seventeen are affected two to four times more often than girls; they are usually obese with underdeveloped genitalia.	Osteotomy with pinning of head of femur. Traction or casting postoperatively with progression to crutches, or a wheelchair if the condition is bilateral.	Child may be overweight, necessitating extra personnel to execute care measures. Treat the affected joint as if it is fractured. Do not attempt to straighten the leg; the traction will do that.
Juvenile rheumatoid arthritis	Chronic synovitis of childhood; thought to be genetically influenced and to involve an antigen-antibody reaction. More common in girls; onset usually in preschool years. May affect more than one joint (polyarthritis). Child holds joint in fixed position or refuses to walk because of the pain.	Balanced program of rest and exercise to maintain joint function and position. Resting the joint decreases inflammation but causes loss of strength and range of motion. The joint is not completely immobilized; it may be splinted, but must be moved several times a day. During remissions, exercises to increase and maintain strength are necessary. Night splints used to prevent contractures of wrists or knees. Aspirin 100 mg/kg/day in four doses for six months to two years, then tapered off.	Apply heat before therapy session to reduce pain and relax the muscles, or use hydrotherapy (whirlpool) for exercises. The water is buoyant and protects joints from the stress of weight bearing. Warn parents of side effects of aspirin: hyperventilation in the young child and tinnitus in the older child. To reduce gastric irritation, give aspirin with meals or milk.

(continued)

Table 28–1. *(Continued)*

Name	*Definition*	*Treatment*	*Special Nursing considerations*
Legg-Calvé-Perthes disease	Avascular necrosis of femoral head. Four stages of disease; initial bone necrosis when the blood supply to the femoral head is interrupted; fragmentation or revascularization with new blood vessels and new but fragile bone at the site; reossification or healing; and residual deformity. The deformity occurs when weight-bearing puts pressure on the new, healing bone, causing it to flatten and not conform to the acetabulum. In addition, there is a tendency toward subluxation whereby the acetabulum is shallow and partial dislocation of the femoral head occurs. Disease course runs two to four years. Seen in child four to eight years of age; affected boys outnumber girls six to one; associated with low birth weight. Tendency to bone age retardation and short stature; some familial tendency. Limp with or without pain in the hip, groin, and/or knee is first symptom; later, there is muscle spasm and limited motion.	Treatment may be conservative, with the use of weight-bearing abduction braces or casts to keep the femur within the acetabulum and maintain its rounded contour. In severe cases, surgery (pelvic osteotomy) may be indicated, in which case the child is placed in a cast postoperatively. After healing (about six weeks) he may return to relatively normal activity.	Stress to child and family the importance of adhering to the prescribed therapy.

internal organs caused by the severe scoliosis predisposes the child to respiratory complications.

Pain is severe after spinal fusion and a narcotic will be needed at regular intervals for the first 24 to 48 hours after surgery. Milder analgesics will be given for several more days.

After surgery, the child remains in traction for a time and then progresses to a body jacket, Risser localizer cast, or Risser turnbuckle cast, all of which encase the trunk.

CLINICAL APPLICATION

Kagan B., twenty-two months old, is admitted to the unit for application of a hip spica cast to correct congenital bilateral dislocated hips.

1. What is a dislocated hip, and why is a hip spica cast necessary to correct it?
2. How will you prepare Kagan and her parents for the cast application?
3. Explain steps you will take in assuring that the cast does not compromise Kagan's skin integrity.
4. How will the immobility effect Kagan's respiratory, cardiovascular, gastrointestinal, and urinary functions?
5. Design a plan of care and nursing intervention that will promote optimal functioning of each of the body systems named in question 4?
6. Describe the effects of immobility on Kagan's development; include steps you will take to minimize these effects.
7. How will you help prepare Mr. and Mrs. B. for Kagan's discharge, knowing she will have to be in the cast for several months?

Bibliography

Barrett, M.J. Surviving Adolescence in a Back Brace: Laura's Experience. *American Journal Maternal-Child Nursing* 2:160, 1977.

Brower, E. Innervations in Nursing: Children Should Be Screened (for Scoliosis). *Nursing '78* 6:16, April, 1978.

Farrell, J. Casts, Your Patients and You. Part I: A Review of Basic Procedures. *Nursing '78* 8:65, October, 1978.

Grass, L.D., Paarlberg, J., Simons, G. Nursing Care of the Orthopedic Patient, in Fochtman, D. and Raffensperger, J.G. (eds). *Principles of Nursing Care for the Pediatric Surgery Patient,* ed. 2. Little, Brown & Co., Boston, 1976, p.225.

Hill, P.M. and Romm, L.S. Screening for Scoliosis in Adolescents. *American Journal Maternal-Child Nursing* 2:156, 1977.

Hilt, N.E. and Schmitt, E.W. *Pediatric Orthopedic Nursing.* St. Louis, C.V. Mosby Co., 1975.

Love-Mignogna, S. Scoliosis. *Nursing '77* 7:50, May, 1977.

Miller, J.J. The Rheumatic Diseases, in Gellis, S.S. and Kagan, B.M. (eds). *Current Pediatric Therapy.* Philadelphia, W.B. Saunders Co., 1978, p. 370.

Salter, R.B. Orthopedic Disorders of the Extremities, in Gellis, S.S. and Kagan, B.M. (eds). *Current Pediatric Therapy.* Philadelphia, W.B. Saunders Co., 1978, p. 435.

Symposium on Common Orthopedic Problems. *Pediatric Clinics of North America* 24:665, 1977.

Tier, L.L. Everybody But Danny Knew How Disabled He Was. *Nursing '78* 8:39, February, 1978.

SECTION SIX

Fluid and Electrolyte Balance

CHAPTER **29**

Body Fluid Regulation

BEHAVIORAL OBJECTIVES

After studying this chapter, you will be able to:

- Discuss normal fluid and electrolyte balance, including components of various body compartments.
- Explain bicarbonate and renal buffer systems.
- Define metabolic acidosis/alkalosis and respiratory acidosis/alkalosis.
- Discuss differences in fluid and electrolyte balance in infants, children, and adults as regards basic metabolism, kidney function, and fluid requirements.
- Calculate oral fluid and caloric needs for a child of a given weight.
- Explain how to use pediatric intravenous equipment.
- Develop a plan of care for a child with a specific fluid and electrolyte imbalance that includes assessment of hydration status and fluid and electrolyte replacement measures.

TERMS AND CONCEPTS

Intracellular fluid (ICF)
Extracellular fluid (ECF)
Interstitial fluid
Intravascular fluid
Electrolytes
Ions
Milliequivalents (mEq)
Hypernatremia
Hyponatremia
Hypertonic dehydration
Hypotonic dehydration
Water intoxication
Isotonic dehydration
Hypokalemia
Hyperkalemia
Acid-base balance
pH
Buffer system
CO_2 content
CO_2 combining power
Metabolic acidosis
Metabolic alkalosis
Respiratory acidosis
Respiratory alkalosis
Nephron
Glomerulus
Glomerular filtration
Hydrostatic blood pressure
Filtration
Filtrate
Tubular reabsorption
Active transport
Obligatory water reabsorption
Acidification
Body surface area (BSA)
Hypodermocylsis
Total parenteral nutrition (TPN)
Fat emulsion

Fluid and electrolyte balance is more precarious in the child than it is in the adult. Changes in this delicate balance may be life-threatening. Responsibility for monitoring fluid and electrolyte status rests primarily with the nurse.

This chapter reviews normal fluid and electrolyte composition within the body; it includes a discussion of the action of various body systems on this composition and offers examples of four basic disturbances: metabolic acidosis, metabolic alkalosis, respiratory acidosis, and respiratory alkalosis. Differences in the child and the adult are discussed and nursing management of the child with a fluid imbalance is stressed. Methods for correcting fluid and electrolyte imbalances are presented.

REVIEW OF FLUIDS AND ELECTROLYTES

Normal Skin

The skin is the largest organ of the body. Normal skin (Figure 29–1) is composed of two layers located above fatty subcutaneous tissue. The most superficial is the epidermis, itself composed of four layers. The deeper layer is the dermis and is also called the "true skin," or corium. The dermis contains collagenous tissue as well as skin appendages—hair follicles, sweat glands, and sebaceous glands. Also located in the dermis at various depths are the heat, cold, pain, pressure, and light touch receptors. Body surface area (skin), measured in square meters, ranges from about 0.25 in the newborn to 1.5 to 2.2 in the normal adult. Injured skin heals by re-epithelialization from the surrounding skin edges or from the skin appendages in the wound itself. Skin thickness varies with age (infants and the aged have thinner skin) and with its location (palms, soles of the feet, posterior aspect of the legs, and buttocks have thicker skin).

Body Fluid

Water is the greatest single constituent of the body and represents about 60 percent of the body weight in adults. In the newborn

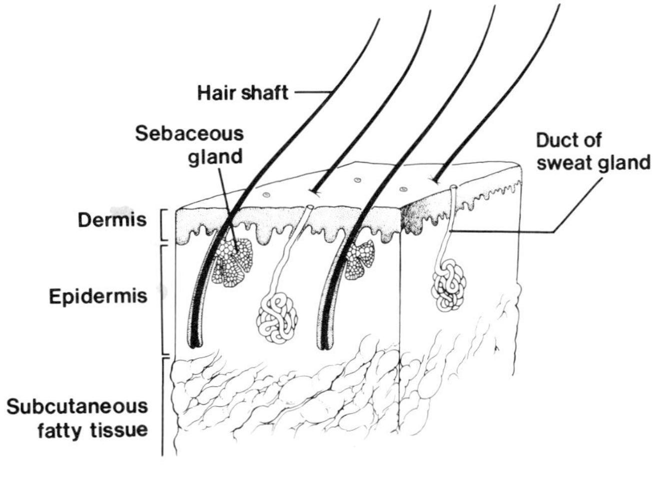

Figure 29–1. *Normal skin.*

infant, 70 to 80 percent of body weight is water; in the premature infant, it is about 90 percent.

Body water and dissolved solutes within the cells make up the *intracellular fluid* (ICF). *Extracellular fluid* (ECF), the body water outside the cells, has a different solute composition. The ECF consists of the *interstitial fluid*, which bathes the cells and blood vessels, and the *intravascular fluid* within the vessels themselves (Figure 29–2).

The body fluid consists primarily of water and *electrolytes*, which separate into electrically charged particles (*ions*) when dissolved in water. Positively charged ions are called *cations*; negatively charged ions are *anions*. Cations and anions exist in equal quantities when measured in *milliequivalents (mEq)*, the unit of chemical activity (Figure 29–3).

The various body fluids differ in their normal composition of water and electrolytes (Figure 29–4). The major electrolytes found in cellular fluid are potassium (K^+), phosphate (HPO_4^{--}), and magnesium (Mg^{++}. Extracellular fluid contains large amounts of sodium (Na^+), chloride (Cl^-), and bicarbonate (HCO^-). The principal cation within the cell is potassium; the principal anion is phosphate. The chief cation in extracellular fluid is sodium; the anion, chloride. Interstitial fluid and plasma (the fluid portion of the blood) have much the same composition with the exception of proteinate, a plasma protein, which prevents excess plasma from seeping into the interstitial fluid.

Electrolytes

Sodium

Sodium is largely responsible for maintaining pressure in the extracellular fluid. Normally, sodium loss from the skin is negligible. However, large amounts may be lost when the environmental temperature rises with fever, exertion, or stress. Perspiration is not a sodium-regulating mechanism; rather, it is a by-product of bodily temperature regulation. Most of the body's sodium is regulated by the kidneys. The sodium concentration in the extracellular fluid influences the amount of fluid and

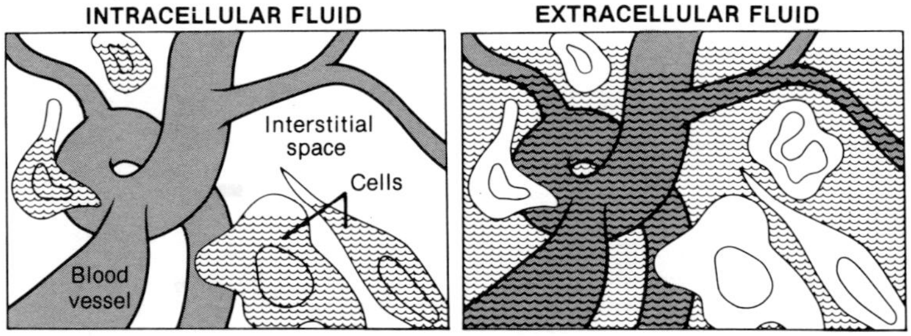

Figure 29–2. *Body fluids. Intracellular fluid is within the cells. Extracellular fluid is outside the cells and includes interstitial fluid (between the cells) and intravascular fluid (within the blood vessels).*

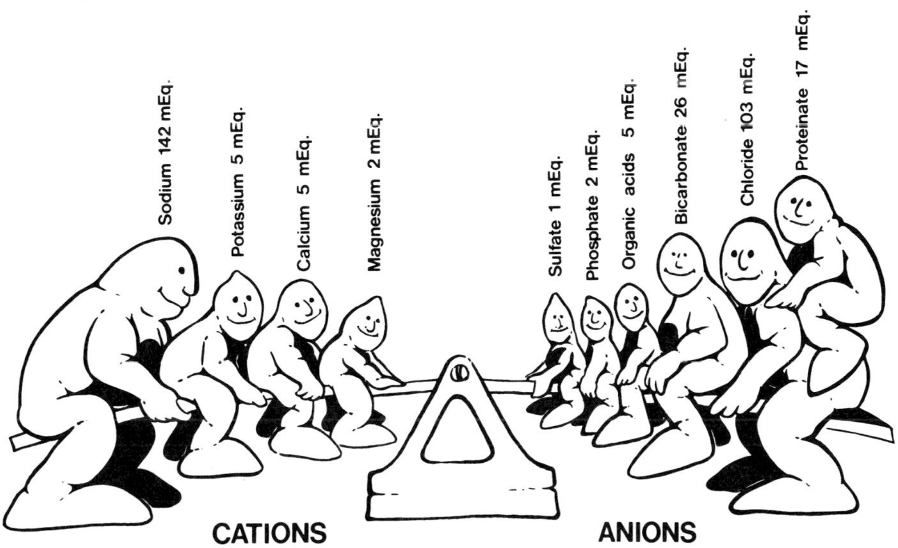

Figure 29–3. *Anions and cations are balanced in body fluid.*

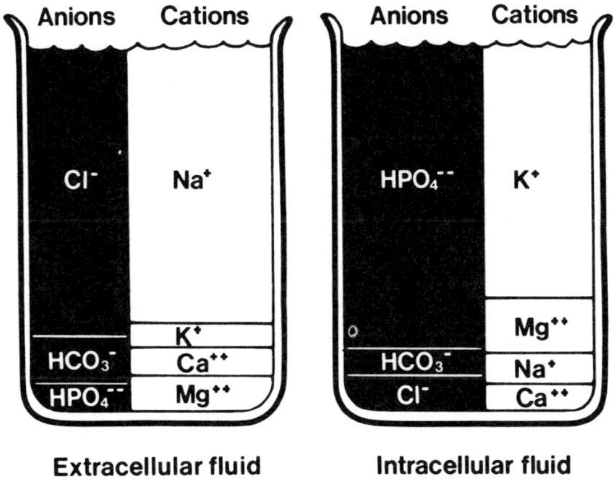

Figure 29–4. *Electrolytes (cations and anions) in body fluids.*

electrolytes excreted by the kidneys. When sodium concentration is high (*hypernatremia*), the kidneys retain water; when it is low (*hyponatremia*), the kidneys excrete more water. Both actions by the kidneys constitute an effort to maintain homeostasis within the extracellular fluid by keeping the sodium concentration level. In order to conserve sodium when body stores are low, the hormone *aldosterone*, secreted by the adrenal cortex, influences the renal tubules to reabsorb sodium and excrete potassium.

Hypernatremia, also known as *hypertonic dehydration*, is a dangerous fluid and electrolyte imbalance in which the serum sodium level rises above 142 mEq/L. Conditions in which there is loss of water greater than that of electrolytes (for example, liquid stools or rapid breathing) may cause hypernatremia. Decreased water intake and increased sodium intake (such as that with excessively salty foods or the administration of concentrated oral electrolyte solutions) may contribute to sodium excess. Symptoms of hypertonic dehydration include flushed skin, elevated temperature, rough, dry tongue, and tachycardia.

Hyponatremia, or *hypotonic dehydration*, is also known as *water intoxication* and results from excessive sodium loss without water loss (for example, as a result of fever, sweating, and exercise) and from a gain of water in excess of sodium (i.e., replacement of fluid deficit with plain water, such as drinking water after vigorous exercise). It also occurs when the hospitalized patient is given repeated tap water enemas or electrolyte-free parenteral fluids. The serum sodium drops below 137 mEq/L. Symptoms of hyponatremia such as abdominal cramps, muscular weakness, headaches, nausea, and vomiting may lead to vasomotor collapse (shock).

Extracellular fluid volume deficit, or *isotonic dehydration*, occurs when water and electrolytes are lost in the same proportions in which they are normally found in the ECF. Severe diarrhea in infancy usually results in isotonic dehydration. Symptoms include weight loss, dry skin with poor tissue turgor, sunken eyeballs and anterior fontanelle (if it is still patent), cool gray skin, lethargy, weak rapid pulse, and oliguria.

Potassium

Potassium is necessary for reassembling amino acids into proteins and for converting carbohydrates into energy. It is needed for normal muscle functioning, including the heart muscle, and for maintaining normal cellular composition. The ECF contains about 5 mEq/L as opposed to 150 mEq/L in the cellular fluid (recall that potassium is the major cation within the cells). Because the intracellular concentration of potassium is not easily determined, *serum* potassium levels are used, although this is an indirect measurement. Normal serum K levels are 3.5 to 5.3 mEq/L.

The kidneys excrete 25 to 120 mEq/L of potassium per day; therefore, in times of decreased potassium intake, *hypokalemia*, or potassium deficit, develops quickly. Administration of diuretics that cause a loss of potassium without potassium replacement, and loss of potassium-rich body fluids (e.g., caused by diarrhea and vomiting) are among other causes of hypokalemia. The chief symptoms of potassium deficit are muscle weakness, abdominal distension, decreased peristalsis, dizziness, and cardiac arrhythmias. Heart block, as well as apnea and respiratory arrest, may occur. Serum potassium levels fall below 3.5 mEq/L.

Hyperkalemia, or potassium excess, occurs when the kidneys are not functioning properly, and potassium intake is accelerated, due to either oral ingestion or to overzealous administration of potassium-containing parenteral fluids. This excess can also be caused by the release of potassium from the cells after crushing injuries or burns. Symptoms include abdominal cramps, nausea and vomiting, oliguria or anuria, and bradycardia. Death in potassium excess results from ventricular fibrillation and cardiac arrest. Serum potassium levels above 5.3 mEq/L indicate potassium excess.

Acid-Base Balance

pH

The acid-base balance of a solution is determined by the number of hydrogen (H^+) ions it contains. Because only minute amounts of hydrogen are found in the ECF (.0000001 gm/L), the symbol pH was devised to simplify the mathematical expression of hydrogen ion concentration. The symbol pH represents the *negative* expression of hydrogen ion concentration and is the power of 1/10. A pH of 5 would be expressed as $1/10^5$ or 1/100,000 gm hydrogen/liter of ECF; a pH of 7, 1/10,000,000 gm/L. The greater the pH, the smaller the number of ions; therefore, as the pH goes up, the solution is more *alkaline* (less hydrogen ions). A lower pH is more *acidic* (a pH of 6 is ten times more acidic than a pH of 7). A pH of 7 is neutral because the hydrogen ions are exactly balanced by the alkaline hydroxyl (OH^-) ions (Figure 29–5). The normal pH of ECF is 7.35 to 7.45. This is a narrow normal range; therefore, seemingly small fractional changes have major implications; death occurs when the plasma pH is below 6.8 or above 7.8.

Buffer System

The ratio of carbonic acid to base bicarbonate determines the hydrogen ion concentration of the ECF. This ratio is the body's most important *buffer system*, and it acts to control body pH by soaking up excess hydrogen ions and releasing them as needed. Strong acids in the body combine with a bicarbonate to form carbonic acid, a weak acid which is then eliminated by the lungs as carbon dioxide and water. Alkalis are neutralized in the body by carbonic acid to form water and bicarbonate. Normally, there are 1.35 mEq of carbonic acid to every 27 mEq of base bicarbonate, or a ratio of 1:20. *Absolute levels* of carbonic acid and base bicarbonate are not as important as their *ratio*. If *both* levels rise or fall, the body has compensated for the problem. However, if the ratio is upset, then the condition is uncompensated, resulting in either acidosis or alkalosis (Figure 29–6).

The status of acid-base balance is determined by measuring the blood pH, the pCO_2 (respiratory component), and the HCO_3 or serum CO_2 (metabolic or renal

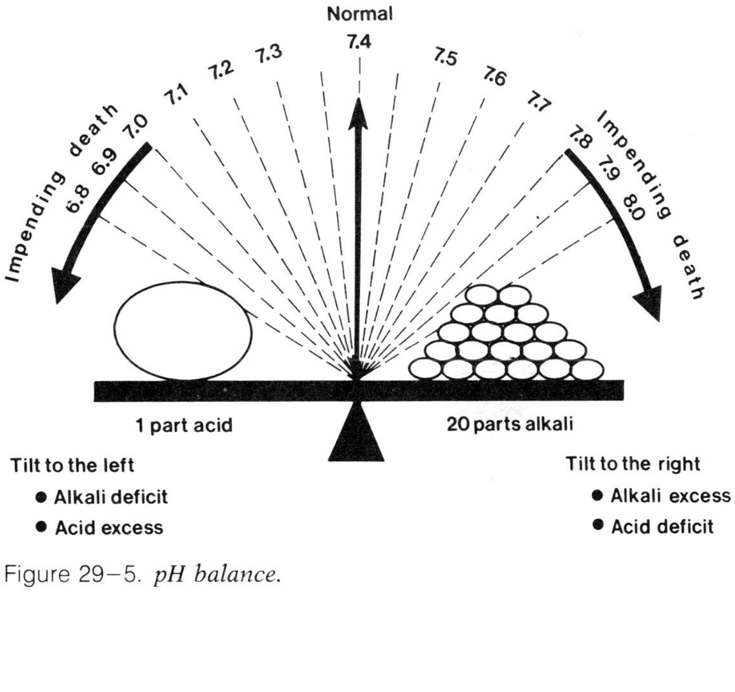

Figure 29–5. *pH balance.*

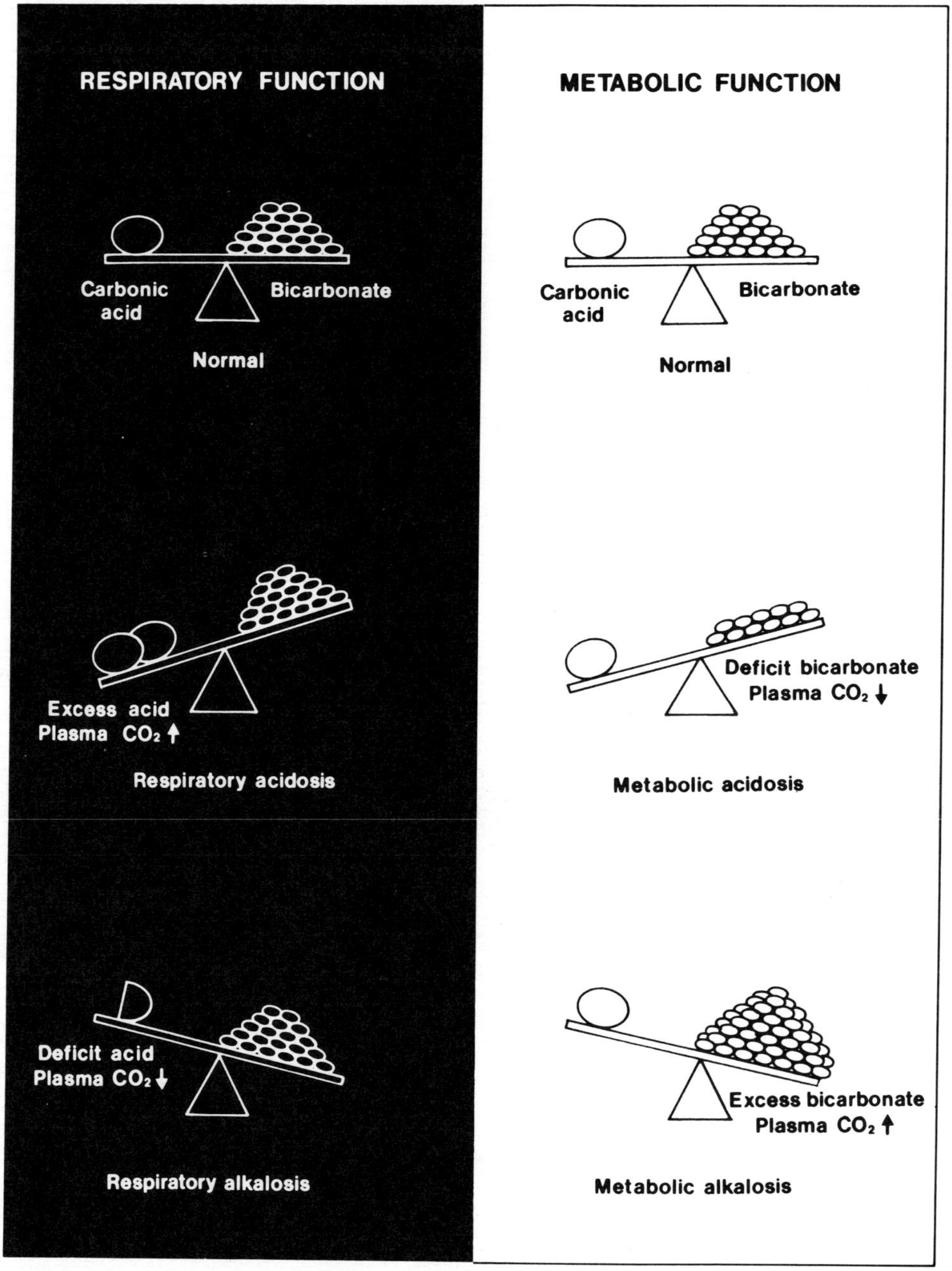

Figure 29–6. *Acidosis and alkalosis.*

component). The bicarbonate level of arterial blood (HCO_3) is determined by the amount of CO_2 dissolved in the blood, commonly referred to as the CO_2 *content*. The normal range for the infant or child is 18 to 27 mEq/L. The serum CO_2 is also called CO_2 *combining power*. It refers to the amount of cations (H^+, N^+, K^+, etc.) available to combine with HCO_3. The normal range is 22 to 32 mEq/L.

Several organ systems within the body help maintain acid-base balance. The lungs excrete carbon dioxide and water, thereby controlling carbonic acid levels. The kidneys excrete acid products of metabolism and either excrete or retain water and various electrolytes. Both the adrenal and posterior pituitary gland regulate the excretion of water and electrolytes by the kidney.

Metabolic acidosis may result from an increase in hydrogen ions (as in ketoacidosis, starvation, or salycilate intoxication) or from a decrease in base bicarbonate (lost in stools and urine) in the extracellular fluid. It also results when the kidneys fail to excrete acid waste products of metabolism. Compensation is accomplished by the lungs as they hyperventilate and blow off carbon dioxide, thus reducing the carbonic acid level and maintaining the buffer ratio closer to 1:20.

Don, sixteen months old, has severe diarrhea of 36 hours' duration. He is restless, has poor skin turgor, flushed skin, and dry mucous membranes. His respirations are deep and he is sighing (i.e., exhaling CO_2). Don has lost sodium ions in his stools, contributing to metabolic acidosis.

Metabolic alkalosis results from an increase of base bicarbonate or loss of a strong acid (such as during vomiting). Compensation is accomplished by hypoventilation as the lungs hoard carbon dioxide, thus increasing the carbonic acid concentration.

Five-week-old Kerry is admitted to the hospital with pyloric stenosis. He has been vomiting for two weeks with increasing intensity. Kerry's skin turgor is poor, and his eyes and anterior fontanelle are sunken. His respirations are shallow and slow (because he is hoarding CO_2). His mouth twitches and he "trembles all over." Kerry has metabolic alkalosis secondary to loss of chloride ions in his vomitus.

Respiratory acidosis is caused by hypoventilation in the lungs whereby the pCO_2 content rises. The kidneys compensate by excreting hydrogen ions and retaining bicarbonate.

Jane, nine months old, has pneumonia. She is in a croup tent, her respirations are labored, and she seems weak and lethargic. Jane is not able to exchange carbon dioxide and oxygen in her lungs (because of the pneumonia). Therefore, her CO_2 level rises; she is in respiratory acidosis.

Respiratory alkalosis results from hyperventilation whereby carbon dioxide is blown off, and the carbonic acid level falls. Compensation is accomplished by kidney excretion of bicarbonate and retention of hydrogen.

Jenny, a fourteen-year-old girl, has an argument with her mother over a party she wants to attend. Jenny swallows 12 five-grain aspirin tablets (60 grains). Her mother finds her in bed, barely conscious. Her respirations are deep and rapid (salicylates cause the respiratory center to be more sensitive to carbon dioxide); her mouth, eyes, and arms are twitching. Jenny is rushed to the hospital in respiratory alkalosis from salicylate intoxication.

Kidneys

The organs of the urinary system include the kidneys, ureters, bladder, and urethra. The kidneys not only remove wastes from the body and maintain fluid and electrolyte balance but also excrete hormones and help with metabolism (Figure 29–7).

The embryologic development of the urinary system begins a few weeks after conception. At three months' gestation, although they are not fully developed, the kidneys begin to secrete urine. At birth, the kidneys are still structurally and functionally immature; thus filtration and tubular absorption are prolonged in the newborn. Functional development of the kidneys is not complete until about the end of the first month of life.

The *nephron* is the functional unit of the kidney (Figure 29–8). Each kidney is composed of about one million nephrons, each capable of forming urine. The nephron is a complex system of tubules, arterioles, and capillaries. Blood is brought to the nephron by the afferent arterioles. As blood flows through the nephron, wastes are removed, and valuable substances are reabsorbed into the bloodstream. The *glomerulus* is a network of capillaries where the filtration process begins.

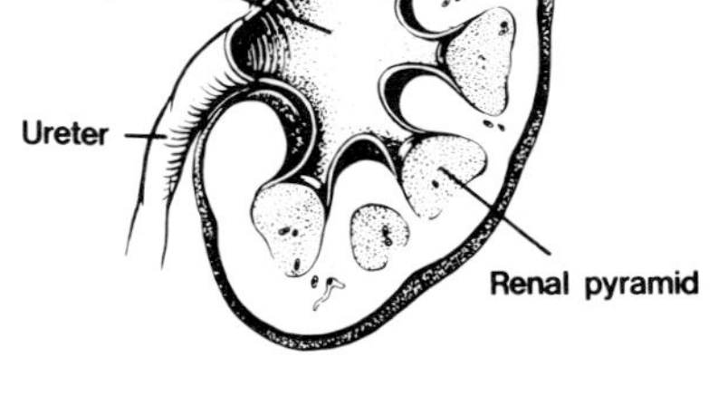

Figure 29–7. *Cross-section of the kidney.*

Glomerular filtration

Hydrostatic blood pressure (produced by the pumping action of the heart) in the afferent and efferent arterioles force *filtration* of fluids from the glomerular capillaries into Bowman's capsule (Figure 29–9). Filtration is the transfer of water and dissolved substances through a permeable membrane from an area of high pressure to an area of low pressure. Formed elements in the plasma have too high a molecular weight to pass through the glomerular membrane. For this reason, the fluid in the capsule, or *filtrate*, resembles plasma except that it lacks formed elements and has a much lower protein content.

Tubular Reabsorption and Secretion

Reabsorption in the renal tubules occurs by osmosis, diffusion, and active transport, and reduces the amount of glomerular filtrate by about 98 percent (Figure 29–10). In addition to waste products, the filtrate also contains substances the body needs. Through the process of *active transport*, these useful substances (such as glucose, amino acids, calcium, sodium, and potassium ions) are retained and the waste products excreted. In active transport, substances are moved by energy from an area of low concentration to an area of high concentration. In the proximal convoluted tubules, 80 to 90 percent of these useful solutes are reabsorbed. Water, also 80 to 90 percent, follows the solutes by osmosis; this is called *obligatory water reabsorption*. Chloride follows the sodium and potassium by diffusion in order to maintain electrical homeostasis.

Aldosterone, a hormone secreted by the adrenal cortex, causes sodium to be reabsorbed in the renal tubules. Water is obliged to follow the sodium (Figure 29–11A). *Antidiuretic hormone* (ADH), secreted by the

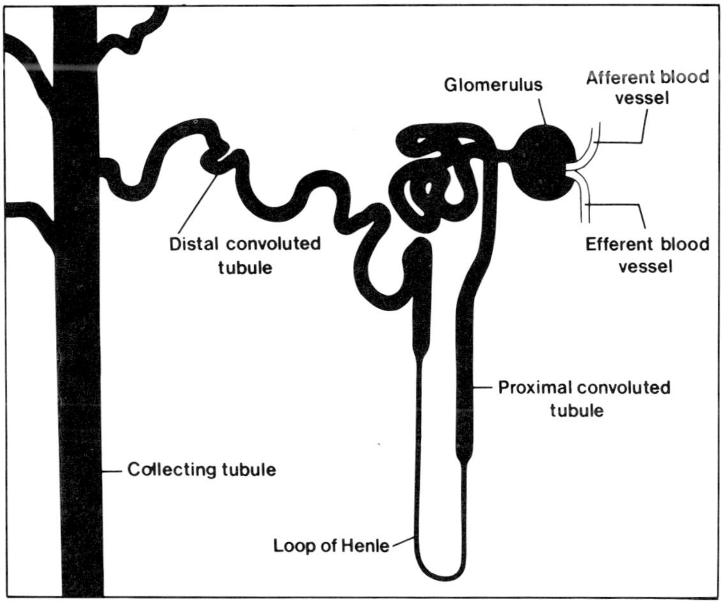

Figure 29–8. *Nephron of the kidney.*

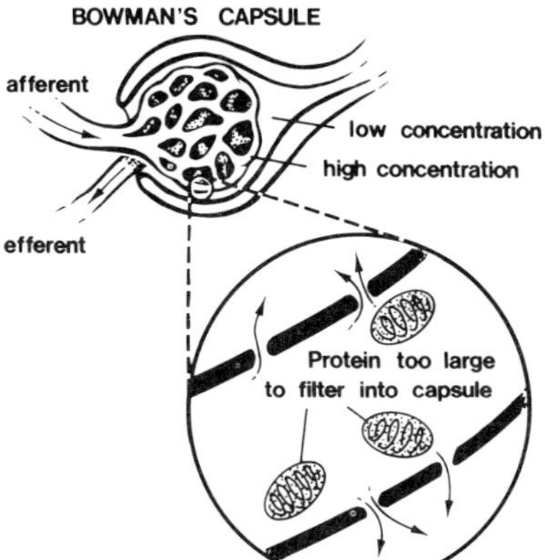

Figure 29–9. *Filtration of fluids from glomerular capillaries into Bowman's capsule.*

hypothalamus and released by the posterior pituitary, forces the distal tubules to reabsorb water. ADH secretion varies with the solute concentration of the blood. If plasma osmotic pressure is increased, ADH is secreted and water is reabsorbed; if plasma osmotic pressure is decreased (as with excess fluid intake), ADH is *not* released and therefore more water is excreted (Figure 29–11B).

Acidification

The pH of urine (5.0 to 7.0) is much lower (more acidic) than that of plasma. In the distal tubules, hydrogen, potassium, and ammonia are secreted into the tubular urine. The hydgrogen in the tubular cells exchanges with the sodium in the tubular urine (present as a sodium salt) and is excreted. The sodium combines in the tubular cell with bicarbonate to form sodium bicarbonate and is reabsorbed into the blood. Ammonia, formed in the renal tubular cells, also aids in the excretion of hydrogen ions. It reacts with hydrogen to form an

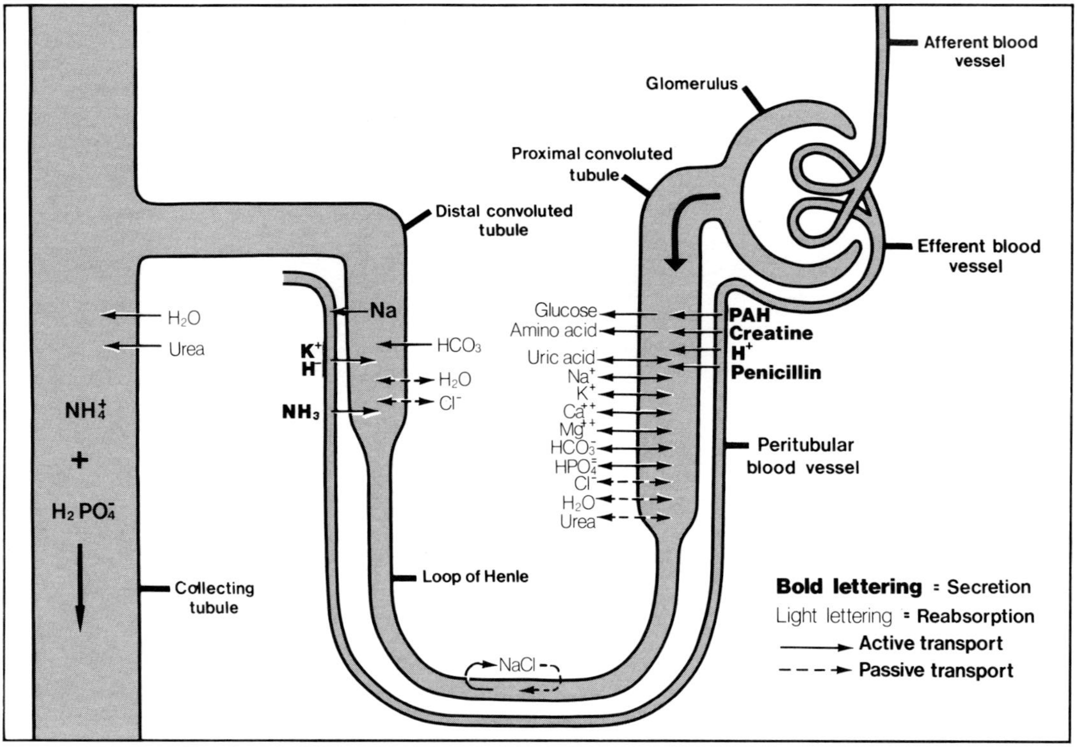

Figure 29–10. *Tubular reabsorption and secretion.*

ammonium ion, which then reacts with an anion and is excreted.

FLUID AND ELECTROLYTE BALANCE IN INFANTS AND CHILDREN

Differences in Children and Adults

Not only is the child smaller than the adult, his body composition and mechanisms for homeostasis are different. The younger the child, the more pronounced the difference. As stated earlier, the premature infant's body weight is about 90 percent water; the newborn's, about 70 to 80 percent, and the adult's, about 60 percent. The infant has more extracellular fluid in proportion to body weight than does the adult—about 40 percent as opposed to 20 percent in the adult (Figure 29–12). After the second year of life, body water approaches adult levels, and at puberty, the adult body water composition is attained.

Body Water Turnover

The infant may exchange as much as half of his ECF daily through ingestion and excretion while the adult exchanges only one-sixth of his (Figure 29–13). The infant's metabolic rate is twice as high per unit of weight than is the adult's. This high metabolic rate produces a large amount of

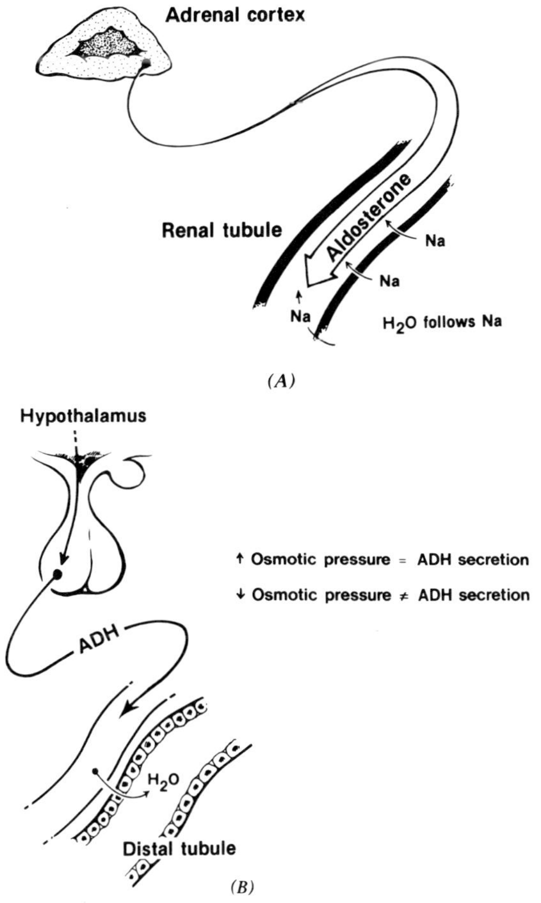

Figure 29–11. *Hormonal influence on body water balance. (A) aldosterone causes reabsorption of sodium (and water) in renal tubules. (B) ADH secretion causes reabsorption of water in distal tubules.*

metabolic waste, which requires a large urinary volume for excretion. Because of the immaturity of the infant's kidneys, he is not able to concentrate urine efficiently, and he loses a great amount of fluid through the kidneys. Premature and newborn infants have five and three times (respectively) the *body surface area* in relation to weight as do older children and adults. The infant's greater body surface area in proportion to weight means that he has more skin surface through which he loses a greater amount of fluid. For these reasons, any disturbances in body fluid balance in the infant can be dangerous.

Kidneys

The infant's kidneys are adequate for his needs when he is healthy. In illness, however, they are unable to excrete larger amounts of solutes and to conserve body water as needed. For example, if salt intake is too high, the kidneys cannot excrete the excess sodium, and therefore the infant may develop hypernatremia (an increase in fluid volume) and edema. The kidneys may not be able to excrete an excess fluid volume. During acidosis, the infant can increase acid excretion only to a modest degree and is therefore more susceptible to acidemia.

Fluid Requirements

The healthy individual (both child and adult) requires about 100 millileters of water for each 100 calories metabolized. The child, because of his greater metabolic rate, requires more calories per kilogram of body weight than does the adult. The infant, who expends 100 calories per kilogram, also requires 100 milliliters of water per kilogram. The adult, expending only 30 to 40 calories per kilogram needs only 30 to 40 milliliters of water. (See Table 29–1 for water and caloric needs at various ages at rest. When using Table 29–1, remember that the figures represent the body's needs in the resting state. Increments are added for normal activity and/or water loss. For a normal, healthy child, use 1.5 times the basal requirements, for a combination of unusual activity, fever, or hyperventilation, figure two times the basal requirements; and for all of these conditions occuring

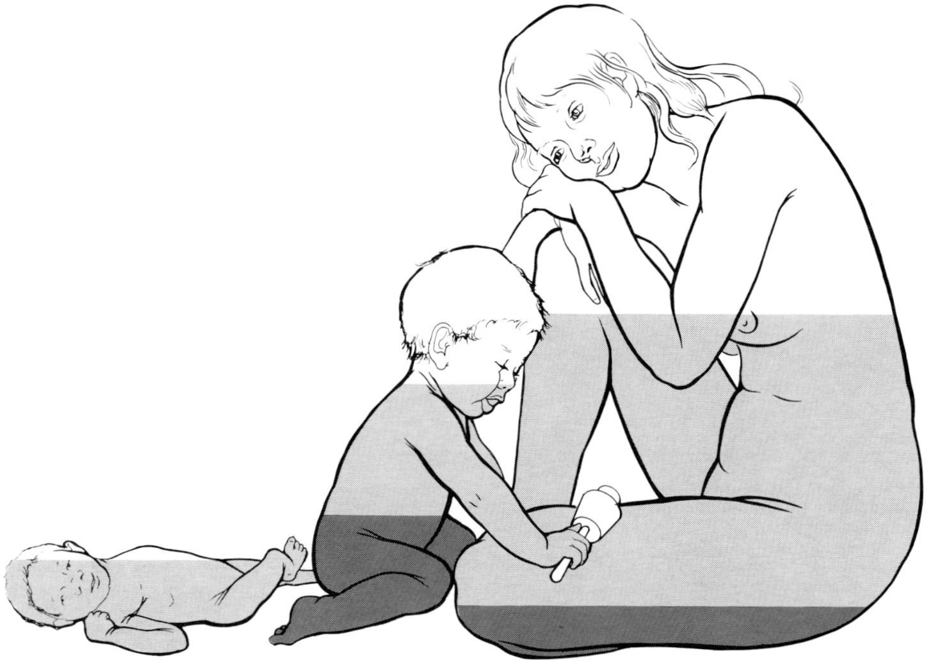

Figure 29–12. *Comparison of total body water in "premie," infant, and adult.*

simultaneously, use three times the basal requirements. The latter is maximum and is theoretical only.) The young infant's need can be met via human milk, diluted cow's milk, or commercially prepared formulas except in times of increased temperature or abnormal fluid loss.

NURSING MANAGEMENT OF THE CHILD WITH A FLUID IMBALANCE

The nurse who is responsible for the child with a fluid imbalance must be especially observant because the child's fluid balance is precarious, and he may not be able to verbalize his problems. Children who are particularly susceptible to fluid imbalances are those with diarrhea and vomiting, pyloric stenosis, diabetes, fever (with excessive sweating), and cardiac anomalies.

Symptoms

History

Ask the mother if she has noticed any change in the child's appearance or behavior. Has

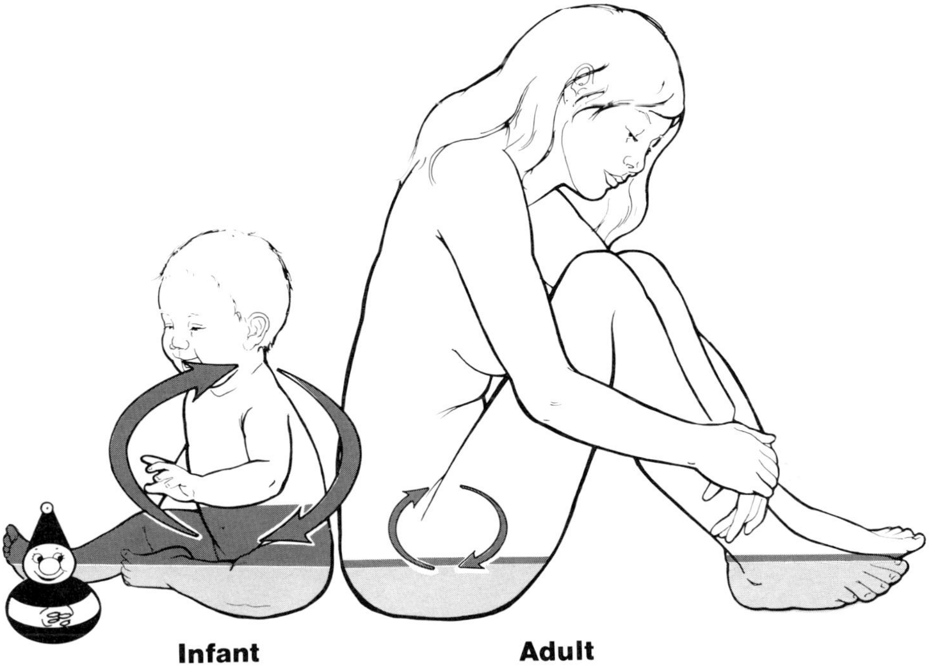

Figure 29–13. *Daily extracellular fluid volume exchange.*

Table 29–1. Basal Water Requirements in Relation to Age, Weight, and Surface Area

Age	Weight (kg)	Surface Area (M^2)	Basal Metabolism (cal/24 hr)	Basal Metabolism (cal/kg/24 hr)	Minimal Basal Water Requirement (ml/24 hr)	Minimal Basal Water Requirement (ml/m^2/24 hr)	Minimal Basal Water Requirement (ml/kg/24 hr)
Newborn	3.3	0.2	150	45	150	750	45
1 week	3.3	0.2	200	60	200	1,000	60
2 months	5	0.25	270	54	270	1,080	54
6 months	8	0.35	400	50	400	1,140	50
12 months	10	0.45	500	50	500	1,110	50
3 years	15	0.60	700	47	700	1,170	47
5 years	20	0.80	900	45	900	1,120	45
8 years	30	1.05	1,100	37	1,100	1,050	37
13 years	60	1.70	1,600	27	1,600	840	27

Adapted from Rudolph, A.M. (ed.) *Pediatrics,* ed. 16. New York, Appleton-Century-Crofts, 1977, p. 198. Used with permission.

she noticed inappropriate responses to people? purposeless movements? Is he lethargic? Irritable? Is his cry shrill and less energetic than normal? All these are signs of illness in the child.

General Appearance

Cool gray skin is a sign of decreased peripheral circulation due to severe fluid volume deficit. In dark-skinned children, check the nail beds, conjunctivae, oral mucosa, and tongue; these areas are normally pinkish-red.

The child's face may be pinched and drawn. His anterior fontanelle, if patent, will be sunken, as will be his eyes. Touch his eyes; if they are soft, he has decreased intraocular pressure.

Neurologic Signs

Smooth-muscle irritability is a sign of potassium deficit. Note any weakness, paralysis, or diminished reflexes. Muscle twitching, a sign of calcium or magnesium deficit, is often mistaken for a sign of a seizure.

Weight Loss

If possible, ascertain the child's weight before his illness. His weight should be taken on admission to the unit and every day thereafter. Always weigh the child naked, before he has eaten, after he has voided, and on the same scale at the same time of day. Minor errors are serious. Weight loss may be due to fluid loss or to catabolism of body fluids, which is a slower process than fluid loss. Mild dehydration occurs with a loss of 3 to 5 percent of normal body weight, moderate dehydration with a 5 to 9 percent loss, and severe dehydration with a loss of 10 percent or more.

Tissue Turgor

In the well-hydrated person, pinched skin falls back into normal configuration when released. When the pinched skin remains raised, the person has poor tissue turgor. In the obese child, the skin may seem deceptively normal. The undernourished child will have poor tissue turgor. Feel the skin on the child's abdomen and medial aspects of the thighs to assess tissue turgor. In sodium excess (hypertonic dehydration), the skin feels thickened and firm.

Mucous Membranes

Mouth breathing, various medications, and fluid volume deficit all cause dry mouth. To determine if the dryness is due to dehydration, run your finger inside the child's mouth where gums and cheek meet. True fluid volume deficit causes dryness in this area.

Thirst

Avid thirst is an indication of dehydration but is hard to determine in a baby. If he has not been vomiting, offer sips of flattened soda frequently.

Tearing and Salivating

Absence of saliva and tears is a sign of fluid volume deficit and should be reported.

Pulse

Pulse rate is always evaluated in sick children. Note rate, regularity, volume, and ease of obliteration. Always take the child's pulse for one full minute and consider variables such as crying, that may influence the pulse. Take the pulse every time the temperature is taken and more often in seriously ill children. Refer to Table 25–2 for the significance of pulse variations.

Table 29–2. **Significance of Pulse Variations**

Symptom	*Imbalance Indicated by Symptom*
Rapid, weak, irregular pulse	Severe potassium deficit
Slowing pulse, weak, irregular	Severe potassium excess
Increased pulse rate	Sodium excess Magnesium deficit
Decreased pulse rate	Magnesium excess
Bounding pulse (not easily obliterated)	Fluid volume excess Interstitial fluid-to-plasma shift
Bounding, easily obliterated pulse	Impending circulatory collapse
Rapid, weak, thready pulse, easily obliterated	Circulatory collapse Sodium deficit Hemorrhage Plasma-to-interstitial fluid shift
Decrease in pulse volume on changing position	Impending circulatory collapse Sodium deficit

Adapted from Metheny, N.M. and Snively, W.D. Jr. *Nurse's Handbook of Fluid Balance,* ed. 2., Philadelphia, J.C. Lippincott Co., 1974, p. 62. Used with permission.

Temperature

Subnormal temperature often accompanies fluid volume deficit and is due to a reduced energy output. Fever, which may be caused by the underlying disease, greatly increases water loss. Even with an elevated temperature, the child's extremities may be cold because of poor peripheral circulation caused by hypovolemia.

Respirations

Note the rate, depth, and regularity of the child's respirations. His water loss may be *doubled* by Kussmaul breathing, or hyperpnea, of metabolic acidosis. Acidosis is frequently due to diarrhea or salicylate poisoning. The child will not always exhibit the obvious overbreathing that is seen in adults, but he will have cherry-red lips. With metabolic alkalosis, the older child will have shallow, irregular respirations. The infant normally has an irregular respiratory rate; therefore, changes in rhythm are not dependable signs of alkalosis in the infant. Note and report changes in respiratory rate and depth since these are significant in evaluating the child's response to therapy.

Blood Pressure.

Blood pressure is not a good indicator of fluid loss in the child. The natural elasticity of young vessels usually keeps the pressure stable until the fluid loss is severe. Cardiovascular collapse will then occur, followed rapidly by severe shock.

Urine Output

The urine output should be measured as accurately as possible. Several methods may be employed to note the child's output. A diaper count, signifying the number of times the child voids, can be used. Diapers can also be weighed before and after the child voids to obtain a gram weight of urine excreted. It may be necessary to apply a urine collection device such as a "wee bag" to catch the urine (Figure 29–14). Note the concentration according to color. With fluid volume deficit, the child's urine output will be decreased and the specific gravity elevated, indicating a more concentrated urine. If the child with a fluid volume deficit has a large urinary output, he may have renal damage. See Table 29–3 for normal urine output for the child.

Table 29–3. **Normal Urine Output for the Child**

Age	*Ml/24 hours*
1–2 days	30–60
3–10 days	100–300
10 days–2 months	250–450
2–12 months	400–500
1–3 years	500–600
3–5 years	600–700
5–8 years	650–1000
8–14 years	800–1400

Adapted from Vaughan, V.C., III, McCay, R.J., and Behrman, R.E. (eds)., *Nelson's Textbook of Pediatrics* ed. 11. Philadelphia, W.B. Saunders Co., 1979, p. 2093. Used with permission.

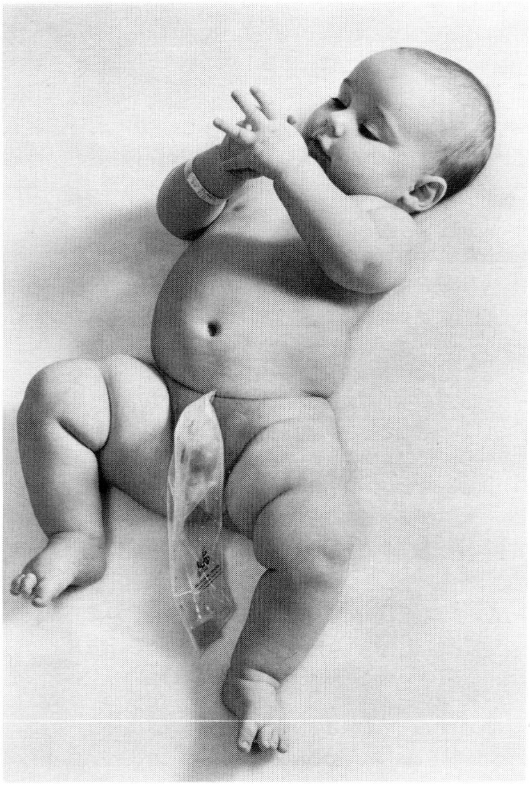

Figure 29–14. *The U-Bag collector by Hollister.*

Stools

In addition to number and amount of stool, the nurse also records their character and consistency. It is important for the physician to know if the stools are normal, if they are diarrheal, or if they contain blood or mucus.

Vomitus

Record the number of times the child vomits as well as the quantity and character. If bile, which is alkaline, is in the vomitus, an alkaline solution should be given for fluid replacement.

Other Losses

Fluids lost by suction, drainage tubes, and fistulas should be noted. Measure these losses if possible; if not, estimate the amount.

Intake

Record the amount and type of fluids the child takes, whether orally or parenterally.

Blood Chemistry Studies

Every 4 to 8 hours, hematocrit, BUN, CO_2, and serum electrolytes should be tested in the child with a fluid imbalance. Baseline arterial blood gas studies, such as pCO_2, pH and pO_2 should also be used to evaluate acid-base status. Calcium studies are done if signs of tetany are noted.

The dehydrated child will have an elevated hematocrit, due to hypovolemia. Other blood studies, such as serum sodium and serum potassium, may be elevated, normal, or low. Elevated BUN and creatinine levels will return to normal within 48 hours after fluid therapy begins; if not, the child may have kidney damage.

FLUID REPLACEMENT THERAPY

Daily Requirements

Basic daily requirements of fluids and electrolytes must be met, and additional amounts must be given to correct preexisting deficits and concurrent losses due to diarrhea, vomiting, and so on. Sodium and potassium, in the amount of 2 to 3 mEq per kg of body weight, are also necessary for maintenance needs. The omission of calories may produce ketonuria within a few hours after the onset of fasting. For this reason, carbohydrates must also be included to meet daily maintenance requirements.

Body Surface Area

Calculations for fluid requirements are based on weight, or on the child's body surface area (BSA), measured in square meters. The BSA is a more accurate gauge because requirements for fluids and electrolytes, as well as therapeutic dosages of many medications, are roughly proportional to the BSA (with the exception of neonates and premature infants). Several nomograms and tables for estimating BSA are available. (The Skills Manual discusses two methods of determining the BSA: a nomogram and a formula that can be used in lieu of the nomogram.) After determining the child's BSA, use Table 29–1 to estimate his minimum fluid requirements. For example, if the BSA is 0.35, column 7 shows that the child will need 1,140 ml/M^2/24 hours to meet his minimum fluid requirements.

Oral Fluid Replacement

When possible, fluids are replaced orally. The oral route has two advantages: orally ingested fluids are absorbed more slowly than are parentally administered fluids, which go directly into the circulatory system (i.e., excessive amounts of oral fluids are less hazardous than excessive amounts of parenteral fluids); and oral fluid replacement permits the child freedom of movement and activity, whereas parenteral therapy often requires long hours of relative immobility.

Even with the safer oral route, it is still possible to overload the child; therefore, care should be taken in calculating and administering oral fluids. Potassium should not be given orally when renal function is impaired (e.g., oliguria or anuria).

The accidental use of salt for sugar in formula preparation, although uncommon, does occur, and produces hypernatremia. Recall that hypertonic dehydration is one of the most dangerous fluid and electrolyte imbalances. The hypertonic formula causes the infant to cry; his mother thinks he is hungry and gives him more of the formula, and his condition worsens. Symptoms of sodium excess include extreme thirst, nuchal rigidity (stiff neck), muscle rigidity, expansion of extracellular fluid with visible edema, and, sometimes, brain damage. The child's daily need for sodium is 2 to 3 mEq per kg of body weight. When one tablespoon of salt is added to one quart of water, its sodium content is 350 mEq. It is easy to see why substituting salt for sugar is so dangerous. The nurse should stress to the parents the importance of avoiding such a mistake in formula preparation.

Tube Feedings

Formulas for tube feeding (gavage), often used for the unconscious child or the child with swallowing problems, may contain large amounts of solutes, in particular, protein. An increase in solute load, accompanied by a decrease in fluid intake, may increase plasma osmolarity. Water will be drawn from the tissues to supply the necessary blood volume to excrete the excess solutes. The apparently normal volume of the resulting urine output is misleading because output exceeds intake when the fluid loss from tissues is taken into account. Dehydration will occur, with an accumulation of nitrogenous waste produces in the bloodstream. Protein excess causes nausea, vomiting, diarrhea, and, eventually, *ileus*, or intestinal obstruction. High fever and disorientation may result.

Diarrhea may follow tube feedings and is usually due to contamination of the feeding material, overconcentration of carbohydrates or fats, or improper administration of the feeding (too rapid administration or too cold a feeding). (Refer to ch. 18 for further discussion of nasogastric tubes and to the Skills Manual for instructions on insertion and use.)

Parenteral Fluid Therapy

Hypodermoclysis

Parenteral fluids may be administered by the subcutaneous or the intravenous route. The subcutaneous administration of fluids is termed *hypodermoclysis*. Clysis is only occasionally used for infants and small children because it is easier to start than intravenous fluids. However, there are disadvantages to the subcutaneous route, and the variety of fluids which can be used is limited. Hypodermoclysis is never used in cases of moderate to severe dehydration because of the danger of precipitating hypovolemic shock. The peripheral circulatory collapse often accompanying severe ECF volume deficit prevents the adequate absorption of subcutaneously administered fluids. In addition, painful swelling may occur at the infusion site, and the fluid-logged tissues are excellent sites for infection. In order to aid absorption of the fluids, an enzyme is often added at the infusion sites. The sites most often used for clysis in the infant are the anteriolateral aspects of the thighs. However, the pectoral region, the lower portion of the abdomen, and the back are also used. Two needles are used at once and the rate of flow is dependent on the rate of absorption. Sterile technique is imperative. After the hypodermoclysis is discontinued, sterile dressings are applied to the infusion sites.

Meet the infant's needs for sucking, love, and security during clysis. With the parents' permission, a pacifier can be used, unless contraindicated, to provide for his sucking needs. However, use one with caution because a pacifier may be too tiring, especially for the weak infant; it may use up his energy and calories. Any time an infant is allowed to suck a pacifier (or his thumb), he should be burped because he will invariably swallow air as he sucks.

Intravenous Fluid Therapy

Intravenous therapy is often used for the child who is unable to take nourishment orally (for example, the child with anorexia or vomiting, or the unconscious child), or for a child who has a fluid and electrolyte imbalance. IVs are also used for the administration of medications that must be given often. For example, an antibiotic that must be given every four hours may be less distressing to the child when given intravenously than when given intramuscularly. The physician may want to rest the gastrointestinal tract of the child with severe diarrhea and thus order intravenous fluids.

The fluid therapy intake is usually calculated in 24-hour blocks to maintain the child's urine output in the normal range for his age. After the physician orders the type of fluid and the amount to be administered, the nurse obtains the desired solution (usually from the hospital pharmacy) as well as the necessary equipment needed to start the infusion. Bottles containing no more than 250 milliliters are used for the child under five years of age. To avoid the hazard of accidental overload, no more than 500 milliliters per bottle is used for any child.

Special pediatric administration sets are used to minimize the possibility of errors. These sets have a small calibrated volume chamber that holds only 100 to 150 milliliters of fluid at a time. The flow rate is easier to control because these set-ups use "micro" or "mini" drops, equal to 1/50 to 1/60 milliliters. They deliver 50 or 60 drops per milliliter as opposed to adult IV set-ups, which deliver 10, 12, or 15 drops per milliliter. The formula for calculation of flow rate is as follows:

$$\frac{\text{Total volume infused}}{\text{number of hours of infusion}} = \text{ml per hour}$$

For example, the physician orders 250 ml of D_5W to infuse in four hours and the microdrip for your equipment delivers 50 drops per ml:

$$\frac{250 \text{ ml}}{4 \text{ hours}} = 62 \text{ ml/hour}$$

To convert this to drops per minute, use the formula:

$$\frac{\text{ml/hour} \times \text{drops/ml}}{\text{minutes/hour}} = \text{drops/minute}$$

$$\frac{62 \text{ (ml/hour)} \times 50 \text{ (drops/ml)}}{60} = 52 \text{ drops/minute}$$

This two-step formula may be combined into one step as follows:

$$\frac{\text{Total volume} \times \text{drops/ml}}{\text{Total infusion time in minutes}} = \text{drops/minute}$$

$$\frac{250 \text{ ml} \times 50 \text{ drops/ml}}{240 \text{ minutes (4 hours)}} = 52 \text{ drops/minute}$$

The disadvantage of using this latter formula is that it does not calculate ml per hour. Because of the difficulty of regulating IV fluids in the child, drops per minute may be difficult to control; you must also know the desired volume per hour, which can be more easily controlled.

It is easier to compute the flow rate using the microdrip adapter, which delivers 60 drops per ml. Because the drop factor (60 per ml) is equal to the number of minutes per hour (60), these two figures cancel each other out, with the result being that "ml per hour" equals "drops per minute." Using the same examples as above:

$$\frac{250 \text{ ml} \times \not{6}0 \text{ drops/ml}}{4 \text{ (hours)} \times \not{6}0 \text{ (minutes)}} = 62 \text{ drops/minute (or 62 ml per hour)}$$

When regulating the flow rate on a crying child, remember that the crying produces vasoconstriction, which slows the infusion rate. As the crying stops, the constriction is lessened and the IV speeds up. For this reason, drops per minute may be difficult to control in the child; milliliters per hour can still be carefully controlled. Overhydration is always a possibility, with pulmonary edema resulting and, consequently, pneumonia.

Automatic infusion-regulator monitors should be used on all children undergoing intravenous therapy. These machines monitor, or count, the drops administered per minute. The IV tubing is connected to the monitor (check manufacturor's instructions for the monitor in your facility) and the flow rate is set according to physician's orders. Should the IV infiltrate, the tubing kink, or the drip chamber empty, an alarm will sound. (Note: infusion *pumps* are sometimes used, rather than monitors. Some pumps will continue to pump the IV solution, even if the needle has infiltrated or the bottle emptied. *Know* your equipment and do not confuse monitors and pumps.) These infusion monitors are no substitute for the nurse, however. Check the child every half hour, paying particular attention to the infusion site itself. At least every hour, record on the pediatric IV infusion record kept at the bedside the amount of solution infused, the amount remaining, the flow rate, and the status of the infusion site (Figure 29–15).

Restrain the child before initiating or assisting with the IV infusion (in some hospitals specially trained nurses may start infusions). Scalp veins are often used for IV therapy in children. They are near the surface and easy to locate and do not infiltrate as readily as do other sites. If a scalp vein is to be used, a mummy restraint is appropriate. The site, usually over the temporal bone, is lathered and shaved. Be careful to shave only enough hair to avoid interference with the infusion site. Parents, who may be worried that the child will be bald, should be told that the hair will grow back quickly. They may be particularly fearful of an IV in this site and may worry that the needle will penetrate the child's brain. Explain that the scalp vein infusion does not infiltrate as readily, meaning less trauma to the child, and that the child will have more freedom of movement than if an arm were used. This will usually allay the parents' fears. After the needle is inserted, it is supported with a small piece of gauze and then taped in place. The scalp vein site may be protected with a small paper cup (Figure 29–16), and the child's arms restrained with a clove-hitch restraint. If a hand or foot is to be used for the infusion, secure it to a padded arm board. (The foot is not used in the walking child unless absolutely necessary). A sandbag may then be taped to the arm board to prevent the child from dislodging the needle (Figure 29–17).

This constant restraint leaves the child frustrated, fretful, and irritable. He may withdraw and become apathetic. A pacifier may be used to help comfort the infant. He should be picked up (condition permitting), cuddled, rocked, and otherwise comforted. The child undergoing such frightening and painful procedures needs the physical presence of his mother.

Of course, therapy of any kind *must* be explained to the older child prior to the procedure itself. If offering a choice of sites can be permitted, allow the child to choose which arm (leg) he would rather use. The child who enjoys fine motor skills with his right hand, for example, would choose his left hand for the infusion. The older child may be mobile after the IV fluids have been started and the infusion site is secured and protected.

A phlebotomy, or *cutdown* (into a vein), may be done on the child who needs IV therapy for a longer period of time. However, a cutdown is not used indiscriminately because cutdown sites are limited,

Time (Hour)	Bottle Number	Solution	Medication Added	Rate Ordered	Drop Chamber Filled to (ml)	Actual Hourly Intake (ml)	Total Intake (ml)	Desired Intake (ml)	Observed Infusion Site	Comments	Initial
8	1	D5 250 ml.		30 ml/hr	40	32	32	30	✓	started 7 a.m.	Lu
9		E/10 mEq KAC			40	32	64	60	OK	left hand	Lu
10					40	28	92	90	OK		Lu
11			Ampicillin		40	30	122	120	OK		Lu
12N			250 mg/5 ml.		40	30	152	150	puffy,	red – IU D/C	Lu
1											
2											
3											
4											
5											
6											
7											
8											
9											
10											
11											
12MN											
1											
2											
3											
4											
5											
6											
7											

Figure 29–15. *Pediatric intravenous infusion record.*

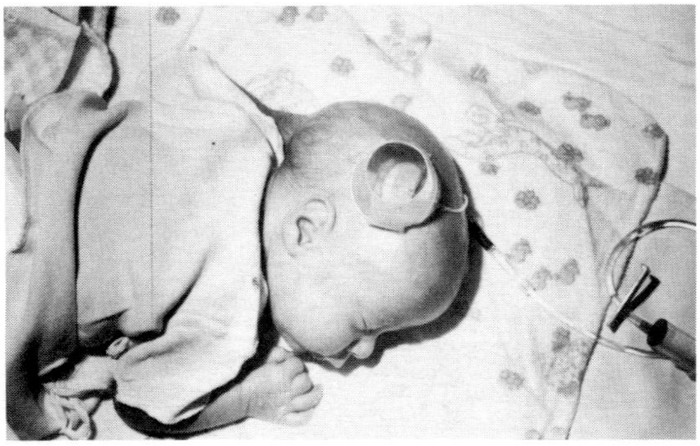

Figure 29–16. *Scalp vein infusion.*

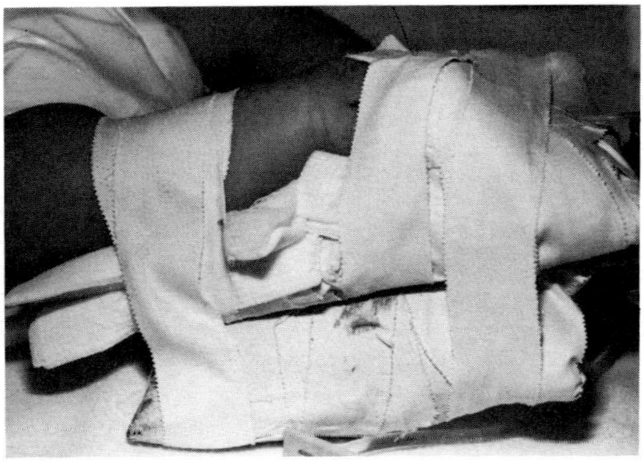

Figure 29–17. *IV secured with use of a sandbag.*

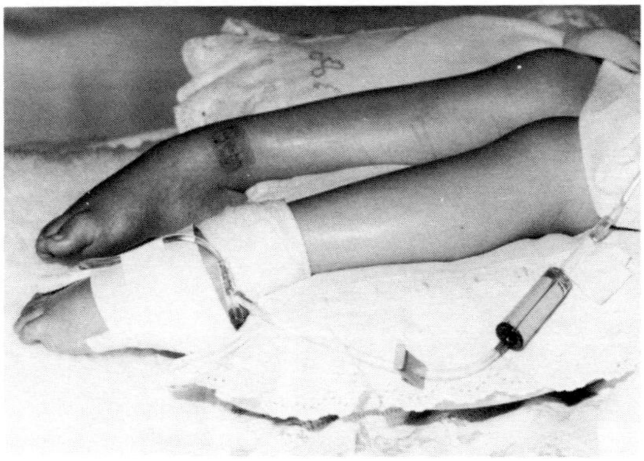

Figure 29–18. *Cutdown in ankle of a comatose child with a progressive nervous system disease. Note old cutdown site in right ankle.*

especially if the child has a chronic illness. A cutdown involves minor surgery, as a catheter is threaded into a vein, then sutured in place (Figure 29–18). There is less likelihood of infiltration and dislodged needles when a cutdown is used. The child can usually move a little more freely, although the site is always secured and protected.

Total Parenteral Nutrition

The newborn needs 50 to 75 calories for each kilogram of weight every 24 hours to maintain his body stores; for maximum growth, he needs additional calories in the amount of 100 to 130 calories per kilogram each 24 hours. Intravenous fluids, even 10 percent glucose, cannot meet these requirements. In order to prevent the permanent reduction in brain size (and consequently, intelligence) that accompanies severe malnutrition in the perinatal period, the neonate needs a source of adequate nutrition if he is unable to take and/or utilize sufficient oral nourishment.

Complete nutrition, adequate to sustain life and promote growth, is possible via the intravenous route. This method of providing nutrition is called *total parenteral nutrition* (TPN) or *hyperalimentation* and may be used for several months. Total parenteral nutrition is used for a variety of conditions; for example, congenital gastrointestinal anomalies, chronic diarrhea, prematurity, extensive burns, aplastic anemia, or cancer. The TPN fluid contains protein (in the form of protein hydrosylate), calories (hypertonic dextrose solution), water (for hydration), vitamins, minerals, and electrolytes. The concentration of this solution is 4 gm/kg/24 hours.

Weekly injections of iron and Vitamin K are given to combat anemia and clotting disorders. Essential fatty acids and trace elements are given as needed via plasma transfusions. However, symptoms of essential fatty acid deficiency may occur as early as seven to ten days after therapy begins with fat-free alimentation. Observe the child for scaly skin lesions, poor wound healing, growth retardation, and thrombocytopenia.

When *central venous hyperalimentation* is necessary, a Silastic catheter is threaded from the jugular vein into the superior vena cava under sterile conditions. The high concentration of the solution is irritating to blood vessels and must enter the body in an area of high blood flow in order to be diluted quickly. The catheter may be tunneled subcutaneously from the vein entry point in the neck to a skin exit site away from the incision. Moving the exit site to a remote point lessens the likelihood of blood contamination from skin organisms. The catheter is secured with subcutaneous sutures. An antibacterial ointment and a sterile dressing are applied to the exit site, and a coil of catheter is included in the dressing to avoid accidental displacement. (See the Skills Manual.) The child is properly restrained so that he can have as much movement as possible without touching the catheter. Insertion sites are limited and can be used only once.

The TPN fluid itself is prepared under the strictest of aseptic conditions in the hospital pharmacy. It may be stored for five days in the refrigerator and should hang at room temperature for no more than 24 hours. The hypertonic solution, rich in nutrients, is an excellent culture medium for fungal and bacterial growth. Sepsis is the chief hazard for the child with an indwelling catheter; therefore, every precaution should be taken to avoid infection in the child undergoing TPN therapy. A millipore filter is placed between the infusion tubing and the Silastic catheter to filter particulate matter and/or microorganisms.

Controversy exists over the administration of medications into the hyperalimentation tubing because of the risk of introducing infection or an air embolus. In institutions that adhere to the policy of avoiding this risk, you will use a separate intravenous infusion for medications. If the institution's policy allows the administration of medications through the tubing, be sure to add them via a T-connector placed between the filter and the Silastic catheter to avoid blocking the filter.

The tubing is connected to a constant infusion pump to ensure an even flow rate and to reduce the possibility of clot formation at the tip of the catheter. The flow rate is calculated for maximum glucose tolerance and should not exceed 10 percent of the ordered rate per hour. The nurse must not attempt to "catch up" on fluids because the high osmolality of the concentrated dextrose will cause hyperglycemia and an osmotic diuresis, which may lead to dehydration, seizures, and coma.

Because of the location of the catheter in the vena cava, a break in the line could cause exsanguination or an air embolism on deep inspiration. A padded Kelly clamp is kept at the bedside to occlude the catheter should a break occur. The break is repaired immediately. Under sterile conditions, the line is cut below the break, air gently withdrawn, a new adapter inserted, the clamp released, and the infusion resumed. If the repair is done quickly with aseptic technique, there is little danger of clot formation.

TPN is begun gradually, with a 10 percent dextrose concentration of hyperalimentation solution to meet the child's basic needs. Blood glucose and urine sugar levels are checked every four hours to determine the child's tolerance for the solution. Blood glucose levels are checked with Dextrostix; Labstix are used to determine urine values. If the Dextrostix levels are consistently 130 mg/100 ml or less and the urine sugar 3+ or less, the physician will order an increase in the concentration of glucose to 15 percent, then 20 percent as the child indicates tolerance. Once the child is able to tolerate this glucose concentration, the fluid volume is gradually increased in 5 to 10 ml increments from the basal level of 100 ml/kg/24 hours to 150 ml/kg/24 hours, which promotes optimal growth. Hyperalimentation is discontinued in the reverse process as the child is able to take and utilize orally administered foods. He should be checked for hypoglycemia for 48 hours after therapy is discontinued.

Nursing management of the child undergoing TPN therapy involves monitoring his response to the therapy and maintaining the strictest aseptic technique to avoid infection, as well as fostering his growth and development.

Routine daily monitoring includes the measurement of blood sugar levels with Dextrostix, urine and stool Labstix, daily weight, and accurate intake and output measurements. Dextrostix testing is done every 4 to 24 hours, or as ordered. Findings above 175 mg/100 ml or below 45 mg/100 ml are abnormal and should be reported. If the level is elevated, the alimentation setup is checked, and a blood sugar sample obtained. Hyperglycemia may be due to an increase in infusion rate and, if not, it usually indicates sepsis. Hypoglycemia can be caused by a decrease in infusion rate or a leak in the tubing.

Urine output is monitored hourly. Diapers are weighed before and after use. A pH of 5 to 6 is normal, but a pH of 8 or more indicates a loss of electrolytes (alkalines) and possible sepsis. A stool pH of 8 (especially important in infants with diarrhea) indicates possible acidosis.

The child's growth is monitored by measuring his weight daily, head and chest circumference weekly, and length bimonthly. The child's weight should increase by 15 to 20 grams a day.

Lab tests are routinely scheduled to further monitor the child's response to therapy. Studies include a complete blood count, serum electrolyte content and osmolarity, and blood sugar concentration; these tests indicate the child's nutritional progress and readily detect the occurrence of osmotic diuresis or abnormal fluid retention, as well as electrolyte or acid-base imbalances. Blood specimens and central venous pressure (CVP) should *not* be obtained via the hyperalimentation catheter, as this exposes the system to infection. Only when the catheter itself is suspect as a source of infection is it permissible to obtain a specimen from it.

All equipment is changed daily with the exception of the Silastic catheter. The dressing is changed when the equipment is changed, using strict aseptic technique. (See the Skills Manual.)

When changing the infusion tubing, clamp the catheter with the padded Kelly clamp to prevent the introduction of air into the vena cava. Filters are cultured weekly to determine if infection is present before clinical symptoms appear. All joints in the infusion circuit are wiped with Betadine b.i.d. to remove any traces of the nutrient solution and to aid in preventing infection. Antibiotics are given only if the child's underlying condition warrants.

Promoting the child's growth and development is an important part of nursing care for the child on TPN. Age-appropriate motor and perceptual skills are fostered within the limits of the child's overall condition. The child's needs can best be met by his family. For this reason, the parents should be taught how to manage the child's care and supported in their attempts to help.

TPN prevents stimulation of the gastrointestinal tract. For this reason, the infant on TPN does not experience normal hunger, and therefore does not associate sucking, swallowing, and food intake with its relief. He misses the opportunity to learn taste, touch, and temperature sensations in his mouth. It is important to foster the development of these sensations in the infant. This can be accomplished through the use of simulated feedings. The infant is held, cuddled, rocked, and talked to for 15 to 20 minutes every four hours. A pacifier is offered, and eye-to-eye contact, as well as hand and finger play, is encouraged. The child learns to associate sucking (pacifier) with pleasant human interaction.

The infant also needs help in learning to swallow as he sucks. This may be facilitated by dropper/pacifier feedings. Liquids are given by a dropper while the infant sucks the pacifier. Gradually he is weaned to a premie nipple and then a regular nipple.

Peripheral hyperalimentation therapy may be more advantageous at times than central venous hyperalimentation. TPN can be offered with a 10 percent glucose concentration via peripheral infusions for short periods of time (several weeks). The nursing management and monitoring are essentially the same, although no dressing changes are needed. Careful observation of the infusion site is necessary because of the irritating properties of hyperalimentation fluids. Infiltration may cause sloughing of the skin severe enough to require skin grafts. If the IV infiltrates, remove it at once, and notify the physician.

Fat emulsions (lipids) may be used to supplement therapy with hypertonic dextrose solutions. Because fat is a more concentrated form of energy, it supplies more calories in a smaller amount of water. Fat emulsions are isotonic and are thus less hazardous than hypertonic dextrose solutions. Intralipid 10 percent is a fat emulsion made from egg yolk, soybean oil, phospholipids, and glycerin, and is best given peripherally. No more than 4 gm/kg/24 hours should be administered.

No drugs, other fluids, or electrolytes can be added to fat emulsions, nor can an in-line filter be used because it breaks up the emulsion. Hypertonic dextrose solutions can be given through a separate line that connects with the fat emulsion via a Y-connector *only* at the site of infusion (see the Skills Manual). Two infusion pumps are required to administer both fat emulsion and hypertonic dextrose solution. Transient side effects that may occur are vomiting, shivering, fever, chills, flushing, and pain in the chest and back. Delayed reactions are also possible.

CLINICAL CONDITIONS CAUSING FLUID AND ELECTROLYTE IMBALANCES

A number of clinical conditions can cause fluid and electrolyte imbalances in the child. Among them are diarrhea, vomiting, salicylate intoxication, and burns.

Diarrhea

Diarrhea is a common cause of fluid and electrolyte disturbances in the child. A large loss of liquid stools can rapidly deplete the child's extracellular fluid volume, especially if the diarrhea is accompanied by vomiting. Usually water and electrolytes are lost in isotonic proportions; that is, the same proportions in which they are normally found in the ECF, thus the term *isotonic dehydration*. Isotonic dehydration or ECF volume deficit occurs in 70 percent of children with severe diarrhea. However, water may be lost in excess of electrolytes (hypertonic dehydration), and electrolytes may be lost in excess of water (hypotonic dehydration), affecting 20 percent and 10 percent, respectively, of children with severe diarrhea. Recall that intestinal fluids are alkaline; therefore, losses may result in metabolic acidosis, as well as potassium deficit.

The child with metabolic acidosis will have increased rate and depth of respiration (usually absent in the infant) and may have an acetone odor on his breath if ketosis of starvation is present. With potassium deficit, the child will exhibit muscle weakness, anorexia, vomiting, excessive flatus, and flabby muscles.

Ask the mother about the child's usual bowel habits and when she noticed an increase in the number of stools. Ask her the character and quantity of the stools as well as the amount of fluids the child has been taking. Has the child been vomiting? Has there been excessive sweating or polyuria? Has there been any blood in the child's stools? (See chapter 18 for a discussion of the nursing care of the child with diarrhea.)

Vomiting

The child who vomits loses, in addition to fluids, hydrogen, potassium, sodium, and chloride, all plentiful in gastric secretions. Consequently, he suffers from fluid volume deficit, metabolic alkalosis, potassium deficit, and sodium deficit. With the loss of chloride ions, another anion, bicarbonate, increases to maintain electrical balance. Thus, not only does the child lose acids but the bicarbonate level rises; metabolic alkalosis results. The child's respirations are shallow and slow in an attempt to retain carbon dioxide and increase the carbonic acid level in the blood. Calcium ionization is decreased in an alkaline pH; therefore, tetany may accompany alkalosis. (Nursing care of the child with vomiting is discussed in chapter 18.)

Salicylate Intoxication

The normal child's dose of aspirin is a grain per year of age up to age ten, when the child reaches the adult dose of 10 grains. As little as two to four times this dose will produce toxic effects. Salicylates increase the sensitivity of the respiratory center to carbon dioxide, resulting in an increased loss of carbon dioxide from the lungs. Respiratory alkalosis results. In the older child, this is the major symptom. Calcium deficit accompanies the alkalosis and is manifest by twitching, positive Chvostek's sign, and convulsions.

The child under age five may develop metabolic acidosis following the initial respiratory alkalosis. Symptoms of severe intoxication—hyperpnea, acetone odor on the breath, vomiting, and fluid volume deficit—resemble those of diabetic acidosis. The child's temperature rises, and his skin is flushed and sweaty. Disturbances in clotting may contribute to bleeding.

Gastric contents are removed, and the stomach lavaged with isotonic saline. Since 80 percent of ingested salicylates are excreted through the kidneys, adequate renal function is established with a hydrating solution which also compensates for the excessive amount of fluid lost through the lungs because of hyperpnea. Carbohydrate is given to prevent or combat ketosis, and Vitamin K is administered to prevent excessive bleeding. Calcium gluconate may be given to relieve symptoms of tetany.

Burns

Burns are a major cause of fluid and electrolyte imbalance and will be discussed in detail in chapter 31.

SUMMARY

The child's fluid and electrolyte composition differs from that of the adults. The balance is more precarious and therefore even seemingly small deviations can be crucial. A variety of conditions affects this delicate balance. It is the nurse's responsibility to recognize and report subtle changes in the child that may be indications of fluid or electrolyte deviations. Parenteral fluid administration is the primary mode of treatment, and its success depends on meticulous nursing care.

Bibliography

Alfin-Slater, R.B. and Jelliffe, D.B. Nutritional Requirements with Special Reference to Infancy. *Pediatric Clinics of North America* 24:3, 1977.

Bode, H.H. and Warshaw, J.B. (eds). Parenteral Nutrition in Infancy and Childhood, in: *Advances in Experimental Medicine and Biology*, vol. 46. New York, Plenum Press, 1974.

Borgen, L. Total Parenteral Nutrition in Adults. *American Journal of Nursing* 78:224, 1978.

Conway, A. and Williams T. Parenteral Alimentation. *American Journal of Nursing* 76:574, 1976.

Finberg, L. Water and Electrolyte Physiology, in Rudolph, A.M. (ed). *Pediatrics*, ed. 16. New York, Appleton-Century-Crofts, 1977, p. 260.

Fischer, J.E. (ed). *Total Parenteral Nutrition*. Boston, Little, Brown & Co., 1976.

Ghadimi, H. (ed). *Total Parenteral Nutrition Premises and Promises*. New York, John Wiley & Sons, Inc., 1975.

Guyton, A.C. *Textbook of Medical Physiology*, ed. 5. Philadelphia, W.B. Saunders Co., 1976.

Kee, J.L. *Fluids and Electrolytes with Clinical Applications: A Programmed Approach*. New York, John Wiley & Sons, Inc., 1978.

Kee, J.L., and Gregory A.P. The ABC's (and mEq's) of Fluid Balance in Children. *Nursing '74* 4:28, June, 1974.

Manni, C., Magalini, S.I., Scrascia, E. (eds). Total Parenteral Alimentation, in: *Proceedings of the International Symposium on Intensive Therapy. Rome, May 30*–June 2, 1975. New York, American Elsevier Publishing Co., Inc., 1976.

Metheny, N.M. and Snively, W.D. Jr. *Nurses' Handbook of Fluid Balance*, ed. 2. Philadelphia, J.B. Lippincott Co., 1974.

Vaughn, V.C. III, McCay, R.J., and Behrman, R.E. (eds). *Nelson's Textbook of Pediatrics* ed. 11. W.B. Saunders Co., 1979, p. 2093.

CHAPTER **30**

The Child with a Urinary Deviation

BEHAVIORAL OBJECTIVES

After studying this chapter you will be able to:

- Discuss the relationship between impaired glomerular filtration and edema, identifying nursing care measures for each.
- Explain the effect of changes in electrolyte balance, such as potassium and calcium, have on the child with a urinary deviation.
- Contrast the information received from a urinalysis to that obtained from urine culture.
- Make a teaching plan for a child receiving corticosteroids and diuretics, explaining how the drugs work, possible side effects, and daily care needs.
- Construct a nursing care plan for a child receiving hemodialysis.

TERMS AND CONCEPTS

Glomerular filtration
Tubular reabsorption
Edema
Pitting edema
Ascites
Dependent edema
Proteinuria
Hypertension
Specific gravity
Creatinine clearance
Plasma creatinine
Blood urea nitrogen
Addis count
Suprapubic aspiration
Intravenous pyelogram
Voiding cystourethrogram
Diuretics
Corticosteroids
Dialysis
Hemodialysis
Peritoneal dialysis

The kidneys maintain fluid and electrolyte balance, excrete metabolic waste products, and secrete endocrine substances. The kidneys operate by processes of filtration, reabsorption, and secretion: the glomeruli filter blood plasma as it passes through the kidneys, the tubules reabsorb needed solutes and water, and excess products are excreted as urine.

This chapter is about children with alterations in glomerular filtration and tubular reabsorption. Common problems of edema, hypertension, and proteinuria are discussed along with the necessary nursing care interventions. Table 30–1 lists specific urinary disorders.

COMMON PROBLEMS AND NURSING INTERVENTIONS

Impaired Glomerular Filtration and/or Tubular Reabsorption

The cause of kidney damage in most children is unknown, and may have *no* early symptoms of renal problems. Frequently, much of the child's kidney function is lost by the time symptoms develop, because forces work undetected to impair *glomeruli filtration* or *tubular reabsorption*. Infection and many acquired disorders, such as diabetes mellitus, can drastically reduce the overall number of glomeruli. When this happens, the kidney lacks sufficient functioning nephrons to regulate urine volume and urine composition, and waste products accumulate. Neoplasms or congenital anomalies can obstruct the passage of blood plasma through the kidneys, preventing normal filtration, reabsorption, or secretion.

Drastic changes in blood pressure also can impair glomerular functioning. If the blood pressure drops—as it does during trauma, hemorrhage, or severe dehydration—solutes and water cannot be pushed into the glomeruli. As a result, waste products accumulate and fluid and electrolyte imbalances occur. Heredity plays a role in some glomerular disease. Certain toxic drugs and chemicals can damage glomeruli and tubules, causing a urinary disorder. Lastly, immunologic factors, such as the clumping of antigen-antibody complexes in the glomeruli, can cause lesions and disturbances in glomerular functioning.

Decreased glomerular filtration reduces the amount of salt and water available for processing and excretion. If the child retains too much salt and water, the extracellular fluid expands, causing an increased work load on the heart and may lead to congestive heart failure and pulmonary edema. If the child excretes too much salt and water, large amounts of sodium are lost in the urine. Such children are frequently referred to as "salt wasters" and need diets high in sodium and water. You are far more likely, however, to encounter the child who retains too much salt and water, and who has edema and hypertension.

Edema

Edema is the accumulation of excess fluid between body cells or within a body cavity. Because fluid is displaced and cannot be used to meet body water requirements, edema is a form of dehydration. Edema is a broad term, and there are several specific types. *Pitting edema* is found in body areas where so much fluid has accumulated that a depression remains temporarily if pressure is applied to specific points. *Ascites* is excessive fluid accumulated in the peritoneal cavity, and *dependent edema* is fluid accumulations in areas that are affected by gravity, such as the feet, ankles, or hands. Edema becomes noticeable when the volume of interstitial fluid increases by 10 to 15 percent. It usually is seen first in areas of low tissue tension, such as the eyelids. Edema can inhibit the movement of limbs, alter arterial blood flow to vital organs, (especially in confined areas such as the cranial vault), and ultimately may affect the lungs and internal and external respiratory exchange. The child with edema is uncomfortable. He is fussy, irrita-

Table 30–1. Common Urinary Disorders in Children

Name	*Definition*	*Treatment*	*Special Nursing Considerations*
		Congenital Disorders	
Polycystic kidneys	An autosomal recessive condition causing enlarged spongy kidneys containing many cysts. For the infant, progressive renal insufficiency usually causes death in a period of weeks or months. Older infants and children suffer liver problems, but live longer.	No specific treatment. Use of dialysis and renal transplant for chronic renal failure. Surgery for liver complications.	The risk of having another affected child is one in four. Parents need genetic information and support in deciding about having more children.
Hypospadias	A urethra opening on the underside of the penis, proximal to the normal external orifice, occurring in one of every 125 males. Many boys with hypospadias also have short *chordae*, tough fibrous bands of tissue that cause the penis to bow downward. Infants with hypospadias are not circumcized so the foreskin can be used in the repair procedure. *Cryptorchism* (undescended testes) frequently accompanies hypospadias.	If the hypospadias is minimal, no treatment is necessary. When short chordae are present, they are surgically released, usually by the time the child is two years old. The urethera is repaired (urethroplasty) in a one- or several-step surgical procedure, generally before the boy begins school.	Following a urethroplasty, the child has a foley catheter or suprapubic tube to divert urine away from the operative site. Keep the incision dry and free from trauma. Hypospadias is a difficult diagnosis for parents to accept and explain to friends and relatives. Assure them their son will void normally following the surgery.
Epispadias	The urethra opens on the dorsal side of the penis.	Same as hypospadias.	Same as hypospadias.

Exstrophy of the bladder	The entire bladder to the external urethral meatus is exposed. Urine seeps constantly from the ureters onto the abdominal wall, causing an excoriation of the surrounding skin.	Surgical closure of the bladder and the anterior abdominal wall. If the bladder cannot be saved and must be removed, the ureters are diverted into an ileal loop or ileal conduit. The abdominal wall is then closed. An *ileal conduit* is made by removing a small segment of the ileum from the small intestines. The ends of the ileum are rejoined so the child has a normal digestive tract. One end of the ileal segment is brought through a small opening in the abdomen, forming an *ostomy stoma;* the remaining end of the ileal segment is sutured closed. The ureters are anstomosed to the ileal segment. After the operation, urine drains from the kidneys, through the ureters, and ileal conduit out of the body into the attached pouch. The collecting pouch is emptied at intervals during the day by opening a small valve on the bag.	Cover the exposed bladder with petrolatum-saturated gauze or silver nitrate ointment. Position the child on his side so urine can drain freely. Change the infant's diaper frequently, and wash his feces promptly to prevent the spread of fecal pathogens to the exposed bladder. If ileal conduit surgery is performed, explain and diagram the procedure for the parents, assuring them that the surgery has no effect on the sexual organs or child-bearing. The collecting appliance imposes few limits on the child's activities, and the operation offers an active life for a previously very ill child.
Patent urachus	Continuation of the embryonic connection of the umbilicus to the bladder. Urine is discharged through the umbilicus after birth. A persistently moist or nondrying cord is usually indicative of a patent urachus.	Surgical correction.	

(continued)

Table 30–1. *(Continued)*

Name	*Definition*	*Treatment*	*Special Nursing Considerations*
		Glomerular Disorders	
Nephrotic syndrome	A chronic kidney disease of unknown origin with exacerbations and remissions. The disease usually lasts from 18 months to 2 years. The glomeruli are severely damaged and their permeability to protein is increased, leading to large losses of albumin in the urine. In addition, aldosterone (which acts to conserve sodium) is overproduced, causing massive edema. The child also has high blood cholesterol levels and is susceptible to infection because of losses of gamma globulins.	Steroids during the acute phase and exacerbations, to induce diuresis and reduce edema. Steroids are gradually withdrawn when urine findings are normal. Immunosuppressive drugs (e.g., Cytoxan or methotrexate) may be used if the child does not respond to steroids. Antibiotics prescribed for infection. A diet high in protein helps to compensate for protein loss. Sodium is restricted when edema exists. The child's activity is not restricted unless bedrest is needed for edema or infection.	Protect edematous skin from trauma and infection. Observe for signs of cerebral edema and respiratory difficulties because of ascites. Live vaccines are contraindicated because of steroid therapy. Explain to the parents and child the expected effects of steroid dosage, possible side effects, and special care to minimize exposure to infection.
Glomerulonephritis			
Acute glomerulonephritis (AGN)	Inflammation of the glomeruli caused by an immune response following a group A beta-hemolytic streptococcus infection. As a result of the inflammation, the glomeruli have increased permeability to protein and blood cells, causing proteinuria and hematuria. Symptoms involve the renal	Antibiotics are not indicated since the disease is not an active streptococcal infection. Treatment is directed at symptoms. Acute symptoms of edema, hypertension, and hematuria demand antihypertensive therapy, strict bed rest, and sodium restriction. Acute symptoms last one to two	During the acute phase, observe blood pressure closely and report any elevation. An elevated blood pressure may cause cerebral ischemia. Watch for any cerebral changes, such as headache, irritability, lethargy, or altered mental state. Weight the child daily to assess fluid retention or fluid loss. Main-

	system (hematuria and oliguria), and the cardiovascular system (hypertension, cardiac insufficiency, and congestive heart failure).	weeks almost always followed by a spontaneous recovery.	tain intake and output records. AGN can be prevented with early antibiotic treatment of group A betahemolytic streptococcal infections, which occur frequently as insect bites, impetigo, and sore throats.
Chronic glomerulo-onephritis (CGN)	Progressive renal disease of unknown origin. Problems include proteinuria, hematuria, and hypertension. The disease runs a long course with eventual renal insufficiency or renal failure.	Because the cause in unknown, treatment is directed at symptoms. The child is hospitalized for severe edema, infection, acute or uncontrolled hypertension, oliguria, and electrolyte imbalances. Use of thiazide diuretics and hypotensives for edema and hypertension. Use of corticosteroids and cytotoxic drugs for immunosuppressive effects. Peritoneal dialysis or hemodialysis for renal failure. Kidney transplant.	Measures for edema and hypertension. Precautions against infection during immunosuppressive therapy. Nursing care for dialysis. Close monitoring of vital signs, intake and output, and weight, as discussed under AGN.
Uremia	Renal insufficiency which may be acute or chronic. *Acute Uremia* usually results from infection, hemorrhage, shock, or trauma. The child recovers. *Chronic Uremia* is progressive and is commonly caused by a neoplasm, a congenital or genetic anomaly, a metabolic disorder (such as diabetes mellitus), or recurrent urinary infections resulting from a renal abnormality such as glomerulonephritis. The child has oliguria, excreting less than 15	Use of diet restrictions, diuretics, hypotensives, corticosteroids, and dialysis. Possibly a kidney transplant, depending on the child's degree of kidney impairment. See common treatments section of this chapter.	According to treatments used. Refer to discussion of nursing care in the treatments section of this chapter.

(continued)

Table 30–1. *(Continued)*

Name	*Definition*	*Treatment*	*Special Nursing Considerations*
	ml of urine per kilogram of weight per day. Accumulation of nitrogenous waste causes nausea, vomiting, and anorexia. Glomerular filtration is impaired resulting in edema, proteinuria, hypertension, and electrolyte imbalances.		
Urinary tract infections	Urinary tract infections (UTI) involve an infection of one or more structures in the urinary tract. UTI are more common in females because of the short urethra and closeness of the urinary meatus to the anus. The Escherichia coli (E. coli) pathogen is usually responsible for UTI. Symptoms depend on the infection site.	A sulfonamide antibiotic, usually Gantrisin, is given for at least ten days. Ampicillin may also be used for treatment. The acutely ill child is given intravenous antibiotic therapy. Analgesics are given for fever and discomfort. Lots of clear liquids and noncarbonated beverages to help diuresis.	Because diagnosis and treatment are based on the presence of bacteria in a sterile urine specimen, thoroughly cleanse the external genitals and obtain a midstream urine sample.
Cystitis	Infection in the bladder. The young child suffering from cystitis usually has abdominal pain, low-grade fever, and urinary frequency. The older child has pain and burning with voidings, frequency, and hematuria.		Follow-up urine cultures, at least three sterile specimens, are taken after antiobiotic treatment is finished. In females, 30 to 50 percent have recurrent UTI; of these, over 50 percent are asymptomatic. Since repeated infections can seriously harm kidney function, emphasize to the family the importance of follow-up urine specimens.

Pyelonephritis	Infection of the kidney and pelvis. Symptoms are generally acute, including a high fever, vomiting, and abdominal pain.		Teach all children good perineal hygiene, emphasizing the importance of cleansing from anterior perineum to anal region. Since resideal urine can lead to a UTI, instruct the child to empty his bladder completely with each voiding. Advise minimal use of bubble baths since studies indicate a positive relationship to UTI.
Vesicoureteral reflux	The retrograde flow of urine from the bladder up into the ureters. This flow results from a defective valve at the junction of the bladder and ureters. Reflux occurs at voidings as the urine goes up to the ureters and then returns to the bladder after voiding stops. A residual pool of urine stays in the bladder, causing recurrent UTI. The reflux may be slight or gross, transient or persistent, unilateral or bilateral.	Surgery. The placement of the ureters is corrected to create a normal valve effect.	Following surgery, the child has a suprapubic catheter to keep the bladder empty and two ureteral catheters to drain urine directly from the kidney pelvis. Observe all three catheters for drainage, checking the color and amount of urine. The catheter tips must be kept clean to avoid infection, which could spread to the surgical area of the kidneys.
Hydronephrosis	Enlargement of the kidney pelvis caused by obstruction at the ureter-pelvic junction resulting in back pressure. Continued pressure can interfere with renal tubule function or cause nephron destruction. Hydronephrosis is the most common obstructive deformity in children. Symptoms vary from none to abdominal pain, nausea, vomiting, hypertension, and repeated UTI.	Surgery if the obstruction is complete. If the obstruction is partial with no progressive kidney destruction, surgery is withheld.	

ble, and most probably will try the patience of the parents and the nurse.

Comfort measures begin with skin care. Edematous skin is stretched taut and tends to break down easily. Place soft gauze material between contiguous skin surfaces to help absorb moisture and to prevent skin irritation and breakdown. Edematous tissue does not heal well, and skin breaks are likely to become infected.

If the child is bed-ridden, protect the pressure areas, such as the elbows, sacrum, and knees, by changing his position every 30 minutes to one hour during the day. Remember that prolonged moisture macerates the skin, change the infant's diapers frequently, and be sure that the child's underclothes are dry. For the boy with an edematous scrotum, place a soft pad under his scrotum and secure it in place with a T-binder. This prevents the scrotum from rubbing against the thighs. Bathe the genitals several times a day; then dust liberally with powder. Check to see that the elastic of the child's underpants is not restricting his circulation. If the elastic leaves a pressure mark, it needs loosening.

Never use adhesive tape on edematous skin. If the edematous skin breaks down, stop all powders and ointment. Carefully wash and dry the skin lesion; then expose it to air. A heat lamp may be used with great care. At night and for naps, place the child with edema in a semi-Fowler's position. The elevation of the head will reduce edema around the eyes. If the child sleeps flat, the edema can be so severe by morning that his eyes are swollen shut. Each of these comforting measures is equally as important at home as it is during hospitalization.

The child with edema is frequently anorectic, and if ascites is present, abdominal discomfort may precipitate nausea or vomiting. Nutritional deficiencies can develop quickly. In fact, the edematous child, although he appears obese, may actually be malnourished. Plan a high calorie and protein diet with the parents and child. Proteins are especially important if the child is losing protein in his urine. Because medications are poorly absorbed from edematous skin areas, avoid intramuscular injections and use oral medications as much as possible.

Fluids and salt are commonly restricted during severe edema. Emphasize to the child and his parents how much fluid the child can have during the day, not how little. Fluids served in small colorful cups will not appear restrictive to most children. Draw a chart of stars, balloons, or smiling faces, having each figure represent a number of ounces. Each time fluid is taken, color in a figure. Even young children quickly learn how much fluid is left for the day. This is an amusing method of forming a daily fluid plan. The same idea can be used at home, where the chart can be taped to the refrigerator. Careful measurement and recording of daily fluid intake and output and weight is essential.

This is a difficult time for both the parents and the child. The edematous child may be teased by his siblings and friends. He is uncomfortable and fretful. Meanwhile, his parents are tired, worried, and anxious about his condition. Offer the parents support, acknowledging the stress an ill child places on the family (see ch. 3).

Hypertension

Hypertension may be the primary cause of the kidney damage; severe chronic kidney disease may cause hypertension or contribute to it through sodium retention. It is frequently impossible to know which came first—the hypertension or the kidney disease. Since blood pressure increases from infancy through adolescence, it is difficult to define what is hypertension for any given child. One good criterion is a blood pressure more than two standard deviations above the mean for the child's age. Since a blood pressure value is only as reliable as the technique used in obtaining it, review the procedure carefully (see the Skills Manual). The child with chronic hypertension usually complains of frequent headaches, dizziness, or changes in vision, and these may be the only signs of hypertension. No reliable evidence exists that the hypertensive child should be restricted in activities or diet except in specific circumstances. Antihypertensive drugs usually control hypertensive symptoms; however, severe prolonged hypertension may lead to retinopathy.

Electrolyte Imbalances

Potassium

Changes in the concentration of *potassium* in the plasma are very serious because only a narrow percentage range of potassium in the system is compatible with life. Since 80 percent of the normal intake of potassium is excreted in the urine, the child with polyuria may develop low levels of potassium (hypokalemia), while the child with oliguria is at risk for hyperkalemia. The major life-threatening effect of hyperkalemia is its effect on heart rhythm and rate. Fatal arrhythmias, or cardiac standstill, may occur even with slightly elevated serum potassium levels. For this reason the hyperkalemic child will have a cardiac monitor and will need to have his vital signs carefully observed and recorded.

Calcium

Calcium, an electrolyte crucial for bone development, is absorbed from the intestine in the presence of Vitamin D. Since the most active form of Vitamin D is metabolized by the kidneys, the child with impaired renal function may become hypocalcemic and have bone deformities (such as rickets) or growth failure.

Metabolic Acidosis

Metabolic acidosis is a common problem of children with severely impaired glomerular functioning. Normally the kidneys maintain the body's balance of fixed (nonrespiratory) acid by excreting, in the urine, a quantity of acid equal to that made in the metabolic processes. When glomerular filtration is altered, normal amounts of acid are no longer excreted; the result is metabolic acidosis.

Many children with renal problems tolerate metabolic acidosis without any symptoms if their serum bicarbonate is greater than 15 mEq/liter. As the acidosis worsens, however, the child will probably become anorectic or nauseated. If Kussmaul respirations (the deep sighing respirations used to expell more carbon dioxide and thus reduce acidosis) are present, the child is definitely in metabolic acidosis. Alkali usually is given when the child's bicarbonate level falls below 15 mEq/liter. Given as a solution of sodium citrate and mixed with a favorite beverage, such as Kool-Aid or Tang, the alkali is usually well accepted. The serum bicarbonate level must be checked carefully to be sure alkalosis is not induced. If the acidosis is corrected too quickly, tetany and convulsions can be induced. Be aware of the child's serum bicarbonate level, looking for early respiratory signs of acidosis.

Anemia

Anemia is another common problem of chronic severe kidney disease. Renal failure causes a decrease in the production of red blood cells, as well as a shortened life span for existing erythrocytes. In addition to the inadequate red blood cell production, anorexia and undernutrition caused by metabolic acidosis and edema may also result in iron-deficiency anemia. The child with a urinary disorder and accompanying anemia fatigues easily and may have dyspnea on exertion. Plan energy-saving activities, rest periods, and a diet high in iron. If anemia is a problem, refer to chapter 24.

Proteinuria

Normal healthy children excrete small amounts of protein in their urine. When significant amounts of protein are excreted (*proteinuria*), the cause is *always* an increase in glomerular permeability. Normally, only a small amount of albumin (the smallest protein molecule in the serum) is filtered in the glomeruli; most is reabsorbed in the tubules. Then if large amounts of albumin appear in the urine, there is almost certainly a glomerular disorder.

COMMON DIAGNOSTIC TESTS AND NURSING IMPLICATIONS

Urinalysis

A *urinalysis*, or study of the urine, provides information on the amount and type of formed elements in the urine, as well as a variety of special information. A freshly voided morning specimen is ideal for a urinalysis since the urine is concentrated and acidic. A small amount of urine is centrifuged, and a portion of the sediment is placed on a microscope slide and examined for blood cells, casts, and bacteria. Other specific tests that are part of a urinalysis include: specific gravity, pH, and the examination of color, odor, and the presence of protein, glucose, hemoglobin, and ketones.

Specific Gravity

Specific gravity is a measurement of all particles in the urine, and indicates the concentrating capacity of the kidneys. The normal sp.g. of urine is 1.001 to 1.030, and is measured with a hydrometer or refractometer. If fluids are forced or restricted, the ability of the kidneys to dilute or concentrate the urine is measured by sp.g. A very dilute urine may be an early sign of kidney dysfunction because the kidneys cannot concentrate urine sufficiently to remove normal quantities of waste solutes. To test the kidneys' ability to *concentrate* urine, withhold all fluids from the child for 16 hours, usually from early evening until the following morning. The sp.g. should *rise* to 1.025 or more. For a dilution test, fluids are forced over a short period, and the bladder is emptied at brief intervals. Here the sp.g. should *fall* and water will be excreted.

Certain conditions (such as diabetes mellitus, adrenal insufficiency, hepatic disease, and congestive heart failure) raise the specific gravity of urine. The child with fever, severe or prolonged vomiting, diarrhea, or sweating also has an elevated specific gravity. Another cause of an elevated sp.g. is the contrast medium used in x-ray studies. When you measure and record sp.g., consider the child's condition. Has he had an x-ray using contrast media, been vomiting, or had diarrhea? Does he have a fever? If so, record this information along with the specific gravity.

pH

The pH of urine measures its hydrogen ion concentration. A pH below 7 is acidic urine; a pH above 7 is an alkaline urine. Normal pH varies from 4.5 to 8.0. Freshly voided urine from healthy children on normal diets is acidic. Excessively acidic urine (a pH below 6.0) can be caused by a high protein diet, acidosis, uncontrolled diabetes mellitus, or such medications as ammonium chloride. In contrast, alkaline urine is commonly voided after meals in response to the secretion of hydrochloric acid in gastric juice. When the body puts gastric acid into the digestive process, the kidneys respond with a corresponding amount of bicarbonate. Diets high in vegetables, citrus fruits, and milk can also produce alkaline urine as can certain medications, such as sodium bicarbonate and potassium citrate. The pH is easily measured with nitrazine paper and a color chart.

Color

Urine *color* is another important part of the urine study. A change in urine color may be the first indicator of a renal or metabolic disorder. Always save abnormally colored urine. Normal urine is a pale yellow or amber color. Color intensity usually indicates urine concentration. For example, a pale almost colorless urine is most probably a very diluted urine, while a darker urine is denser. This is not a constant rule, since the urine of a child with diabetes mellitus frequently has a pale color but has a specific gravity is high because of the added presence of glucose as a dissolved solvent.

Always compare urine color to fluid intake. Also, remember that like sp.g. and pH, the color of urine is changed by certain diseases. Bile pigments, an indication of liver disease, can produce a yellow to yellow-brown or greenish urine. Blood released in the upper urinary tract usually turns red-brown in the urine, while bright red blood in the urine is probably from the lower urinary tract, and may be from the kidneys. Of course, red urine can also be caused by menstrual flow or the ingestion of certain foods such as beets or blackberries. Cloudy urine indicates the presence or large particles, such as bacteria, drugs, or cells. Milky urine generally means lipids are present.

Odor

The *odor* of urine is also significant. Fresh urine has a characteristic unoffensive odor. The ammoniacal odor develops as urine decomposes from urea to ammonia. Be aware of other odors. A fruity odor usually means acetone is present. A fecal odor suggests infection with bacteria. Always save urine with a peculiar odor.

The presence of protein, glucose, hemoglobin, and ketones are easily assessed by using a dipstick. Record each value of the urine test along with additional notes on the child's diet, medication, and general health. Each of the tests in a urinalysis is simple, quick, and nonthreatening to the child.

Talk with the child and his family about the purpose of and information yielded from each part of the urinalysis. Urine tests are done frequently, sometimes every hour. Without repeated explanations of the need for these tests, the family and the child may become irritated and anxious.

Volume

The *volume of urine* is important. The amount of urine excreted is not an indication of renal function since failing kidneys can excrete large quantities of urine. Charts of normal urine output for children of different ages are of little value in assessing the importance of volume because output is related to solute intake. It is easier to remember that for a healthy child, urine output should be 40 to 50 percent of his normal fluid requirements (see ch. 29).

Creatinine Clearance Test

Creatinine is an end product of muscle metabolism and is normally excreted into the urine by glomerular filtration. Creatinine is not reabsorbed by the tubules. The *creatinine clearance test* estimates the glomerular filtration rate (GFR). For a creatinine clearance test, all urine voided by the child during a 24-hour period is collected, and one blood specimen is taken. With the use of a special formula, the creatinine clearance ability of the glomeruli is then calculated.

Plasma Creatinine and Blood Urea Nitrogen

Plasma creatinine and *blood urea nitrogen (BUN)* are end products of protein metabolism which are normally excreted in the urine. When the rate of glomerular filtration decreases, the plasma level of creatinine and blood urea nitrogen rise, leading to a condition called *azotemia*, which is an excess of nitrogenous substances in the blood. The child with azotemia is uremic. This condition is discussed in Table 30–1.

The Addis Count

An *Addis count* measures the kidney's ability to concentrate urine. To do an Addis count, the child is given a normal lunch but a dry dinner. No fluids are allowed from after lunch until the following morning. Have the child empty his bladder at bedtime and record the time. This specimen is thrown away. Save all the following urines, including the first morning urination. Record the time of the first morning voiding and the test is complete. Usually the child has only one voiding during the test period.

The 12- or 24-Hour Urine Collection

To determine the quantitative measurement of urine products such as protein, glucose, and electrolytes, a *12- or 24-hour urine* collecting period is necessary. To begin the collection have the child void; or, for an infant, wait until he voids. Discard this urine, and record the time. This time marks the beginning of the 12- or 24-hour collecting period. Save all other voidings, and place them in a collection bottle which is kept refrigerated. Have the child void at the end of the collection period, and add this final specimen to the collection bottle. For the infant and child not potty-trained, you will need a urine collector bag.

Urine Culture

A urinary tract infection is determined by a *urine culture.* Since a bladder catherization can introduce bacteria into the bladder, a clean catch, midstream specimen is preferred for the urine culture. To obtain the specimen, begin by washing the area around the urinary meatus with soap and water. This is done to prevent organisms on the skin from contaminating the voided urine.

For girls, separate the labia, and, using a soapy cotton ball, wash from clitoris to anus on the left side of the urinary meatus. Using a second cotton ball, repeat the procedure, this time washing the right side. With a third cotton ball, wash directly over the meatus. Rinse, using three more cotton balls saturated with sterile water. Then use three more cotton balls to wash with an antiseptic solution. Remember to use the same front-to-back motion for each step. Rinse and dry the perineum using six more cotton balls. Have the girl begin to void into the toilet, then place a sterile urine cup into the stream to obtain the midstream urine.

For a young boy, wash the penis thoroughly, remembering to retract the foreskin if the child is uncircumcised. The older boy can clean his penis independently after he receives instructions. Again, a midstream collection is made. For infants, the genitals are washed as above, and a sterile collector applied. Since a midstream catch for infants is impossible, label the specimen "clean catch."

A clean catch, midstream urine specimen obtained with good technique can almost totally eliminate the need for a catheterization specimen. If the cleansing procedure is not followed, however, the specimen may be contaminated. Explain to the child and his parents why the elaborate cleansing is necessary. For girls, turn the lengthy cleansing procedure into a game, having her hand the cotton balls to you while she keeps count of how many remain. Give the older child a small mirror and use this as a time to teach the child about genital anatomy and hygiene.

Suprapubic Aspiration

A *suprapubic aspiration* (Figure 30–1) is another method frequently used to obtain sterile urine for a culture. When a suprapubic aspiration is done, the anterior abdominal wall is cleansed with an antiseptic; a needle is inserted just above the pubis into the bladder; and urine is withdrawn into a sterile syringe. This procedure can seem very frightening to the child and his parents. Explain that because of the easily accessible position of a distended bladder, the aspiration is a simple procedure that

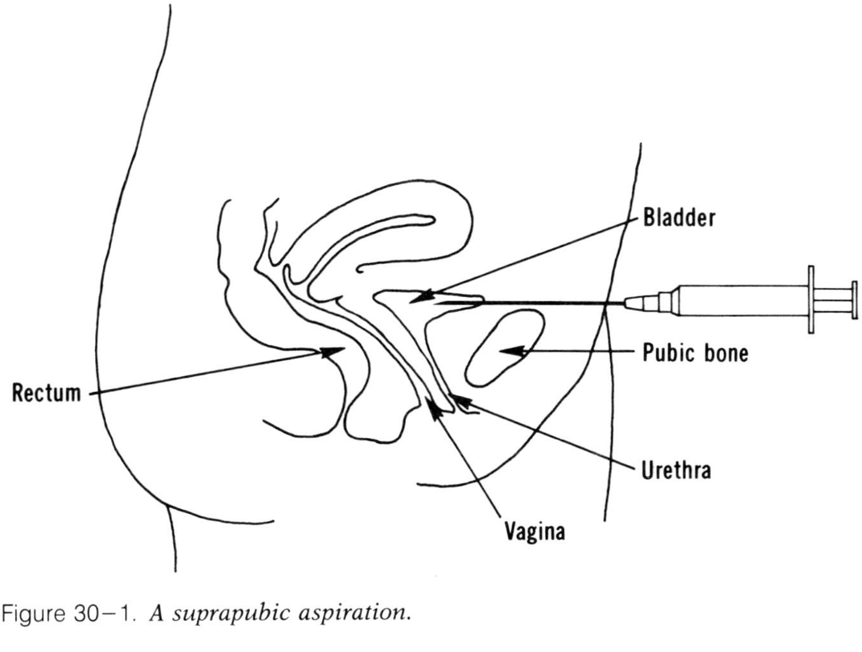

Figure 30–1. *A suprapubic aspiration.*

greatly reduces the risk of bladder infections—a constant worry when a catherization specimen is taken. A small quantity of the urine is then examined under the microscope for the presence of bacteria. If the urine is plated on a culture medium, valuable information can be obtained.

Common Radiographic Tests

Intravenous Pyelogram

An *intravenous pyelogram (IVP)* is a study of the size, shape, position, and integrity of the urinary tract. A radiopaque dye is injected into the antecubital vein. When the dye reaches the kidney, it is filtered into the urine by the glomeruli. A series of x-rays, taken as the dye is filtered, shows the outline of collecting systems in the kidney and of the ureters.

A serious drawback of the IVP is the possibility of an allergic reaction to the dye. Although such reactions are rare, question the family about the child's allergy history, especially to iodine or other radiopaque preparations. For safety, 1 milliliter of contrast medium is injected intravenously before the actual test begins, and the child is observed closely for 30 to 60 seconds.

Voiding Cystourethrogram

The *voiding cystourethrogram (VCUG)* is a study of the size and contour of the urethra and bladder that demonstrates the presence of reflux into the ureters. The child is catheterized and radiopaque dye is slowly injected into the bladder. The size and contour of the bladder are studied. The child is asked to void, and serial x-ray films are taken. Small infants will begin to urinate spontaneously as the bladder becomes distended. It is more difficult for the older child to urinate, especially with people present. Offer your support, reassuring him that you know it is difficult to void with others watching, but that his urinating is an important way he can help to complete the study. The first voiding after a catheterization is frequently painful; warn the child about this. Subsequent urinations usually are not painful. Tell the child this so he will not fear painful voidings and refuse to urinate. Forcing fluids, applying cold compresses to the urinary meatus, or sitting in a warm tub of water are measures that may help to relieve postcatheterization discomfort. A voiding cystourethrogram should not be done if the child has an active urinary tract infection because the procedure may spread the infection to the kidneys, either by reflux or by introducing bacteria. Possible infection can be assessed by knowing the child's most recent clean catch urine results. Some signs of infection are urinary frequency, pain on voiding, or a change in the color, odor, specific gravity, or other urine parameters previously discussed.

Renal Biopsy

A *renal biopsy* involves passing a thin needle into the kidney and removing a small piece of kidney tissue for special microscopic studies. Local anesthesia before the biopsy may be sufficient for the older child, but the younger child, who cannot cooperate, may need general anesthesia. Explain that the child will feel a pin-prick as the local anesthetic is injected to "put his back to sleep," and that he will feel pressure when the biopsy needle is inserted.

Stress that the child must not move during the biopsy. Accompany the child to the biopsy, and keep him informed of the progress as you offer touch and verbal reassurance. A large sterile pressure bandage will be applied after the biopsy. Following this, the child must remain in bed, lying on his back or abdomen, for at least 12 hours.

Assure the child and his parents that although the pressure bandage is large, the incision is only a tiny nick, the size of a pencil lead. Check the bandage site frequently for any bleeding. Monitor the child's pulse and blood pressure as often as the physician directs—usually every fifteen minutes for two hours; then every half hour for two hours; then once every four hours; then every three hours for a 24-hour period. Force fluids for 24 hours to maintain urine flow and to prevent blood clotting. Check all his urine both visually and with a dipstick for hematuria. The child is likely to feel some flank tenderness for 24 to 48 hours after the biopsy. The major concern following a renal biopsy, however, is bleeding. For this reason, a renal biopsy is *not* done if the child has only one kidney or a tendency to hemorrhage. Additional contraindications include small kidneys, advanced renal failure, and severe hypertension.

COMMON TREATMENTS AND NURSING IMPLICATIONS

Diet

Dietary management can help to reduce the production of nitrogenous wastes, ensure proper nutrition, foster physical growth, and minimize fluid and electrolyte imbalances. To reduce nitrogenous waste, reduce the intake of protein; however, much controversy exists about how much dietary protein to decrease. A reduction of protein lowers the BUN (blood urea nitrogen) but also reduces needed potassium, phosphate, and hydrogen ions. Normally, a child takes in from 2 to 4 gm/kg/day of protein; typically, the diet will be lowered to contain 1.0 to 1.3 gm/kg/day of protein. The *type* of protein offered on a restricted diet is very important. Protein provides essential amino acids that cannot otherwise be made by the body; but these amino acids are best found in animal protein such as milk, eggs, and meat, not vegetable protein such as beans and grains. To grow normally, children must have sufficient protein. To maintain growth, yet restrict excessive protein intake, the child with a urinary disorder may be given prepared balanced mixtures of essential amino acids. Although these preparations are generally well accepted, their high cost limits their usage. Their cost will decrease, however, as they are used more. When protein is restricted, the child's diet must still remain abundant in total calories. He will need adequate calories to use the protein and foster growth. Children with kidney disease often fail to grow because they do not consume enough calories. Most children with renal impairment are anorectic, and many of them suffer from daily deficits in protein, fats, and carbohydrates. This is a complex problem that requires working closely with families both to explain the need for nutrients and to help them plan and offer menus that are enticing.

Sodium is another element that is frequently restricted in diets of children with a urinary disorder. (Figure 30–2 shows foods that are high in sodium.) Retaining too much sodium—which is a common problem in glomerular and advanced renal disease—can lead to fluid retention, peripheral edema, pulmonary edema, hypertension, and congestive heart failure (see Figures 30–3 and 30–4). If sodium is restricted and a negative sodium balance results, the child's glomerular filtration

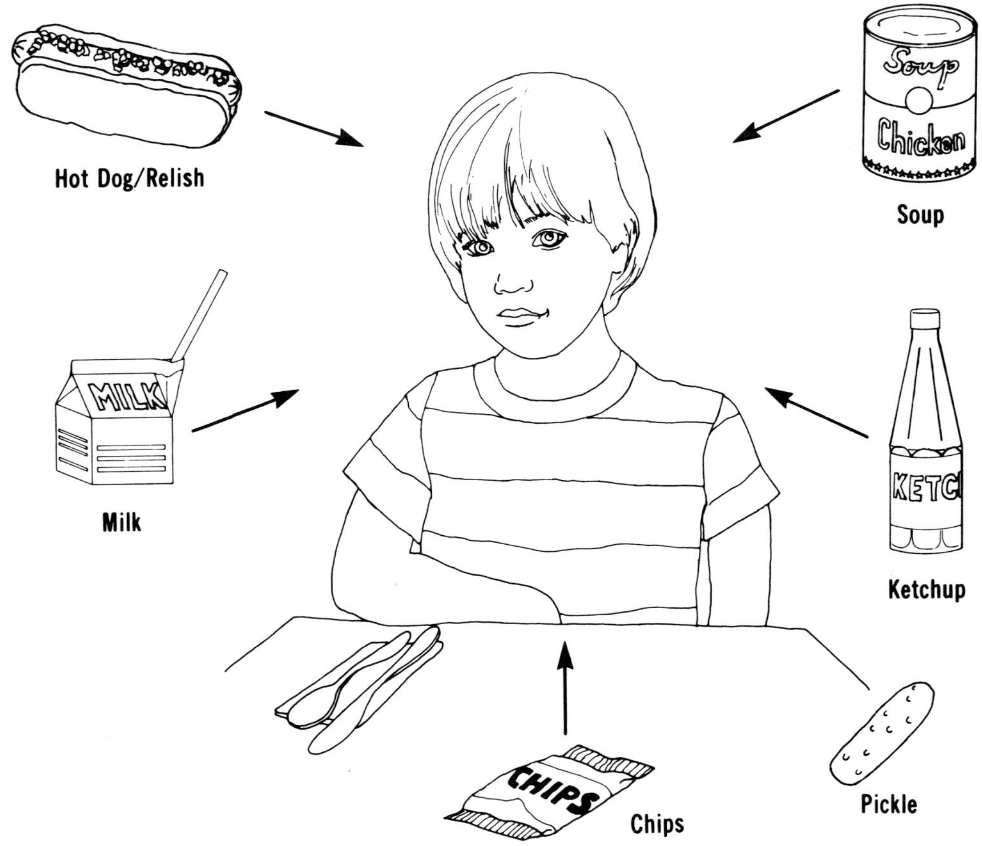

Figure 30–2. *Foods that are high in sodium.*

rate may decrease and renal function may deteriorate further. Daily weighing, and observing for signs of edema, are essential for determining the child's necessary sodium intake.

Fluid regulation is another essential treatment for the child with a urinary disorder. If he receives too much fluid, circulatory overload, edema, and water intoxication may result. Conversely, if too little water is ingested, dehydration, hypotension, and a deterioration in renal function can occur. To determine the child's fluid needs, watch his daily weight and his intake and output records. Remember that both sodium and fluid must be regulated for fluid balance.

Medications

Diuretics

Diuretics impair sodium reabsorption in the renal tubules, causing increased sodium and water excretion and an overall increase in urine production (*diuresis*). Diuresis is accomplished by the diuretic's specific site of action in the nephron or by blocking hormonal mechanisms that aid in the reab-

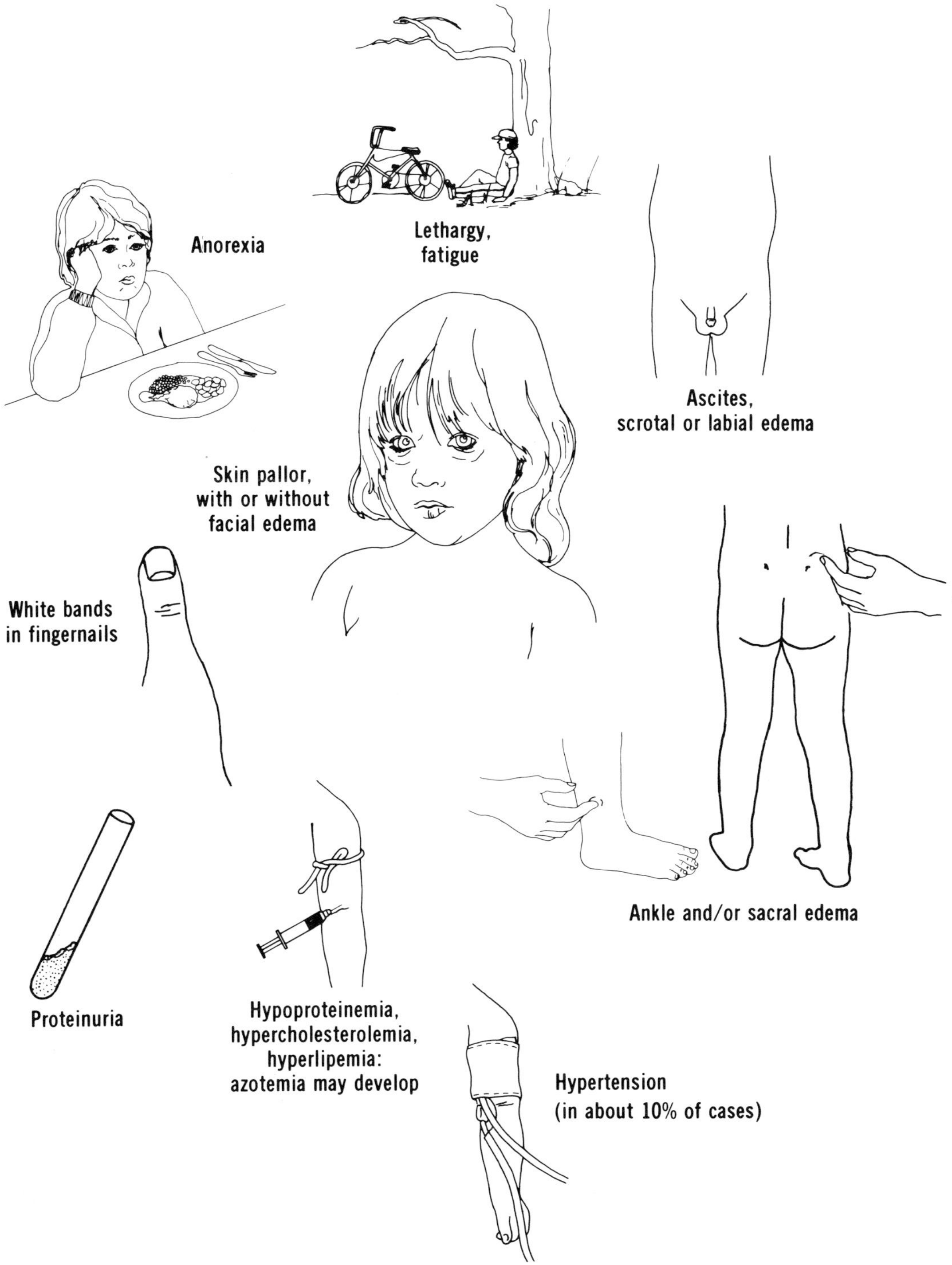

Figure 30–3. *The child with nephrotic syndrome.*

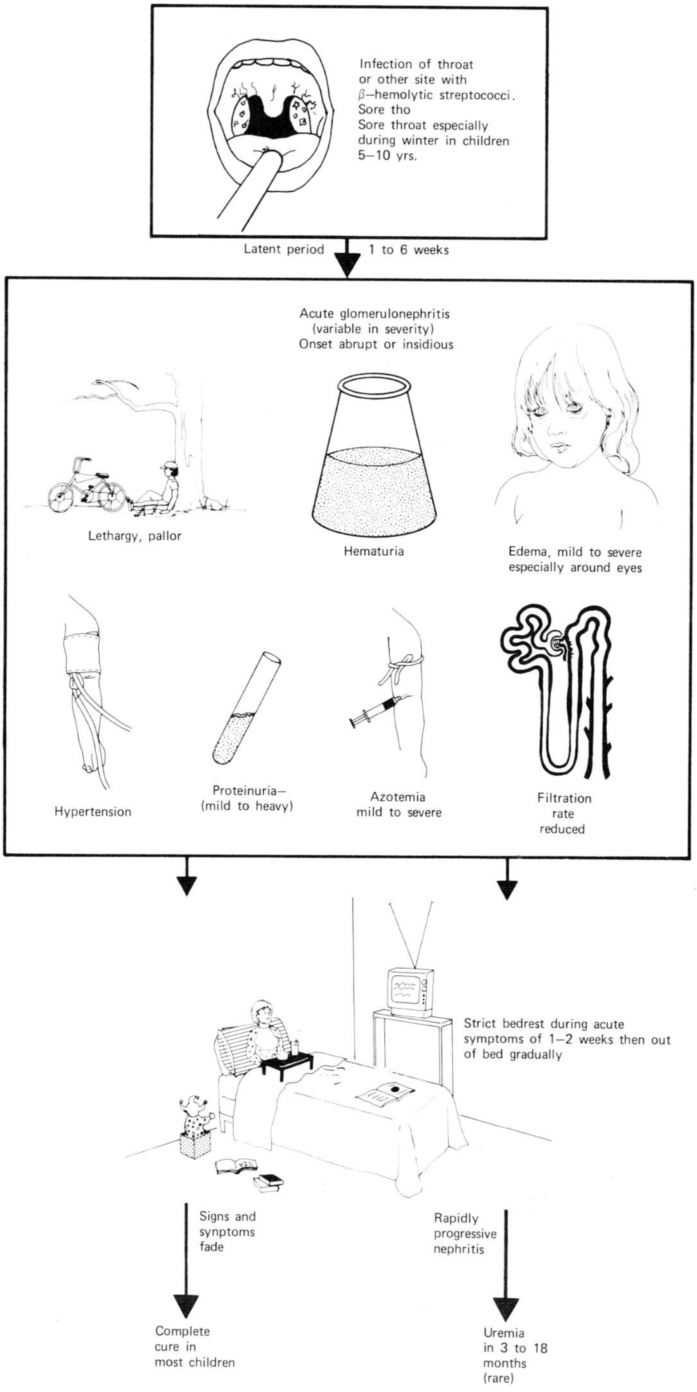

Figure 30–4. *The child with acute glomerulonephritis.*

sorption of sodium. Normally, most of the filtered sodium is reabsorbed in the proximal tubules; then that portion of the glomerular filtrate not reabsorbed passes into the descending loop of Henle where more sodium is reabsorbed. The most frequently prescribed diuretics are the thiazides, such as Diuril (chlorothiazide) and Hydro-Diuril (hydrochlorothiazide). The thiazides act in the loop of Henle and distal tubules to decrease the reabsorption of sodium.

The loop diuretics, Lasix (furosemide) and Edecrin (ethacrynic acid), block active chloride transport in the ascending limb of Henle's loop, thus interfering with passive sodium reabsorption.

The potassium-sparing diuretics act in the distal tubules to remove fluid and sodium from the body without potassium depletion. Aldactone (spironolactone) and Dyrenium (triamterene) are drugs in this potassium-sparing group which are usually given with a thiazide or loop diuretic.

Both the loop diuretics and the thiazides are used for hypertension and edema. Thiazides are often ineffective when the glomerular filtration rate is greatly reduced; in this situation loop diuretics are prescribed. Additional antihypertensive drugs are used for acute and chronic hypertension. For dosage regulation, parents may be asked to check the child's blood pressure at home during certain times of the day. (Before teaching the family how to monitor and record the blood pressure, carefully review the Skills Manual.)

When diuretics are prescribed, explain to the child and his family that the desired effect is to increase the number of voidings. For the child just beginning mastery over bladder elimination, this is a very difficult period. Just as he attains self-control, the diuretic produces frequent urinations and a tendency for "accidents." If possible, give the diuretic in the morning so that diuresis will occur during the day and not disturb the child's sleep. If the child is hospitalized, place the call light and urinal or bed pan within his reach, and reassure the child that if his undergarments or linens become soiled, they can be changed easily.

The child's body weight indicates if he is losing weight too quickly or retaining the fluid. Always measure body weight using the same circumstances: same time of day, same scale, and same clothing. Since unrestricted sodium intake is a primary reason for a poor response to diuretic therapy, a low sodium diet is frequently prescribed along with the diuretic therapy. Explain to the parents and child the relation of sodium to kidney action, and the need for diuretics and a sodium restricted diet. Relating this treatment to reducing edema, which the child knows is uncomfortable, can greatly increase his and the family's cooperation.

Corticosteroids

Corticosteroid preparations, such as cortisone, hydrocortisone, and prednisone, have a wide array of effects in the body. Among the benefits of corticosteroids for the child with a urinary disorder are: an increase in glomerular filtration rate and diuresis; better protein breakdown and inhibited protein synthesis; and—of special importance to the child with a renal transplant—suppression of inflammation by blocking allergic responses and decreasing the number of leukocytes and the size of lymphatic tissue.

The child receiving prednisone begins diuresis after one to two weeks of treatment and has a gradual loss of weight and an increase in urinary output. Proteinuria decreases, the child's appetite, activity, and general health improve. An initial daily dosage is usually followed by a maintenance every-other-day program. This intermittent therapy decreases the incidence of side effects from the drug, offers better maintenance of the child's own adrenal functioning, and makes the transition of corticosteroid withdrawal easier. Every-other-day treatment may be difficult for the family to understand. They will ask, if the medicine is so effective in relieving the discomforts of edema, why is the child restricted to every-other-day treatment? Explain the desired effects of the steroid and why the dosage is tapered. Steroid dosage is based, in part, on nursing assessment of the child's weight, intake, output, and urine test.

Side effects of steroids include the typical features of Cushing's syndrome—rounding of the face, abdominal distention, increased hair growth, a pad of fatty tissue over the base of the neck, and increased appetite with subsequent weight gain. The child may develop a huge appetite, stuffing himself with candy, cookies, and snack foods. Prepare the family and the child for this side effect, planning low-calorie snack foods, such as cheese and crackers, celery and carrot sticks. Suggest substituting low fat for whole milk, serving fewer concentrated sugar foods, and planning an exercise schedule and interesting activities to help to divert the child's attention away from eating. Emphasize that all side effects of steroid treatment are temporary and will disappear in two to three months after the therapy stops. Unfortunately, no explanation exists for the Cushing's syndrome.

A more serious side effect of steroid therapy is an increased susceptibility to infections. The problem is heightened because the steroid masks the common signs of infection such as fever, redness, pain, and swelling. Limit the child's contact with infectious agents, including his contact with crowds and persons with infections. Be certain that all family members wash their hands carefully.

Another possible consequence of prolonged steroid therapy is adrenal suppression and insufficiency, and sudden, fatal adrenal insufficiency is possible if the child suffers the stress of infection, surgery, or trauma. Although adrenal suppression is unlikely with every-other-day therapy, both the child and his parents should carry an identification card that includes the child's diagnosis, name, and dosage of steroid therapy, as well as the attending physician's name and contact phone number, and emergency care instructions.

Growth suppression, cataracts, intracranial hypertension, and peptic ulceration are additional side effects of steroid therapy. If a peptic ulcer occurs, it heals very slowly because of the anti-inflammatory effects of the steroids. As a precaution, offer the steroid drug with food or milk. An antacid may also be prescribed.

Dialysis

Dialysis is the diffusion of solutes and water through a porous membrane from one fluid area to another. *Hemodialysis* and *peritoneal dialysis* are the two major dialysis techniques; both procedures diffuse solutes and water *from* the child's blood plasma *to* a dialysis solution. The diffusion works because of the difference in concentration between the child's blood and the dialysis solution.

In both types of dialysis, the child's blood is on one side of a semipermeable membrane, and the dialysis bath, or *dialysate,* is on the other. Dialysis depends on the principle that substances always move from a high to a lower concentration. Using a dialysis solution containing the important electrolytes in concentrations normal for healthy children, the concentration of these electrolytes can be corrected in the blood of the child with a renal disorder.

Figure 30–5 shows a child whose blood potassium level is high. The potassium level in the dialysis bath is low, so potassium moves out of the child's blood into the dialysis bath. Notice that protein, blood cells, and bacteria are too large to pass through the pores of the dialysis membrane. In peritoneal dialysis, the peritoneum is the semipermeable membrane. In hemodialysis, a hemodialyzer uses cellophane or Cuprophane for the semipermeable membrane. Different types of dialyzers exist, but they all use the same principle of diffusion.

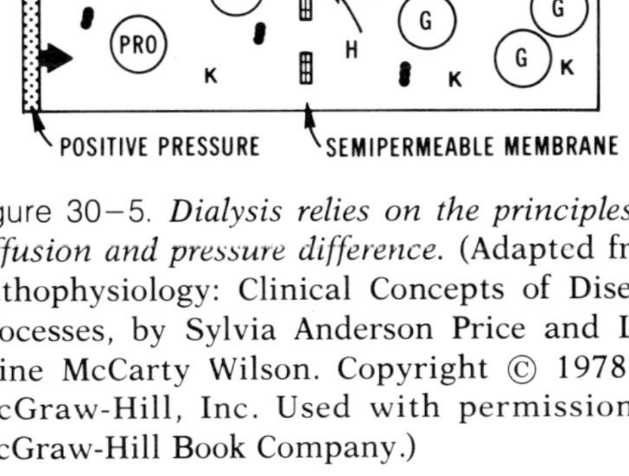

Figure 30–5. *Dialysis relies on the principles of diffusion and pressure difference.* (Adapted from Pathophysiology: Clinical Concepts of Disease Processes, by Sylvia Anderson Price and Lorraine McCarty Wilson. Copyright © 1978 by McGraw-Hill, Inc. Used with permission of McGraw-Hill Book Company.)

Peritoneal Dialysis

Peritoneal dialysis can be quickly begun and does not require the specially trained personnel and expensive equipment necessary for hemodialysis. Peritoneal dialysis can provide supportive treatment for the child with acute renal failure resulting from sudden illness, trauma, poisoning, or drug intoxication; and for problems of chronic renal failure.

Begin by preparing the child and his family for the dialysis procedure. Peritoneal dialysis tends to be lengthy, taking as long as 24 to 72 hours. Since the child must remain in bed throughout the procedure, boredom is a major problem. Explain to the child and his family that the peritoneal fluid acts like a filter which removes materials that make him sick from the child's body. Needles and catheters are needed in the dialysis procedure, and all children voice fear and resentment about injections. Show the child the dialysis fluid, the catheter that will drain the fluid into his abdomen, and where he will be injected with an anesthetic so that the catheter insertion is not felt. A doll or puppet can be used to demonstrate.

To minimize the possibility of nausea or vomiting during the dialysis, the child will be given a liquid diet; this is usually not a problem since the pressure of the peritoneal fluid causes a feeling of fullness, and the child does not feel hungry.

Before beginning peritoneal dialysis, record the child's weight and vital signs. These data provide a base against which subsequent values can be checked as the procedure progresses. Have the child empty his bladder. This precaution minimizes the chance of accidental perforation of the bladder. If the child cannot urinate, catheterization is necessary. Next, the child's abdomen is cleansed with an anesthetic solution and covered with a sterile drape. Since peritoneal dialysis is a minor operative procedure, the physician will wear a mask and gown. Strict asepsis is important because peritonitis is the most serious and common complication of the procedure. Be alert for possible peritonitis, and carefully watch the child's temperature, quickly reporting any elevation.

The infusion process is less uncomfortable and the procedure is more efficient if the dialysis fluid is at body temperature. Place the bottles of fluid in a basin of warm water to warm them. For convenience, keep the warming basin at the bedside. Have the first bottle of warmed fluid and dialysis administration set at the bedside ready for use.

After the abdomen is draped, a local anesthetic is injected into the abdominal wall, and an 18-gauge needle is inserted into the peritoneal cavity. If ascitic fluid is in the abdomen, it is removed; otherwise the warm hypertonic dialysis solution is allowed to flow by gravity into the peritoneal cavity. Then the peritoneal catheter is inserted, sutured, and firmly taped in place. The catheter will remain in place for the entire dialysis period. The infusion set is connected to the catheter, and the remaining fluid flows into the peritoneal cavity.

Continue your flow sheet, on which you've already recorded the base line weight and vital signs. Systematically record the starting time of each dialysis bottle, how much dialysis fluid infuses, and how much drains. Carefully calculate the difference between infused and drained amounts. More fluid is usually drained than was infused because the dialysis process diffuses excessive fluid across the peritoneum. Also include on the flow sheet any medications given, hourly vital signs, and comments about the child's apparent comfort or discomfort. The average volume of dialysis fluid infused is about 60 to 80 ml/kg of body weight. Each bottle of dialysis fluid is run in over a 15-minute period, allowed to diffuse for 45 to 60 minutes, then drained over 10 to 15 minutes. Heparin is usually added to at least the first bottle to keep small clots from plugging drainage holes in the catheter. Dialysis continues for from 24 to 72 hours, depending on the electrolyte concentrations and levels of urea and creatinine.

Hemodialysis

Hemodialysis, or extracorporeal hemodialysis, uses an artificial kidney outside the child's body to perform the dialysis. Three basic types of dialyzers exist: the *coil dialyzer,* the *parallel plate dialyzer,* and the *hollow fiber,* or *capillary, dialyzer.* Each dialyzer has two circuits—one for blood and one for dialysis fluid. During dialysis, blood flows *from* the child's arterial circulation in a plastic tube; through the fibers of the dialyzer, and back to the child's venous circulation. Heparin is placed in the arterial tubing to prevent clotting. A clot and bubble trap in the venous tubing prevent air or blood clots from entering the child's venous circulation. The dialysis bath forms the second circuit. The dialysis bath is very similar to normal blood, except that it is modified to correct the child's fluid and electrolyte disorders. Maintenance dialysis (as opposed to emergency acute care dialysis) is usually done three times a week and takes four to six hours. As during peritoneal dialysis, keep a flow sheet to record base line weight, vital signs, and subsequent assessments.

The AV Shunt

Long-term, intermittent hemodialysis requires a ready access route to the circulation. In 1960, Scribner devised an external arteriovenous (AV) cannula made of Teflon. His AV shunt involves placing one cannula in an artery (usually the radial) and inserting a second cannula into a nearby vein. The cannula tips are connected to form a bridge (Figure 30–6A). For dialysis, the external cannula is separated and connected to the dialyzer. Blood flows from the arterial tube, through the dialyzer, back into the vein.

Because the shunt is outside the body, infection and clotting are constant possibilities. As a result, the shunt must be kept covered with a dry, sterile dressing. Swimming is impossible for the child with an AV shunt, and tub or shower baths are possible only if a plastic cover is placed over the shunt to keep it dry.

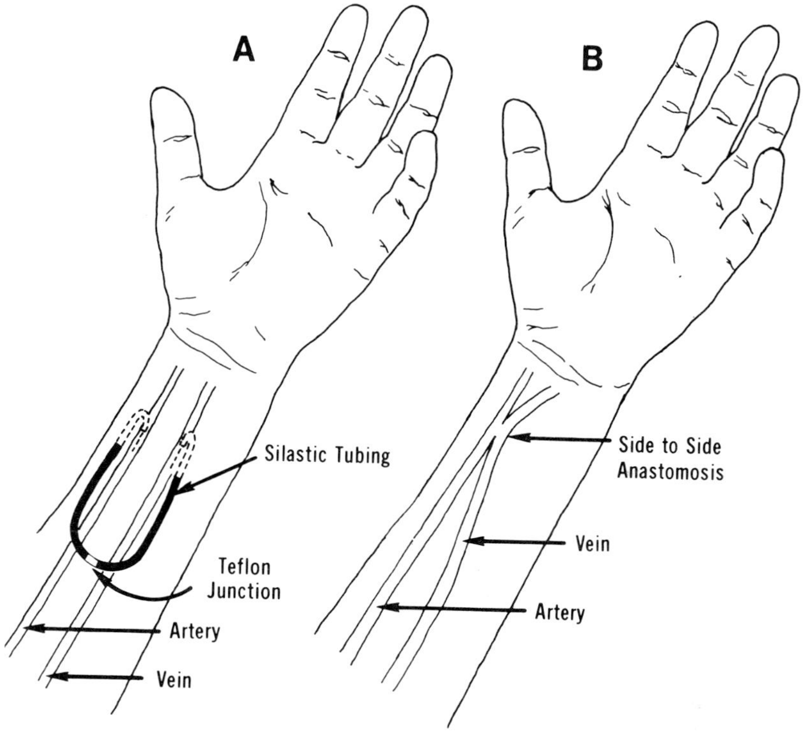

Figure 30–6. *A. External AV shunt or cannula. B. Internal AV fistula.* (Adapted from Pathophysiology: Clinical Concepts of Disease Processes, by Sylvia Anderson Price and Lorraine McCarty Wilson. Copyright © 1978 by McGraw-Hill, Inc. Used with permission of McGraw-Hill Book Company.)

Inspect the AV shunt daily for signs of infection such as redness, tenderness, edema, or drainage. Immediately notify a physician if signs of infection are present. Several times a day check the appearance of the blood in the plastic cannula. The blood should always be red. If the blood clots or appears separated into two layers, inform the physician immediately. If the shunt should ever separate (a rare possibility), immediately apply a tourniquet above the shunt, unwrap the sterile dressing, clamp both sides of the shunt, reconnect the shunt, and remove the clamps and then the tourniquet. Rewrap the dressing and notify the physician. Keep clamps on the shunt dressing at all times.

If one of the shunts pulls out of the skin, immediately apply a tourniquet above the shunt. This is an emergency situation. If the child is at home and a tourniquet is not available, have a parent or the child apply enough pressure to the area to stop the bleeding. To keep the AV shunt functioning well, the child must avoid all strenuous exercise, making sure no pressure is placed on the shunt at any time. It is extremely difficult to keep an AV shunt functioning in a child. His small blood vessels makes cannula insertion very tedious, and the dialysis procedure must be specially adapted to expose the child's circulating blood to dialysis safely without reducing the total circulating volume to a dangerously low level. Children with external AV cannulas can experience complications of anemia, convulsions, hypertension, and bone disease. The cannula generally needs replacement every six to nine months.

AV Fistula

A major breakthrough in pediatric hemodialysis is the development of an internal arteriovenous (AV) fistula. The AV fistula is made by connecting an artery directly to a vein (usually the radial artery and cephalic vein at the wrist) (Figure 30–6B). As blood is shunted from the artery to the vein, the vein enlarges. As a result, in a few weeks large needles can be used for easy venipuncture access to the rapidly flowing blood. An internal fistula avoids the problems of infection, clotting, and possible hemorrhage. Since there are no skin openings, although the large dilated vessel is visible, activity is *not* restricted. There are *no* daily dressing changes, restrictions from water, or close monitoring of activity, and the fistula usually lasts four years. Venipuncture is necessary for dialysis, however, and even with an initial anesthetic injection, the venipuncture is traumatic. If the first venipuncture misses the fistula, repeated venipunctures are necessary. Movement is severely limited during the actual dialysis. The internal fistula makes both aneurysms and ischemia of the hand (steal syndrome) dangerous possibilities.

To maximize their use for dialysis, both the AV internal fistula and AV external fistula must be protected. The fistula or shunt extremity is *never* used for intravenous therapy or taking blood specimens or blood pressure. Check the patency of either shunt daily by feeling for a thrill over the incision and by listening with a stethoscope for a swishing sound.

Home Dialysis

Families trained to complete dialysis at home are able to maintain a more normal schedule in that home dialysis affords the family more independence and flexibility. On the other hand, home dialysis requires the family to spend hours learning about machinery parts; composition and concentration of the dialysis bath; and the actual process of starting, infusing, and ending the dialysis. This instruction is involved and difficult. Venipunctures are the major trauma for children with an AV fistula, and they frequently are more accepting of a puncture which can be done by the older child himself or his parent. If home dialysis is decided upon, the family must have constant professional help available to provide technical assistance, medical care, and psychological support. Home dialysis, with its advantages, thrusts a heavy burden of responsibility on the family. Often family roles change: a mother may need to stop working or to curtail other pursuits; siblings may be needed to assist during dialysis and will have to limit time away from home; and each family member feels the financial burden. Dialysis may continue for years with no improvement. In short, dialysis creates families in stress, families who need time, support, and encouragement. (Refer to chapter 3 for a description of the family experiencing the stress of chronic illness.)

Ileal Conduit Surgery

An *ileal conduit* is created surgically in order to make it possible for urine to drain from the kidneys into a collecting pouch, thereby bypassing the bladder completely. Ileal conduit surgery is discussed further in Table 30–1 (under Extrophy of the Bladder), and is illustrated in Figure 30–7.

Kidney Transplant

A successful kidney transplant is the preferred method of treatment for children with serious renal failure, who have been on hemodialysis for extended periods, perhaps years.

The actual surgical procedure for kidney transplant is simple. A donor kidney is placed in the iliac fossa of the receiving

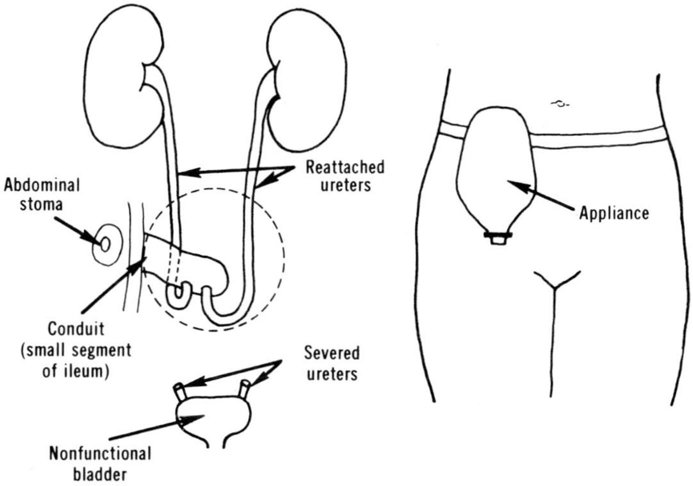

Figure 30–7. *An ileal conduit and collecting bag in place.*

child. The main renal artery and vein are connected to the iliac vessels, and the ureter is implanted into the child's bladder.

The major difficulty encountered in transplantation is the body's own immunologic response that initiates a natural rejection of the implanted kidney. Rejection may be *cell-mediated* when T-lymphocytes produced in response to antigens in the donor's kidney invade the transplanted kidney and destroy it; or it may be *humoral-mediated* when antibodies against antigens in the donated kidney are produced, and the child's plasma cells recognize them as foreign. Rejection can occur within hours or as long as several years after the transplant. The survival of the transplanted kidney depends on minimizing the action of the child's own natural defense mechanisms. To suppress the child's immune system, Imuran (azathioprine) and prednisone are given; both drugs, however, make the child very susceptible to infection.

Almost every child with a kidney transplant acquires some type of infection. Bacterial infections are common immediately after the transplant, while fungal and viral infections tend to occur later. (The immunosuppressive drugs administered to transplant patients makes these children highly susceptible to infection, and the nursing measures discussed in chapter 20, under immunosuppression, are applicable for the child with a kidney transplant.) If the infection is serious, immunosuppressive therapy may be halted long enough to allow the child's immune system to rebound. If the corticosteroids are stopped or decreased, however, the risk of losing the kidney increases. If the kidney is rejected, it is removed, and the child resumes dialysis.

Another common complication of a renal transplant is the reoccurrence of the primary renal disease in the transplanted kidney. If the child originally had chronic glomerulonephritis, the transplanted kidney may also succumb to glomerulonephritis. In the immediate posttransplant period, the child also may suffer from hypertension caused by high dosages of corticosteroids, fluid and salt retention, or the rejection process.

Following surgery, vital signs, weight, and intake and output are strictly monitored. Within one to three days, the child begins taking liquids and then, gradually, solid foods. His protein, fluid, and sodium are restricted according to physical and laboratory data, which indicate how well the transplanted kidney is working. When the transplanted kidney is felt to be functioning well, the child can begin eating a normal diet.

Until the sutures are removed, daily care includes cleansing the incision site with half-strength hydrogen peroxide, rinsing with sterile water, and application of an antiseptic solution. Routine catheter and intravenous care is needed until each is removed.

Because of the need for long-term use of corticosteroids, side effects such as obesity, hirsutism (excessive growth of hair), growth failure, acne, and Cushingnoid facies are inevitable. As a result, almost all children experience some emotional and social problems. Other children ridicule them, making them even more self-conscious and embarrassed about their appearance. Prepare the child for these side effects and likely changes in his appearance. Repeatedly explain why the treatment is necessary and the possible consequences of noncompliance.

Kidney transplants are most effective if

the kidney is taken from a close relative, such as a twin, sibling, or parent. Tissue studies can help to determine the best donor. The selection of a suitable donor places a great deal of stress on both child and the donor. Much ambivalence surrounds the matter of the source of the kidney, whether the kidney is from a relative or a cadaver. Potential donors feel guilty if they turn out to be unacceptable donors, and the selected donor faces the anxiety of surgery and the prospect of life with only one kidney.

The child, having suffered months and perhaps years of illness, is anxious and worried. Dialysis, medications, and dietary regimens alter his self-concept and change the family's roles and functions. The child considered for a kidney transplant has a chronic kidney illness that may be terminal. Families need to know the advantages and disadvantages of dialysis and renal transplant. They need to know the risk of surgery, the effects of immunosuppressive therapy, and the possibility of kidney rejection. These families need *facts*; and, equally important, they need *hope*. A successful transplant offers the hope of normal kidney function. With it, usually no dietary or fluid restrictions are necessary. No further dialysis is needed, and none of the problems of dialysis or chronic kidney failure exists.

SUMMARY

Healthy kidneys respond to antidiuretic hormone, maintain an adequate rate of glomerular filtration, and reabsorb the majority of the glomerular filtrate in the proximal tubules. The end product is a concentrated urine composed of dissolved solids and water. Fluid and electrolytes are kept within a healthy balance. If this balance is upset by congenital deformities, infection, acquired disorders or other forces, the child either retains too much fluid and electrolytes or loses excessive amounts of them. Edema, hypertension, and proteinuria are the most common problems of the child with a urinary disorder.

Simple procedures, such as the urinalysis and urine culture, as well as more elaborate x-ray studies, such as the intravenous pyelogram (IVP) and the voiding cystourethrogram (VCUG) are used to diagnose urinary disorders. Some children can be treated successfully with temporary changes in diet—especially restrictions of sodium, protein, and fluid—while other children require diuretics, corticosteroids, and hypotensives. For the child with a progressive kidney disease, dialysis or even a kidney transplant may be necessary.

Urinary disorders and accompanying electrolyte imbalances affect almost all the body's systems. The child is likely to be undernourished and anemic, and his growth and development will be delayed. Immunosuppressive therapy changes his body image, altering his self-concept. Children with a chronic urinary disorder and their families experience the problems of acute and chronic physical and emotional stress.

Bibliography

Altshules, A., Meyer, J., Butz, M. Even Children Can Learn to Do Clean Self-Catheterization. *American Journal of Nursing* 77:97, 1977.

Brundage, D. *Nursing Management of Renal Problems.* St. Louis, C.V. Mosby Co., 1976.

Cameron, E. and Kentzel, J. Chronic Renal Failure, in Kintzel, K.C. (ed). *Advanced Concepts in Clinical Nursing,* ed. 2. Philadelphia, J.B. Lippincott Co., 1976.

Carey, M. A Child's Struggle for Independence Following Kidney Transplantation. *American Journal Maternal-Child Nursing* 5:45, 1976.

Gordillo-Paniagua, G. and Velasquez-Jones, L. Acute Renal Failure. *Pediatric Clinics of North America* 23:829, 1976.

Greenill, A. and Gruskin, A. Laboratory Evaluation of Renal Function. *Pediatric Clinics of North America* 23:661, 1976.

Juliani, L. Assessing Renal Function. *Nursing '78* 8:34, 1978.

Juliani, L. and Reamer, B. Kidney Transplant: Your Role in After Care. *Nursing '77* 7:46, 1977.

Kemp, G. and Kemp, G. Diuretics, *American Journal of Nursing* 7:1007, 1978.

Lewy, P. and Hurley, J. Chronic Renal Insufficiency. *Pediatric Clinics of North America* 23:829, 1976.

Malekzadeh, M., Pennisi, A., Uittenbogaart, D.H. et al. Current Issues in Pediatric Renal Transplantation. *Pediatric Clinics of North America* 23:857, 1976.

Mendelco, B. Nursing Assessment of Children Undergoing Kidney Biopsy. *American Journal Maternal-Child Nursing* 5:151, 1976.

Margileth, A., Pedeira, F., Hirschman, G., et al. Urinary Tract Bacterial Infections. *Pediatric Clinics of North America* 23:721, 1976.

Mauer, S. and Lynch, R. Hemodialysis Techniques for Infants and Children. *Pediatric Clinics of North America* 23:843, 1976.

McIntosh, R., Lum, G., O'Brien, D. Kidney and Urinary Tract, in *Current Pediatric Diagnosis,* ed. 5. Los Altos, Ca., Lange Medical Publications, 1978.

Melick, M.E. Nursing Interventions for Patients Receiving Corticosteroid Therapy, in Kintzel, K.C. (ed). *Advanced Concepts in Clinical Nursing,* ed. 2. Philadelphia, J.B. Lippincott Co., 1978.

Neff, J. Autonomy Concerns of a Child on Dialysis. *American Journal of Maternal-Child Nursing* 4:101, 1975.

Rance, C., Arbus, G., Balfe, W. Management of the Nephrotic Syndrome in Children. *Pediatric Clinics of North America* 23:735, 1976.

Wheeler, D. Teaching Home-Dialysis for an Eight-Year-Old Boy. *American Journal of Nursing* 77:273, 1977.

———. Understanding Corticosteroids. *Nursing '77* 7:28, 1977.

Wilson, L.M. Normal Renal Function and Renal Pathophysiology, in Price, S.A. and Wilson, L. (eds). *Pathophysiology: Clinical Concepts of Disease Processes.* New York, McGraw-Hill, 1978.

CHAPTER **31**

The Child with Burns

BEHAVIORAL OBJECTIVES

After studying this chapter, you will be able to:

- Teach children and parents standard safety measures aimed at preventing burn injuries.
- Discuss the problems of body image, isolation, and immobility for the child with burns, identifying nursing measures for the management of these problems.
- Explain complications most often seen in children who are burned, including the nursing interventions to prevent and minimize these complications.
- Identify diagnostic studies used to monitor the status of the burned child, including nursing interventions for each study.
- Explain three techniques or methods for treating burn wounds, the advantages and disadvantages of each, and the nursing implications for each.
- Discuss three types of topical chemotherapy used for the treatment of burn wounds, explaining the appropriate use for each, and the nursing implications.
- Design a plan of care for a child hospitalized with burns of the chest and right arm.
- Explain the pathophysiology of symptomatic hypovolemia (shock) and circulatory overload in the burned child, stating the circumstances of occurrence, clinical manifestations, and nursing implications.

TERMS AND CONCEPTS

Thermal burns
Chemical burns
Electrical burns
Irradiation burns
Neurogenic shock
Hypovolemic shock
Septicemia
Eschar
Escharotomy
Remobilization
Adynamic ileus
Curling's (stress) ulcer
Contracture
Partial-thickness burns
Superficial-partial-thickness burns
Deep partial-thickness burns
Full-thickness burns
Plasma-to-interstitial fluid shift
Fluid resuscitation
Titration
Hydrotherapy
Debridement
Homograft

Heterograft
Autograft
Sheet grafting
Mesh graft

Burns are a major cause of morbidity and mortality in infants and children. From birth to four years of age, burns are the leading cause of accidental death in the home. They are second only to vehicular accidents as a cause of death from birth to 12 years of age. In the United States, an estimated 20,000 people die each year from burns, and another 100,000 are burned seriously enough to warrant hospitalization. Boys are burned five times more often than girls. Eighty percent of all burns occur within the home; three fourths of these could be prevented with the adequate use of standard safety measures.

Burns may be caused by thermal, chemical, electrical, and irradiation exposure. *Thermal burns* are moist (from steam or boiling water) or dry (from flames, hot grease, hot metal, or hot-water bottles). *Chemical burns* are caused by strong acids or strong alkalies. *Electrical burns* are seen both where the current enters and where it leaves the body. Systemic changes may accompany electrical injury and involve the cardiovascular, respiratory, and/or central nervous system. *Irradiation burns* may be caused by the sun (ultra-violet rays) and by x-rays and radium, whose effects develop slowly. (See chapter 20 for a discussion of irradiation burns.)

The majority of burns in children are the result of scalds in infants six months to two years of age. As a child begins to crawl and then toddle, his innate curiosity places him in dangerous situations. Pulling pots off the stove, attempting to taste mother's coffee, and climbing up on a chair to help stir the soup all cause scalds from hot liquids. A young child, left alone in the bathtub for only a minute, can turn on the faucet and scald himself with hot water.

Inconsistencies in the environment confuse the child and contribute to burns. If the child is permitted to touch a burner on the stove when it is cool, or walk barefoot across the nonfunctioning floor furnace in the summer, he is likely to attempt these feats when the burner or furnace is on.

Children may sneak away to a closet or storage room equipped with a gas water heater or a spare gas can to experiment with matches or cigarettes. The result may be severe burns sustained, if their clothing catches on fire, or death, if the gasoline ignites and explodes.

Running when clothing is on fire fans the flames and increases the severity of burns, especially on the anterior torso. Children's sleepwear should be flame *retardant,* which does *not* mean the garment will not burn; flame-retardant materials are more difficult to ignite and burn more slowly, and the flames die out when the source of heat is removed. Federal law requires that sleepwear, sizes 0 to 14, be flame retardant.

Parents should be instructed to follow safety rules and should teach the child simple measures to prevent burns, such as falling to the ground and rolling to extinguish clothing flames. Young children should never be left alone. When newspapers carry a story of a fire in a home in which young children died, the parents often are quoted as saying, "I only ran next door." Each family should plan what to do in case of fire. They should have an emergency escape route and practice using it during regularly scheduled fire drills. Home smoke alarms are available at a nominal cost; their use should be encouraged.

Burn care requires a team approach, with the physician, nurse, physical therapist, occupational therapist, dietitian, play therapist, and social worker all contributing their individual skills toward a common goal.

This chapter focuses on the child with burns. Problems common to all burned children, and frequently seen complications are discussed, along with the nursing implications to minimize or prevent these problems and complications. Diagnostic studies used to monitor the child's status are described. Common treatment regimens for the burned child are explained, along with their special nursing considerations. A number of tables are included for fast and easy reference to such topics as burn-wound characteristics, topical therapy, burn dressings, types of grafts, and so on.

COMMON PROBLEMS AND NURSING IMPLICATIONS

Tissue Damage

Damage to normal, healthy skin creates a break in the body's first line of defense. The severity of tissue damage in the burned child has a direct bearing on the child's reaction to, and survival of, burns. The tissue destruction itself causes pain, shock, and an altered body image.

Pain

The child who is burned may experience great pain. Even if his burns are full-thickness (painless), the surrounding areas are likely to have partial-thickness burns, which can be extremely painful. Exposed nerve endings are sensitive to cool, moving air. Covering the child with a dry, sterile sheet can help decrease the pain.

Children react differently to pain, but keep in mind that certain nonverbal and verbal expressions of pain are common (ch. 2). Explain *all* treatments beforehand and permit the child to cry if he is in pain. Screaming, shouting, and many other responses are all permitted when the child is in pain. Offer him your hand to squeeze—as hard as he can—in an attempt to distract him from the pain. Analgesics should be given (per order) about 20 minutes prior to painful treatments (e.g., dressing changes). Permitting the child to change a bandage on his doll or teddy bear, or even on himself, often helps him to cope with his own dressing change.

Shock

The burned child is in danger of *neurogenic shock* immediately after suffering a burn. Most children, even with severe burns, are alert. Fright, coupled with the severe pain caused by irritation of nerve endings, can produce a cerebral-autonomic reflex response and a precipitous fall in blood pressure. This stage of shock can be lethal, especially in children. (See chapter 25 for care of the child in shock.) Sedatives are given frequently in *very* small doses and always intravenously. Medications given IM will not be readily absorbed, and later may be released suddenly in large doses, when the circulatory blood volume is normal, and the peripheral vasoconstriction is lessened.

Hypovolemic shock may occur within 15 to 30 minutes after the burn injury. Massive amounts of fluid and sodium can shift from the circulation to the burn wound itself. Watch for a drop in blood pressure, increased pulse (as the heart tries to compensate for the decreased blood volume), restlessness, and disorientation. Extreme thirst may be present as a result of dehydration, and shock (symptomatic hypovolemia) may occur. Thirst is a cardinal clinical sign of hypovolemia. The hematocrit is elevated due to the hemoconcentration.

Body Image

The child's body image varies as he grows and develops. There is an abrupt interruption in this process when the child is burned, the degree and duration of the interruption is proportional to the resultant deformity in a previously well-developed body part. As long as the burn wounds are covered with dressings, the child, the family, and the burn team do not have to deal objectively with disfigurement. As the dressings are removed, they first see the extent of the wounds. Because the young child tends to use fantasy to help him cope, he may fantasize that his body is dreadfully mutilated, or is unchanged, despite visible evidence to the contrary. He may try to "wish back" his former appearance, and thus completely ignore reality. The nurse's role is to help the child recognize reality without destroying appropriate coping mechanisms. Assessment of his progress is important, and you must be aware of both verbal and nonverbal responses. Set aside a time to talk with him each day. Permit him to express his anger and fears, and to grieve for his lost body image. Specific questions that may be used to help assess his progress are: "Tell me about (child's name). How is he today? Fine? Tell me about being fine." Questions, such as "How do you look? How will you look to your brother/sister?" are considered hostile, attacking questions that too brutally orient the child to reality. Having him draw pictures and tell you about them may help him to express his feelings. Remember to note the child's nonverbal responses as well. Does he refuse to look at you? Does he hang his head when he answers? Touch him; let him know you are interested in him as an individual. Acknowledge his right to his own feelings and disappointment. *Actively* listen to him, and do not ignore or belittle his feelings. Rather, acknowledge these communications. Note his interaction with other children and adults. Does he refuse to brush his teeth and hair or to dress attractively? As he experiences anger and grief, the older school child and adolescent may deliberately expose himself in order to show off both his disfigurement and his intact parts. This is a test of how others will react to him, and also serves to confirm of deny his own feelings about his body.

How his family accepts his disfigurement is important to the child. Factors influencing their acceptance, as well as the child's, include which body parts are burned (Figure 31–1); the success of skin grafting; which body parts are deformed; the amount of contracture or loss of function; and the child's overall appearance. Parents, along with the child, have many questions regarding both the short- and long-term course of the illness. Will he be able to run and play? Can he write or paint? How will he take care of himself? Grief is evident as the child and his family hear answers to these questions. Depression is common, and anger is often directed toward the staff. (See chapter 3 for a discussion of grief). The parents' guilt seems to be a major factor in how they relate to their child, the staff, the diagnosis, and the treatment.

Dealing with the emotional and psychological reaction to injury is a challenge for the nursing staff. Each child and his family must be dealt with in an individualized manner. The child may draw pictures which are revealing and give the staff a clue as to his feelings.

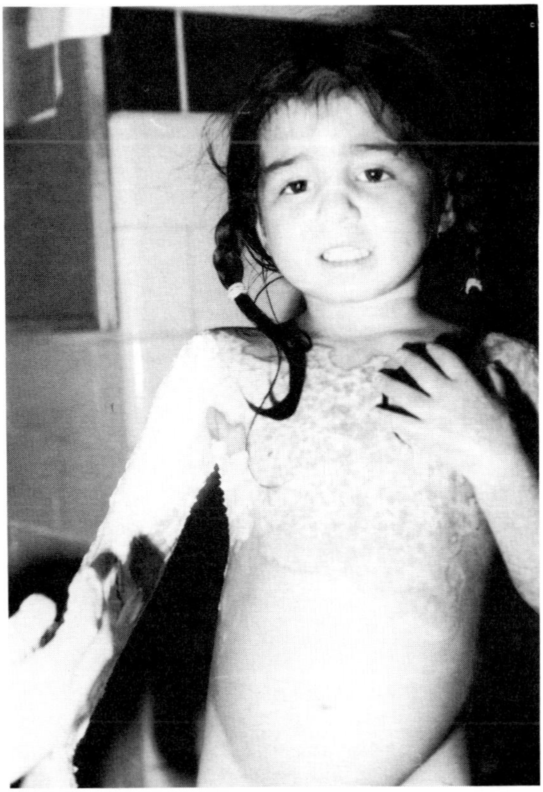

Figure 31–1. *Burns to anterior chest, arms, and hands.*

Terry, aged six, was severely burned on both legs. After several weeks, he was asked by his student nurse to draw a picture of a man. Terry drew a sad man without legs sitting in a chair. This drawing helped the student to understand Terry's distorted body image and his feelings of loss of control over his legs.

Play therapy may also be used to help the child express and work through his feelings. (See chapter 2.)

The older girl may need help with makeup, styling her hair, and the use of cologne and hair ribbons. Covermark is a commercial cosmetic that can be used to disguise overt scars. For boys, baseball caps, "mod" T-shirts, and after-shave lotion may help. (Sometimes girls simultaneously want baseball caps and gloves and a new bra.) Help reinforce the child's sexuality through the use of masculine or feminine clothing, for example, football jerseys for boys, and frilly pajamas for girls (if they like these things). It is even more important to let the child select the clothing that best expresses himself.

Suggest ways for the parents to help the child disguise his scars. Long-sleeve shirts, caps, wigs, and long pants are all appropriate. Help the parents *gradually* expose the child to others to avoid bombarding him with reactions. The parents should also notify the child's teacher so that classmates can be prepared for his appearance. This return to school may be fraught with danger. The child with burns must be treated normally. Teasing is unacceptable and should be dealth with promptly and sternly.

Nutrition

Nutrition may be a severe problem for the burned child, not only because of the physical changes, but because of the emotional stress (anorexia). Following injury, protein is lost from the burn wound, and protein catabolism begins as the body attempts to provide fuel for the abruptly elevated metabolic rate. Energy requirements are increased because the damaged skin no longer prevents the loss of extracellular fluid, and evaporative heat losses are markedly increased. If an infection develops, the loss of the skin's antibacterial function contributes to the energy drain.

The burned child needs about 180 calories and 3 grams of protein per kg per day. This is about twice the normal requirement, and is necessary for tissue repair and for increased metabolic demands. The goal of nutritional therapy is to establish a positive nitrogen balance, or anabolism, in order to promote healing. The resultant diet is high in calories, protein, carbohydrates, and vitamins. The rule-of-thumb is to encourage the child to eat what he wants, as much as he wants, when he wants, and then to encourage him to eat more. This rule is easy to recite but far more difficult to achieve.

The child is often NPO during the first few days of therapy. Intravenous fluids supply nutrients during this time, and occasionally total parenteral nutrition (TPN) may be employed. An oral diet should be started as soon as possible. The child maintained on intravenous feedings has had no responsibility for accepting his therapy. With the introduction of oral feedings, he is given the responsibility for accepting the nutrients to restore him to optimal health. The burned child is anorectic for a variety of reasons, ranging from the physical trauma and pain, to the emotional impact of his injury, to the inactivity of bedrest or isolation. The burned child's anorexia is a real challenge to his nurses. Forcing him to eat may cause vomiting and create hostility. Calorie-rich feedings may cause nausea, vomiting, abdominal distention, and diarrhea. An acceptable compromise for a time is to offer milk every two hours. It is isotonic, and does not cause diarrhea even in large quantities. Milk contains 20 calories per ounce, and enough electrolytes per liter to maintain normal serum electrolyte levels in most cases. However, much attention must be given to the child's total nutrition, and he should be encouraged to eat as soon as possible.

The volume of food required by the child often seems staggering to him and he begins to resent and dislike the persons who force him to eat. In addition to the nursing responsibilities for anorexia discussed in chapter 18, the following ideas may aid you in maintaining the nutritional status of the child with burns. Have an afternoon "tea party" for the child and his teddy bear or doll. He can serve punch (kool-aid or coke) to his "guests" in medicine cups, then drink all the punch himself. He may pretend he is at a baseball game (or actually "be there" via TV) and have a hotdog and coke. Try pouring *more* fluids or medicine than the child needs and tell him he "only has to drink down to here." This "bargaining" may help him to maintain some control and still fosters adequate intake. However, in some cases, the extra amount of fluid may overwhelm the child.

These and any other ideas you may employ are helpful in providing adequate nourishment for the burned child. Failure to ingest adequate nourishment invariably leads to gavage feedings. Since this diet is high caloric and often sweet, the child may become obese as his convalescence continues. He may acquire eating habits that are much too selective and expensive for his family to satisfy. For these reasons, the child should return to his family's eating habits as soon as possible, assuming they are nutritionally sound. Permitting the family to participate in the child's nutrition during hospitalization may make adaption to his family's nutrition easier after discharge.

Evaluation of the child's nutritional status requires accurate monitoring and recording of his daily weight, intake, output, and calorie count.

Isolation

The child with burns is often placed on reverse isolation, limiting his contact with his family, peers, and therapists. While isolation is said to cut down on infection, it also cuts down on the child's interest in living. The child on isolation misses the sensation of touch, which is available only through a gloved hand. The only faces he sees are perched above a wrinkled gown and hidden behind a mask. The eyes are the only human feature about these creatures with muffled voices who poke him, turn him, hurt him, and keep him separated from his parents. He may have a cradle over the bed, with the siderails up and no pillow; or, worse yet, he may be strapped to a CircOlectric bed or Stryker/Foster frame. In either case, he cannot see who is coming into his room until they are standing over his bed. The bed itself is strange, frightening, and uncomfortable. Your assessment will tell you if he sleeps alone at home or with several siblings in the same room and/or bed (ch. 2). His hospital sleeping conditions are different from those at home, and the child will not be able to sleep well.

The isolation room may be strange and frightening with a lack of clocks and calendars, and the usual bland color of the walls and curtains. The air conditioner may hum and for a little while, provides an auditory stimulus, which may later contribute to the child's disorientation. The familiar sounds of childhood—children laughing and playing, dogs barking—are missing. Also absent are the stimuli that orient one to time and place, such as the rumble of the school bus, the ringing doorbell, the mailman's daily delivery, the town clock striking the hour, and the slam of Daddy's car door.

The child's sleep patterns are disturbed because he no longer goes to bed and arises at a set time. He is awakened by the nurse for a check of vital signs, by the lab technician for blood work, and by the cleaning lady who has to mop his room. All these factors totally destroy the young child's immature sense of time. Orient him to time and place every time you enter the room. "Billy, I am Ms. Barnes. I told you I would be back after lunch. Lunchtime is over. It is now time for a nap," or "Today is Saturday, Billy, cartoon day on TV. After your breakfast, we'll turn on the TV so you can watch your favorite shows."

The child may feel that isolation is punishment for real or imagined wrongdoing (see Ch. 2). If he was burned while playing with forbidden matches, his guilt is accentuated. The small child does not understand the reasons for his isolation and therapy. The toddler or preschool child often equates the isolation with moral or psychological issues. In simple terms, explain his treatment and/or isolation to him, thus helping to alleviate his guilt by permitting him to verbalize and deal with it in a realistic way.

The child on isolation may be totally dependent on others to meet his basic needs. He may not even be able to scratch his own nose. His head may face the wall, or he may alternate two hours of looking at the ceiling with two hours of staring at the floor from his CircOlectric bed. He may not be able to see his parents when they visit unless they lay on the floor under him. He feels completely helpless, and should be permitted to cry or to express his frustration. The child in this situation may regress in his behavior. Whining, screaming, thumbsucking, and refusal to cooperate with treatment are all displayed. And such behavior may well be appropriate and necessary.

Isolation is detrimental to children at every age and stage of development. The toddler, learning to use his large muscles, may miss learning to ride his tricycle in warm weather. The preschool child may miss group play at the park; the schoolage child may miss the spring camping trip with his scout troop; and the adolescent, the annual spring dance.

Radio, TV, and cassette recordings are all useful in providing the child with the stimulation of music, voices, and communication with family and peers. For the child on long-term therapy, a bulletin board may be necessary to help keep him abreast of school activities and to orient him to seasons and time. Recall that the child needs to assume some control over his environment in order to overcome his feelings of helplessness. Permit him to participate in the planning and implementation of his care. Give him choices, when possible. Let him plan his own menu from foods he can and should eat; let him choose the chaser to follow his medications, such as coke, juice, or water. Choosing whether or not to take his medicine is not permitted (with the exception of pain medication), but, if possible, allow him to choose the preparation (liquid, tablet, or IM) of his medication. Permit him to choose his bath time. If he bathes at night at home, permit this in the hospital. Encourage visitors to sit (or lie) so that he can see them, maintain eye-to-eye contact with them, and read their nonverbal communication. Assign the same group of personnel to him to maintain continuity of care. Encourage him to talk and express his feelings. Permit him to cry and to be depressed at times. Statements such as "It really must be tough," are often useful as cues to the child that you appreciate what he is going through and are willing to listen to him, if he wants to talk.

Immobility

The child who is immobile because of burns or grafts is a good candidate for developing pressure sores. The turning and positioning done to prevent contractures also aids in preventing these pressure sores. Common sites for decubitus formation in the child are the back of the head, elbows, sacrum, heels, and iliac crests. Destroyed tissues, such as burn wounds, are excellent sites for pressure sores and should be given careful attention. Healing burn wounds are often itchy; the child must be reminded not to scratch or pick at the wounds. Sometimes bulky gloves are useful. Restraints may be necessary as a last resort. If restraints are applied, they should be removed when someone is with the child.

Routine care for decubitus ulcers should not be used on the burned child without the consent of a physician. Ointments can interfere with the burn therapy, and exposing the area to heat and light can aggravate the burn. Often, the treatment of choice is to keep the area clean and exposed to air. Remember to avoid putting pressure on the involved site.

Remove jewelry, such as bracelets, which may cause constrictions and pressure sores. If the child is particularly fond of the jewelry, pin it to his pillow or attach it to the siderails.

Mobility has a special significance during every stage of childhood, and curtailment of activity produces a high level of frustration. The mobile child can work off his frustrations through active body movement, but the immobilized child cannot reduce his anxiety level through action. His self-expression, a primary function of movement, is limited, and he is thus unable to let off steam. His frustration mounts and a vicious cycle ensues. In addition, the immobilized child is dependent on others for his basic needs, and is thus very vulnerable. Refer to Chapter 2 for nursing intervention with the immobilized child.

Comfort

The child who has been burned is anxious and frightened. He has been rushed to the hospital, separated from his family (assuming they have survived the burn accident), and subjected to painful and frightening treatments and procedures. He needs your support and concern. Show him that you are interested in him. Foster personal communication by telling him your name and calling him by his name. Orient him to his surroundings, and explain the various steps in his treatment and the reasons for them. Verify that he understands the procedures before you begin preparing him for them. Let him know what you will do and what is expected of him (see Ch. 2). Routine care measures are frightening, as are the sensations he will feel. Explain the cold, the pain, and the thirst to help him understand the sensations he will experience.

Fatigue often is present during the immediate postburn period. Plan for periods of uninterrupted rest, even though this is very difficult to do, especially after meals and during the night. Visitors may be limited to the immediate family, and they should be encouraged not to tire the child.

Provide comfort measures at regular intervals and p.r.n. Keep the sheets clean, dry, and wrinkle-free. A daily bath, including a shampoo, is essential for comfort. Mouth care should be offered before meals. Perineal care should be given twice a day and after each elimination.

Tell the child when you are leaving, when you will return, and the name of the nurse relieving you. Introduce her to the child. This continuity of care will help provide security for the otherwise frightened and very insecure burned child.

COMPLICATIONS OF BURNS AND NURSING IMPLICATIONS

Infection

Infection, beginning in the burn wound itself, is the most devastating complication of burns in children. It is a threat that persists until the wound is completely healed. An active bacterial infection can cause graft rejection, or convert a partial-thickness wound to full-thickness. It also results in delayed healing, scars, contractures, prolonged hospitalization, septicemia, and death.

The primary source of infection is the child's own intestinal tract. In addition, he may be autocontaminated by bacteria on his unburned skin, in hair follicles, and in his respiratory tract. The child's environment is also a source of infection. His room, the linen and equipment used in his care, and his visitors and nurses all harbor potentially dangerous bacteria.

An aseptic technique, using gowns, gloves, and masks, is imperative when giving wound care, inserting IVs or urinary catheters, injecting medications both IV and IM, clearing the airway, and instilling eye drops.

Septicemia accounts for half of the deaths of burned children who survive the first few days postburn. Infection begins slowly in the burn wound and may not evidence itself for four or five days. An early diagnosis and treatment of septicemia is imperative. If septic shock develops, the mortality rate is close to 80 percent. The nurse must observe carefully for signs of septicemia. Be alert to any sudden changes in behavior. The cooperative and pleasant child may abruptly become lethargic, sullen, and withdrawn. Note hyperventilation, with both increased rate and depth of respiration. Arterial blood gases show a decreased pCO_2 an increased pH, and a normal or decreased pO_2. Jaundice may occur. A sudden increase of 25 percent or more in the white blood cell count, or a decrease below 5,000 may indicate sepsis. Because of the high incidence of stress ulcers in burned children with septicemia, you must watch for the presence of blood in the vomitus and stools.

Early systemic antibacterial treatment with carbenicillin/clindamycin, Keflin/Kantrex, or penicillin/Chloromycetin is routinely used prophylactically against wound invasion by gut organisms. Unless respiratory injury is suspected, systemic antibiotics are seldom used for more than three days. Effects of antibiotic treatment are monitored by frequent blood and wound cultures. Other antibiotics are used as necessary, depending on the organisms involved. Sensitivity to antibiotics is determined prior to administration.

Respiratory Complications

Respiratory involvement occurs both as a result of direct thermal injury, such as burns to the face and neck, and from inhalation of smoke, which often occurs when the burn is sustained in an enclosed space, such as a car or small room. Always ask where the burn occurred, and how long the child was confined in the enclosed space. Look for singed nasal hair and reddened, blackened, or edematous nasal and oral membranes. Inflammation of the upper airway can obstruct ventilation within 6 to 36 hours. Watch for signs of inhalation injury, such as hoarseness, croupy respirations, and soot or blood-stained sputum. Expiratory wheezing may be heard on auscultation. Usually, endotracheal intubation is done early for any of these clinical signs. Diminish the stress of breathing by elevating the head of the bed, and providing humidified oxygen via a T tube (a plastic adapter to deliver high humidity to patients with tracheal intubation) or croup tent. Suction the airway and nasopharynx as needed, using a strict aseptic technique. Have the child cough and breath deeply every 20 minutes, and turn him every hour.

Mechanical, volume ventilation with CPAP (continuous positive airway pressure) and PEEP (positive end expiratory pressure) may be used to lessen the work of breathing and provide adequate ventilation. A tracheostomy is a very high-risk procedure and is performed *only* if endotracheal intubation is not possible.

Steroids (30 mg per kg) may be administered early postburn to prevent or relieve bronchospasm and decrease the inflammatory response. Prolonged use of steroids is avoided with the burned child because of the constant threat of infection.

Antibiotics are given to combat infection in the respiratory tract. Sputum cultures are obtained to monitor bacterial contamination, and blood gases are checked frequently to assess treatment. An arterial cannula is useful in avoiding multiple "sticks" for blood.

The bronchioles and alveoli are involved when the burn occurred in an enclosed space, or when superheated gas or smoke was inhaled. Without the above measures, the result is early pulmonary interstitial edema, which necessitates prolonged ventilatory support. This often causes pneumonia and sometimes culminates in death.

The *eschar* is the coagulated protein of the skin produced after a thermal, chemical, electrical, or irradiation injury. The child with a circumferential burn of the neck or thorax may experience respiratory difficulty, if the eschar creates a tourniquet effect. The arms, fingers, and legs are also subject to circumferential burns. The edema creates pressure, which impairs circulation. The underlying tissue becomes anoxic, and gangrene follows. The physician will perform an *escharotomy* (an incision of the eschar) to relieve the constriction.

Pulmonary edema and congestive heart failure caused by fluid overload during the remobilization phase may occur (see below). Digitalis, diuretics, and oxygen are given, if these pulmonary complications develop.

Bronchopneumonia is also seen in children with burns and is evidenced by fever, leukocytosis, and malaise without overt signs of sepsis. (See ch. 23 for care of the child with pneumonia.)

Acute Renal Failure

Acute renal failure is manifested by a urine volume of less than 0.5 ml/kg/hr. In the first few days after burns are sustained, however, oliguria is more commonly the result of inadequate fluid replacement than of acute renal failure. Hemoglobinuria and/or myoglobinuria, evidenced by black or "port wine"-colored urine, occurs when hemoglobin is released by damaged RBCs and/or muscle and is usually seen with deep wounds and/or electrical injury. Renal failure may occur when kidney tubules are plugged by the free pigment. The kidneys are flushed immediately with IV mannitol, the IV rate is speeded up, and the urine is alkalinized with sodium bicarbonate. Recovery is possible with early detection.

Circulatory Overload

Remobilization of edema fluid, from interstitial spaces to the plasma, begins two to five days after the burn, and lasts from 24 to 72 hours. This sudden increase in blood volume produces large amounts of urine, unless renal damage has occured. Be alert for increasing urine volume, and notify the physician when it occurs.

The volume of edema fluid may equal the total, normal plasma volume. This tremendous increase in blood volume places a strain on the heart that may lead to fluid backup into the lungs, resulting in pulmonary edema and congestive heart failure. Note signs of respiratory distress, moist rales, frothy sputum, and cyanosis.

Continuing IV fluids at this stage can be disastrous because they contribute to the circulatory overload. The amount of fluids is reduced drastically, but is maintained rather than discontinued in case IV medication is needed. A high-protein, high-caloric diet, if tolerated, can supply adequate nutrition during this phase. After diuresis is completed, and the diet well tolerated, IV fluids are discontinued.

Gastrointestinal Complications

Gastroduodenal ulceration and *adynamic ileus* (a lack of peristalsis leading to intestinal obstruction), are physiological responses to fluid overload or stress. They frequently are seen in the burned child and are often associated with septicemia. Immediately after the injury, acute gastric dilatation may occur. Gastric acid secretion, anxiety, and inadequate nutrition may contribute to the formation of stress ulcers of the stomach and duodenum (*Curling's ulcer*).

The nurse should be alert to clinical manifestations of gastrointestinal disturbances. Note any abdominal distention. Check vomitus, nasogastric drainage, and stools for the presence of blood. "Coffee-ground" vomitus and gastric aspiration (via the nasogastric tube), accompanied by large amounts of air, may be caused by hemorrhagic gastritis, often a precursor of Curling's ulcer.

Contractures

Contractures are a frequent complication of burns, usually resulting from the development of scar tissue. It is impossible to prevent all contractures, but it is possible to limit contractures by meticulous nursing care, especially in relation to positioning. The tendency of the child to place his body in the least painful position contributes to the development of contractures, and to consequent surgery.

Methods used to prevent contractures consist of the frequent changing of the child's position, while maintaining good body alignment and the use of a footboard, pillows, sandbags, and splints, as necessary. Static splints are used to keep the body part stationary in a normal position. Dynamic splinting is especially useful if the child cannot exercise or otherwise control the part involved. It is a form of traction applied with rubber bands (to the fingers, e.g.). This type of splinting permits movement of the body part involved, yet helps prevent contractures (see Color Plate 5). Early splinting in the position of function is vital, especially for the hands. Static splints are removed for whirlpool treatments, dressing changes, and exercise, and then reapplied. Remember to check the splinted areas for adequate circulation and decubitus-like pressure points.

Position changes include moving the child from his back to his side to his abdomen, and moving the head of the bed up and down. If the child has burns of the anterior neck, do not use a pillow. If he has a fresh tracheostomy, respiratory difficulties, or edema of the face and neck, do not place him on his abdomen. (See Table 31–1 for positions that prevent deformity).

Passive and active exercise is necessary for body parts not immobilized by skin grafting. Getting the child to exercise his burned extremities can be accomplished with the use of games and toys that require his participation. Songs and nursery rhymes that require hand and arm movements, such as "Deep and Wide," "Inky Dinky Spider," and "I'm a Little Teapot," are fun for both the child and the staff. The cardinal rule is that everybody claps after each song, which is often a painful but necessary process for the burned child. Sculpting exercises strengthen burned fingers. Make the child's own private supply of sculpting material (play dough) daily by mixing three cups flour, 3/4 cup salt, one cup water with food coloring of his choice, and one tablespoon of oil. Discard it daily, since it can easily become contaminated. Make a boat with a plastic bowl or cup, equip it with a tongue blade mast and paper sail, and let him sail it during his bath. Put a washable doll in the tub with him, and let him bathe and shampoo it. Drying and dressing the doll also exercises burned hands and arms. Permit the child to feed himself and to brush his hair and teeth. Place wanted articles within his reach, but

Table 31–1. **Positions That Prevent Deformity**

Area Burned	*Resulting Deformity*	*Position of Prevention*
Neck:		
Anterior aspect or circumferential	Flexion contracture of neck	No pillow under head.
Posterior aspect only	Extensor contracture of neck	Prone–pillow under upper chest to flex cervical spine. Supine–small pillow under neck.
Axilla:		
Anterior	Adduction and internal rotation	Shoulder joint in abduction (100° to 130°) and external rotation.
Posterior	Adduction and external rotation	Shoulder in forward flexion and 100° to 130° abduction.
Pectoral region	Shoulder protraction	No pillow. Shoulders abducted and externally rotated.
Chest or abdomen	Kyphosis	As above and hips neutral (*not* flexed).
Lateral trunk	Scoliosis	Supine, affected arm abducted.
Elbow:		
Anterior surface or circumferential	Flexion and pronation	Arm extended and supinated.
Wrist:		
Total or volar surface	Flexion	Splint in 15° extension.
Dorsal surface	Extension	Splint in 15° flexion.
Hip:		
(Includes inguinal and perineal burns)	Internal rotation, flexion and adduction, possible joint subluxation if contracture severe.	Neutral rotation and abduction, and maintain extension by prone position or pillow under buttocks.
Knee:		
Popliteal surface or cirumferential	Flexion	Maintain extension, using posterior splints, or suspend heels with plastic heel protecting boots. *No pillows* under knees while supine, or under ankles while prone.
Ankle	Plantar flexion if foot muscles are weak or their tendons are divided.	90° dorsiflexion with splint, if possible, rather than footboard.

Adapted from Jones, C.A. and Fellar, I. Burns: Avoiding and Coping With Complications Before and After Grafting. *Nursing 77*, 7:72, 1977. Reprinted with permission from the November issue of *Nursing '77*. Copyright 1977, Intermed Communications, Inc.

do not hand them to the child — encourage him to reach for them. All of these activities will help to prevent deforming contractures, give him some control over his environment, contribute to his well-being, and hopefully shorten the period of rehabilitation.

Burn Encephalopathy

Burn encephalopathy, or central nervous system dysfunction, is a frequent complication of burns in the child. It is seen with both large and small burns and is attributed to hypoxia, cerebral edema, and hypovolemia, among other factors. The clinical manifestations are personality changes, hallucinations, delirium, seizures, and coma. Emotional stress is increased; when the child realizes he is confused, his anxiety is heightened. Explain these changes both to the child and to his family, assuring them that these symptoms are anticipated and are only temporary. Full neurological recovery is the rule, even after prolonged and serious manifestations.

DIAGNOSTIC STUDIES FOR THE CHILD WITH BURNS AND NURSING IMPLICATIONS

Burns are obvious wounds and need no laboratory studies to confirm or deny their existence. However, some studies are imperative for monitoring the status of the child who is burned.

Vital signs are taken on admission. Both blood pressure and pulse are monitored frequently. Temperatures over 38.3° C (101° F) or under 36.1°C (97°F) are reported.

Weight and height are also recorded on admission; thereafter, weight is monitored daily. Include the previous weight when you record the present weight, for the physician's quick reference.

After the Foley catheter is inserted, the first urine is measured for specific gravity, sugar, acetone, and albumin; these measurements are used as a baseline for future renal function. Monitor the volume and specific gravity hourly. Test the urine with Hematest tabs or Combistix for the presence of hemoglobin, and record all of this information on the chart.

Hemoglobin and hematocrit are checked every 4 to 6 hours during the first 48 hours, and daily thereafter to provide information about the child's fluid status. Recall that these values are elevated during hemoconcentration and will fall as blood volume is restored by parenteral fluids, and as autolysis of red blood cells occurs.

Typing and cross-matching of the blood is also done in the event the child needs a transfusion. Serum electrolyte levels and blood gases are monitored every 4 to 6 hours during the first 48 hours, and daily thereafter to aid in determining replacement needs and to help assess the child's respiratory status. Remember that these studies deplete blood volume and may lead to anemia.

Blood and wound cultures are done routinely in an effort to diagnose and treat infection. Laboratory technicians or nurses may obtain blood samples. Wound cultures are obtained by the physician or the nurse.

Stool and gastric aspirate are examined for the presence of blood (if they contain blood, they are called "coffee-ground"). To distinguish this from bile, place a drop on a Hematest tab. Gastric and duodenal ulcers manifest themselves through gastrointestinal hemorrhage, and any evidence of blood should be reported.

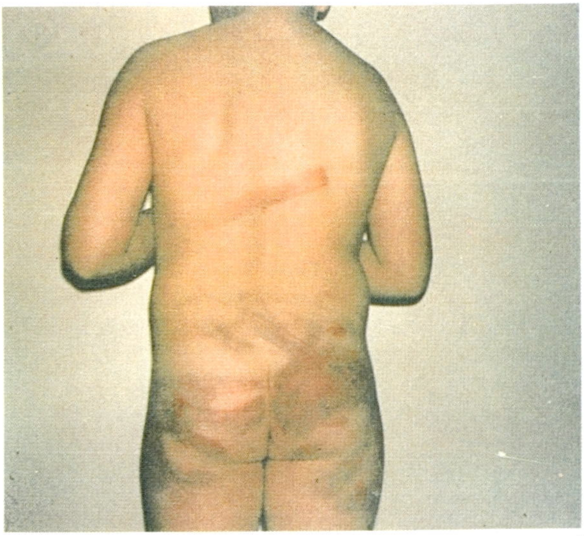

1

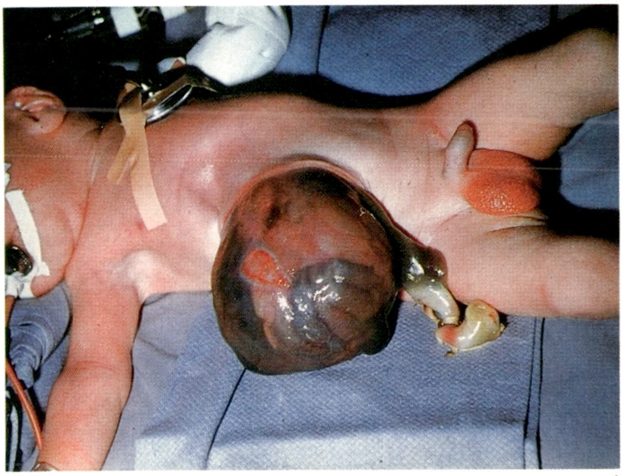

4

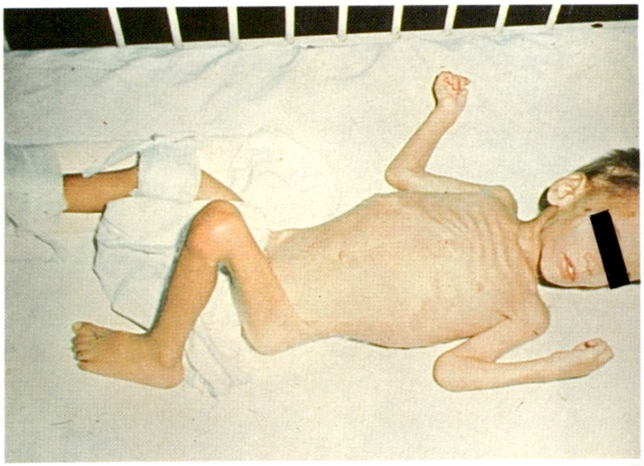

2

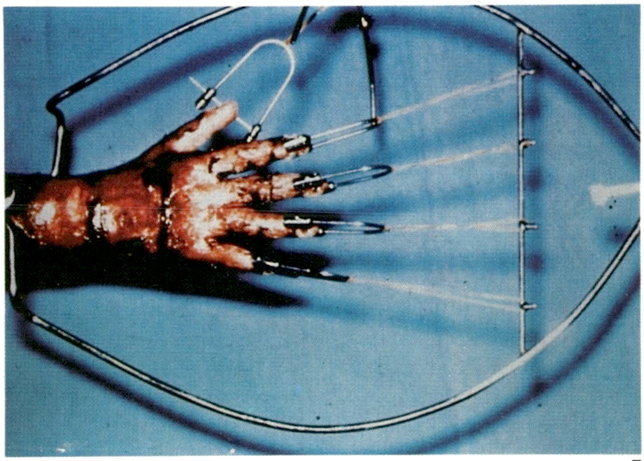

5

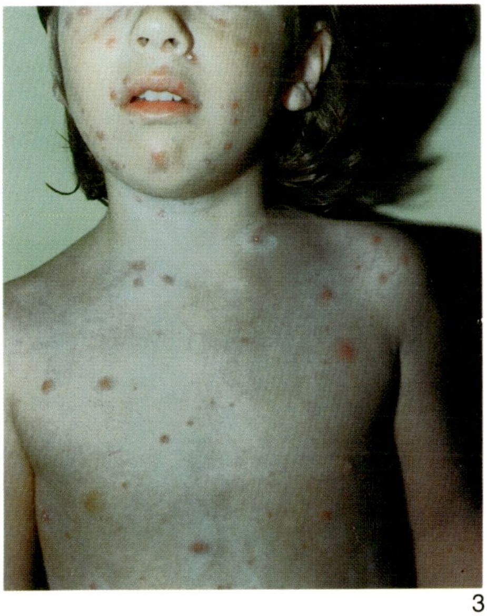

3

Plate 1. *A nine-year-old boy with strap marks left from a beating by his father.*

Plate 2. *Severe malnutrition and skin abrasions in a three-year-old child. Weight on admission was 17 pounds; ten days later, after proper nutrition and loving care, the child weighed 27 pounds.*

Plate 3. *Varicella, note lesions in various stages.*

Plate 4. *Omphalocele.*

Plate 5. *Dynamic splinting of the fingers.*

Plates 1 and 2. *Courtesy of ten Bensel, R.W. "The Battered Child Syndrome."* Famous Teachings in Modern Medicine. *New York, Medcom, Inc., 1971.*

Plate 4. *Courtesy of Earle L. Wrenn, Jr., M.D., Pediatric and Cardiovascular Surgery, Le Bonheur Children's Hospital, Memphis, Tenn.*

Plate 5. *Courtesy of Shriners Burns Institute, Galveston, Texas.*

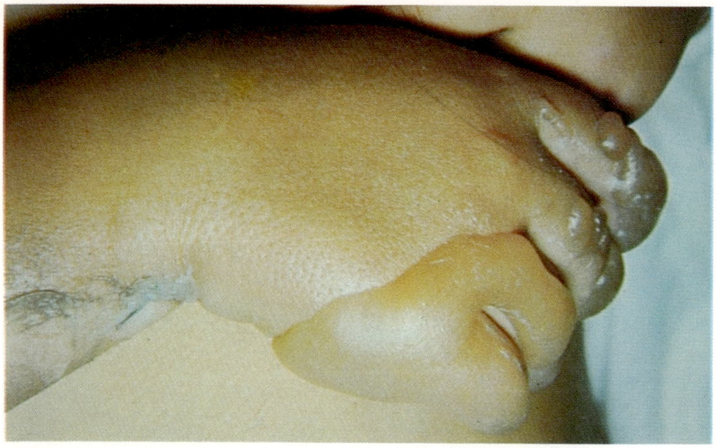

6

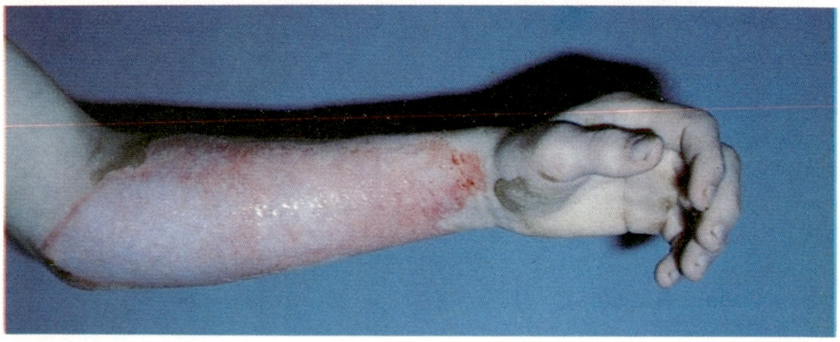

7

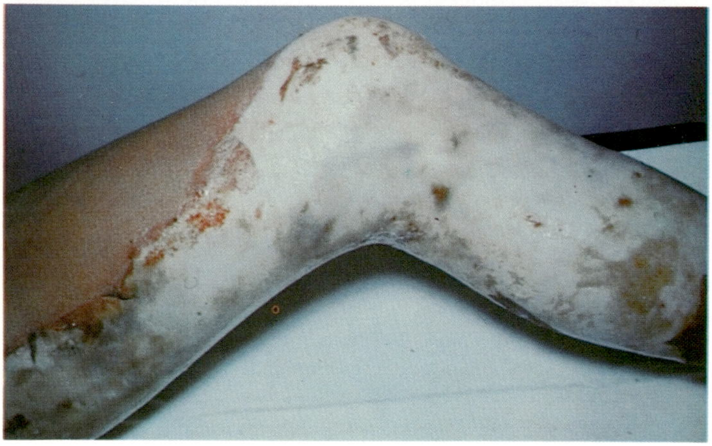

8

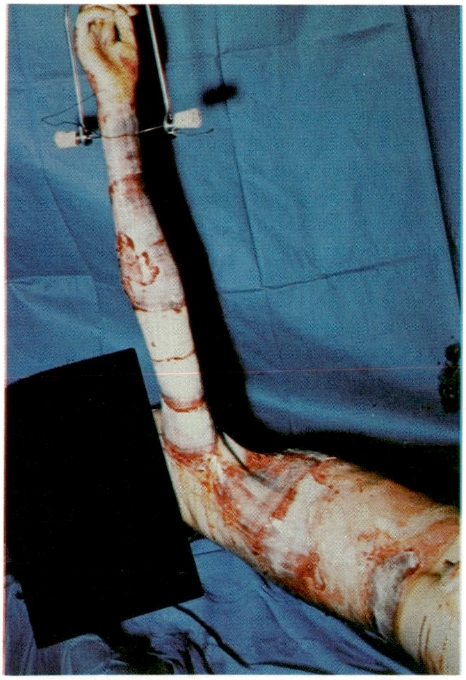

9

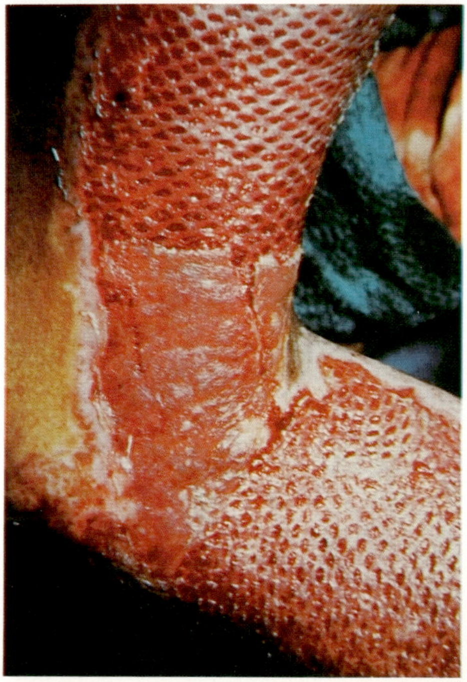

10

Plate 6. *Superficial partial-thickness burn of the hand.*

Plate 7. *Deep partial-thickness burn of the arm.*

Plate 8. *Full-thickness burn of the leg.*

Plate 9. *Sheet graft.*

Plate 10. *Mesh graft.*

Plates 6 to 10. *Courtesy of Shriners Burns Institute, Galveston, Texas.*

COMMON TREATMENTS AND NURSING IMPLICATIONS FOR THE CHILD WITH BURNS

First Aid

Emergency first-aid measures for the child with burns may save his life or diminish the injury. First, remove the child from the source of the burn and take off his clothes. If scalding water is the cause of the burn, ice water or towels soaked in ice water will help to decrease the pain and the amount of local edema for small burns. Do not put ice on the burn wound because it may inflict further thermal damage. If the clothes are on fire, throw the child to the ground and roll him to extinguish the flames. If necessary, grab a blanket or rug to smother the fire. Irrigate chemical burns with large amounts of water, or have the child stand in a shower or running bath. Irrigate the eyes with cool, clean water. Remove constricting jewelry and clothing. Wrap the child in a clean dry cloth, such as a sheet, and have him lie down to await transport to the hospital. *Give no oral fluids*, even if the child complains of thirst.

Emergency care

On admission to the hospital, the child's clothes are removed, his height, weight and vital signs are recorded, and he is placed between sterile sheets while his treatment is being explained to him. Therapy is begun simultaneously by the burn team. Intravenous therapy is begun, respiratory status is evaluated, a Foley catheter is inserted, and blood specimens are withdrawn for hematocrit, type, and cross-matching, serum electrolytes, and blood gas analysis. The child needs someone to comfort and care for *him*, not just his body, during this stressful and frightening time.

Airway

When a child is burned, the primary concern is pulmonary injury. The first objective of the burn team during the emergency period immediately postburn is to establish a patent airway. Signs of smoke inhalation and direct thermal injury to the face and neck point to pulmonary involvement. The burn team is alert to these signs and institutes measures to assure unobstructed breathing (see Respiratory Complications, pg. 752).

Assessment

An estimate of the depth and extent of the burn wounds is made after an initial wound cleansing. Burn wounds are classified as either partial-thickness or full-thickness, depending on their depth (see Table 31–2 and Figure 31–2). *Partial-thickness* wounds correspond to the old classifications of first- and second-degree burns. They may be either superficial or deep. *Superficial partial-thickness burns* may involve the epidermis and/or the intradermis. If such a burn involves the epidermis—as in a sunburn—it will be characterized by erythema and pain. It will heal in two to three days and may peel. If the burn is intradermal, it is characterized by erythema, pain, blister formation, and edema (Color Plate 6). Healing is often spontaneous in seven to fourteen days. *Deep partial-thickness burns* extend into the dermis (Color Plate 7). The skin appendages remain intact. Healing may occur without grafting, unless these wounds convert to full-thickness as a result of edema and/or infection. These burns are edematous and extremely painful. Healing occurs in 3 to 4 weeks from the epidermis at the edge of the wound and from skin appendages within the wound. Scarring may be severe.

Table 31–2. **Evaluation of Burn Depth**

Classification	*Skin Involvement*	*Cause*
Superficial Partial-thickness (first-degree)	Epidermis	Sunburn Low-intensity flash
Superficial or Deep Partial-thickness (second-degree)	Dermis	Scalds Flash flame Fire
Full-thickness (third-degree)	Subcutaneous tissue	Fire Prolonged exposure to hot liquids

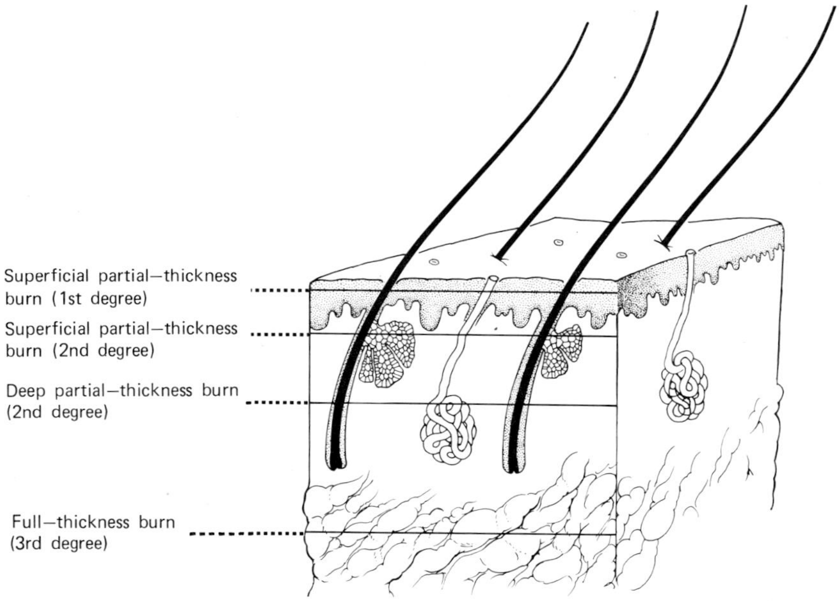

Figure 31–2. *Burn depth.*

Symptoms	Appearance	Course
Tingling Hyperesthesia Painful Soothed by cooling	Reddened; blanches with pressure Minimal or no edema	Complete recovery within a week Peeling
Painful Hyperesthesia Sensitive to moving air	Blistered, weeping Edema	Recovery in 2 to 3 weeks Some scarring and depigmentation Infection may convert to third degree
Painless Symptoms of shock Hematuria and hemolysis of blood likely	Dry; pale white, translucent or charred Mahogany; thrombosed veins visible Broken skin with fat exposed Edema	Eschar sloughs Grafting necessary Scarring and loss of contour and function

Full-thickness (third-degree) burns (Color Plate 8) involve the dermis, skin appendages, and subcutaneous tissue. There is often marked skin rigidity as a result of edema beneath the heat-tanned skin. The surface is translucent, and coagulated blood vessels are visible. These wounds are painless to the touch. Full-thickness burns will not heal without skin grafting.

The extent of total body surface area (TBSA) involved is estimated in children with the use of the chart shown in Figure 31–3. This chart allows for the change of body surface area of various body parts as the child grows.

Any child with a total area burned equal to or greater than 10 percent of his TBSA, or with third-degree burns of greater than 5 percent of the TBSA should be hospitalized. Burns of less than 10 percent TBSA but involving the face, hands, feet, or perineum also warrant hospitalization, as do burns of greater than 5 percent in the child under two years of age (Figure 31–4).

The prognosis depends on the depth and extent of the burns, as well as the age and general condition of the child. The child over the age of five has a better chance of survival than does the younger child (Figure 31–5).

The initial examination of the child also includes assessment of systemic consequences of the burn and any other injuries or disease. A thorough history is essential, and includes not only how and where (in an open space or enclosed space; recall that burns sustained in an enclosed space contribute to respiratory involvement) the child was burned, but also his general state of health, including his weight, prior to the burn.

Hypovolemia leading to shock is an immediate threat to life following a thermal injury. Therefore, immediate care must in-

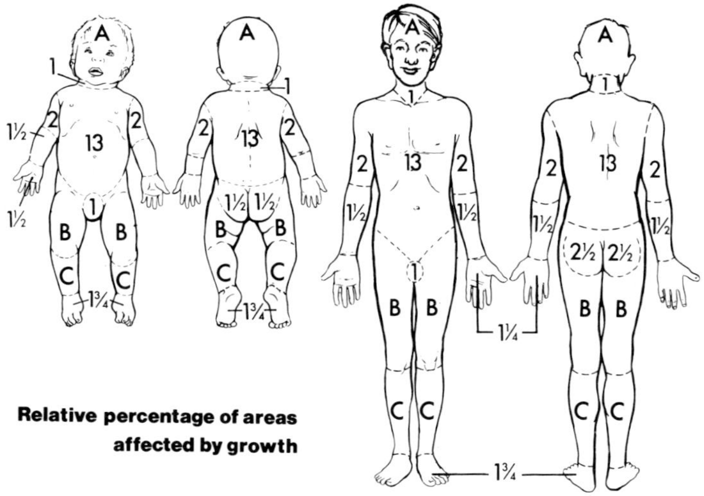

	Age in years					
	0	1	5	10	15	adult
A—½ of head	9½	8½	6½	5½	4½	3½
B—½ of one thigh	2¾	3¼	4	4¼	4½	4¾
C—½ of one leg	2½	2½	2¾	3	3¼	3½

Total per cent burned ____ 2°+ ____ 3°= ____

Figure 31–3. *Estimation of total body surface area burned (TBSA), according to age.*

vólve assessment of the cardiovascular system. Blood pressure and pulse are monitored frequently during the first few hours of treatment.

Within an hour postburn, damaged and dilated capillaries at the burn site permit intravascular fluid, electrolytes, and protein to move from the circulatory system into the tissues. This *plasma-to-interstitial fluid shift* results in edema at the burn site and is in direct proportion to the depth and extent of the burn wound itself. Recall that the amount of this edema fluid may equal the total normal plasma volume. Proportionately more water is lost than protein. The large size of protein molecules prevents them from shifting as rapidly as does the fluid. This concentrated plasma protein causes an increase in oncotic pressure, which draws fluid from undamaged tissues in the body and results in a generalized dehydration. In addition, evaporation occurs from the burned surface. These physiological processes cause a decrease in circulating blood volume, which leads to less efficient circulation. Unless there is adequate fluid replacement, circulation to vital organs, especially the brain and kidneys, is compromised.

This stage is manifested by an elevated

Figure 31–4. **Classification of burn severity**

A burn should be considered *Minor* if
the child is between 2 and 5 years of age *and*
less than 15 percent of TBSA is involved, *or*
if full-thickness burn, less than 2 percent of TBSA is involved.
Area involved: any except face, hands, feet, or perineum.

A burn should be considered *Moderate** if
the child is between 2 and 15 years of age *and*
15 to 30 percent of TBSA is involved, *or*
if full-thickness burn, 2 to 10 percent of TBSA is involved.
Area involved: any except face, hands, feet, or perineum.

A burn should be considered *Severe** if
The child is less than 2 years of age, and more than 5 percent of TBSA is involved, or any percent of TBSA affected by full-thickness burns, or burns of any severity affect face, hands, feet, or perineum; *or* if child is between 2 and 15 years of age, and more than 30 percent of TBSA is involved, or more than 10 percent of TBSA affected by full-thickness burns, or burns of any severity affect face, hands, feet, or perineum.

*Hospitalize.

Figure 31–5. **Survival Rate in Relation to Age (Assuming 50 Percent of Body Burned)**

Age	*Survival Rate*	*Mortality Rate*
5 and under	66%	34%
5–14	80%	20%

hematocrit, lowered blood pressure, increased pulse, thirst, and disorientation, (see Table 31–3). This massive shift of fluids cannot be stopped, but they can and must be replaced. The replacement of fluids is termed *fluid resuscitation*. Various formulas, based on the amount of TBSA burned and the child's weight, have been devised to estimate fluid replacement. This *titration*, or assessment of fluid replacement, is designed to maintain the child's hourly urinary output at a predetermined level (10 to 30 ml per hour) or 0.5 to 10 ml per kg per hour, and requires careful monitoring of all intake and output, vital signs (including CVP), weight, and hematocrit. This period is critical; the child requires constant nursing attention. A Foley catheter is inserted, and hourly checks are made for urine volume and specific gravity. Notify the physician if the volume falls below 10 ml indicating inadequate fluid resuscitation or kidney failure, or rises above 30 ml, indicating pulmonary edema or water intoxication (manifested by nausea, diarrhea, salivation, tremors,

Table 31–3. Plasma-to-Interstitial Fluid Shift (edema at burn site)
Water and electrolyte changes in the first 48 hours after major burns
Fluid Accumulation Phase or Shock Phase

Water and Electrolyte Changes	*Explanation*
Generalized dehydration	Plasma leaks from damaged capillaries to burn site; undamaged tissues lose fluid to plasma to help maintain plasma volume.
Decreased blood volume	Caused by loss of plasma; blood pressure falls, and cardiac output decreases.
Decreased urinary output	Secondary to: Decreased renal blood flow. Sodium and water retention caused by stress. Hemolysis of RBCs, causing hemoglobinuria, and possibly severe renal damage.
Potassium excess	Massive cellular trauma causes release of potassium into extracellular fluid.
Sodium deficit	Large amounts sodium lost in edema fluid (recall that sodium is chiefly extracellular, and is lost when extracellular fluid is lost.)
Metabolic acidosis (Base Bicarbonate Deficit)	Accumulation of fixed acids released from injured tissues; bicarbonate ions lost with Sodium.
Calcium deficit	Occurs in 12 to 24 hours in extensively burned children.
Hemoconcentration (elevated hematocrit)	Fluid portion of blood lost into burn wound.

Adapted from Metheny, N.M., and Snively, W.D. Jr. *Nurse's Handbook of Fluid Balance* ed. 2. Philadelphia, J.B. Lippincott Co., 1974, p. 178. Used with permission.

twitching, and disorientation), or if hematuria is present. The specific gravity will be elevated initially (1.025 to 1.040), and will fall gradually with adequate fluid replacement. Central venous pressure (CVP) should range from 2 to 10 cm H_2O. The hematocrit is measured frequently and will be elevated immediately postburn due to hemoconcentration. If it is normal or low on admission, the child is anemic. The hematocrit should not be permitted to rise above 50 percent. It will also fall to normal levels with fluid replacement. However, due to dilution, loss, and destruction of RBCs, the hematocrit will frequently fall below normal as the child becomes anemic several days to a week postburn. Blood transfusions often will be necessary (see ch. 25). The child receiving adequate fluid resuscitation will usually be alert, exhibit a sense of well-being, and complain of pain appropriately, *unless* he has suffered a head injury, has been over-sedated, or suffers from hypoxia caused by pulmonary complications.

Neurogenic shock may be fatal to the burned child and is complicated by fright, anxiety, and pain. The recumbent position is often therapeutic. Considerate, gentle care is necessary to support the child during the immediate postburn period. Small doses of a sedative, usually morphine, are given intravenously at short intervals (0.25 to 3 mg every 15 to 60 minutes). If the child has a respiratory injury, the dosage is 0.05 mg/Kg and is adjusted to keep him comfortable. If he is intubated, respiratory depression need not be a deterrent to sedation.

Gastric Decompression

As stated earlier, gastric dilatation occurs shortly postburn in many children, particularly those with burns over 30 percent TBSA. Preventing stress ulcers is always easier than treating them. A Sump-type nasogastric tube is passed in the emergency room, and gastric contents are aspirated. The tube should be left on continuous suction until bowel sounds are heard, usually within 24 hours.

Controlling the child's anxiety, neutralizing gastric acid, and maintaining good nutrition are all deterrents to stress ulcer formation. Diazepam is given to control anxiety, and it also decreases gastric acid secretion in many children. Cimetidine is also a useful antacid. Permitting the parents to visit and provide comfort and security to their child also aids in combatting anxiety, provided the parents are aided in coping with their own anxieties, guilts, and/or other psychosocial responses. After bowel sounds are heard, milk or Maalox is given hourly to neutralize the acid and provide good nutrition. If the child cannot or will not take milk orally, a size 8 Fr feeding tube may be passed to allow installation of these agents.

If Curling's ulcer does develop, it is treated with gastric decompression, iced saline gastric lavage, and blood transfusions. About 30 percent of Curling's ulcers require surgical intervention.

Renal Function

An indwelling urinary catheter is inserted to monitor urinary volume and specific gravity every hour. Intravenous resuscitation is planned according to the volume of urinary output. (See ch. 30 for nursing care in relation to urine collection and reporting).

Prophylactic Therapy

Because burns are contaminated wounds, initial treatment of the child with a thermal injury must include tetanus prophylaxis. If the child has been immunized previously, he is given a booster dose of 0.5 ml of tetanus toxoid. If he has never been immunized or has not had a booster in four years, he is given human tetanus hyperimmune globulin (Homo-tet, Hutet) 250 units IM to provide passive immunity, in addition to the 0.5 ml of tetanus toxoid. These are the only intramuscular injections given in the first 24 hours postburn. Prior to discharge from the hospital, active immunization is begun. Wound cultures are done at the time of initial examination and are repeated every three to five days until healing is complete. Burn wounds are readily infected by organisms constantly present in the GI tract (*Pseudomonas, Klebsiella, Escherichia coli,* aerobacter, fungi, and viruses). Systemic antibiotic therapy does not prevent or control burn wound infection indefinitely because the destruction of the protein in the wound provides an excellent pabulum (food) for bacterial culture, and because the immune mechanisms are compromised by the injury. Local care of the wound should include the application of topical antibacterial cream. Systemic antibiotics are given intravenously early in an attempt to prevent gut bacteria from depositing in the burn wound.

Wound Care

After the systemic crises have been dealt with, the burn team treats the wound itself. Treatment begins with a thorough cleansing of the wound, using a mild soap, such as Ivory Liquid, and water. All debris and loose, sloughing skin is gently removed. Scrubbing must be avoided because the friction will increase the injury. The treatment regimen of choice is then initiated. There are three basic methods of topical therapy: open, multiple dressing changes, and closed. All have advantages and disadvantages (see Table 31–4).

Open or Exposure Method

Exposing the burn to air, with or without medications, promotes drying. If the burn is partial-thickness, epithelialization will occur under the eschar; if the burn is full-thickness, a dry eschar forms. The open method may require a sterile environment (sheets, masks, gowns, gloves, etc.), as well as carefully regulated room temperature and humidity. A bed cradle is used for warmth. Microdon sheeting (3M Co.) helps prevent the child's wounds from adhering to the linen. Heat lamps are used to provide extra warmth.

Multiple Dressing Changes

When done meticulously, the semi-open, or multiple dressing change method speeds debridement and enables earlier grafting than the other methods. The wound is covered with topical agents, with or without the use of dressings. The wound is cleansed once or twice a day either at the bedside or in hydrotherapy. This dressing change removes exudate and prevents a "soupy" wound. Removal of the fine-mesh gauze in direct contact with the wound mechanically debrides the surface and is extremely painful. Dressing changes are done using careful aseptic technique. Note that pain medication is given 20 minutes prior to dressing changes and hydrotherapy.

Closed or Occlusive Method

Occlusive dressings are used to prevent two body surfaces from touching, such as fingers or toes, ear and scalp, genital folds, and breast to chest. Bulky dressings are applied over a topical agent and left in place, sometimes for several days. Functional body alignment is easily maintained with this method, but infection is a problem because the wounds cannot be readily inspected. This is the least desirable method of burn-wound care.

Topical Chemotherapy

Silver Nitrate

Silver nitrate solution is effective against most organisms which invade burn wounds (Table 31–5). Bulky gauze dressings are saturated with a 0.5 percent solution of silver nitrate and kept wet. Dressings are changed several times a day with the aid of hydrotherapy. Debridement is necessary with each dressing change because silver nitrate cannot penetrate the burn eschar. Nursing the child on silver nitrate therapy is a demanding task. Evaporative heat loss through wet dressings is lessened, predisposing the child to a one-to-three-degree (F) temperature rise. Electrolyte loss may be marked because sodium and potassium in particular, are drawn from the body fluids into the silver nitrate dressing while water enters the body. Serum electrolyte levels

Table 31–4. **Methods of Topical Therapy for Burn Wounds**

Method	*Areas*	*Advantages*	*Disadvantages*
Open, exposed	Face, neck, perineum, extensive areas of trunk	No painful dressing changes. Less equipment is used. The wound can be observed, thus infection can be detected early. Large numbers of patients can be treated at once.	Proper alignment and elevation are difficult to maintain; thus, it is sometimes not suitable for hands and feet. Unsuitable when the child must be transported a great distance (from home to burn center). Less effective when other injuries require frequent turning. Topical agents do not stay in place; child's surroundings become messy.
Semi-open/multiple dressing-change	Any area	Wound is cleaned once or twice a day, allowing frequent inspection. Removal of cream and/or dressing hastens debridement. Promotes earlier grafting.	Painful dressing changes.
Closed/occlusive	Feet and hands	Relatively easy to maintain proper alignment (hands and feet).	Prevents frequent wound inspection. Encourages infection beneath the eschar. Painful dressing changes.

are obtained every two to four hours in the early stages of treatment, and Ringer's lactate is administered intravenously. Silver nitrate compounds housekeeping chores because it stains everything that it touches black. Wear rubber gloves to protect your hands when working with silver nitrate. Donor sites will require additional preparation prior to grafting if they have been stained black.

Mafenide Acetate

Sulfamylon is spread over the clean burn wound in an ⅛-inch thick layer. It diffuses through the eschar and is effective against a wide range of gram-positive and gram-negative organisms. Dressings are changed once or twice daily in conjunction with hydrotherapy. Sulfamylon is a carbonic anhydrase inhibitor which may reduce the buffering capacity of the blood, thus pre-

Table 31–5. **Topical Chemotherapy: Advantages, Disadvantages, and Nursing Implications**

Agent	*Advantages*	*Disadvantages*	*Nursing Implications*
Silver nitrate 0.5%	Effective antibacterial action. Isolation not necessary.	Cannot penetrate eschar, frequent debridement necessary. Bulky dressings restrict movement. Stains everything black. Marked loss of electrolytes, causing alkalosis.	Clean technique; mask and sterile gloves for handling child. Keep dressings saturated with use of bulb syringe or catheters incorporated into dressings. Frequent turning. Wear rubber gloves. (Providone iodine applied to fresh silver nitrate on hands and clothes, followed by clear water rinse prevents staining.)
Mafenide acetate 10% (Sulfamylon)	No isolation. Penetrates eschar. Effective against subeschar organisms. Permits open-wound treatment. Easy-to-use; no housekeeping problems.	Painful on application. 10%–15% hypersensitivity (pruritic, erythematous, maculopapular rash), requires antihistamines. May cause metabolic acidosis. Delayed eschar separation and grafting.	Clean technique for dressing changes. Administer analgesics prior to application. Debride in hydrotherapy. Spread 1/8-inch layer over wound. Apply fine-mesh gauze strips (or leave open, according to orders). Observe for signs of metabolic acidosis. (Tachypnea earliest sign.)
Silver sulfadiazine 1% (Silvadene)	Painless. Effective against wide range of organisms. Does not disturb acid-base balance, electrolytes, or renal function. No isolation.	Probably penetrates eschar, but in limited amounts.	Apply with gloved hand b.i.d. or t.i.d. May use light dressing.

disposing the child to metabolic acidosis. You must be alert to the tachypnea (28 to 40 respirations per minute) that signals this complication. In addition, the application of Sulfamylon to second-degree burns produces a painful, burning sensation which lasts for 20 to 30 minutes. For this reason, administer an analgesic to the child about 20 minutes prior to the application of Sulfamylon. Eschar separation, and subsequent grafting, is frequently delayed with the use of mafenide acetate, and the wound may require aggressive surgical debridgement. Adherence of this agent to the wound makes debridement painful.

Silver Sulfadiazine 1%

Silvadene currently is the agent of choice for treating burn wounds. Like Sulfamylon, it is applied with a gloved hand or impregnated gauze rolls (Figure 31–6). Silvadene is effective against a wide range of organisms and is not painful on application. It does not disturb the acid-base balance, electrolytes, or renal function. It softens the eschar and permits less painful debridement, as well as increased joint mobility. Hydrotherapy, debridement, and reapplication are done two or three times daily.

Gentamicin Cream

Gentamicin cream is effective against some strains of *Pseudomonas* and is used when burn wounds are invaded by these organisms.

Subeschar Antibiotics

Subeschar antibiotics are employed if colonization of organisms in the wound reaches 10^5 organisms or more per gram of tissue. Wound cultures provide information on the particular organisms. Antibiotics specific for the organisms are mixed with

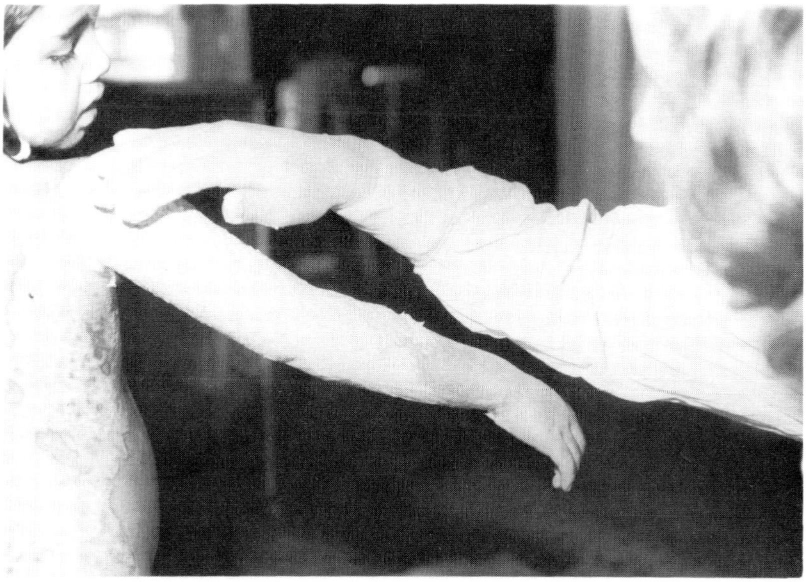

Figure 31–6. *Application of silvadene cream.*

saline and given by needle clysis into the wound itself.

Dressing Changes

Dressing changes are painful and frightening to the child. Tell him exactly what you are going to do, the reason for doing it, and what you expect him to do. Be honest; tell him it will hurt, but that you will be as gentle as possible. Avoid chilling him by covering him with a sterile sheet or bath blanket, and exposing only the part you are dressing. Remember that he is losing body heat through evaporation. Room temperature should be at least 23°C (75°F), and overhead infrared lamps may be used.

Give the child analgesics as ordered and make him as comfortable as possible. The wound is soaked via *hydrotherapy*, either in a whirlpool or a standard bathtub (Figure 31–7), which facilitates wound cleaning and is relatively painless. It can be relaxing and refreshing. However, if the child was burned by a hot liquid, he may be terrified of the whirlpool and must be introduced to it gradually, with concern for his psychological well-being. The child naturally enjoys water play. Utilize the whirlpool with this in mind. Provide boats, sponges, squirt guns, and a washable doll, and so on to help make this a playtime rather than a treatment. If a hose is attached to the faucet, permit the child to squirt his wounds, and thus help with his therapy. (Beware, though, because small hands may turn the hose on you!) The room temperature should be warm enough to decrease chilling. The water is usually kept at 35° to 37°C (95° to 98.6°F). Before the child goes to the whirlpool, offer him his diet and medication. Take his vital signs and measure his intake and output. If he has a Foley catheter, maintain a closed system during the bath. Regulate the IV so that it will not run out. If the child shows any signs of complications, such as changes in pulse, respiration, and blood pressure, or a temperature below 36.7°C (98°F) or above 39.4°C (103°F), or electrolyte imbalance, report this to the physician before placing him in the tub. Wound care is still imperative, however, and should be carried out at the bedside if the tub is not used.

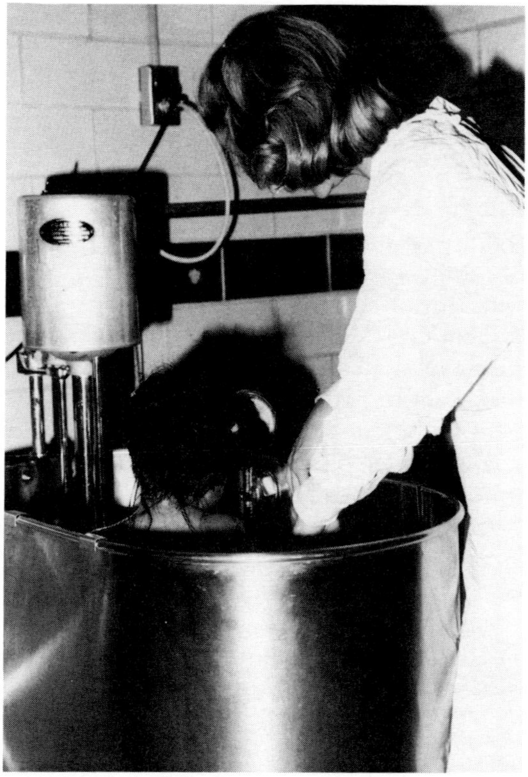

Figure 31–7. *Whirlpool hydrotherapy.*

If hydrotherapy is contraindicated, soak the dressings with a warm, sterile, saline solution. Allow at least 20 minutes for soaking before attempting to remove the dressings. They will then be easier and less painful to remove. Gently remove the inner dressing with gloved fingers and forceps. When the wound is exposed, begin cleaning off exudate, topical ointments, and loose eschar.

Debridement is the process of removing the dead eschar from the viable tissue beneath it. After hydrotherapy, the wound is carefully inspected for loose, sloughing tissue or infection (see Table 31–6). This tissue is trimmed away, and the wound is carefully examined for abcesses which may pocket under the eschar. If the eschar appears to compress when palpated, an incision is made into the eschar, and the exudate is drained. When debridement is complete, place the body part between sterile towels while you prepare a fresh dressing (see Table 31–7).

Skin Grafting

Full-thickness burns must be grafted in order to heal. Wound care prior to grafting is designed to prepare the granulation tissue to receive a graft; this takes from 7 to 21 days. As the time for grafting approaches, the wound is soaked in a warm, saline solution, and the debris is gently removed. When the surface is free of debris, it is ready for grafting.

Grafting is seen as a sign of progress. After the donor site has healed and the graft has taken, the decreased size of the open burn wound reduces the body's metabolic response to stress. Prior to healing, the donor site is equivalent to a partial-thickness wound, and it increases the body's metabolic demands. When the wound has been reduced to less than 20 percent of the TBSA, the child is much less vulnerable to life-threatening burn complications. Physiologic dressings, such as *heterografts* and *homografts* (see Table 31–8), may be used to temporarily cover a wound that is not ready for autografting. These grafts do not last but are important in reducing the size of the wound, limiting the loss of electrolytes, and forming a barrier against infection.

Autografts are usually taken from the child's extremities or trunk. The skin is removed with a dermatome and is placed, dermal side down, on the granulation bed. The use of full strips of skin is called *sheet grafting* (Color Plate 9). A special instrument can be used to create a *mesh graft* or split graft, in which the skin is expanded so that it can cover a larger area (Color Plate 10).

The donor sites usually heal within 10 to 14 days and can be reused many times. Sometimes, on the day before grafting, neomycin dressings are applied to the recipient site, or burn wound, to decrease bacteria on the granulation tissue surface. The donor site is washed with soap and rinsed thoroughly. It is shaved in the

Table 31–6. Burn Wound Characteristics

Appearance	*Probable Indication*
Clean, pinkish, faintly shiny; free from exudate	Healthy granulation (notify physician of any deviation)
Very dry	Dehydration
Wet, soupy, malodorous	Infection
Greenish-grey exudate	Psuedomonas or Proteus infection
Bluish-black discoloration at wound edge	Possible septicemia
Redness and swelling at wound edge	Cellulitis

Table 31–7. **Burn Wound Dressings**

Body Part	*Method*	*Rationale*	*Nursing Implications*
Face	Open	Vascular area, subject to large amount of edema. Difficult to maintain dressings and permit sight, breathing, and oral intake	Sterile technique.
Eyes	Consult Ophthalmologist	Burns of cornea are rare, but lid burns are common. All precautions are taken to preserve sight.	May cover lids with dressing saturated in saline. If eyes are swollen shut, may leave alone or instill antibacterial eye drops q.i.d.
Ears	Semi-open	Delicate cartilage and thin skin may adhere to scalp. Protect whatever tissue is left for possible reconstruction.	Place layer of fine-mesh gauze behind ear to prevent webbing. Saturate another fine-mesh gauze and 4 × 4's with topical agent, place over ear. Wrap securely with Kerlix.
Hands and feet	Splinting and physical therapy or Open or Wire fingers in extended position	Preserve function, prevent infection. Prevent webbing.	Good wound care to prevent infection. Wrap with layer of Kerlix for padding. Anchor to splint in functional position with Kerlix wrap.
Perineum	Open	Wounds are contaminated with urine and feces. Dressings create warm, moist environment which fosters bacterial growth.	Shave perineum on admission and once a week thereafter. Wash with soap and water twice a day and after each elimination. Indwelling catheter will help to keep area clean; change catheter once a week.
Exposed bone and tendon	Keep moist with saturated, sterile, saline dressings	If tissue dries, it dies.	Gently cleanse area and rinse well. Keep dressings saturated with sterile saline.

Trunk	Open Semi-open Closed	Physician's preference.	
New graft	Fine-mesh gauze dressing or Open	Dressings changed only by physician or experienced nurse during first 24 hours to prevent mechanical loss of newly laid grafts. After 72 hours, dressings can be changed by others.	Do not permit child to lie on new grafts; do not disturb graft when giving care. When time to change or remove dressings, soak with normal saline; remove slowly — *do not disturb graft.* Remove loose crusts or gauze threads. Carefully replace fine-mesh gauze, (do not rearrange once it has been laid down). Gauze must not be wrinkled or folded.
Donor site	Dressing of physician's choice applied to donor site in surgery	Separates when healing is complete. When topped by Kerlix saturated with saline and peroxide, drainage by capillary action into the moist outer dressing.	Change Kerlix dressings two or three times a day.

Savedra, M.K. Coping with Pain: Strategies of Severely Burned Children. *Canadian Nurse* 73:28, 1977.

Steele, S. (ed.). *Nursing Care of the Child With Long-Term Illness*, ed. 2. New York, Appleton-Century-Crofts, 1977, p. 415.

Wagner, M.N. Emergency Care of the Burned Patient. *American Journal of Nursing* 77:1788, 1977.

Zitomer, M.M. Protecting Children From the Tragedy of Burns. *American Journal of Maternal-Child Nursing* 2:129, 1977.

INDEX